Fertility and Sterility

A Current Overview

This book has been published with the financial support of
ZENECA Pharmaceuticals

Fertility
and
Sterility

A Current Overview

Proceedings of the 15th World Congress
on Fertility and Sterility

Montpellier, France, 17–22 September 1995

Edited by
B. Hedon, J. Bringer and P. Mares

Hôpital Universitaire, Faculté de Médecine
Montpellier-Nîmes, France

The Parthenon Publishing Group
International Publishers in Medicine, Science & Technology

NEW YORK   LONDON

Editorial Note

THESE PROCEEDINGS INCLUDE ALL THE KEYNOTE ADDRESSES AND OFFICIAL IFFS SCIENTIFIC SESSIONS OF THE 15TH WORLD CONGRESS ON FERTILITY AND STERILITY THAT WERE RECEIVED BY THE ORGANIZERS BY JULY 10TH, 1995.

British Library Cataloguing-in-Publication Data
Fertility and Sterility: A Current Overview: Proceedings of the 15th World Congress on Fertility and Sterility, Montpellier, France, 17–22 September 1995.
I. Hedon, B.   II. Series
616.692
ISBN 1-85070-694-8

Library of Congress Cataloging-in-Publication Data
World Congress on Fertility and Sterility (15th : 1995 Montpellier, France)
  Fertility and sterility today: proceedings of the 15th World Congress on Fertility and Sterility, Montpellier, France 17–22 September 1995 / edited by B. Hedon, J. Bringer and P. Mares.
   p. cm.
  Includes bibliographical references and index.
  ISBN 1-85070-694-8
  1. Infertility–Congresses.   2. Fertility–Congresses.
  3. Contraception–Congresses.
I. Hedon, B. II. Bringer, Jacques. III. Mares, P.
IV. Title.
  [DNLM: 1. Fertility–congresses. 2. Infertility–congresses.   WP 565 W927f 1995]
RC889.W6 1995
616.6'92–dc20
DNLM/DLC
for Library of Congress   95-23865
                                                              CIP

Published in the UK and Europe by
The Parthenon Publishing Group Limited
Casterton Hall, Carnforth
Lancs. LA6 2LA

Published in North America by
The Parthenon Publishing Group Inc.
One Blue Hill Plaza
PO Box 1564, Pearl River
New York 10965, USA

Copyright © 1995 The Parthenon Publishing Group

First published 1995

Typeset by AMA Graphics Ltd., Preston, UK
Printed and bound by
Butler & Tanner Ltd., Frome and London, UK

Contents

Section 9:   Research

List of principal contributors

M. Aboulghar
10 Geziret El Arab Street
Mohandeseen-Cairo
Egypt

A.A. Acosta
FLASEF
Eligio Ayala 1263, 7 Piso
Asuncion
Paraguay

E.Y. Adashi
Department of Obstetrics and Gynecology
University of Maryland School of Medicine
405 W Redwood Street, Third Floor
Baltimore, Maryland 21201
USA

M. Auroux
CHU Bicetre
Biologie de la Reproduction et du
    Developpement
78 rue du General Leclerc
94275 Kremlin Bicetre
France

G. Benagiano
World Health Organization
Department of Human Reproduction
20 Ave Appia
1211 Geneva
Switzerland

P. Boulot
Services de Gynécologie–Obstétrique
Hôpital A de Villeneuve
Faculté de Médecine
Université Montpellier 1
271 Av. doyen G. Giraud
34295 Montpellier
France

J. Bringer
Hôpital Lapeyronie
Service d'Endocrinologie
Route de Ganges
34295 Montpellier Cedex
France

I.A. Brosens
Universität Ziekenhuis St. Rafael
Department of Obstetrics and Gynecology
Herestraat 49
3000 Leuven
Belgium

M. Bygdeman
Karolinska Hospital
Department of Obstetrics and Gynecology
PO Box 140
171 76 Stockholm
Sweden

S. Campbell
King's College Hospital
Department of Obstetrics and Gynecology
Denmark Hill
London SE5 8RX
UK

S.A. Carson
Baylor College of Medicine
Department of Obstetrics and Gynecology
7th Floor – Smith Tower
6550 Fannin – Suite 701
Houston, TX 77030
USA

J. Cohen
8 Rue de Marignan
75008 Paris
France

J. Collins
McMaster University
1200 Main St West
Room 4D9
Hamilton
Ontario L8N 3Z5
Canada

F. Comhaire
University Hospital UZ
185 De Pintelaan
B-9000 Gent
Belgium

I.D. Cooke
Jessop Hospital for Women
Department of Obstetrics and
    Gynecology
Leavygreave Road
Sheffield S3 7RE
UK

S. Daya
McMaster University
Department of Obstetrics and
    Gynecology
1200 Main Street West
Hamilton
Ontario L8N 3Z5
Canada

Ma. del Carmen Cravioto
Inst. Nacional de la Nutricion
'Salvador Zubiran'
Vasco de Quiroga 15
Mexico City 14000
Mexico

M. Desclozeaux
Biochimie CNRS
INSERM
B.P. 5051
34033 Montpellier Cedex
France

J. Donnez
Department of Gynecology
Catholic University of Louvain
Cliniques Universitaires St-Luc
Avenue Hippocrate 10
1200 Brussels
Belgium

M. Elstein
University of Manchester
St. Mary's Hospital
Whitworth Park
Manchester M13 0JH
UK

J.L.H. Evers
Academisch Ziekenhuis Maastricht
Department of Obstetrics and Gynecology
PO Box 5800
6202 AZ Maastricht
The Netherlands

M.F. Fathalla
The Rockefeller Foundation
PO Box 30
Assiut
Egypt

I.S. Fraser
Queen Elizabeth II Research Institute
Department of Obstetrics and Gynecology
University of Sydney
Sydney, NSW 2006
Australia

S. Gordts
Catholic University of Louvain
Clinique St Luc – IVF Unit
Avenue Hippocrate 10
B-1200 Brussels
Belgium

J.E. Griffin
UT Southwestern Medical Center
Department of Internal Medicine
5323 Harry Hines Blvd
Dallas, TX 75235 8857
USA

L. Hamberger
University of Göteborg
Department of Obstetrics and Gynecology
Sahlgrenska sjukhuset
S-413 45 Göteborg
Sweden

C.M. Harrison
Department of Human Assisted Reproduction
Rotunda Hospital
Royal College of Surgeons
Dublin 1
Ireland

B. Hedon
Services de Gynécologie-Obstétrique
Hôpital A de Villeneuve
Faculté de Médecine
Université Montpellier 1
271 Av. doyen G. Giraud
34295 Montpellier
France

J.C. Herr
University of Virginia Health Sciences Center
    for Recombinant Gamete Contraceptive
    Vaccinogens
PO Box 439
Charlottesville, VA 22908
USA

R. Homburg
Golda Medical Center
Infertility Unit
7 Keren-Kayamet Street
Petah-Tikva 49372
Israel

M.G.R. Hull
University of Bristol
Department of Obstetrics and Gynecology
St. Michael's Hospital
Southwell Street
Bristol BS2 8EG
UK

B. Jégou
GERM/INSERM U 435
Université de Rennes 1
Campus de Beaulieu
35042 Rennes Cedex
France

G. Kovacs
Monash University
Box Hill Hospital
Department of Obstetrics and Gynecology
Nelson Road
Box Hill
Victoria 3128
Australia

P.A.L. Lancaster
School of Public Health and Tropical
    Medicine
AIHW Perinatal Statistics Unit
Edward Ford Building (A27)
University of Sydney
NSW 2006
Australia

I. Liebaers
Center for Medical Genetics
Academisch Ziekenhuis VUB
Laarbeeklaan 101
1090 Brussels
Belgium

E. Loumaye
Ares Serono
Medical Affairs Department
15 bis, Chemin des Mines
1211 Geneve 20
Switzerland

T. Makino
School of Medicine – Tokai University
Department of Obstetrics and Gynecology
Bohseidai, Isehara City
259-11 Kanagawa Prefecture
Japan

J. Mandelbaum
Hôpital Necker
INSERM U 173
149 rue de Sèvres
75743 Paris Cedex 15
France

I. Maral
Yali Caddesi 170/6
Saadet Apt. Karsiyaka
Izmir 35600
Turkey

P. Mares
Services de Gynécologie-Obstétrique
Hôpital Caremeau
Faculté de Médecine Montpellier-Nîmes
Rue de professeur Robert Debré
30029 Nîmes
France

P.G. McDonough
The Medical College of Georgia
Department of Obstetrics and Gynecology
1120 Fifteenth Street
Augusta, GA 30912-3360
USA

Y. Menezo
IRH/Foundation Merieux
1 Rue Laborde
69500 Bron
France

L. Mettler
University of Kiel
Department of Obstetrics
Michaelisstrasse 16
24105 Kiel
Germany

K.S. Moghissi
Division of Reproductive Endocrinology
Wayne State University
Hutzel Hospital
Detroit
Michigan
USA

S. Munné
The Institute for Reproductive Medicine and
    Science
Saint Barnabas Medical Center
101 Old Shorts Hills Road
Suite 501
West Orange, NJ 07052
USA

F. Petraglia
Department of Obstetrics and Gynecology
University of Pisa
Via Roma 35
56100 Pisa
Italy

L. Pinsky
The Sir Mortimer B. Davis Jewish General
    Hospital
Lady Davis Institute for Medical Research
3755 Cote Ste-Catherine Road
Montreal, Quebec H3T 1E2
Canada

C. Piquet-Pellorce
GERM/INSERM U 435
Université de Rennes 1
Campus de Beaulieu
35042 Rennes Cedex
France

G. Ragni
University of Milan
Department of Obstetrics and Gynecology
Via Commenda 12
20122 Milan
Italy

D. Reinprayoon
WHO CCR
Department of Obstetrics and Gynecology
Faculty of Medicine
Chulalongkorn University
Bangkok 10330
Thailand

R. Rey
Ecole Normale Supérieure
INSERM U 293
1 rue Maurice Arnoux
92120 Montrouge
France

S. Rimbach
Ruprecht-Karls Universität Heidelberg
Frauenklinik
Vosstrasse 9
69115 Heidelberg
Germany

O. Rodriguez-Armas
Central University of Venezuela
Centro Medico de Caracas 8A
Anexo B
San Bernardino
1196 Caracas
Venezuela

R. Ron-El
Infertility & IVF Unit
Department of Obstetrics and Gynecology
Assaf Harofeh Medical Center
70300 Zerifin
Israel

W.H.-B. Schill
Justus-Liebig Universität Giessen
Zentrum fur Dermatologie & Andrologie
Gaffkystrasse 14
35385 Giessen
Germany

M. Seppälä
Department of Obstetrics and Gynecology
Helsinki University Central Hospital
Haarmaninkatu 2
00290 Helsinki
Finland

J.L. Simpson
Baylor College of Medicine
7th Floor – Smith Tower
6550 Fannin – Suite 701
Houston, TX 77030
USA

S.H. Sohn
New England Medical Center Hospital
750 Washington Street
Box 324
Boston, MA 02111
USA

C. Sultan
Centre de Recherche INSERM
60 Rue de Navacelles
34090 Montpellier
France

S. Tabacova
National Center of Hygiene, Ecology and
    Nutrition
Boulevard D. Nestorov 15
1431 Sofia
Bulgaria

S. Tabibzadeh
University of South Florida
Sciences Center and Moffitt Cancer Center
Department of Pathology
12902 Magnolia Drive
Tampa, FL 33612
USA

B.C. Tarlatzis
Aristotle University
1st Department of Obstetrics and Gynecology
'Geniki Kliniki'
2 Gravias St.
546 45 Thessaloniki
Greece

W. Thompson
The Queen's University of Belfast
Department of Obstetrics and Gynecology
Grosvenor Road
Belfast BT12 6BJ
Ireland

R.I. Tozzini
Presidente Roca 890
10 Piso A
2000 Rosario
Argentina

A. Van Steirteghem
Center for Reproductive Medicine
AZ-Vrije University Brussels
Laarbeeklaan 101
1090 Brussels
Belgium

A. Veiga
Instituto Dexeus,
Reproductive Medicine Service
P/Bonanova 89–91
08017 Barcelona
Spain

Foreword

Once every 3 years the World Congress on Fertility and Sterility is the occasion for an overview of all that is going on in this fast-growing field. More and more physicians and researchers choose to devote their professional lives to the understanding and mastering of human fertility which is now officially recognized as being essential for any human being. Fertility must be understood as a whole, and so must encompass knowledge of the basic mechanisms involved in the making of a new life, understanding of human psychology which is so important in this field, prevention of unplanned pregnancies, and treatment of all disorders which can prohibit men and women from becoming parents.

Each one of the papers included in this book has been carefully chosen by the International Scientific Committee of the IFFS (International Federation of Fertility Societies), with Professor Sakamoto as President, as addressing an important topic. Some of the papers are very practical, in their aim to improve the efficiency of diagnostic and therapeutic procedures. Others are Review papers – up-to-date summaries of the current knowledge about a particular subject, which emphasize the future perspectives that can be developed. Yet other papers are related more to research.

Whether you are a gynecologist, an endocrinologist, a biologist, an andrologist, or a basic scientist, or whatever is your own interest – reproductive surgery, assisted medical procreation techniques, the manufacture of new drugs, contraception, reproductive endocrinology, or perhaps all of these – you will find that this book, the Proceedings of the 15th World Congress on Fertility and Sterility, held in Montpellier, France, September 1995, contains the appropriate answers.

The editors would like to acknowledge the efforts of every author in providing their eminent contribution, each of which will be of benefit to us all.

July 1995

B. Hedon
J. Bringer
P. Mares

1

Contraception

Population concerns for the next century

1

M. F. Fathalla

Introduction

'And God blessed them, and God said unto them, Be fruitful, and multiply, and replenish the earth, and subdue it: and have dominion over the fish of the sea, and over the fowl of the air, and over every living thing that moveth upon the earth.'

Genesis 2:28

And so they did. It took them some time though, but recently they have been very good at it. They needed thousands of years to reach the first billion. But it took only 123 years for the world population to pass from the first billion around 1804 to the second in 1927[1]. The next increment of 1 billion took 33 years (the world population reached 4 billion at the time of the United Nations World Population Conference at Bucharest in 1974). Only 13 years elapsed before the world population reached 5 billion (in 1987) and it is estimated that it will take only 11 years more for it to reach 6 billion (in 1998).

They have now subdued the earth and had dominion over every living thing upon it. Many are those who believe that they have even overdone it, that the health of the planet is now being compromised, and that the biological diversity on the earth is seriously threatened.

Now that the earth has been replenished and subdued, and the mission has been accomplished, they are left with no further explicit divine instruction. They have to steer their way, on their own, into the future.

To continue to be fruitful and multiply is no longer an option. World population growth, we can confidently assert, is bound to come to a halt. Its sustenance in the long term is clearly untenable. It has been calculated that, if present levels of fertility, country by country, remain constant indefinitely, the global population could exceed 100 billion by early in the twenty-second century[2]. On the global level, the world population must eventually come to a stop: it must stabilize.

Homo sapiens is already bracing up for the change. Human reproductive behaviour is evolving fast to adapt to new dramatic realities. Fertility has been declining at an unprecedented steep rate, and is continuing to decline. Side by side with this fertility decline, and although it may seem paradoxical, world population will continue to grow, more than ever before, for at least another century, before finally stabilizing, probably towards the end of the twenty-second century.

The twenty-first century will witness major upheavals in world population, which will have an impact on a world that will never again be the same. The world will have to cope with a long-drawn and agonizing transition, characterized by rapid population growth, before population finally stabilizes. The world will have to prepare for the accommodation of almost double its current population size by making serious and painful adjustments for sustainability and equity, in prevailing patterns of consumption and production. The reproductive evolution to a small family norm will have far-reaching implications that need to be addressed. Women, finally emancipated from the heavy reproductive burden, will emerge as final winners in this major upheaval but only after an uphill struggle. A population-21 agenda for science will be

3

critical to guide the passage of humanity through a difficult next century.

Curbing rapid population growth

More attention is given in the population debate to consequences of population growth, while less attention is given to the components of population growth. To act effectively to curb rapid population growth, it is important to differentiate between its various components. One component of population growth, resulting from mortality decline, is in fact desirable and should be encouraged. Another major component, resulting from the population momentum of the young age structure, can be considered inevitable. A third component, resulting from wanted fertility, should be accepted as a penalty for the inequity in this world, until socioeconomic conditions inducive to a small family norm prevail. A fourth component, resulting from coerced motherhood by denying women any choice in life beyond child-bearing, is unacceptable, and should not be allowed to stand. A fifth component, resulting from unwanted pregnancies and an unmet need for fertility regulation is, by definition, undesirable, unacceptable and should be corrected.

Mortality rates are projected to continue their decline in the twenty-first century in developing countries. This trend is to be encouraged and cannot be manipulated to curb population growth.

It has been estimated that the population momentum will be responsible for about one-half of the population growth in the next century[3]. Record numbers of young people will enter the childbearing years, and even if they adopt a small family norm, the number of births will still be large.

A desire for more than two children is still a norm in most of the developing world. The desire is completely rational where socioeconomic conditions make the 'cost' of children less than their 'value'. The ideational change for a small family norm appears, however, to be spreading in the developing world, with even small improvements in socio-economic conditions. The success of family planning in Bangladesh is a case in point[4].

When societies allow women only one choice in life, child-bearing and child-rearing, and make children the only goods they can produce and are expected to deliver, fertility cannot be a real choice. It is only recently that the world is realizing the heavy price it is paying for not empowering women to make decisions in their lives, including reproductive decisions. The Cairo International Conference on Population and Development (ICPD) upheld the principle that 'Advancing gender equality and equity and the empowerment of women, and the elimination of all kinds of violence against women, and ensuring women's ability to control their own fertility, are cornerstones of population and development-related programs.'

The unmet need for family planning

A recent analysis of data derived from Demographic and Health Surveys, using conservative estimates for the unmet need for limiting fertility and for spacing births, estimated the unmet need to be 24% in sub-Saharan Africa, 13% in Asia and North Africa, and 16% in Latin America. The same study concluded that the total unmet need for contraception could be close to or in excess of 100 million[5].

There will be a major expansion in the need for family planning in the coming decades[6]. It should be a responsibility of the whole international community to ensure that women, wherever they are, are given a choice in their lives and are given the means to implement their choice. Even the poorest people in the world should make these choices. There is no justification in denying poor people access to family planning.

Coping with numbers

In 1803, Malthus wrote the following parable on social entitlements:

'A man who is born into a world already possessed, if he cannot get subsistence from his parents on whom he had a just demand, and if the society do not want his labour, has no claim of right to the smallest portion of food, and, in fact, has no business to be where he is. At nature's mighty feast there is no vacant cover for him. She tells him to be gone, and will quickly execute her own orders, if he does not work upon the compassion of some of her guests. If these guests get up and make room for him, other intruders immediately appear demanding the same favour. The report of a provision for all that come fills the hall with numerous claimants. The order and harmony of the feast is disturbed, the plenty that before reigned is changed into scarcity; and the happiness of the guests is destroyed by the spectacle of misery and dependence in every part of the hall, and by the clamorous importunity of those who are justly enraged at not finding the provision which they had been taught to expect. The guests learn too late their error, in counteracting those strict orders to all intruders, issued by the great mistress of the feast, who, wishing that all her guests should have plenty, and knowing that she could not provide for unlimited numbers, humanely refused to admit fresh comers when her table was already full'[7].

Malthus was right on at least one account and was wrong on at least one account. He was right in that there is going to be a limit on the number that can be seated on 'Spaceship Earth', and in fact people have already heeded the message and are already changing their reproductive patterns to meet the new reality. He was wrong on how big that number can be. At the time Malthus made this statement, the population of the world was an estimated one billion. 'Nature's mighty feast', now accommodates, and serves, at least as well, 5.7 billion. Within the next two centuries, it is projected that this number will, probably inevitably, double.

Population growth

It may seem paradoxical that the world population continues to grow in spite of the continued fertility decline. Because of the fertility decline,

Table 1 Crude birth rate (per 1000 population). Estimates and medium-variant projections (source: reference 26)

	1950–55	1990–95	2020–25
World total	37.5	26.0	17.9
More developed regions	22.6	14.2	11.9
Less developed regions	44.7	29.4	19.1

birth rates will continue to decline in the twenty-first century (Table 1). The annual average number of births will, however, continue to increase, mainly as a consequence of the increasing number of women of reproductive age, which itself resulted from the high fertility of the past. The increase in the number of births, together with the effects of declining mortality, will continue to fuel the increments in population size despite the decline in fertility rates.

World population growth will not stop in our lifetime. It is also unlikely to stop in the lifetime of our grandchildren. It may not even make the ultimate stop in the lifetime of our grandchildren. In recent United Nations long-range population projections, it is assumed that fertility will ultimately stabilize at the replacement level (i.e. when the two parents produce only two children to replace them) around the year 2100[1]. Population will continue to grow for some time, even after fertility rates drop to simple replacement levels. It is thus projected that the world population will increase by 89 per cent between 1990 and 2050, reaching a size of 10 billion, then expand by 12 per cent during the following 50 years (2050-2100) to a size of 11.2 billion, and by 3 per cent during the next 50 years (2100-2150) to a size of 11.5 billion. The world population may stabilize ultimately at 11.6 billion shortly after the year 2200[1]. World population will thus continue to grow for another two centuries from now, and our crowded planet will have to accommodate about twice its current population.

Many are those who believe that these numbers are beyond the carrying capacity of planet earth. Others, including the writer of this paper, believe that it is our caring capacity, for others and for future generations, that will make the difference. As stated in the Programme of Action of the Cairo ICPD, 'Recognizing the longer term realities and implications of current actions, the development challenge is to meet the needs of present generations and improve their quality of life without compromising the ability of future generations to meet their own needs'[8]. There is no question that current consumption and production patterns are unsustainable. They must change to foster sustainable resource use and to prevent environmental degradation. In this major challenge for the twenty-first century, as reaffirmed by the Cairo ICPD Programme of Action, 'Developed countries should take the lead in achieving sustainable consumption patterns and effective waste management.'

In addition, the large numbers will bring new realities that need to be faced. The world demographic map will be redrawn. The world will become more urban. 'Mega cities' will increase in size and number. More people will be on the move than ever before.

Adapting to the reproductive evolution

The biological potential of human reproduction can be great. According to the Guinness Book of Records, 'A 32nd child was born to Raimundo Carnauba and his wife Madelena of Ceilandria, Brazil. In May 1972, the mother said "They have given us a lot of work and worry but they are worth it".' The father, typical to his limited investment in the big enterprise, said 'I don't know why people make such a fuss.'

A dramatic change in people's reproductive behavior began in the nineteenth century in the North of our globe. During the second half of the twentieth century, the change has been sweeping the South. The world is experiencing an unprecedented decline in fertility. Fertility level is measured by demographers as the total fertility rate (TFR), which reflects the average total number of children that a woman would have by the end of her reproductive life if current fertility patterns remain unchanged. The total fertility rate continued to decline in all of

Table 2 Total fertility rates. Estimates 1950–90 and medium variant projections 1990–2025 (source: reference 26)

	1950–55	1985–90	2020–25
World total	5.00	3.43	2.36
More developed regions	2.83	1.92	1.90
Less developed regions	6.19	3.90	2.44

the world regions in recent decades, and is expected to continue to do so in the coming years and to drop to 2.36 by the years 2020–2025 (Table 2).

To put the rate of fertility decline in developing countries in perspective, a recent study compared the time taken for fertility to decline from 6.5 to 3.5 in different countries. What took 58 years in the USA took 27 years in Indonesia, 15 years in Colombia, 8 years in Thailand, and merely 7 years in China[9].

The adoption of a smaller family norm, with consequent decline in total fertility, should not be viewed only in demographic terms. It means that people, and particularly women, are empowered to take control of their fertility and to plan their lives; it means that more children are born by choice, not by chance, and that births can be planned to take place at optimal times for child-bearing to ensure better health for women and children; and it means that families are able to invest relatively more in a smaller number of beloved children, trying to prepare them for a better future[10–12].

What we are witnessing is a major evolutionary jump that is science-mediated, rather than brutally imposed by Nature. Our reproductive function is being voluntarily adapted to dramatic new realities. *Homo sapiens* has escaped the grip of Nature in evolution to become a self-evolving animal. The recent dramatic evolution in human reproductive behavior is not followed or accompanied by a change in the anatomy and/or function of the reproductive system, as would have been expected in other major evolutionary jumps mediated by Mother Nature. As a consequence, *Homo sapiens* has to accomplish its reproductive evolution while retaining a reproductive system geared to high fertility. Women, or their partners, have to use contraception. Women have a span of about 30 reproductive years, during which they were meant by Nature to get pregnant. If women are to bear only one or two children, they will spend only 1–3 years in child-bearing. For the remaining years, they, or their partners, will have to lead a contraceptive life if they are to remain sexually active. Contraceptive technology, from now on, will play a crucial role in reproductive life.

With the adoption of a small family norm, the demand for quality in births will substitute the demand for quantity. New developments in reproductive technologies can help more people to have the healthy babies they want, but they can also be abused. Sex, as a tool for reproduction, is evolving into an expression of love, with consequent changes in sexual behavior.

As a consequence of changes in age structure, low fertility societies will experience the 'graying' of their populations. Adolescence, as an age group, will not increase, but the widening biosocial gap in reaching maturity will have important implications.

Contraceptive life

The change to contraceptive life has been sweeping the world. Levels of contraceptive use are estimated as percentages of currently married women of reproductive age (15–49), including where possible, those in consensual unions. According to the latest United Nations estimates, of the 899 million currently married women of reproductive age in the world, 57% are using contraception at any one time[13]. The prevalence among developing countries as a whole is 53%, and in the more developed countries 72% (Table 3). The date to which these estimates pertain is approximately 1990, according to data available during 1993. Considering the lag between the time of data collection and the current period, the level of contraceptive use in the developing countries is likely to have been about 55% in 1993[8].

Regional differences in levels of use remain large. While there remain many countries in Africa and several in other regions where the level of contraceptive use is still very low, most developing countries that have available data on trends have experienced a substantial increase in the level of contraceptive use. Even in sub-Saharan Africa, recent surveys show an increase in levels of use in several countries: Botswana, Cameroon, Kenya, Lesotho, Namibia, Rwanda, Swaziland, South Africa and Zimbabwe.

In view of the major worldwide expansion in the use of modern methods of contraception by healthy women over prolonged periods of time, contraceptive safety has become an important issue in women's health. In developed countries, where the number of women using contraceptives is much larger than the number of those who are pregnant, and where maternal mortality rates are very low, reproductive mortality attributable to contraceptive use assumes a relatively large dimension[14]. In developing countries, reproductive mortality attributable to contraceptive use is still insignificant compared with maternal mortality.

Table 3 Contraceptive use in the world (source: reference 13)

	Couples in reproductive age, 1990 (millions)	Level of contraceptive use (%)
World	899	57
Less developed regions	710	53
Africa	97	18
Asia and Oceania	545	58
Eastern Asia	236	79
Other countries	309	42
Latin America and the Caribbean	67	58
More developed regions	189	72

The contraceptive technology revolution

A scientific revolution in contraceptive technology in the past few decades has helped these hundreds of millions of people to achieve their aspirations to regulate and control their fertility. The fruits of science have been enjoyed by people living in the most varied circumstances, in the skyscrapers of Manhattan, in peri-urban slums in Latin America, in rural communities of the Indian subcontinent; people in all socio-economic strata; people with different cultures, religious beliefs and value systems; and people postponing a first pregnancy, spacing their children or putting the limit on child-bearing.

Until the middle of the present century, contraceptive choice was limited to either coitally-related methods which lacked in effectiveness, or permanent methods. Contraceptive choices have now been broadened[15]. Contraception was moved outside the bedroom by the development of systemic methods such as the pill. People no longer had to make the choice between a method to be used at every coitus or a permanent method; long-acting reversible methods now offer protection ranging from 1 month to several years. Also, highly effective but reversible methods became an available option. Technical developments have allowed sterilization to be performed as an out-patient procedure and without the need for general anesthesia.

But perhaps the most significant development, brought about by the contraceptive technology revolution, has been the empowerment of women. For the first time, women had at their disposal effective methods that they can use to regulate and control their fertility, without being too dependent on co-operation of the male partner. Methods used by women now make up about two-thirds of contraceptive practice worldwide, and such methods have been increasing their share in total contraceptive use.

The embryos they ask for

'The Predestinators send in their figures to the Fertilizers, who give them the embryos they ask for. And the bottles come in here to be predestinated in detail, after which they are sent down to the Embryo Store'.
Aldous Huxley, 1932, *Brave New World*

Aldous Huxley's vision of a brave new world, where people get *the embryos they ask for*, is not too far away. New frontiers of science have opened the way for hitherto unimaginable reproductive technologies that have made possible artificial insemination, *in vitro* fertilization, embryo transfers, surrogate motherhood, cryogenic storage of sperm and ova, genetic selection and prenatal diagnosis, including sex determination.

With the adoption of a small family norm, demand for quality of births has substituted for quantity of births. To seek the birth, through the use of these new technologies, of only healthy babies is a legitimate request. The new technologies may, however, be abused to seek babies with certain demographic characteristics.

Although most of these technologies have as yet no significant demographic impact, there is already serious concern about possible alterations in sex composition of populations, when the desire for quality is translated as a desire for a son.

In a number of countries, the practice has taken on a large dimension. In 1988–89 the sex ratio for first-born children was 104.9 in China and 107.2 in Korea, but for the fourth child or higher birth order, it was 131.7 and 199.1, respectively[16] (Table 4). In India, the practice

Table 4 Reported sex ratios* at birth by birth order in China and South Korea (source: reference 16)

Year	Country	Birth order				All births
		1st	*2nd*	*3rd*	*4th +*	
1988	Korea	107.2	113.5	170.5	199.1	113.6
1989	China	104.9	120.9	124.6	131.7	113.8

*, (number of male infants/number of female infants) × 100

became so prevalent that the government felt the obligation to introduce legislation to make it punishable by law.

Sex: a duty became a pleasure

In the evolution of *Homo sapiens*, the temporal relationship between sex and reproduction has been severed. It must have taken our ancestors such a long time to realize any relationship between the act and the event, probably not until they began to observe domesticated animals. In our fellow mammals, the female will only be attractive to the male and receptive to his advances if she is ovulating and ready to conceive. In our fellow primates, the female never fails to advertise the fact that she is ovulating; external sexual organs undergo a change in size or color that is clearly visible and that makes her sexually attractive to the male. At other times, she will have little or no appeal for him. The sexual receptivity of the human female has been completely emancipated from hormonal control. The human female has also succeeded through evolution to hide completely all external evidence of ovulation.

The dissociation of the act of sex from reproduction was an ingenious mechanism for reproductive efficiency. Mother Nature was not as much keen on our pleasure, as on ensuring the survival of the species. Making sex perpetually available encouraged the pair bond and favoured the development of the family institution, as an essential mechanism for care of the children. Other mammals produce infants who are able to run sufficiently well to keep up with the herd less than 30 min after birth. The human newborn, on the other hand, has a long period of years of extreme dependence and helplessness during which it needs to be taken care of, preferably by two parents, before being able to survive on its own.

With reproduction receding further into the background, the role of sex in our lives is going to continue to evolve. It will sublime into an expression of love. As such, sex will increasingly be an important component in our psychosocial well-being, and less and less a tool of reproduction. We are beginning to witness the implications of this evolution for sexual behavior.

Graying of the world

'Altogether, Methuselah lived 969 years, and then he died.'

Genesis 5:27

The record of Methuselah remains unbroken. The world, however, has recently been making good progress. People are now living longer almost everywhere, and life expectancy is expected to continue to increase. With proportionately less people born and proportionately more people living longer, the 'graying' of the world will continue in the twenty-first century.

It is estimated that as of mid-1990, about one out of every three persons on the earth was a child, one out of five was a person in the late teens or early twenties and one out of 16 was aged 65 or older[17,18]. The median age was 24 years, indicating that the world population is still relatively young, This is rapidly changing. The world is getting older.

The size of the world elderly population is currently considerably smaller than the size of the child population. The projected speed of relative increase of the world elderly population, however, is substantially faster than that of the world child population. The number of persons aged 65 or over in the world was estimated to be 328 million in 1990. It is projected to grow to 828 million in 2025, more than 2.5 times its current size[17,18].

In 1950–55 only five countries (Denmark, Iceland, Netherlands, Norway and Sweden) belonged to what is called the 'Over-70s Club', that is, the countries in which life expectancy at birth is more than 70 years. By 1980–85, the number of these countries had increased to 47, with nine in Latin America, six in Asia, 32 in Europe, North America and Oceania, and none in Africa. In 2020–25, the Club's membership is projected to grow to 102, including the currently industrialized countries[19].

The growing proportion of aged people imposes new demands. Societies have to make difficult decisions on allocation of resources, and to struggle with a formula to establish a reasonable degree of 'intergenerational equity'.

Adolescence and the widening biosocial gap

Nature has delayed the onset of puberty in the human species more than in any other mammal, to ensure physical and mental maturity in the mother (and father) and to allow enough time for the transmission of intergenerational knowledge and skills, before taking on the responsibility of parenthood.

During the period of adolescence, defined as the period of transition from childhood to adulthood, three developments take place. Biological development progresses from the point of the initial appearance of the secondary sex characteristics to that of sexual maturity; psychological processes and cognitive and emotional patterns develop from those of a child to those of an adult; and a transition is made from the state of total socioeconomic dependence to one of relative independence. Two trends are taking place in almost every society, though at different paces: a trend towards an earlier onset of biological maturation and a trend towards delay in socio-economic maturation, with a resultant wider biosocial gap in human development. Today, girls everywhere are becoming sexually mature at an earlier age than previous generations. Genetic, health and socioeconomic factors influence the wide variations in age of menarche between different countries. Since boys and girls have now to spend more years in school, learning and training, before they can enter the complex labor market, the period of socioeconomic dependence is prolonged. The biosocial gap will continue to widen for other world regions, where the gap is still narrow.

Adolescents are left with difficult choices in sexual behavior: premarital sex, early marriage or abstinence. The different patterns predominate in different countries, and patterns of transition exist.

Adolescence and the widening biosocial gap are not a problem in themselves. The problem is in the need to come to grips with the new realities of adolescence. Misconceptions are contributing to turning what should be a normal positive phase in growth and development into a problem.

The winners: women

'But first we must ask: what is a woman? "Tota mulier in utero", says one, "woman is womb".'
Simone de Beauvoir[20]

In this upheaval in population and reproductive behavior, there is one clear winner to emerge: women. They deserve to be the winners. They were the ones who made the sacrifices in the battle for survival of our species. They still make these sacrifices, unnecessarily, even today, as evidenced by the world estimates of maternal mortality[21]. It may not be sufficiently realized that only for the birth of the 5.7 billion people who are now living, replenishing the earth and subduing it, more than 25 million women had to die, not to mention those who suffered but survived.

With the adoption of the small family norm, and with the ability of women to regulate and control their fertility, the woman is finally emerging from behind the mother. Hitherto, womens' potential has been suppressed to serve the survival needs of humanity. It is high time they were permitted to take their chances, in their own interest and in the interest of all. Child-bearing is becoming *a* function of women, and not *the* function of women. Women are becoming producers, and not only reproducers. The world is making the discovery that women are not mobile wombs. They are human beings, in their own right. There will continue to be, for some time, those who cannot accept a role for women, other than being satellites that have to move around men. Women still have an uphill struggle, but there is no turning back[22].

Population-21: an agenda for science

Success in replenishing the earth was largely an accomplishment of science. It was not brought about by increased fertility, but by decreased mortality. With more people surviving to reproductive age, more children were born. Now that the battle for survival has been won, science has the challenge to guide humanity in the new era.

Unprecedented changes in world population, on a hitherto unknown scale, are taking place and will continue to gather momentum in the twenty-first century. Science has not yet kept pace with the changes, and research is needed in almost all disciplines.

In the field of reproductive biology, a research agenda is needed to help the world to adapt to the reproductive evolution. New contraceptives are needed in the twenty-first century. The female reproductive system has to cope with new reproductive patterns. The mature woman has new biological needs that must be addressed.

Contraception-21

Current contraceptive 'hardware' (methods) used with improved software (service delivery approaches), together with a few developments now at the end of the research pipeline, can carry us through the end of this century but will fall far short of meeting the agenda for the twenty-first century. According to current population projections, the next few decades will witness the emergence of more new contraceptive users than in any comparable time in human history, past or future.

The need for new contraceptive methods is not because currently available methods are not good, but because they are not adequate to meet the widely diverse needs of all the hundreds of millions of people using contraception now and in the future. There is not, and there probably will never be, an ideal method of contraception for all users, but there can be a variety of 'ideal methods' for the needs of different users[23].

Science is ripe for a Contraception-21 initiative to launch a second contraceptive techno-logy revolution[15]. While advances in cell and molecular biology and in biotechnology have opened new frontiers for medical and biological sciences, the field of contraceptive research and development is yet to benefit from the opportunities provided by these new advances.

There are four main events in the reproductive process that can be targeted in contraceptive approaches: ovulation; production and maturation of sperm; meeting of the ovum and sperm (fertilization); and implantation of the fertilized ovum. Only the process of ovulation has been so far successfully targeted by modern science. New frontiers now opening up in science can provide novel ways to target the other events in the process that have not yet been exploited and to provide women and men with a broader choice of better state-of-the-art contraceptives.

The second contraceptive technology revolution should not be demographic-driven or completely science-driven. It should be driven by a woman-centered approach, to provide women and men with the contraceptive technologies which they need and which they miss in currently available methods[15,24].

Is the female reproductive system becoming obsolete?

The human female was well equipped, through evolution, with a reproductive system geared to high fertility and efficient reproduction. It has served her well in the past. It may become more of a burden in the future.

In primitive human societies, a woman was meant to menstruate only a few times in her life. The rest of her child-bearing years were to be spent either in pregnancy or lactational amenorrhea. In the modern reproductive evolution, the uterus may be utilized for child-bearing only once or twice in a lifetime. The breast may or may not be used at all for its physiological function. Ovulations and menstrual cycles will continue when there is no chance or desire to conceive.

Strong evidence links incessant ovulation to the occurrence of the common ovarian epithelial, benign and malignant, tumors[25]. The relationship of endometrial cancer to nulliparity is well-established. A protective effect of breastfeeding on the development of breast cancer has been reported. The length of the interval between menarche and child-bearing has been incriminated in the etiology of breast cancer.

Contraceptives of the future will not only have to protect women against conception, but also help the reproductive system to adapt to the changing role. An example is the protective effect of the oral contraceptive pill on ovarian and endometrial cancer, which has now been established.

Biology and the mature woman

Women live, on average, longer than men, in both developed and developing countries. United Nations projections indicate that this trend will continue in the twenty-first century. This advantage of women is variously attributed to an inherent biological advantage, a more healthy life-style behavior (less consumption of alcohol and tobacco), and to environmental factors (more dangerous work activities performed by men).

The human female was not well equipped in evolution for this extended longevity. Cessation of ovarian function, and the menopause, was probably imposed by Nature on the human female, on the basis of life expectancy assessment. To ensure that a newborn gets good care from a living and healthy mother, Nature put a limit to the ability of women to bear children after a certain age, by stopping ovarian function. Women in many countries now, and in more countries in the twenty-first century, can confidently expect to lead a healthy life for more than 20 years after the menopause.

The human female will now have to lead a long period of life without the benefit of the endogenous production of estrogen, making her more liable to bone fragility and cardiovascular disease, apart from other impact on quality of life. Hormone replacement therapy is becoming available to correct this hormonal deficiency. Scientific progress is still needed to develop hormonal preparations which target tissues where the beneficial effect is needed, and which avoid tissues where the exogenous therapy can have adverse effects.

References

1. United Nations (1994). *Experiences Concerning Population and Development Strategies and Programmes. Fourth review and Appraisal of the World Population Plan of Action*, A/Conf.171/4. (New York: United Nations)
2. Demney, P. (1994). *Population and Development.* (Belgium: IUSSP (International Union for the Study of Population) Distinguished Lecture Series)
3. Population Council (1994). Population growth and our caring capacity. *The Population Council Issues Papers*, pp. 1–13. (New York: The Population Council)
4. Larson, A. and Mitra, S. N. (1992). Family planning in Bangladesh: an unlikely success story. *Int. Fam. Plann. Perspect.*, **18**, 123–9
5. Bongaarts, J. (1991). The KAP gap and the unmet need for contraception. *Population Dev. Rev.*, **17**, 293–313
6. Fathalla, M. F. (1992). Family planning: future needs. *Ambio*, **21**, 84–7
7. Malthus, T. R. (1803). An essay on the principle of population. In *The Works of Thomas Robert Malthus*, 2nd edn., vol. 3, pp. 697–8. (London: William Pickering, 1986)
8. United Nations (1994). *Report of the International Conference on Population and Development*, Cairo, 5–13 September 1994 A/CONF.171/13. (New York: United Nations)
9. UNFPA (United Nations Population Fund) (1991). *The State of World Population.* (New York: UNFPA)

10. Fathalla, M. F. (1993). Contraception and women's health. *Br. Med. Bull.*, **49**, 245–51

11. Fathalla, M. F. (1994). Family planning and reproductive health – a global overview. In Graham-Smith, F. (ed.) *Population – the Complex Reality. A Report of the Population Summit of the World's Scientific Academies*, pp. 251–70. (Colorado: The Royal Society, London and North American Press)

12. Fathalla, M. F. (1994). From family planning to reproductive health. In Mazur, L. A. (ed.) *Beyond the numbers – A Reader on Population, Consumption and the Environment*, pp. 143–9. (Washington DC: Island Press)

13. United Nations (1994). *World Contraceptive Use 1994*, United Nations Department for Economic and Social Information and Policy Analysis, ST/ESA/SER.A/143, New York

14. Beral, V. (1979). Reproductive mortality. *Br. Med. J.*, **2**, 632–4

15. Fathalla, M. F. (1994). Mobilization of resources for a second contraceptive technology revolution. In Van Look, P. F. A. and Peres-Palacios, G. (eds.) *Contraceptive Research and Development 1984 to 1994. The Road from Mexico City to Cairo and Beyond*, pp. 527–42. (Bombay: Oxford University Press on behalf of The World Health Organization)

16. Zeng, Yi, Ping, Tu., Baochang, Gu., Yi, Xu., Bohua, Li. and Yongping, Li. (1993). Causes and implications of the recent increase in the reported sex ratio at birth in China. *Population Dev. Rev.*, **19**, 283–302

17. United Nations (1992). *World Population Monitoring 1991*. United Nations Department of International Economic and Social Affairs, Population Studies No.126, ST/ESA/SER.A/126, New York

18. United Nations (1992). *Concise Report on the World Population Situation in 1991, with a Special Emphasis on Age Structure*. United Nations Department of International Economic and Social Affairs, ST/ESA/SER.A/126, New York

19. United Nations (1989). *World Population at the Turn of the Century*. United Nations Department of International Economic and Social Affairs, Population Studies No. 111, ST/ESA/SER.A/111, New York

20. Beauvoir, S. de (1947). *The Second Sex*, p. 13. (London: Pan Books Ltd)

21. World Health Organization (1991). New estimates of maternal mortality. *Weekly Epidemiol. Record*, **66**, 345–8

22. United Nations (1991). *The World's Women 1970–1990. Trends and Statistics*, p. 83. (New York: United Nations)

23. Fathalla, M. F. (1990). Tailoring contraceptives to human needs. *People*, **17**, 3–5

24. Fathalla, M. F. (1994). Fertility control technology: a women-centered approach to research. In Sen. G., Germain, A. and Chen, L. C. (eds.) *Population Policies Reconsidered – Health, Empowerment and Rights*, pp. 223–34. (Boston, MA: Harvard University Press)

25. Fathalla, M. F. (1971). Incessant ovulation – a factor in ovarian neoplasia. *Lancet*, **2**, 1963

26. United Nations (1992). *World Population Prospects: The 1992 Revision*, Annex Tables. (New York: United Nations)

The evolution of contraceptive methods and practices to the year 2000

2

G. Benagiano and I. Shah

Thirty years of progress

Contraceptive technology, utilized to exercise reproductive choices, has moved forward very rapidly over the last 30 years and a number of very useful, effective and safe methods are now available and in widespread use throughout the world.

An area which has witnessed major progress, as well as renewed interest by many groups, is that of the natural regulation of fertility. The development of a purely observational method of detecting ovulation[1] has greatly simplified the utilization of periodic abstinence, although – in field experience – failure due to non-compliance remains high[2]. A number of gadgets and kits are now being developed to enable a precise determination to be made of the beginning and end of the fertile period, and one such device (known as the Personal Contraceptive System (PCS) and made by Unitpath) is being introduced widely on the market[3].

Significant progress has also occurred in the field of hormonal contraception: low-dose monophasic, as well as triphasic combined oral contraceptives have gone a long way towards minimizing adverse effects, while retaining efficacy and acceptability[4]. Progestogen-only mini-pills have been found to be particularly useful for lactating, postpartum women[5], whereas long-acting progestogen-only injectables[6] and implants[7] are gaining momentum.

More recently, the Special Programme of Research in Human Reproduction, a United Nations research program, co-sponsored by UNDP, UNFPA, WHO and the World Bank, has led to the development of monthly injectable estrogen–progestogen contraceptives that greatly reduce the incidence of menstrual bleeding-related disturbances[6]. Two such preparations are being introduced in selected national family planning programs using a new conceptual framework developed by the Special Programme[8].

After the rediscovery in the 1960s of intrauterine contraception with the development of the Lippes loop, better intrauterine devices (IUDs) have also been produced. Efficacy, safety and continuation rates have been greatly improved following the discovery by Zipper that copper has an anti-fertility effect[9]. Large, multi-center clinical trials conducted by the Special Programme have satisfactorily proven the superiority of 'medicated' (copper impregnated) devices over 'non-medicated' ones[10].

The initial drawback of copper-releasing IUDs, the limited duration of action, has now been overcome: an ongoing long-term study conducted by the Special Programme has convinced the US Food and Drugs Administration (FDA) progressively to expand the 'approved' duration of action of copper-releasing devices from 3 years, stipulated when these were initially marketed, to 10 years[11].

After the development of a progesterone-releasing IUD[12], which had a life span of only 1 year, IUDs releasing synthetic progestins are now being developed. One such device, which releases levonorgestrel[13], has reached the marketing stage.

The HIV/AIDS pandemic and the resurgence of sexually transmitted diseases in many areas of the world provided a compelling reason for a re-evaluation of both male and female barrier methods, a modality somewhat neglected because of high failure rates. Barrier methods are especially being promoted by women's health advocates, who argue that they place the decision on contraceptive use squarely in the hands of the users, contrary to the long-acting and provider-controlled methods[14].

Male and female methods of sterilization are becoming more and more acceptable in a number of settings and situations. Although surgical contraception must be selected only after careful consideration of existing options, new techniques, like the non-scalpel vasectomy[15] or the mini-laporotomy route of access to the Fallopian tubes[16], have greatly simplified these procedures.

Non-surgical sterilization remains a very sound alternative, although the recent re-introduction of quinacrine as a pharmacological approach to female sterilization[17] has created great debate, because of a lack of supporting toxicological data on this technique[18]. The World Health Organization has now made public its view that, until a proper preclinical evaluation of quinacrine pellets for intrauterine instillation has been carried out, no further large-scale clinical trials using quinacrine should be undertaken[19].

Trends in contraceptive practice and current use by specific method

Contraceptive practice, measured in terms of its prevalence, i.e. the percentage 'currently' using contraception among couples in which the woman is of childbearing age, has been estimated for 1960–65 at 30% for the world as a whole and below 10% for the less developed regions[20]. In 1990, however, 57% of couples in the world were using a contraceptive method (Figure 1). The rise in contraceptive practice has been most spectacular in developing countries, where 53% of couples were utilizing a method of family planning in 1990. Contraceptive practice was already high in the more developed regions in 1960–65 (67%) and it increased to 72% in 1990.

Global averages, however, mask the great variation in contraceptive practice by region and sub-region, and among countries. For example, in 1990 contraceptive prevalence was only 18% in Africa, as compared to 58% in other developing regions of Asia, Oceania, Latin America and the Caribbean[21]. Within Africa, the use was 31% in the northern part and 13% in sub-Saharan Africa. Among developing countries, contraceptive practice is highest (79%) in eastern Asia (China, Hong Kong and the Republic of Korea).

Female sterilization (tubectomy) has continued to be the single most frequently used method worldwide as well as in the less developed regions, where it accounted for 38% of all use in 1990. Among the 513 million couples in the world using a method in 1990, 153 million relied on female sterilization and 45 million on male vasectomy; 108 million women used IUDs, 72 million the pill and 18 million injectable or vaginal methods; 45 million men used condoms; and the remaining 72 million couples used traditional methods.

In 1990, the three methods more commonly used by couples in the more developed regions were: the pill (16%), the condom (14%) and withdrawal (13%). In the same year, the main methods used in the less developed regions were: tubectomy (20%), the IUD (14%), the pill (6%) and vasectomy (5%). Female sterilization accounts for most of the recent growth in prevalence in developing countries; IUDs have also grown in prevalence. On balance, in developing countries, pill use shows little recent change; the same is true for condom use, at least as reported by women in a marital or stable sex union. New information from interviewing men shows that they often report much higher levels of current condom use than do women. This is especially so for unmarried men; in sub-Saharan Africa, even married men usually report substantially more condom (and rhythm) use than do women. It is plausible that the results are due primarily to a tendency for condoms to be used mainly outside marriage. This also suggests that there could be significant trends in condom use

16

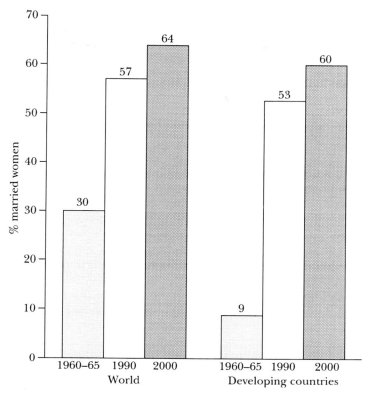

Figure 1 Estimated percentage of married women using contraceptives in the years 1960–2000

outside marriage without a corresponding increase within marriage.

Future demand for contraceptives

Projecting the future trends in contraceptive use and the demand for various methods is not straightforward, as they are likely to be influenced by trends in urbanization, educational attainment, marriage patterns, breast-feeding, induced abortion and the availability of new and/or improved contraceptive methods. Whatever the future trends in these factors may be, one can safely conclude that the demand for contraceptives will continue to increase for at least the next 3 decades. Solely by meeting the existing potential demand of at least 120 million women in the developing world who say that they want to avoid pregnancy but are not using any contraceptive, the prevalence in the developing world would rise from 53% in 1990 to over 60% and the number of users would increase from 384 million to 501 million. Even with no increase in contraceptive prevalence, an additional 100 million couples in the year 2000 will require family planning compared to 1990, due to the increasing number of women of reproductive age.

With fertility below replacement level in much of the more developed regions, the estimation of future demand focuses on the less developed regions, where 536 million couples are expected to be using a contraceptive method in the year 2000 (Table 1). It is predicted that among them, in 235 million couples (44% of all users), one partner will be sterilized (male or female); in 129 million the woman (24%) will have an IUD and in 65 million (12%)

17

Table 1 Estimated and projected number of contraceptive users (in millions), by method, year and region. From references 21 and 22

Method	1990		2000	
	Total	Less developed regions	Total	Less developed regions
All methods	513	384	689	536
Modern methods	441	348	591	474
tubectomy	153	142	213	190
vasectomy	45	36	54	45
the pill	72	43	108	65
injectable	18	7	16	14
intrauterine device	108	99	144	129
condom	45	21	56	31
Traditional methods*	72	36	98[†]	62[†]

*Includes rhythm and withdrawal; [†]includes vaginal methods, Norplant® and traditional methods

she will use the oral pill; in 31 million the man will utilize the condom (6%), and the remaining 76 million will use other methods including female injectables[22]. It is estimated that, in the year 2000, 60% of all couples in the developing world will be using a method. This is an increase of seven percentage points over the prevalence of 53% in 1990.

In conclusion, we can look back at the achievements of the second half of the 20th century and acknowledge with satisfaction the new reality of the expansion in the choice of contraceptive methods enabling couples to exercise their reproductive rights. With over 50% of couples using a contraceptive method in 1990, contraception – a 'novelty' three decades ago – has become a reproductive norm in much of the world. Only in sub-Saharan Africa does the prevalence remain below 18% in most countries. However, it is expected to rise to 26% in the year 2000.

Tubectomy, the IUD and the pill account for much of the contraceptive use in the world. Although 90% of all use is accounted for by modern methods, the use of traditional methods (rhythm and withdrawal) is non-negligible in some more developed countries with high prevalence and in some countries of sub-Saharan Africa with low prevalence. Tubectomy is the method most commonly used, especially in Latin America and in some countries of Asia

(for example, India, Pakistan, Philippines, Republic of Korea, Sri Lanka and Thailand). The IUD is the leading method in China, Egypt, Tunisia and Viet Nam while the oral pill is the main method in Bangladesh, Indonesia and Mauritius. The wide variety of contraceptive patterns shows that the choice of a particular method is affected by the needs and preferences of individual couples, their sociocultural environment and the availability of alternative methods in family planning programs.

Where do we go from here?

The available information suggests that the future family planning trajectory will be characterized by a rapid growth in the number of contraceptive users in the developing world, from 384 million in 1990 to 536 million in the year 2000. The rate of increase in the prevalence is compatible with the changes observed in recent years. However, to meet the existing potential demand and the anticipated demand of the increasing number of couples, the provision of services poses new challenges and will remain a priority issue for policy-makers and agencies concerned with the improvement of the quality of life.

Nearly half of all couples in the developing world do not utilize any of the methods theoretically available, though many would wish to use them if modern contraceptive modalities were to be made accessible. Information on available methods, a prerequisite to exercise reproductive rights, is still lacking in some parts of the world. The concept of reproductive health developed and defined by the WHO has now been accepted by the International Conference on Population and Development (ICPD), held in Cairo in September 1994. ICPD called for a greater emphasis on people, not on methods; on quality of services, not just distribution[23]. The realization that reproductive health goes beyond the use of contraceptive technology to achieve demographic goals, calls for attention for the preferences of people and their changing needs to guide technology development and introduction. The provision of reproductive health services within the new framework has made the challenge even more profound, albeit more rewarding. Can the international community assist in broadening family planning options and provide methods and services to those couples who have little or no choice; to people not yet reached by services or to whom services are provided in an inappropriate manner; to people who are unable to cope with the side-effects of existing methods or worry about their health impact; to people who do not believe that family planning is a personal or social necessity; to people who cannot afford to buy a method or to spend time and money getting to a service delivery point?[24] This question is vital in setting the agenda for further activities in the field of contraception.

References

1. Billings, E. L., Billings, J. J., Brown, J. B. and Burger, H. G. (1972). Symptoms and hormonal changes accompanying ovulation. *Lancet*, **1**, 124–5
2. Benagiano, G. and Bastianelli, C. (1989). Clinical trials of the ovulation method. *Int. J. Gynecol. Obstet.* (Suppl. 1), 91–8
3. Roberts, I., Catt, M. and Jacobs, J. E. (1994). The relationship between a new rapid method of detecting hormonal markers of the fertile period and NFP signs. In *Natural Contraception through Personal Hormone Monitoring*. A satellite symposium, Abstr. 1056. *Abstracts, XIVth World Congress of Gynecology and Obstetrics*, Montreal, September
4. Rivera, R. (1994). Oral contraceptives: the last decade. In Van Look, P. F. A. and Pérez-Palacios, G. (eds.) *Contraceptive Research and Development 1984 to 1994*, pp. 23–36. (New Delhi: Oxford University Press)
5. McCann, M. F. and Potter, L. S. (1994). Progestin-only oral contraception: a comprehensive review. *Contraception*, **50** (Suppl. 1), S1–S195
6. Garcia-Flores, J., Cravioto, M. C. and Pérez-Palacios, G. (1994). Contraceptive research and development today: injectables. In Van Look, P. F. A. and Pérez-Palacios, G. (eds.) *Contraceptive Research and Development 1984 to 1994*, pp. 53–68. (New Delhi: Oxford University Press)
7. Than, R. and Robbins, A. (1994). New implant systems for men and women. In Van Look, P. F. A. and Perez-Palacios, G. (eds.) *Contraceptive Research and Development 1984 to 1994*, pp. 91–106. (New Delhi: Oxford University Press)
8. Spicehandler, J. and Simmons, R. (1994). Contraceptive introduction reconsidered: a review and conceptual framework, WHO/HRP/ITT/94.1, pp. 1–34. (Geneva: The World Health Organization)
9. Zipper, J. A., Tatum, H. J., Medel, M., Pastene, L. and Rivera, M. (1971). Contraception through the use of intrauterine metals. I. Copper an adjunct to the 'T' device. *Am. J. Obstet. Gynecol.*, **109**, 771–6
10. World Health Organization (1982). A randomized multicentre comparative trial of the Lippes Loop D, TCu 220C and Copper 7. *Contraception*, **26**, 1–22
11. Special Programme of Research, Development and Research Training in Human Reproduction (1992). *Annual Technical Report 1992*, WHO/HRP/ATR/92/93, pp. 132–3. (Geneva: World Health Organization)
12. Scommegna, A., Geeta, N., Pandya, M. R., Christ, M., Lee, A. W. and Cohen, M. R. (1970). Intrauterine administration of progesterone by a slow releasing device. *Fertil. Steril.*, **21**, 201–10
13. Sivin, I., El Mahgoub, S., McCarthy, T., Mishell, D. R., Shoupe, D., Alvarez, F., Brache, V., Ji-

menez, E., Diaz, J., Faundes, A., Diaz, M. M., Coutinho, E., Mattos, C. E. R., Diaz, S., Pavez, M. and Stern, J. (1990). Long term contraception with the Levonorgestrel 20 mcg/day (LNg 20) and the Copper T 380Ag intrauterine devices: a five-year randomized study. *Contraception*, **42**, 361–78

14. Germain, A., Nowrojee, S. and Pyne, H. H. (1994). Setting a new agenda: sexual and reproductive health rights. In *Population Policies Reconsidered*, pp. 27–46. (Boston: Harvard University Press)

15. Li, S. Q., Goldstein, M., Zhu, J. B. and Huber, D. (1991). The no-scalpel vasectomy. *J. Androl.*, **145**, 341–4

16. Wilson, E. W. (1995). The evolution of methods of female sterilization. *Int. J. Gynecol. Obstet.* (Suppl.), in press

17. Hieu, D. T., Tann, T. T., Tan, D. N., Nguyet, P. T., Than, P. and Vinh, D. Q. (1993). 31 781 cases of non-surgical female sterilization with quinacrine pellets in Vietnam. *Lancet*, **342**, 213–17

18. Berer, M. (1994). The quinacrine controversy one year on. *Reprod. Health Matters*, **4**, 99–103

19. Benagiano, G. (1994). Sterilisation by quinacrine. *Lancet*, **344**, 689

20. Shah, I. (1994). The advance of contraceptive revolution. *World Health Stat. Q.*, **47**, 9–15

21. United Nations (1994). *World Contraceptive Use 1994*. (New York: United Nations)

22. United Nations Population Fund (1994). *Contraceptive Use and Commodity Costs in Developing Countries, 1994–2005*, Technical Report Number 18. (New York: United Nations Population Fund)

23. United Nations (1994). *Report of the International Conference on Population and Development*, A/CONF.171/3. (New York: United Nations)

24. Benagiano, G. (1994). Availability for everyone. In Senanayake, P. (ed.) *The Reproductive Revolution*, pp. 126–35. (Carnforth, UK: Parthenon Press)

Advances in oral hormonal contraception

3

M. Elstein and H. A. Furniss

Introduction

With over 60 million users of 'the pill' worldwide, the safety of combined oral contraceptive (COC) agents has advanced considerably since their introduction just over 30 years ago. In Britain, by the age of 25, more than 95% of sexually active women have been exposed to combined oral contraceptives[1]. In view of their widespread usage, any associated effects carry important public health implications and this has results in the oral contraceptive (OC) probably being the most thoroughly researched and monitored pharmacological agent[2]. In addition to the well proven efficacy, there have been continuing improvements in the clinical profile over the last 30 years, enhancing the acceptability and safety of oral contraceptive preparations. The coverage of the lay press often emphasizes the rare, but sometimes significant, individual risk that may be present, without regard for the general benefits afforded to women who use OCs. Pregnancy alone offers far greater risks to women than the OC in appropriate cases. Its usage has, by many, been proven to provide significant health benefits, including a reduction of 50% in the incidence of ovarian and endometrial carcinoma[3], reduced iron deficiency, less benign breast disease, fewer functional ovarian cysts and a lower incidence of pelvic inflammatory disease[1].

Lowering the estrogen content of the 'pill'

Enovid®, the first 'pill', marketed from May 1960, contained 150 μg of mestranol, but with over 300 reported cases of thromboembolism by 1963 in the USA alone, the risks associated with its usage and high estrogen content were quickly appreciated. The late 1960s and 1970s saw the widespread usage of OCs containing 50 μg ethinylestradiol with the gradual elimination of the higher estrogen containing products once the dose of estrogen was implicated as the cause of thromboembolism[4]. Subsequently, even lower-dose pills were introduced in the 1970s[5]. In 1980, a striking reduction in the occurrence of vascular events in users of a COC containing 30 μg compared with one containing 50 μg was demonstrated[6]; this was reinforced by Bottiger and colleagues[7], also in 1980, who observed a decrease in thromboembolic risk paralleling the decline in estrogen dose. By 1984, only 4.6% of women using OCs were taking preparations containing 50 μg of estrogen or more[8] and by 1987 this figure had fallen to 2.7% in the UK[9]. The basic pharmacological principle of employing the least dose of agent for the desired effect was thereby being followed.

In 1982, Kay[10] provided evidence from the Royal College of General Practitioners' study that reports of cardiovascular diseases showed a significant trend in relation to the dose of progestogen as well. The risk of thromboembolism in users of low-dose COCs was assessed by Lidegaard[11], more recently, in 1993. It was found that pills containing 50 μg estrogen were associated with an odds ratio for cerebral thrombotic attack of 2.9, those containing 30–40 μg estrogen with an odds ratio of 1.8 and those with progestogen only had an odds ratio of 0.9. There was a 50% increase in the risk of a cerebral thrombotic attack among cigarette smokers, independent of OC status and age. There was no change in the odds ratio with increasing age or duration of OC usage, which agrees with Vessey's data[12] from 1986, which also distinguished the increased risk as being associated with current use only.

The association between OC usage and myocardial infarction (MI) has been demonstrated in several studies[4,6,13,14], but there is no evidence from the Nurses' Health Study[15] or the Royal College of General Practitioners' oral contraception study[16] to suggest an increased risk of cardiovascular disease among past users, even with prolonged previous use. The adverse effect of smoking on MI risk in young women is emphasized in all these studies and indeed remains a far more potent risk factor than COC use in young women[1,16]. In 1991, Engel[17] reported on the angiographic findings after MI in women under 50 years of age and their relationship to COC usage. Sixty per cent of those women sustaining an MI during OC medication did not have coronary atherosclerosis angiographically, whereas in the non-OC users 80% had angiographically demonstrable atherosclerosis. Therefore, it may be suggested that the mechanism of cardiovascular disease in pill users is more likely to be a thrombotic pathogenetic process rather than one of atherogenesis. This theory is supported by the fact that previous use of OCs does not increase the risk factor for cardiovascular disease; atherogenesis, if initiated by OCs would persist after discontinuation of such medication.

Effects on coagulation

The use of the gonane progestogens has enabled the further decrease in estrogen dosage within newer COCs thereby also reducing cardiovascular risks attributable to thromboembolic processes. In 1993, Petersen and co-workers[18] found that the dynamic balance between generation and resolution of fibrin was maintained during treatment with both desogestrel and gestodene containing preparations. A review of nine studies addressing the coagulation effects of gestodene-containing OCs[19] revealed that eight of these found increases in several coagulation promoting factors and four observed that some blood clotting indices remained unchanged. The clinical consequences of these changes are unknown. There are no significant changes in the levels of coagulation or anticoagulation factors after the use of norgestimate COCs in either monophasic or triphasic preparations. The highest risk factor for cardiovascular disease in women remains that of smoking, indeed some believe the 'pill' to be merely an association[20].

Winkler's model[21] of OC usage and changes in hemostatic mechanisms supports the thrombogenic theory of the association of OCs with vascular events. He found that changes in the dosage of ethinylestradiol within OCs alters the hemostatic balance of the coagulation and the fibrinolytic system; a reduced dose leads to a reduction in the imbalance, but the thromboembolic risk which persists may be a manifestation of an idiosyncratic response to synthetic ovarian steroids in some women. The Northwick Park Heart Study[22] also concluded that the biochemical disturbance leading to cardiovascular disease may lie at least as much within the coagulation system as in the metabolism of cholesterol. Specific defects of blood coagulation such as anticoagulation protein C (APC) and protein S deficiency occur in between 1 in 500 and 1 in 5000 women and activated protein C resistance (factor V Leiden) can be present in up to 7% of caucasian populations[23]. In subjects with such disorders thromboembolic events occur before the age of 40 years[24]. These are obviously high-risk cases who should not be prescribed OCs which may further disturb the hemostatic balance. Perhaps screening tests should be implemented to identify such women, where there is a family history or background of thromboembolic disease. Research in this area is urgently required in order to develop a screening test to identify such at risk women, for whom the 'pill' should be contraindicated.

Ethinylestradiol 20 μg instead of 30 μg

In the ongoing search for yet safer OCs, and with the introduction of new progestins, the dosage of ethinylestradiol has been further reduced to 20 μg and even 15 μg. The initial problems encountered with cycle control appear to have diminished. A recent comparative study[25] has demonstrated both 20 μg ethinylestradiol with 75 μg gestodene and 20 μg ethinylestradiol with 150 μg desogestrel to be effective in suppressing ovulation. Intracyclic bleeding was reported in approximately half the women during the first cycle of pill-taking (desogestrel, 53%; gestodene, 47%), but improved in the subsequent studied cycles. There is more residual ovarian activity with the lower-ethinylestradiol-dose pills, but the efficacy is unaffected.

Long-term studies are awaited with regard to the improved safety of these 20 μg formulations. A study[26], reported in 1994, has observed that in reducing the dose of ethinylestradiol from 35 to 20 μg, there is a decrease in the changes in coagulation profile induced by the OC in both smokers and non-smokers.

In some women, the low steroid levels in these preparations may lead to insufficient anti-gonadotropic effect, partial inhibition and therefore development of cyst-like structures in the ovaries. The protective effect of older high-dose OCs with regard to ovarian epithelial carcinoma has been well documented, but the degree of protection afforded by low-dose preparations may well be lessened[27]. However, most benefits from OC usage result from suppression of ovulation, and are not dose dependent[28].

In 1989, the FDA recommended that there should be no upper age limit for the prescription of COC to healthy non-smoking women. As pills are developed with lower total steroid dosage, women may be able to continue using them up to a higher age and to the menopause.

Triphasic regimes

In the 1960s and early 1970s, OC development was directed towards decreasing the estrogen dose as well as that of the progestogen. This led to the development of the triphasic preparations. These have the maximum steroid concentration coinciding with the artificial mid-cycle. They have a dosage profile closely resembling that of the physiological state[29], but allow the total hormone content, particularly the progestogen, to be decreased from the previously marketed monophasic 50 μg estrogen preparations, which were rarely prescribed. Better cycle control was demonstrated with the triphasic formulation, but with the same contraceptive efficacy as with the monophasics. Recent data of usage in the UK from Medical Data Index (Intercontinental Medical Statistics Ltd., UK) extending that reported by Thorogood and Vessey[30] has demonstrated a continued uptake of triphasics in spite of pressure to reduce the usage of these more expensive products.

However, triphasic preparations are consistently reported more frequently with regard to COC failures[31,32]. It is debatable whether this is due to the overall lower dosage of many of the preparations, or because of the increased complexity of taking the preparation, especially when pills are missed. Nevertheless, although suppression of ovarian activity may be incomplete with incorrect pill-taking, secondary mechanisms of contraception, e.g. cervical mucus hostility, remain operational[33].

Triphasic preparations have been proven to be effective, with good cycle control and tolerance. Additionally, these characteristics may be enhanced in those pills with newer progestins, e.g. gestodene[34]. They are particularly suitable for intelligent and motivated women, where estrogen dominance is required and when cycle control has been a problem.

The role of the 'selective' gonane progestins

In the 1960s, little consideration was given to the potent progestins and their interaction with estrogens, but by decreasing the estrogen content of COCs, the adverse androgenic properties of some synthetic progestins have been revealed. These include the potential for atherogenesis effected through changes in cholesterol and lipoproteins, changes in carbohydrate metabolism and enhanced androgenic effects by reduction in sex hormone binding globulin. Indeed, some studies[6,13,35,36] implicate the progestogenic component, both in the nature of the progestogen and its dose, in the adverse effect of OCs on clotting and arterial disease. Also, reducing the dose of OCs, has resulted in adverse effects on cycle control. Hence more recent research has focused on the development of more selective progestins.

The desired biological effect of the progestin component of COCs is its progestational activity. Its androgenic pharmacological properties are unnecessary for contraception and increase the potential for adverse effects. Therefore, selective progestins have progestational activity at relatively low concentrations or doses and their potential for androgenic effects only becomes manifest at relatively high concentrations or doses. The measure of their selectivity is the ratio of the affinity for progesterone receptors to the affinity for androgen receptors; the selectivity index[37]. These progestins – gestodene, desogestrel and norgestimate – are all chemically related to levonorgestrel (i.e. are gonanes), but are more selective in their action on reproductive function, which can be specifically directed towards inhibiting ovulation with lower doses of ethinylestradiol, than levonorgestrel and the estrane progestogen norethisterone, without any significant adverse androgenic-related metabolic effects at the therapeutic dose.

All of these latter gonane progestins are well tolerated, with reduced rates of weight gain, headache and nausea commonly reported with preparations containing older progestogens.

Cycle control

A large comparative study of cycle control of low-dose combined oral contraceptives, reported in 1991, demonstrated statistically significant lower rates of breakthrough bleeding, in the same time frame, with the gestodene preparation (13.7%) compared with the desogestrel (19.8%) and norgestimate (20.1%) pre-parations[38]. With all these products the tendency is for cycle control to settle after 6 months. Gestodene preparations are found to provide better cycle control than those containing desogestrel in several comparative studies[25,39,40] and those containing norgestimate[41]. Further large comparative studies are awaited, as poor cycle control remains the major non-medical reason for discontinuation of pill usage[39].

What is the significance of the lipid profile?

The progestogenic component of COCs has been implicated as a factor in the genesis of cardiovascular disease with regard to its effect on lipid profile. As long ago as 1978, Bradley and colleagues[42] questioned the significance of the effect of OCs on lipid profiles, noting the natural variation that is found in concentrations of high-density lipoproteins (HDL) associated with weight, alcohol intake, exercise and age. Indeed, the low-dose gonane progestins have had positive beneficial effects attributed to them[19], with the potential for protection against cardiovascular disease. This is an important factor when we consider that cardiovascular disease remains the leading cause of death in women in the developed world[43]. High-density lipoprotein levels are increased in formulations containing desogestrel and gestodene[44-46], and norgestimate preparations result in a lowering of the low-density lipoprotein/high-density lipoprotein (LDH/HDL) ratio[47]. However, the clinical significance of these changes of lipoprotein metabolism remains conjectural since they are slight and their impact with regard to the pathogenesis of cardiovascular disease will only be determined by new and extensive epidemiological studies which are currently underway.

Overall risks and benefits of oral contraceptive use

Those women at risk of deleterious effects from OC use are largely those already having a predisposition to the development of cardiovascular disease, i.e. those with hypertension, diabetes mellitus, obesity, a family history of thromboembolic disease and particularly those who smoke[16]. With regard to the protective effect against ovarian and endometrial cancers, this appears to persist, even with the new lower-dose formulations[27]. Any associations with breast or cervical carcinoma remain controversial. The Royal College of General Practitioners' study[48] suggested that pill usage in young nulliparous women, or those delaying a family could reveal a predisposition to breast carcinoma in an already at risk woman. The facts regarding cervical cancers are difficult to interpret, with separation of contributory factors being difficult. There is probably an increase in cervical intraepithelial neoplasia, though this may be a reflection of the increased frequency of smears in pill users or the sexual activity of the subjects studied. Of most concern is the possible increased incidence of adenocarcinoma of the cervix[49].

The benefits of COCs are not inconsiderable (e.g. reduction in ovarian and endometrial cancer, fewer ovarian cysts, less benign breast disease, lower incidence of pelvic inflammatory disease and menorrhagia), as well as providing a convenient, reversible method of contraception, independent of the timing of intercourse[28].

New regimes with 20 μg ethinylestradiol

In reducing the dosage of ethinylestradiol, some loss of cycle control results. In addition to this, residual ovarian activity may become significant should pills be missed thereby lessening the efficacy of such a preparation.

New regimes currently being researched involve shortening of the pill-free interval (i.e. 23- and 24-day regimes) to reduce follicular ripening which may occur during this time. Alternatively, priming with ethinylestradiol during the traditional pill-free phase, might help both to inhibit any follicular ripening and reduce breakthrough bleeding. Indeed, current research looks at 23- or 24-day regimes of 15 μg as well as 20 μg ethinylestradiol. Results from such studies are eagerly awaited, with particular reference to effective suppression of ovarian activity and cycle control which are the critical factors in determining acceptability and continued use of these newer formulations.

Estradiol instead of ethinylestradiol

The use of estradiol instead of ethinylestradiol may be possible with one of the new regimes being investigated presently. In 1993, Wenzl and co-workers[50] reported on a study combining 1 mg estradiol with 150 μg desogestrel. Although ovulation inhibition was complete in all the studied cycles, the bleeding profile was unacceptable, probably due to the progestogen dominance of the preparation. An increased dose of estradiol (2 or 3 mg) may provide an improved clinical profile, maintaining endometrial proliferation as well as ovulation inhibition. Whether such a relatively high dose of estrogen would be acceptable is the crucial issue to be resolved.

Progestins with specific effects

Antiandrogenic, cyproterone acetate

As many as 10% of the female population may have mild polycystic ovarian disease, with androgenic effects such as hirsutism and acne. Combined formulations containing the antiandrogen cyproterone acetate with ethinylestradiol have been highly successful and well tolerated for some time. Newer lower-dosage formulations are being investigated which may continue to provide beneficial antiandrogenic effects for appropriate women in addition to their reconfirmed contraceptive efficacy.

Antimineralocorticoid, dihydrospirenone or drospirenone

In the second half of the natural menstrual cycle, physiological levels of progesterone exert an antimineralocorticoid effect resulting in natriuresis. Virtually all synthetic progestins used as constituents of COCs are devoid of antimineralocorticoid activity. COCs, even in low-dose formulations, may lead to sodium retention and increased blood pressure; susceptible women can develop hypertension while taking OCs. The ethinylestradiol also has sodium retaining properties, unopposed by the progestogen component. In this regard progestogens are being developed with pharmacodynamic profiles more similar to that of progesterone, e.g. drospirenone.

Drospirenone is a progestogen that suppresses ovulation in normal women at a daily dosage of 2 mg as well as preventing endometrial receptivity and producing cervical mucus hostility. It is an aldosterone antagonist which is eight times as potent as spironolactone in the rat. A study assessing the effects of drospirenone[51] concludes that it is a suitable 'partner' of ethinylestradiol as a COC and should lessen side-effects. It should be well tolerated, indeed weight loss was greater after drospirenone treatment than with placebo in this study. It blocks androgen receptors and thereby inhibits sebum production. It could provide an effective OC for those women with problems of weight gain, hypertension and significant premenstrual symptoms, with acne or seborrhea[52].

Antiprogestins in contraception

The antiprogestogen RU 486 has been shown to be well tolerated and most effective as a post-coital contraceptive[53,54]. The WHO is currently conducting a dose-finding study to determine what level of mifepristone can be given to achieve this post-coital effect, which has less side-effects than other currently used methods. Recent studies have also shown that antiprogestogens, e.g. mifepristone (RU 486), effectively block the mid-cycle gonadotropin surge[55]. The development of such agents for contraception may provide an estrogen-free contraceptive.

New regimes are currently under investigation, with mifepristone (RU 486)[56] and onapristone, the latter of which may have a more specific genital tract function. Mifepristone, depending upon when it is administered, has an effect on the menstrual cycle. The aim is to counter any potential of implantation, depending on the time of administration. It would have little contraceptive effect in the proliferative phase, since it does not interfere with the development of the follicle, only delaying its maturation. In the secretory phase, immediately postovulation, it impairs endometrial development and later on in the cycle causes extravasation of blood and destruction of the endometrium, hastening shedding. Therefore 50 mg mifepristone, administered continuously, prevents ovulation and causes amenorrhea with a risk of endometrial proliferation. This is also apparent with 25 mg mifepristone. There is therefore a need for a progestogen to ensure shedding and prevent endometrial hyperplasia. Even lower continuous doses of mifepristone, down to 2 mg, result in ovulation inhibition. A dose of 1 mg has a variable effect on ovarian function, but does result in cycle disruption. The unfortunate aspect of mifepristone is the marked individual variability.

A study by Gemzell-Danielsson and colleagues[57] in 1993 reported effective contraception with mifepristone 200 mg when administered at LH surge plus 2 days. A pregnancy rate of only one in 124 cycles has been demonstrated. The limiting factor would be the detection of the LH surge. There is therefore a need to evaluate the contraceptive potential of these antiprogestogens.

Conclusions

The oral contraceptive pill has become one of the world's most used pharmacological agents since it was first marketed in 1960. Research continues 30 years on, constantly seeking safer effective preparations. Whilst providing women with a convenient, reversible method of contraception, newer and better accepted formulations free of minor side-effects would promote significant health advantages and retain the established benefits and lessen the risks for those who are susceptible.

References

1. Thorogood, M. and Villard-Mackintosh, L. (1993). Combined oral contraceptives: risks and benefits. *Br. Med. Bull.*, **49** (Suppl. 1), 124–39

2. Tyrer, L. B. (1993). Current controversies and future direction of oral contraception. *Curr. Opin. Obstet. Gynecol.*, **5**, 833–8

3. Thorneycroft, I. H. (1992). Non-contraceptive benefits of modern low-dose oral contraceptives. *Adv. Contracept.*, **8** (Suppl. 1), 5–12

4. Inman, W. H. W., Vessey, P. H., Westerholm, B. and Engelund, A. (1970). Thromboembolic disease and the steroidal content of oral contraceptives. A report to the committee of safety of drugs. *Br. Med. J.*, **2**, 203–9

5. Bye, P. and Elstein, M. (1973). A clinical assessment of a low-oestrogen combined oral contraceptive. *Br. Med. J.*, **2**, 389–92

6. Meade, T. W., Greenberg, G. and Thompson, S. G. (1980). Progestogens and cardiovascular reactions associated with oral contraceptives and a comparison of the safety of 50 and 30 mcg oestrogen preparations. *Br. Med. J.*, **280**, 1157–61

7. Bottiger, L. E., Boman, G., Eklund, G. and Westerholm, B. (1980). Oral contraceptives and thromboembolic disease: effects of lowering oestrogen content. *Lancet*, **1**, 1097–101

8. Vessey, M. (1988). Presented at *XII World Congress of Obstetrics and Gynaecology*, Rio de Janeiro

9. Thorogood, M. and Vessey, M. P. (1990). An epidemiological survey of cardiovascular disease in women taking oral contraceptives. *Am. J. Obstet. Gynecol.*, **163**, 274–81

10. Kay, C. R. (1982). Progestogens and arterial disease – evidence from the Royal College of General Practitioners' study. *Am. J. Obstet. Gynecol.*, **142** (6 pt 2), 762–5

11. Lidegaard, O. (1993). Oral contraception and risk of a cerebral thromboembolic attack: results of a case-control study. *Br. Med. J.*, **306**, 956–63

12. Vessey, M.P., Mant, D., Smith, A. and Yeates, D. (1986). Oral contraceptives and venous thromboembolism: findings in a large prospective study. *Br. Med. J.*, **292**, 526

13. Meade, T. W. (1988). Risks and mechanisms of cardiovascular events in users of oral contraceptives. *Am. J. Obstet. Gynecol.*, **158** (6 pt 2), 1646–52

14. Thorogood, M., Mann, J., Murphy, M. and Vessey, M. (1991). Is oral contraceptive use still associated with an increased risk of fetal myocardial infarction? Report of a case-control study. *Br. J. Obstet. Gynaecol.*, **98**, 1245–53

15. Stampfer, M. J., Willett, W. C., Colditz, G. C., Speizer, F. E. and Hennekens, C. H. (1988). A prospective study of past use of oral contraceptive agents and risk of cardiovascular diseases. *N. Engl. J. Med.*, **319** (Suppl. 20), 1313–17

16. Croft, P. and Hannaford, P. C. (1989). Risk factors for acute myocardial infarction in women: evidence from the Royal College of General Practitioners' oral contraception study. *Br. Med. J.*, **298**, 165–8

17. Engel, H. J. (1991). Angiographic findings after myocardial infarctions in young women: role of oral contraceptives. *Adv. Contracept.*, **7** (Suppl. 3), 235–43

18. Petersen, K. R., Sidelmann, J., Skouby, S. O. and Jespersen, J. (1993). Effects of monophasic low-dose oral contraceptives on fibrin formation and resolution in young women. *Am. J. Obstet. Gynecol.*, **168** (1 pt 1), 32–8

19. Speroff, L. and De Cherney, A. (1993). Evaluation of a new generation of oral contraceptives. The Advisory Board for the New Progestins. *Obstet. Gynecol.*, **81** (Suppl. 6), 1034–47

20. Thorogood, M. and Vessey, M. P. (1991). Oral contraceptive prescribing in the presence of risk factors. *Br. J. Fam. Plann.*, **16**, 30–3

21. Winkler, U. H., Koslowski, S., Oberhoff, C., Schindler, E. M. and Schindler, A. E. (1991). Changes in the dynamic equilibrium of hemostasis associated with the use of low-dose oral contraceptives: a controlled study of cyproterone acetate containing oral contraceptives combined with either 35 or 50 mcg ethinylestradiol. *Adv. Contracept.*, **7** (Suppl. 3), 273–84

22. Meade, T. W., Brozovic, M., Chakrabarti, R. R., Haines, A. P., Imeson, J. D., Mellows, S., Miller, G. J., North, W. R. S., Sterling, Y. and Thompson, S. G. (1986). Haemostatic function and ischaemic heart disease: principle results of the Northwick Park Heart Study. *Lancet*, **2**, 533–7

23. Svensson, P. J. and Dahlback, B. (1994). Resistance to activated protein C as a basis for venous thrombosis. *N. Engl. J. Med.*, **330**, 517–22

24. Rabe, Th. and Runnebaum, B. (1993). Update on oral contraceptive. *Eur. J. Obstet. Gynecol. Reprod. Biol.*, **49**, 10–12

25. Fitzgerald, C., Feichtinger, W., Spona, J., Elstein, M., Ludicke, F., Muller, U. and Williams, C. (1994). A comparison of the effect of two monophasic low-dose oral contraceptives on the inhibition of ovulation. *Adv. Contracept.*, **10**, (Suppl. 1), 5–18

26. Fruzzetti, F., Ricci, C. and Fioretti, P. (1994). Haemostasis profile in smoking and nonsmok-

ing women taking low-dose oral contraceptives. *Contraception*, **49** (Suppl. 6), 579–92

27. Rosenblatt, K. A., Thomas, D. B. and Noonan, E. A. (1992). High-dose and low-dose combined oral contraceptives: protection against epithelial ovarian cancer and the length of the protective effect. The WHO Collaborative Study of Neoplasia and Steroid Contraceptives. *Eur. J. Cancer*, **28A** (Suppl. 11), 1872–6

28. Drife, J. (1990). Benefits and risks of oral contraceptives. *Adv. Contracept.*, **6** (Suppl.), 15–25

29. Lachnit-Fixson, U. (1984). Progress in oral contraception. Advantages of a levonorgestrel-containing 3-stage preparation over low-dose levonorgestrel and desogestrel containing monophasic combination preparations. *Fortschr. Med.*, **102** (Suppl. 33), 825–30

30. Thorogood, M. and Vessey, M. P. (1990). Trends in the use of oral contraceptives in Britain. *Br. J. Fam. Plann.*, **16**, 14–53

31. Ketting, E. (1988). The relative reliability of oral contraception – findings of an epidemiological study. *Contraception*, **37**, 343–8

32. Guillebaud, J. (1993). *Contraception: Your Questions Answered.* (Singapore: Churchill Livingstone)

33. Hamilton, C. J. and Hoogland, H. J. (1989). Longitudinal ultrasonographic study of the ovarian suppressive activity of a low-dose triphasic oral contraceptive during correct and incorrect pill intake. *Am. J. Obstet. Gynecol.*, **161** (Suppl. 5), 1159–62

34. Weber-Diehl, F., Lehnert, J. and Lachnit, U. (1993). Comparison of two triphasic oral contraceptives containing either gestodene or norethindrone: a randomized, controlled trial. *Contraception*, **48** (Suppl. 4), 291–301

35. Meade, T. W., Chakrabarti, R., Haines, A. P., Howarth, D. J., North, W. R. S. and Stirling, Y. (1977). Haemostatic, lipid, and blood pressure profiles of women on oral contraceptives containing 50 mcg or 30 mcg oestrogen. *Lancet*, **2**, 948–51

36. WHO – Task force on oral contraceptives (1991). A multicentre study of coagulation and haemostatic variables during oral contraception: variations with four formulations. *Br. J. Obstet. Gynaecol.*, **98**, 1117–28

37. Collins, D. C. (1994). Sex hormone receptor binding, progestin selectivity, and the new oral contraceptives. *Am. J. Obstet. Gynecol.*, **170** (5 pt 2), 1508–13

38. Brill, K., Muller, C., Schnitker, J. and Albring, M. (1991). The influence of different modern low dose oral contraceptives on intermenstrual bleeding. *Adv. Contracept.*, **7** (Suppl. 2), 51–61

39. Rosenberg, M. J. and Long, S. C. (1992). Oral contraceptives and cycle control: a critical review of the literature. *Adv. Contracept.*, **8** (Suppl. 1), 35–45

40. Kirkman, R. J., Pedersen, J. H., Fioretti, P. and Roberts, H. E. (1994). Clinical comparison of 2 low-dose oral contraceptives, Minulet and Mercilon, in women over 30 years of age. *Contraception*, **49** (Suppl. 1), 33–46

41. Affinito, P., Monterubbianesi, M., Primizia, M., Regine, V., Di Carlo, C., Farace, M. J., Petrllo, G. and Nappi, C. (1993). Efficacy, cycle control and side effects of two monophasic combination oral contraceptives: gestodene/EE and norgestimate/EE. *Gynecol. Endocrinol.*, **7** (Suppl. 4), 259–6

42. Bradley, D. D., Wingerd, J., Petitti, D. B., Krauss, R. M. and Ramcharan, S. (1978). Serum high density lipoprotein cholesterol in women using oral contraceptives, estrogens and progestins. *N. Eng. J. Med.*, **299** (Suppl. 1), 17–20

43. Kaffrissen, M. E. (1992). A norgestimate-containing oral contraceptive: review of clinical studies. *Am. J. Obstet. Gynecol.*, **167** (Suppl. 4), 1196–202

44. Benagiano, G. (1989). Comparison of two monophasic oral contraceptives: gestodene/ethinyl estradiol versus desogestrel/ethinyl estradiol. *Int. J. Fertil.*, **34** (Suppl.), 31–9

45. Gevers Leuven, J. A., Dersjant-Roorda, M. C., Helmerhorst, F. M., De Boer, R., Neymeyer-Leloux, A. and Havekes, L. M. (1990). Effects of oral contraceptives on lipid metabolism. *Am. J. Obstet. Gynecol.*, **163** (Suppl. 4), 1410–13

46. Fotherby, K. and Caldwell, A. D. (1994). New progestogens in oral contraception. *Contraception*, **49** (Suppl. 1), 1–32

47. Phillips, A., Hon, D. W. and McGuire, J. L. (1992). Preclinical evaluation of norgestimate, a progestin with minimal androgenic activity. *Am. J. Obstet. Gynecol.*, **167** (Suppl. 4), 1191–6

48. Kay, C. R. and Hannaford, P. C. (1988). Breast cancer and the pill – further report from the Royal College of General Practitioners' oral contraception study. *Br. J. Cancer*, **58**, 675–80

49. Fitzgerald, C. and Elstein, M. (1995). The oral contraceptive pill and cervical neoplasia. *Br. J. Fam. Plann.*, in press

50. Wenzl, R., Spona, J., Bennink, H. C., Huber, J. and van Beek, A. (1993). Ovulation inhibition with a combined oral contraceptive containing 1 mg micronized 17β-estradiol. *Fertil. Steril.*, **60** (Suppl. 4), 616–19

51. Oelkers, W., Berger, V., Bolik, A., Bahr, V., Hazard, B., Beier, S., Elger, W. and Heithecker, A. (1991). Dihydrospirorenone, a new progestogen with antimineralocorticoid activity: effects

of ovulation, electrolyte excretion, and the renin-aldosterone system in normal women. *J. Clin. Endocrinol. Metab.*, **73** (Suppl. 4), 837–42

52. Foidart, J. M., Dombrowicz, N., Heithecker, A. and Oelkers, W. (1994). Clinical tolerance and impacts on blood pressure, the renin-aldosterone system, glucose and lipid metabolism of a new oral contraceptive containing an anti-mineralocorticoid progestogen-drospirenone. *Int. J. Gynecol. Obstet.*, **46** (Suppl. 3), 11

53. Webb, A. M. C., Russell, J. and Elstein, M. (1992). Comparison of Yupze regimen, danazol and mefipristone (RU 486) in oral postcoital contraception. *Br. Med. J.*, **305**, 927–31

54. Glasier, A., Thong, K. J., Dewar, M., Mackie, M. and Baird, D. T. (1992). Mifepristone (RU486) compared with high dose estrogen and progestogen for emergency post-coital contraception. *N. Eng. J. Med.*, **327** (Suppl. 15), 1041–4

55. Lobo, R. A. and Stanczyk, F. Z. (1994). New knowledge in the physiology of hormonal contraceptives. *Am. J. Obstet. Gynecol.*, **170** (5 pt 2), 1499–507

56. Baird, D. T. (1993). Antigestogens. *Br. Med. Bull.*, 73–87

57. Gemzell-Danielsson, K., Swahn, M. L., Svalander, P. and Bygdeman, M. (1993). Early luteal phase treatment with mifepristone (RU486) for fertility regulation. *Hum. Reprod.*, **8** (Suppl. 6), 870–3

Advances in intrauterine device technology

4

D. Reinprayoon

Introduction

Advances in intrauterine device (IUD) technology have led to the development of highly effective, safer and long-lasting devices. The IUD releasing 20 µg levonorgestrel (LNG-20 IUD) is one of the most effective IUDs with a cumulative pregnancy rate of 1.1 per 100 woman-years at 7 years of use[1]. The Copper (Cu) T 380A is more effective, safer and has an even longer life-span[2,3]. However, the reduction in other problems related to the use of currently available IUDs, namely, expulsion, bleeding and pain, has been less impressive. Therefore, efforts continue to develop new IUDs such as the Cu-Fix® IUD, Cu-Safe 300® IUD and other devices[4–6]. One of the major advances in the field of IUD technology, in an attempt to minimize the problem of expulsion, is an implant technology[7,8].

The purpose of this paper is to review the recent important findings with regard to the safety and efficacy of the long-lasting and newly developed IUDs.

Efficacy and safety of currently available long-lasting IUDs

Consistent findings have proven that the long-lasting copper IUDs having a relatively larger surface area (TCu 380A/Ag® and the Multiload 375 (ML 375)® IUDs) are more effective than the TCu 200® and ML 250® IUDs and non-medicated devices such as the Lippes Loop and Chinese stainless steel ring (SSR)[5,6,9,10].

The World Health Organization (WHO) study showed that the pregnancy rates after 5, 7, 9 and 11 years of use for the TCu 380A were 1.5,

1.6, 1.8 and 2.3, respectively[3,11]. The rates were consistently and significantly lower than those of the TCu 220C at all durations of use. The ectopic pregnancy and pelvic inflammatory disease (PID) rates were low for both devices, indicating the long-term efficacy and safety of the IUDs. Based largely on the results of this study, the TCu 380A was approved by the US Food and Drug Administration for extended use up to 10 years[12].

Chi's recent reviews[13,14] demonstrated that the MLCu 375 IUD seems to be slightly less effective in preventing pregnancies than the TCu 380A. Its efficacy is comparable to that of the Nova-T® by 2–3 years of use. Very low perforation rates ranged from 0 to 0.2 per 1000 Multiload IUD insertions[13]. No consistent differences were detectable between the Multiload IUDs and comparative Copper T IUDs in expulsion rates or in removal rates for bleeding/pain, PID and ectopic pregnancy risks[13,14].

A WHO multicenter study[11] showed that the cumulative pregnancy rates at 3 and 5 years of use for the Nova-T were 6.6 and 12.3, respectively, which were significantly higher than those of the TCu 220C. In a recent study[15], the accidental pregnancy rate at 3 years for the ML 375 was 2.9 per 100 woman-years, significantly higher than the corresponding rate of 1.6 for the TCu 380A.

A Population Council study[1] reported cumulative 7-year gross pregnancy rates of 1.1 and 1.4 per 100 woman-years for the LNG-20 IUD and the TCu 380Ag IUD, respectively. However, the continuation rate of the LNG-IUD was lower than that of the TCu 380Ag. The lower continuation rate in LNG-IUD acceptors was because of removals for amenorrhea/abnormal uterine bleeding and/or other hormonal side-effects[1]. The particularly important characteristic of the LNG-IUD is its effectiveness in reducing the menstrual blood loss with women who experienced menorrhagia. It has been reported that the LNG-IUD has a protective effect against PID and myoma or subsequent hysterectomy. No ectopic pregnancies were experienced with the LNG-20 IUD[1].

Efficacy and safety of newly developed IUDs

The Cu-Fix IUD (FlexiGard®, GyneFix®) has six copper sleeves on a single nylon thread with a copper surface area of 330 mm[2]. Recent data from a WHO multicenters study indicated that the 2-year pregnancy rate for the FlexiGard was higher than that of the TCu 380A (1.2 vs. 0.6 per 100 woman-years)[2]. However, with an improved inserter, the cumulative pregnancy rate is 0.6 and there is a removal rate for medical reasons of 3.2 at 3 years[7]. The cumulative expulsion rate is 0.6 per 100 woman-years at 3 years and is not significantly higher in the nulligravid/nulliparous group[7,8]. There are no reports of serious complications such as PID, ectopic pregnancies or perforation in either study.

The Cu-Fix PP 330 device is identical to the FlexiGard except for a small cone of biodegradable plastic at the end of the thread[2]. The preliminary results for immediate postplacental insertion (IPPI) from a WHO pilot study are encouraging in that only one expulsion has occurred in 55 insertions. This study will be expanded to include at least 16 centers[2].

The Gyne T 380 Slimline® differs from the TCu 380A in that the copper sleeves are placed at the recessed end of the arm and have the same diameter as the plastic. Recent findings[16] showed a lower pregnancy rate (0.3 vs. 1.5 per 100 woman-years) but a significantly higher expulsion rate than those of the TCu 380A (8.6 vs. 4.4 per 100 woman-years) at 4 years of use.

The Cu-Safe 300®[4,6] is lightweight, flexible and smaller than other copper IUDs. Clinical data from a multicenter study[4] have been favorable with a 12-month pregnancy rate of 0.6, expulsion 0.6, removal for bleeding 4.2 and for pain 1.5. The clinical performance of other IUDs[4,6] such as Fincoid®, Ombrelle®, Dimelys® and the Chinese IUD releasing indomethacin[5] are quite impressive. However, long-term, multinational, randomized comparative studies are needed to provide definite results.

Discussion

The acceptability of intrauterine device use can be increased by good counseling, screening and good clinical management[17]. The World Health Organization is compiling a list of eligibility criteria for initiating the use of selected methods of contraception for improving access to quality care in family planning. As a choice for intrauterine device use, the recommended device may be the TCu 380A. Its low initial cost and long life-span make the intrauterine device highly cost-effective compared with other reversible contraceptive methods. Pelvic inflammatory disease usually occurs within the first 20 days after intrauterine insertion[18], so the shorter the permitted duration of use, the greater the number of insertions and re-insertions, with corresponding increases in the risk of infection and other use-related events such as pain, bleeding and perforation. Moreover, the longer lifespan of TCu 380A would reduce the frequency of clinic visits, which decreases the costs in providing family planning for women in developing countries. Hence, this intrauterine device will steadily become one of the most popular intrauterine devices used in family planning programs worldwide.

References

1. Sivin, I., Stern, J. and International Committee for Contraception Research (ICCR) (1994). Health during prolonged use of levonorgestrel 20 µg/d and the Copper TCu 380 Ag intrauterine contraceptive devices: a multicenter study. *Fertil. Steril.*, **61**, 70–6

2. UNDP/UNFPA/WHO/World Bank/Special Programme of Research, Development and Research Training in Human Reproduction (1994). Challenges in reproductive health research. *Biennial Report 1992–1993*. (Geneva: World Health Organization)

3. UNDP/UNFPA/World Bank/WHO/Special Programme of Research, Development and Research Training in Human Reproduction (1995). Long-term effective and safe contraception with the TCu 380A: results from a comparative trial with the TCu 220C at seven, nine and eleven years of use. *Contraception*, in press

4. Boating, J., Chi, I.-C. and Jones, D. B. (1994). An evaluation of six new intrauterine devices. *Adv. Contracept.*, **10**, 57–70

5. Zhuang, Liu Qi (1994). Research on intrauterine devices in China in the 1990s. Presented at a *Symposium on Intrauterine Devices*, Nanging, China, August

6. Rowe, P. J. (1994). Clinical performance of Copper IUDs. In Bardin, C. W. and Mishell, D. R. (eds.) *Proceedings from the Fourth International Conference on IUDs*, pp. 13–31. (Boston: Butterworth-Heinemann)

7. Wildemeersch, D., Van Kets, H., Van der Pas, H., Vrijens, M., Van Trappen, Y., Temmerman, M., Batar, I., Barri, P., Martinez, F., Iglesias-Cortit, L. and Thiery, M. (1994). IUD tolerance in nulligravid and parous women: optimal acceptance with the frameless CuFix implant system (GyneFix). Long-term results with a new inserter. *Br. J. Fam. Plann.*, **20**, 2–5

8. Van Kets, H., Wildemeersch, D., Van der Pas, H., Vrijens, M., Van Trappen, Y., Delbarge, W., Temmermen, M., Batar, I., Barri, P., Martinez, F., Wu Shang-chung, Cao Xiao Ming, Feng Zuan Chong, Wu Ming Hui, Pizarro, E., Andrade, A. and Thiery, M. (1995). IUD expulsion solved with implant technology. *Contraception*, **51**, 87–92

9. Farr, G. and Amatya, R. (1994). Contraceptive efficacy of the Copper T 380A and Multiload Cu 250 intrauterine devices: results from a multinational comparative clinical trial. *Adv. Contracept.*, **10**, 137–49

10. World Health Organization (1987). Mechanism of action, safety and efficacy of intrauterine devices. *Technical Report Series 753*, p. 91. (Geneva: World Health Organization)

11. World Health Organization (1990). The TCu 380A, TCu 220C, Multiload 250 and Nova-T IUDs at 3, 5, 7 years of use – results from three randomized multicenter trials. *Contraception*, **42**, 141–58

12. The Population Council (1994). Copper T 380A intrauterine device is effective for 10 years. News Release, The Population Council, New York, September

13. Chi, I.-c. (1992). The Multiload IUD. US researcher's evaluation of a European device. *Contraception*, **46**, 407–25

14. Chi, I.-c. (1993). The TCu 380A (Ag), MLCu 375, and Nova-T IUDs and the IUD daily releasing 20 µg levenorgestrel – four pillars of IUD contraception for the nineties and beyond? *Contraception*, **47**, 325–47

15. UNDP/UNFPA/WHO/World Bank/Special Programme of Research, Development and Research Training in Human Reproduction: IUD Research Group (1994). A randomized multicenter trial of the Multiload 375 and TCu 380A IUDs in parous women: three-year results. *Contraception*, **49**, 543–9

16. Sivin, I., Diaz, J., Alvarez, F., Brache, V., Diaz, S., Parez, M. and Stern, J. (1993). Four-year experience in a randomized study of the Gyne T380 Slimline and the Standard Gyne T380 intrauterine devices. *Contraception*, **47**, 37–42

17. Reinprayoon, D. (1992). Intrauterine contraception. *Curr. Opin. Obstet. Gynecol.*, **4**, 527–30

18. Farley, T. M., Rosenberg, M. J., Rowe, P., Chen, J. H. and Meirik, O. (1992). Intrauterine devices and pelvic inflammatory disease; an international perspective. *Lancet*, **339**, 785–88

Recent advances on the path to a contraceptive vaccine

5

J. C. Herr, A. B. Diekman, S. A. Coonrod and A. J. Freemerman

Introduction

This paper discusses several recent advances in the development of a contraceptive vaccine, based upon antigens derived from sperm. It focuses attention on technical milestones that have been reached in understanding the nature of a sperm antigen (SP-10) used in making a contraceptive vaccine and discusses an *in vitro* mechanism of contraceptive action of antibodies to SP-10. In addition, an oral method for contraceptive vaccine delivery is discussed and recent results from fertility testing of a peptide contraceptive vaccine based on the testis-specific isozyme, LDH-C$_4$, is reviewed. The data presented are derived from small animal and non-human primate studies.

The advances described have not yet been applied to human subjects. No contraceptive vaccine is currently on the market in any country and development of a contraceptive vaccine has many hurdles to overcome, not the least of which is achieving efficacy that will match that of contraceptive products currently in the marketplace – products that deliver 95% efficacy or better (over-the-counter birth control pills).

Sperm antigen-based contraceptive vaccines: general concerns

Pre-fertilization vaccine for females The principal focus is on a vaccination model in which the vaccine recipient is a female and the objective of immunization is to induce infertility at a stage prior to completion of fertilization. This type of vaccine, in contrast to vaccines that are directed against antigens of the trophoblast or early embryo (e.g. human chorionic gonadotropin (hCG)), has been termed a 'pre-fertilization vaccine'. This contraceptive strategy is deemed to have the highest likelihood of widespread acceptance by individuals of varied religious, ethical and political persuasions.

The pathway to a sperm vaccine To reach the goal of a pre-fertilization contraceptive, candidate antigens for inclusion in the vaccine must be identified and undergo extensive analysis and characterization, including understanding of not only primary structure, but also tissue specificity and analysis of the major immunogenic regions of each molecule. The most attractive candidate vaccinogens then require synthesis as peptides or scaled-up production using genetic engineering methods prior to being incorporated into vaccine formulations for small animal, non-human primate and human testing.

A strategy for developing several sperm antigens for mixture in a multideterminant formulation It is probable that the vaccine formulation with the highest efficacy will ultimately consist of a mixture of several sperm immunogens. This 'ideal sperm vaccine' may be conceived to contain sperm-specific immunogens that induce antibodies to all sperm surface domains accessible to antibody: head, midpiece and tail plasmalemma, including the inner acrosomal membrane, which forms a major part of the anterior surface of the sperm head following the acrosome reaction. Antibodies to these domains, if present in cervical mucus, uterine and oviductal fluids, might act to agglutinate or lyse (complement-mediated immobility) sperm during cervical and uterine transport, coat key sperm receptors necessary for the acrosome reaction, thus preventing zona penetration, block sperm/zona interaction by inhibiting the zona receptor(s), block sperm/oolemma interaction and prevent gamete fusion.

Immunogenicity   In order for a sperm antigen to be potentially useful as a contraceptive vaccine agent, the antigen must be a strong immunogen capable of inducing antibody-mediated (humoral, B cell) and/or cell-mediated immune responses (e.g. T helper cells, macrophages, natural killer (NK) cells). Because sperm represent cells that do not normally differentiate in the female body, sperm-specific proteins may prove to be powerful immunogens in female animals.

The importance of surface accessibility of sperm antigens chosen for contraceptive vaccine development   In the case of antibody-mediated events, the sperm antigen targets chosen for contraceptive development must be accessible on the sperm surface, so that immune events such as sperm agglutination, sperm lysis, antibody coating of surface antigens, or phagocytosis of opsonized sperm might proceed. Certain cell-mediated processes, such as NK cell lysis of targets, also require interactions between the NK cell and sperm surface antigens; however, other cell-mediated events, such as release of cytokines inhibitory to sperm function, do not necessarily require the target antigens to be exposed on the sperm surface. Whether B cell or T cell immune effectors are considered, delivery of antibodies, cytokines or phagocytic and lytic cells will be through the vehicle of the secretions of the female reproductive tract (oviductal fluid, uterine fluid (milk) and cervical mucus).

Mechanisms of contraceptive action in vivo   As sperm progress through the female reproductive tract, immune effectors in female secretions may exert contraceptive effects that act in various regions. Thus, anti-sperm antibodies present in cervical mucus might agglutinate or lyse sperm in the vagina prior to sperm passage through the cervix. Sperm, coated with surface antibody, might be prevented from swimming through and penetrating cervical mucus. Clinically, this condition is often referred to as the 'shaking phenomenon' and is well described in the literature on sperm–cervical mucus interaction. In the uterus sperm might be trapped or lysed by antibodies present in uterine secretions and thus be prevented from reaching the oviduct. Antibodies present in oviductal fluid might likewise bind to sperm antigens and prevent key steps in the fertilization process from occurring in the oviduct. At the level of sperm–egg interaction, penetration of the cumulus mass or zona pellucida, zona binding, capacitation, induction of the acrosome reaction, shedding of the acrosomal ghost, penetration of the zona pellucida, binding to the oolemma or internalization of the spermatozoan by the egg represent stages of fertilization where antibodies bound to sperm might inhibit key functions.

Immunoglobulins embedded within the zona pellucida   When considering these possible immunocontraceptive events in the oviduct, it is important to appreciate that the zona pellucida is itself permeable to immunoglobulins. Anti-sperm antibodies may become embedded in the zona pellucida during differentiation of the oocyte within the ovarian follicle, where the oocyte is bathed in immunoglobulins present in the follicular fluid. Passage of the egg through the oviduct may also result in antibody equilibrating within the layers of the zona pellucida. If such antibody were directed against sperm antigens and sufficient antibody were present in the oviductal fluids and tissues surrounding the egg, fertilization might be blocked.

Two categories of sperm antigens may be distinguished on the basis of surface accessibility   It is useful to consider the target sperm antigens for use in contraceptive vaccines in two groups:

(1) antigens that are present on the sperm surface plasma membrane; and (2) antigens that are present in the acrosomal membranes and matrix (e.g. acrosin, SP-10) and that remain associated with the sperm surface after the acrosome reaction. It is to be remembered that the acrosome reaction results in remodelling of the anterior portion of the sperm head, so that the inner acrosomal membrane becomes the limiting membrane over the sperm nucleus when the acrosome reaction is complete. Antigens associated with the inner acrosomal membrane may be made accessible to antibodies after they 'decloak'.

Some proteins, such as hyaluronidase (PH-20)[1], may bridge both categories by having dual localizations, both on the sperm plasma membrane and within the acrosome. Such antigens are accessible to antibody at many stages of sperm transport within the female tract. However, proteins that are restricted to the acrosomal membranes and matrix afford a much narrower window of opportunity for immunological interdiction and contraceptive action. Such antigens within the acrosomal compartment become accessible to antibody as the acrosome reaction is initiated, fusion pores form, hybrid vesicles develop and the acrosomal membranes and matrix are exposed to the surrounding medium.

Recent advances in sperm antigen-based contraceptive vaccines

Advance 1: Oral immunization with attenuated Salmonella expressing the human SP-10 antigen induces antibodies in serum and the reproductive tract

Introduction to the SP-10 protein SP-10 is an intra-acrosomal protein known to be conserved across various mammalian species including humans, baboons, macaques, pigs, foxes and mice[2,3]. In humans, the protein is 265 amino acids in length and contains a typical signal sequence of 17 amino acids at its amino-terminus. Human SP-10 is encoded by a single gene

consisting of four exons located on human chromosome 11 at band q23-24. In mature human sperm, SP-10 is localized to the acrosomal matrix and is also associated with acrosomal membranes[4]. The World Health Organization Taskforce on Contraceptive Vaccines has designated SP-10 as a 'primary vaccine candidate'[5].

The concept of oral vaccines based on live attenuated Salmonella S. typhimurium strains with deletions of the adenylate cyclase (*cya*) and cyclic AMP receptor protein (*crp*) genes are avirulent and immunogenic while retaining their ability to colonize gut-associated lymphoid tissue (GALT) and internal organs[6]. The advent of recombinant DNA technology has enabled foreign genes to be expressed in *Salmonella*, thus converting this bacterium into an efficient delivery system for the induction of immune responses to the expressed antigens. Since *S. typhimurium* naturally invades and persists in GALT[7], oral immunization with attenuated *Salmonella* expressing foreign antigens stimulates antigen-specific secretory, humoral and cellular immune responses (for a review see reference 8). Such a system may be particularly advantageous in eliciting an immune response against a gamete-specific antigen in the female reproductive tract for the purpose of developing a contraceptive vaccine.

S. typhimurium expressing the human SP-10 sperm antigen induces a secretory immune response in the mouse female reproductive tract. A cDNA sequence encoding human SP-10 was cloned on an *asd* + vector and expressed to a high level in an avirulent Δ-*cya*, Δ-*crp* and Δ-*asd* vaccine strain of *S. typhimurium*. Oral immunization of female BALB/c mice with this recombinant *Salmonella* elicited high-titer anti-SP-10 IgG antibodies in serum and IgA antibodies in vaginal secretion. Anti-SP-10 antibody titers could be increased by secondary and tertiary oral administration of the recombinant *Salmonella*. Induction of sperm-specific antibodies in the reproductive tract, following oral administration of a recombinant *Salmonella*, could lead to the development of a simple, safe, efficient and easy-to-use anti-fertility vaccine[9].

Advance 2: A mechanism of contraceptive action of antibodies against SP-10 has been clarified in vitro

SP-10 is exposed on the sperm surface following the acrosome reaction Electron microscopic immunocytochemical observations of epididymal, ejaculated and capacitated sperm have revealed colloidal gold labelling of SP-10 to be most abundant within the principal segment and posterior bulb of the equatorial segment of the acrosome, while the colloidal gold labelling of SP-10 was sparse in the anterior equatorial segment of the acrosome[10]. Following a follicular fluid-induced acrosome reaction, SP-10 was detected on the inner acrosomal membrane, in the equatorial segment and associated with hybrid vesicles[10]. With completion of the acrosome reaction, the entire anterior portion of the sperm head becomes remodelled as the inner acrosomal membrane becomes the limiting membrane over the anterior portion of the sperm nucleus. The persistence of SP-10 on this inner acrosomal membrane makes it an attractive candidate for blocking interactions between the inner acrosomal membrane and the egg investments. This localization of SP-10 after the acrosome reaction is consistent with the hypothesis that this protein is involved in sperm–zona binding or penetration. This hypothesis has been directly addressed with the use of bovine *in vitro* fertilization (IVF), as discussed in the following section.

Antibodies to SP-10 inhibit bovine IVF by affecting sperm prior to sperm–zona secondary binding[11]
Anti-SP-10 antibodies are cross-reactive with bovine sperm and reduce bovine fertilization rates *in vitro* by affecting both sperm motility and the ability of sperm to complete the acrosome reaction and sperm motility. To characterize bovine SP-10, sonicated bovine sperm extracts were analyzed by Western blot using three monoclonal antibodies (mAbs) previously developed to human SP-10 and a polyclonal

antibody to recombinant baboon SP-10 (rbSP-10). Under denaturing and reducing electrophoretic conditions, the 6C12 mAb reacted with proteins of 30–35 kDa and the polyclonal antibody reacted with numerous proteins of 18–35 kDa. Under non-denaturing and non-reducing (native) electrophoretic conditions, both the 6C12 and MHS-10 mAbs reacted with proteins of 35–40 kDa and the polyclonal antibody reacted strongly to a single protein band of 33–38 kDa. The 3C12 mAb did not recognize proteins from bovine sperm extracts in western blot analysis under either condition. Indirect immunofluorescence revealed that the MHS-10 mAb, 6C12 mAb and polyclonal antibody were reactive with the acrosomal region of methanol-fixed bovine sperm, but not live sperm.

Several IVF experiments were performed with bovine oocytes and sperm. The first IVF experiment revealed that fertilization rates of bovine oocytes were significantly reduced ($p < 0.01$) from 83.2 and 86.5% in the null ascites and control lacking antibody, respectively, compared with 47.7 and 7.5% in groups treated with 1 : 20 and 1 : 10 dilution of a cocktail containing the three SP-10 mAbs. In the next experiment, MHS-10 mAb ascites was added to the fertilization medium, followed by immediate absorption of the antibody with the use of recombinant SP-10 protein. The resulting fertilization rate (81.3%) was no different ($p > 0.10$) from either the control lacking antibody (85.3%) or the null ascites (87.6%). However, unabsorbed MHS-10 mAb ascites reduced ($p < 0.01$) fertilization rates to 16%, thus demonstrating that the reduction in fertilization rates was due to SP-10 antibodies and not to another component of the ascites. In another IVF experiment, the addition of SP-10 polyclonal antisera to fertilization medium resulted in a 44.3% fertilization rate, which was significantly lower ($p < 0.01$) than that out of the control lacking antibody (79%) and the pre-immune sera (84%). Functional assays were performed to study the possible stage of sperm–egg interaction at which the antibodies were exerting their effect. The SP-10 mAB cocktail was shown significantly to reduce ($p < 0.05$)

sperm–zona secondary binding during IVF. The MHS-10 mAb reduced the ability of capacitated sperm to undergo the acrosome reaction while having no effect ($p > 0.10$) on sperm viability. The MHS-10 mAb significantly reduced ($p < 0.01$) both the motility and rapid motility of capacitated sperm but did not reduce the motility parameters of non-capacitated sperm. Together, these data indicate that antibodies to SP-10 block sperm–egg interaction by preventing secondary binding. This blockage of bovine fertilization appears to be due to an effect of antibodies on sperm motility and on the ability of sperm to complete the acrosome reaction[11].

Advance 3: The molecular basis of SP-10 micro-heterogeneity has been shown to involve alternative splicing

A single-copy gene with multiple protein isoforms

The intra-acrosomal protein SP-10 is a particularly interesting example of a sperm protein that, although encoded by a single gene, gives evidence of considerable micro-heterogeneity. Analyzed by one-and two-dimensional sodium dodecyl sulfate-polyacrylamide gel electrophoresis (SDS-PAGE) and Western blot, human SP-10 presents as a series of immunoreactive peptides ranging from 18 to 32 kDa (Figure 1), the majority of which have isoelectric points of 4.9[12]. The relationship between the immunoreactive peptides and the amino acid sequence of SP-10 deduced from cDNAs has been determined. Amino-terminal sequence analysis of the eight immunoreactive SP-10 peptides seen in Figure 1 shows that each of the peptides can be aligned along the deduced 265 amino acid sequence of SP-10 (Figure 2). Thus, portions of the amino-terminal region of SP-10 are absent in the lower molecular weight SP-10 peptides observed in ejaculated sperm[13].

Western blots of SP-10 in testis extracts and epididymal sperm suggest that the pattern of immunoreactive SP-10 peptides is established in the testis and modified in the epididymis and upon ejaculation[10]. Analysis of the stability of the immunoreactive SP-10 peptides after ejacu-

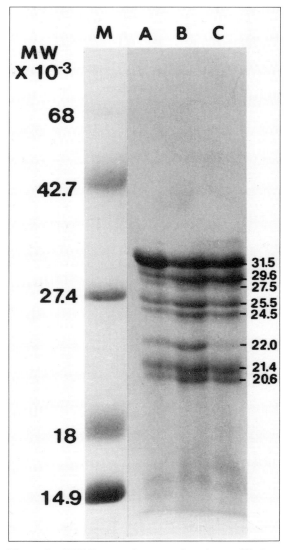

Figure 1 PVDF membrane showing affinity-purified human SP-10 stained with Brilliant Blue. The molecular weight markers are on the left and the relative molecular weight of each SP-10 peptide is on the right

lation with and without protease inhibitors indicates that most of the SP-10 peptides are quite stable[12].

Cloning of alternatively spliced human SP-10s[13]

Human testis poly A+ RNA was isolated from four separate individuals. Each mRNA was reverse transcribed, creating single-stranded

```
M   N   R   F   L   L   L   M   S   L   Y   L   L   G   S   A   R   G   T   S      20
S   Q   P   N   E   L   S   G   S   I   D   H   Q   T   S   V   Q   Q   L   P      40
G   E   F   F   S   L   E   N   P   S   D   A   E   A   L   Y   E   T   S   S      60
G   L   N   T   L   S   E   H   G   S   S   E   H   G   S   S   K   H   T   V      80
                                            (31.5 kD) - H   T   V -

A   E   H   T   S   G   E   H   A   E   S   E   H   A   S   G   E   P   A   A     100
A   E   H   T   S   G   E   - (31.5 kD)
        (29.6 kD) - G   E   H   A   E   E   E   H   A - (29.6 kD)
                            (27.5 kD) - G   E   P   A   A

T   E   H   A   E   G   E   H   T   V   G   E   Q   P   S   G   E   Q   P   S     120
        (25.5 kD) - G   E   H   T   V   G   Q   Q   P   S - (25.5 kD)
                        (24.5 kD) - E   Q   P   S   G   E   Q   P   S -

G   E   H   L   S   G   E   Q   P   L   S   E   L   E   S   G   E   Q   P   S     140
G   E - (24.5 kD)
            (22.0 kD) - E   Q   P   L   S   E   L   E   S   G   E   Q   P   S -
                            (21.4 kD) - E   Q   P   S
                                    (20.6 kD) - S

D   E   Q   P   S   G   E   H   G   S   G   E   Q   P   S   G   E   Q   A   S     160
D - (22.0 kD)
D - (21.4 kD)
D   E   Q   P   S   G   E   H   G   S   G - (20.6 kD)

G   E   Q   P   S   G   E   H   A   S   G   E   Q   A   S   G   A   P   I   S     180
S   T   S   T   G   T   I   L   N   C   Y   T   C   A   Y   M   N   D   Q   G     200
K   C   L   R   G   E   G   T   C   I   T   Q   N   S   Q   Q   C   M   L   K     220
K   I   F   E   G   G   K   L   Q   F   M   V   Q   G   C   E   N   M   C   P     240
S   M   N   L   F   S   H   G   T   R   M   Q   I   I   C   C   R   N   Q   S     260
F   C   N   K   I  TER                                                           265
```

Figure 2 Comparison of N-terminus amino acid sequences from isolated SP-10 peptides with the amino acid sequence deduced from cDNA cloning and sequencing. Amino acids are presented according to the single-letter code from data published by Herr and colleagues[14]

cDNAs. SP-10 was then amplified via reverse transcriptase polymerase chain reaction (RTPCR) and the resulting products were separated on a 2% agarose gel containing ethidium bromide (100 ng/ml). The DNA was visualized by ultraviolet light transillumination (Figure 3). The oligonucleotide primers utilized in the PCR amplification flanked the one previously charac-terized alternatively spliced variant of human SP-10[15]. The primers mapped to the beginning of exon 2 and the middle of exon 4; the intervening sequence accounted for 85% of the open reading frame of SP-10. The same banding pattern was seen when the entire open reading frame was amplified (data not shown). Between seven and ten discrete DNA bands were

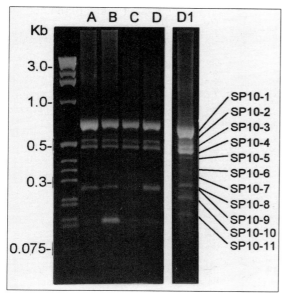

Figure 3 Agarose gel stained with ethidium bromide showing 30% of the SP-10 RTPCR products from four individuals (A, B, C and D). Lane D1 is over-loaded with loading 100% of an RTPCR amplification and the bands corresponding to SP-10-1 through SP-10-11 are labelled. The PCR products were amplified 40 cycles from reverse transcribed testis mRNA. A DNA ladder is located in the left lane

observed in the four individuals tested. The highest two migrating DNA bands corresponded in mass to the two previously reported SP-10 cDNAs[15]. As seen in the right lane of Figure 3, these two DNA bands resolved poorly, due to the greater amount of DNA in the upper band. All other bands observed were considered potentially novel alternatively spliced SP-10 variants.

In order to determine the relatedness of each DNA band observed in the RTPCR amplification to the previously sequenced SP-10 open reading frame, 11 distinct bands were isolated, subcloned into pBluescript, and sequenced. The two highest mass RTPCR products proved to be identical to the SP-10 cDNAs previously characterized[14]. The other nine subclones proved to be unique splice variants of SP-10 (Figure 4). Each contained in-frame deletions of sequence present in the largest SP-10, which encodes a 265 amino acid protein. The novel

splice variants all contained either one or two in-frame deletions located within exons 2 and/or 3 of the coding region. The 5′ border of the first (and sometimes only) in-frame deletion was shared amongst the nine splice variants and was located between amino acids 40 and 41. The 3′ border of the first deletion and, in some cases, the location of a second deletion varied for each of the nine SP-10 transcripts.

Each deletion was defined by a 5′ and 3′ donor splice junction. All but one of the splice junctions creating the deletions conformed to the GT–AG consensus splice sequence[17]. The exception, the second 3′ donor splice junction of SP-10-7, had GT–TG as the first and last two nucleotides of the excised sequence. Also, the second 5′ donor splice junction of SP-10-9 appeared not to follow to GT–AG rule. However, the splice probably utilized the GT sequence found at the beginning of intron 2 and the AG sequence at the end of exon 3, splicing out all of intron 2 and exon 3, thus conforming to the consensus splice rule. Therefore, due to the fact that the splices were in-frame and conformed to the GT–AG rule, the SP-10 RTPCR products were not artifacts of the amplification, but represented authentic alternatively spliced SP-10 mRNAs.

Quantitative competitive RTPCR[13]   Quantitative competitive RTPCR (QCRTPCR) was utilized to determine the relative abundance of each of the SP-10 splice variants in four different individuals. In theory, the most abundant SP-10 mRNAs would, following the reverse transcription reaction, be represented as the most abundant SP-10 cDNAs. In an RTPCR amplification, the most abundant SP-10 cDNAs, on a semi-logarithmic scale, should accumulate in a co-linear fashion and the relative abundance of each SP-10 splice variant could then be quantitated. The PCR amplifications utilized were the same as before, with the exception that the 3′ oligonucleotide primer was end-labelled with γ-ATP. In order to determine the appropriate time points for quantitative sampling, aliquots of the RTPCR amplifications were taken after cycles 18, 20, 22, 24, 26, 28, 30, 35 and 40. These aliquots were

```
                    EXON 1                  |                        EXON 2                                     *               *
SP10-1:   MNRFLLLMSLYLLGSARGTSSQPNELSGSIDHQTSVQQLPGEFFSLENPSDAEALYETSSGLNTLSEHGSSEHGSSKHTVAEHTSGEHAE
SP10-2:   MNRFLLLMSLYLLGSARGTSSQPNELSGSIDHQTSVQQLPGEFFSLENPSDAEALYETSSGLNTLSEHGSSEHGSSKHTVAEHTSGEHAE
SP10-3:   MNRFLLLMSLYLLGSARGTSSQPNELSGSIDHQTSVQQLP.........................................
SP10-4:   MNRFLLLMSLYLLGSARGTSSQPNELSGSIDHQTSVQQLP.........................................
SP10-5:   MNRFLLLMSLYLLGSARGTSSQPNELSGSIDHQTSVQQLP.........................................
SP10-6:   MNRFLLLMSLYLLGSARGTSSQPNELSGSIDHQTSVQQLP.........................................
SP10-7:   MNRFLLLMSLYLLGSARGTSSQPNELSGSIDHQTSVQQLP.........................................
SP10-8:   MNRFLLLMSLYLLGSARGTSSQPNELSGSIDHQTSVQQLP.........................................
SP10-9:   MNRFLLLMSLYLLGSARGTSSQPNELSGSIDHQTSVQQLP.........................................
SP10-10:  MNRFLLLMSLYLLGSARGTSSQPNELSGSIDHQTSVQQLP.........................................
SP10-11:  MNRFLLLMSLYLLGSARGTSSQPNELSGSIDHQTSVQQLP.........................................

          *           *                           EXON 3          *      *  *
SP10-1:   SEHASGEPAATEHAEGEHTVGEQPSGEQPSGEHLSGEQPLSELESGEQPSDEQPSGEHGSGEQPSGEQASGEQPSGEHASGEQASGAPIS
SP10-2:   SEHASGEPAATEHAEGEHTVGEQPSGEQPSGEHLSGEQPLSELESGEQPSDEQPSGEHGSGEQPSGEQASGEQPSGEQASGEQPS......
SP10-3:   ....GEPAATEHAEGEHTVGEQPSGEQPSGEHLSGEQPLSELESGEQPSDEQPSGEHGSGEQPSGEQASGEQPSGEHASGEQASGAPIS
SP10-4:   ........GEQPSGEQPSGEHLSGEQPLSELESGEQPSDEQPSGEHGSGEQPSGEQASGEQPS......
SP10-5:   ........GEQPSGEQPSGEHLSGEQPLSELESGEQPSDEQPSGEHGSGEQPSGEQASGEQPS......
SP10-6:   ....................GEQPSDEQPSGEHGSGEQPSGEQASGEQPSGEHASGEQASGAPIS
SP10-7:   ....GEPAATEHAEGEHTV.......................................GEHASGEQASGAPIS
SP10-8:   ............GEQPSGEQPS.......................GEHASGEQASGAPIS
SP10-9:   ....GEQPSGEQPSGEHLSGEQPLSELESGEQPSDEQPSGEHGSGEQPSGEQASGEQPSGEHASGEQASGAPIS
SP10-10:  ..........................................................
SP10-11:  ..........................................................

          |                          EXON 4
SP10-1:   STSTGTILNCYTCAYMNDQGKCLRGEGTCITQNSQQCMLKKIFEGGKLQFMVQGCENMCPSMNLFSHGTRMQIICCRNQSFCNKI   265
SP10-2:   ...GTILNCYTCAYMNDQGKCLRGEGTCITQNSQQCMLKKIFEGGKLQFMVQGCENMCPSMNLFSHGTRMQIICCRNQSFCNKI   246
SP10-3:   STSTGTILNCYTCAYMNDQGKCLRGEGTCITQNSQQCMLKKIFEGGKLQFMVQGCENMCPSMNLFSHGTRMQIICCRNQSFCNKI   210
SP10-4:   STSTGTILNCYTCAYMNDQGKCLRGEGTCITQNSQQCMLKKIFEGGKLQFMVQGCENMCPSMNLFSHGTRMQIICCRNQSFCNKI   195
SP10-5:   ...GTILNCYTCAYMNDQGKCLRGEGTCITQNSQQCMLKKIFEGGKLQFMVQGCENMCPSMNLFSHGTRMQIICCRNQSFCNKI   176
SP10-6:   STSTGTILNCYTCAYMNDQGKCLRGEGTCITQNSQQCMLKKIFEGGKLQFMVQGCENMCPSMNLFSHGTRMQIICCRNQSFCNKI   170
SP10-7:   STSTGTILNCYTCAYMNDQGKCLRGEGTCITQNSQQCMLKKIFEGGKLQFMVQGCENMCPSMNLFSHGTRMQIICCRNQSFCNKI   165
SP10-8:   STSTGTILNCYTCAYMNDQGKCLRGEGTCITQNSQQCMLKKIFEGGKLQFMVQGCENMCPSMNLFSHGTRMQIICCRNQSFCNKI   155
SP10-9:   STST.......................GGKLQFMVQGCENMCPSMNLFSHGTRMQIICCRNQSFCNKI   155
SP10-10:  STST.......................GGKLQFMVQGCENMCPSMNLFSHGTRMQIICCRNQSFCNKI   120
SP10-11:  ....GTILNCYTCAYMNDQGKCLRGEGTCITQNSQQCMLKKIFEGGKLQFMVQGCENMCPSMNLFSHGTRMQIICCRNQSFCNKI    81
```

Figure 4 Amino acid sequence comparisons of alternatively spliced human SP-10. SP10-1 through SP10-11 are arranged in decreasing molecular mass. The amino acids are overscored to delineate the coding region of each of the four exons of the human SP-10 gene[13]. Gaps in the sequence represent the in-frame deletions, and the total number of amino acids in each SP-10 variant is located at the end of each sequence. Amino acids overscored with an asterisk delineate the N-terminal residue of SP-10 peptides previously microsequenced after isolation on PVDF membrane[14]

separated on a 2% agarose gel with ethidium bromide; the gel was then dried and placed on X-ray film. The log of the counts per minute (CPM) vs. the increasing PCR cycle number was plotted. It was apparent that the proper sampling time points were between cycles 18 and 25; beyond 25, the increase of RTPCR products was no longer linear. The experiment was repeated and aliquots of the RTPCR amplifications were taken after cycles 18, 19, 20, 21, 22, 23, 24, 25 and 30. Again, the aliquots were separated on an agarose gel, dried and placed on film. The SP-10 DNA bands were subsequently quantitated with a phosphoimager and the experiment was repeated three times for each individual. Bands corresponding to SP-10-1 and SP-10-2 were the first to appear, followed by bands corresponding to SP-10-3 and SP-10-4. The log of the CPM of these four bands left the linear scale (cycles 18–23) prior to the appearance of any other SP-10 variants. The relative abundance of each of the four major SP-10 mRNAs was determined by plotting the log CPM vs. the increasing PCR cycle number and drawing a regression line through those points. Quantitation showed that more than 99% of the SP-10 mRNA was accounted for by SP-10-1 through SP-10-4, while the rest of the SP-10 splice variants accounted for the remaining > 1% of the SP-10 message. The relative abundance of the four major SP-10 mRNAs was similar in three of the four individuals tested. SP-10-1 accounted for just over 50% of the SP-10 mRNA in individuals A, C and D, but over 70% in individual B. SP-10-2 was the next most abundant transcript, accounting for between 15.5 and 31.7% of the message, while SP-10-4 and SP-10-3 accounted for 8.7–12.5% and 3.4–8.3% of the SP-10 mRNA, respectively.

Significance for SP-10 micro-heterogeneity Four of the 11 SP-10 mRNAs, designated SP-10-1 through SP-10-4, accounted for over 99% of the SP-10 message in each individual tested. The four SP-10 mRNAs, comprising > 99% of the mRNA, each possess an identical first exon (which mediates ribosomal attachment) and translate into proteins consisting of 265, 246,

210 and 195 amino acids, respectively. The translational efficiency of the four mRNAs should be directly proportional to the relative abundance of each mRNA. Thus, significant amounts of all four SP-10 proteins should be present in the developing spermatid.

Foster and associates[10] showed that proteolytic processing of SP-10 is initiated in the testis. Due to alternative splicing, there should exist four different SP-10 protein precursors available for proteolytic processing. Each SP-10 protein could have one or two exposed proteolytic sites that would be cleaved, forming a stable product. Indeed, the relative abundance of SP-10-2 is much greater than believed previously and, when combined with SP-10-3 and SP-10-4, these alternatively spliced SP-10s may account for nearly 50% of the SP-10 protein. This helps explain the existence of multiple immunoreactive SP-10 peptide bands observed on western blots of sperm extracts. Also, there appears to be some heterogeneity or variability amongst individuals in the relative abundance of each of the four mRNAs. This agrees with our observations that there exist qualitative differences in the banding pattern of SP-10 on western blots between individuals.

In summary, we have demonstrated the existence of 11 alternatively spliced SP-10 mRNAs and quantitated the relative abundance of the four major SP-10 mRNAs that account for > 99% of the SP-10 message in four individuals. We propose that all four SP-10 mRNAs are translated and that a combination of alternative splicing and proteolytic processing of the four SP-10 precursors is the major cause of SP-10 micro-heterogeneity observed on western blots, as seen in Figure 1.

Advance 4: Infertility in female baboons has been demonstrated with a vaccine consisting of peptides derived from LDH-C$_4$

Introduction to lactate dehydrogenase-C$_4$ The testis-specific isozyme lactate dehydrogenase-C$_4$ (LDH-C$_4$) described by Goldberg and colleagues is perhaps the most extensively characterized sperm antigen[18]. Homotetrameric LDH-C$_4$ functions in lactate metabolism and glycolysis of developing and mature sperm[19]. The LDH-C subunit is an independent gene product expressed only in spermatogenic cells[20,21] and is immunologically distinct from the LDH-A and LDH-B subunits[22]. Identification of this tissue-specificity led to the investigation of LDH-C$_4$'s antigenicity and its potential as an immunocontraceptive. Active immunization with LDH-C$_4$ suppressed fertility in a variety of mammalian species, including primates. The observed effects were attributed to multiple immunological mechanisms[19,22–29].

Although the somatic lactate dehydrogenases are cytoplasmic, LDH-C$_4$ is localized both intracellularly and extracellularly[30]. LDH-C$_4$ is not actively transported to the sperm surface; apparently, disruption of the cytoplasmic droplet in the epididymis permits non-specific binding of LDH-C$_4$ to the sperm surface. Beyler and co-workers[30] identified LDH-C$_4$ on the surface of human and murine sperm, using a solid-phase radioimmunoassay with rabbit anti-mouse LDH-C$_4$ antisera. Biochemical analyses[31] demonstrated that 10% of LDH-C$_4$ enzymatic activity was associated with the plasma membrane. Furthermore, the agglutinating and cytotoxic effects of anti-LDH-C$_4$ antibodies implicated their binding to the sperm surface[24].

Reversible contraception has been shown in female baboons immunized with a synthetic epitope of LDH-C$_4$ The immunodominant B cell epitope of mouse LDH-C$_4$ (designated mC5-16) and of human LDH-C$_4$ (designated hC9-20) have been identified and synthesized. Native mouse LDH-C$_4$, peptide mC5-16 coupled to diphtheria toxoid and peptide hC9-20 conjugated to diphtheria toxoid have each been shown to suppress the fertility of female baboons by 70–75% compared to controls. The contraceptive effect is reversed within 1 year after the last immunization[24,32]. It is thought that, since serum antibody levels were not directly correlated with infertility in these studies, cell-mediated immunity rather than humoral immunity may be the critical effector mechanism.

Summary

This paper has reviewed five recent technical advances toward developing a contraceptive vaccine for humans.

(1) *Oral delivery of SP-10* Oral immunization of female BALB/c mice with a human sperm antigen (SP-10) expressed in recombinant *Salmonella* elicited high-titer anti-SP-10 IgG antibodies in serum and IgA antibodies in vaginal secretions. Anti-SP-10 antibody titers could be increased by secondary and tertiary oral administrations of the recombinant *Salmonella*.

(2) *Fate of SP-10 after the acrosome reaction* Following a follicular fluid-induced acrosome reaction, SP-10 was detected by immunoelectron microscopy on the inner acrosomal membrane, in the equatorial segment and associated with hybrid vesicles. The persistence of SP-10 on this inner acrosomal membrane makes it an attractive candidate for blocking interactions of the inner acrosomal membrane and the egg investments. The localization of SP-10 after the acrosome reaction is consistent with the hypothesis that this protein is involved in sperm–zona binding or penetration.

(3) *In vitro mechanism of contraceptive action of antibodies to SP-10* Antibodies to SP-10 blocked bovine sperm–egg interaction by preventing secondary binding. This blockage of fertilization appeared to be due to an effect of antibodies on the ability of sperm to complete the acrosome reaction and on sperm motility.

(4) *Source of SP-10 micro-heterogeneity defined* The existence of 11 alternatively spliced SP-10 mRNAs has been elucidated. Four major SP-10 mRNAs were found to account for > 99% of the SP-10 message in four individuals. We propose that all four SP-10 mRNAs are translated and that a combination of alternative splicing and proteolytic processing of the four SP-10 precursors is the major cause of SP-10 micro-heterogeneity.

(5) *Peptide vaccine based on LDH-C$_4$ induced infertility in baboons* A synthetic epitope of human LDH-C$_4$ suppressed the fertility of female

baboons by 75% compared to controls. The contraceptive effect was reversed within 1 year after the last immunization.

Acknowledgements

This work was supported by NIH HD 23789, U54 HD 29099, a grant from the Andrew W. Mellon Foundation, and CSA-93-125 from the CON-RAD program of USAID.

References

1. Lin, Y., Mahan, K., Lathrop, W. F., Myles, D. G. and Primakoff, P. (1994). A hyaluronidase activity of the sperm plasma membrane protein PH-20 enables sperm to penetrate the cumulus cell layer surrounding the egg. *J. Cell Biol.*, **125**, 1157–63
2. Freemerman, A. L., Wright, R. M., Flickinger, C. J. and Herr, J. C. (1994). Tissue specificity of the acrosomal protein SP-10: a contraceptive vaccine molecule. *Biol. Reprod.*, **50**, 615–21
3. Herr, J. C., Wright, R. M., John, E., Foster, J., Kays, T. and Flickinger, C. J. (1990). Identification of human acrosomal antigen SP-10 in primates and pigs. *Biol. Reprod.*, **42**, 377–82
4. Foster, J. A. and Herr, J. C. (1992). Interactions of human sperm acrosomal protein SP-10 with the acrosomal membranes. *Biol. Reprod.*, **46**, 981–90
5. Anderson, D. J., Johnson, P. M., Alexander, N. J., Jones, W. R. and Griffin, P. D. (1987). Monoclonal antibodies to human trophoblast and sperm antigens: report of two WHO-sponsored workshops. *J. Reprod. Immunol.*, **10**, 231–57
6. Curtiss, R. III and Kelly, S. M. (1987). *Salmonella typhimurium* deletion mutants lacking adenylate cyclase and cyclic AMP receptor protein are avirulent and immunogenic. *Infect. Immun.*, **55**, 3035–43
7. Carter, P. B. and Collins, F. M. (1974). The route of enteric infection in normal mice. *J. Exp. Med.*, **139**, 1189–203
8. Curtiss, R. III (1990). Attenuated *Salmonella* strains as live vectors for the expression of foreign antigens. In Woodrow, G. C. and Levine, M. M. (eds.) *New Generation Vaccines*, pp. 161–88. (New York: Marcel Dekker)
9. Srinivasan, J., Tinge, S., Wright, R., Herr, J. C. and Curtiss, R. III (1995). Oral immunization with attenuated *Salmonella* expressing human sperm antigen induces antibodies in serum and the reproductive tract. *Biol. Reprod.*, **53**, 462–71
10. Foster, J. A., Klotz, K., Flickinger, C. J., Thomas, T. S., Wright, R. M., Castillo, J. R. and Herr, J. C. (1994). Human SP-10: acrosomal distribution, processing, and fate after the acrosome reaction. *Biol. Reprod.*, **51**, 1222–31
11. Coonrod, S. A. and Herr, J. C. (1995). SP-10 is present in bovine sperm and antibodies to SP-10 inhibit bovine fertilization *in vitro*. *Am. J. Reprod. Immunol.*, **33**, 442
12. Herr, J. C., Flickinger, C. J., Homyk, M., Klotz, K. and John, E. (1990). Biochemical and morphological characterization of the intra-acrosomal antigen SP-10 from human sperm. *Biol. Reprod.*, **42**, 181–93
13. Freemerman, A. J., Flickinger, C. J. and Herr, J. C. (1995). Characterization of alternatively spliced human SP-10 mRNAs. *Mol. Reprod. Devel.*, **41**, 100–8
14. Herr, J. C., Klotz, K., Shannon, J., Wright, R. M. and Flickinger, C. J. (1992). Purification and microsequencing of the intra-acrosomal protein SP-10. Evidence that SP-10 heterogeneity results from endoproteolytic processes. *Biol. Reprod.*, **47**, 11–20
15. Wright, R. M., John, E., Klotz, K., Flickinger, C. J. and Herr, J. C. (1990). Cloning and sequencing of cDNAs coding for the human intra-acrosomal antigen SP-10. *Biol. Reprod.*, **42**, 693–701
16. Wright, R. M., Suri, A. K., Kornreich, B., Flickinger, C. J. and Herr, J. C. (1993). Cloning and characterization of the gene coding for the human acrosomal protein SP-10. *Biol. Reprod.*, **49**, 316–25
17. Mount, S. M. (1982). A catalogue of splice junction sequences. *Nuc. Acids Res.*, **10**, 459–72
18. Anderson, D. J. and Alexander, N. J. (1983). A new look at antifertility vaccines. *Fertil. Steril.*, **40**, 557–71
19. Goldberg, E. (1990). Lactate dehydrogenase C4 as an immunocontraceptive model. In Alexander, N. J., Griffin, D., Spieler, J. M. and Waites, G. M. H. (eds.) *Gamete Interaction: Prospects for Immunocontraception*, pp. 63–74. (New York: Wiley-Liss)

20. Cooker, L., Brooke, C. D., Kumari, M., Hofmann, M.-C., Millán, J. L. and Goldberg, E. (1993). Genomic structure and promoter activity of the human testis lactate dehydrogenase gene. *Biol. Reprod.*, **48**, 1309–19

21. Edwards, Y., West, L., Van Heyningen, V., Cowell, L. and Goldberg, E. (1989). Regional localization of the sperm-specific lactate dehydrogenase, LDHC, gene on human chromosome 11. *Ann. Hum. Genet.*, **53**, 215–19

22. Goldberg, E. and Shelton, J. (1986). Immunosuppression of fertility by LDH-C$_4$. In Talwar, G. P. (ed.) *Immunological Approaches to Contraception and Promotion of Fertility*, pp. 219–30. (New York: Plenum Publishing)

23. Goldberg, E. (1973). Infertility in rabbits immunized with lactate dehydrogenase-X. *Science*, **181**, 458–9

24. Goldberg, E., Gonzales-Prevatt, V. and Wheat, T. E. (1981). Immunosuppression of fertility in females by injection of sperm-specific LDH-C$_4$ (LDH-X): prospects for development of a contraceptive vaccine. In Semm, K. and Mettler, L. (eds.) *Human Reproduction, Proceedings of the IIIrd World Congress*, pp. 360–3. (Amsterdam: Excerpta Medica)

25. Kille, J. W. and Goldberg, E. (1980). Inhibition of oviductal sperm transport in rabbits immunized against sperm-specific lactate dehydrogenase. *J. Reprod. Immunol.*, **2**, 15–21

26. Lerum, J. E. and Goldberg, E. (1974). Immunological impairment of pregnancy in mice by lactate dehydrogenase-X. *Biol. Reprod.*, **11**, 108–15

27. Shelton, J. and Goldberg, E. (1986). Local reproductive tract immunity to sperm specific lactate dehydrogenase-C$_4$. *Biol. Reprod.*, **35**, 873–6

28. Tung, K., Goldberg, E. H. and Goldberg, E. (1979). Immunological consequence of immunization of female mice with homologous spermatozoa: induction of infertility. *J. Reprod. Immunol.*, **1**, 145–58

29. Goldberg, E., Wheat, T. E., Powell, J. E. and Stevens, V. C. (1981). Reduction of fertility in female baboons immunized with lactate dehydrogenase-C$_4$. *Fertil. Steril.*, **35**, 214–17

30. Beyler, S. A., Wheat, T. E. and Goldberg, E. (1985). Binding of antibodies against antigenic domains of murine lactate dehydrogenase-C$_4$ to human and mouse spermatozoa. *Biol. Reprod.*, **32**, 1201–10

31. Alvarez, J. G. and Storey, B. T. (1984). Assessment of cell damage caused by spontaneous lipid peroxidation in rabbit sperm. *Biol. Reprod.*, **30**, 323–31

32. O'Hern, P. A., Bambra, C. S., Isahakia, M. and Goldberg, E. (1995). Reversible contraception in female baboons immunized with a synthetic epitope of sperm-specific lactate dehydrogenase. *Biol. Reprod.*, **52**, 331–9

Combined injectable preparations and introduction as a new method

6

Ma. del Carmen Cravioto

Introduction

Injectable contraceptives constitute a valuable component in any successful birth control 'cafeteria', since they are highly effective and safe methods for fertility regulation, simple to use, non-invasive, unrelated to coitus and relatively inexpensive. The most widely used are those that contain only a progestin: the 3-monthly depot-medroxyprogesterone acetate (DMPA), currently used by over 9 million women, and the 2-monthly norethisterone enanthate (NET-EN), used by 1 million women worldwide. They produce marked menstrual cycle disruptions and amenorrhea, which, besides a delayed return to fertility, represent their major disadvantage and the main obstacle to large-scale acceptability.

Combined once-a-month injectable contraceptives were first developed by Siegel, in 1963, to overcome the problem of irregularities in menstrual bleeding patterns produced by the progestin-only injectables[1]. Since then, a number of formulations have been tested, but only four of them are of practical relevance (Table 1).

First generation of once-a-month injectable contraceptives

Until 1976, there were only two once-a-month injectable contraceptive formulations available for general use: a combination of 150 mg dihydroxyprogesterone acetophenide (DHPA) and 10 mg estradiol enanthate, initially named Deladroxate® (Squibb) and mostly used in Spain and Latin America, and a combination of 250 mg 17α-hydroxyprogesterone caproate and 5 mg estradiol valerate, named Injectable No. 1, available in China. It is estimated that about 2 million women currently use them.

Deladroxate is highly effective, as has been demonstrated by a number of studies that included a total of 3017 women with 32 857 woman-months of use, in which no pregnancies were reported[2]. However, since animal toxicity studies showed a high incidence of breast cancer in dogs and pituitary hyperplasia in rats, and studies in humans have suggested a possible accumulation of its components over time[3], the original manufacturer withdrew this preparation from further studies, and therefore uncertainties still remain as regards its safety. A half-dose formulation is also available, having the same efficacy.

Table 1 Currently available once-a-month combined injectable preparations

Progestogen	Dose (mg)	Estrogen	Dose (mg)
17α-Hydroxyprogesterone caproate	250	Estradiol valerate	5
Dihydroxyprogesterone acetophenide	150	Estradiol enanthate	10
Dihydroxyprogesterone acetophenide	75	Estradiol enanthate	5
Medroxyprogesterone acetate	25	Estradiol cypionate	5
Norethisterone enanthate	50	Estradiol valerate	5

Injectable No. 1 is manufactured and distributed only in China. It has been found to be acceptable, even though it produces short cycles, and it is relatively free from side-effects. Under a strict once-a-month schedule of administration, its efficacy is lower than the second generation of monthly injectables.

Second generation of once-a-month injectable contraceptives

In response to the request from a number of countries for once-a-month injectables which are effective, safe and thoroughly studied, extensive pharmacokinetic and pharmacodynamic studies and clinical trials were carried out by the Special Programme of Research, Development and Research Training in Human Reproduction of the World Health Organization (WHO/HRP) and other institutions over the last 20 years. As a result, two new and improved monthly injectables were developed: Cyclofem® (Concept Foundation) (previously named Cycloprovera® (Upjohn), and HRP 112), which is a combination of 25 mg DMPA and 5 mg estradiol cypionate, and Mesigyna® (Schering AG) (previously coded HRP-102), which contains 50 mg NET-EN and 5 mg estradiol valerate.

As a consequence of the large availability of Cyclofem and Mesigyna, a potential expansion of demand and use of monthly injectables is envisaged in the near future. It prompted WHO/HRP to convene a meeting of experts to review the information, collected over three decades, on all once-a-month combined injectable contraceptives. In their conclusions it is pointed out that both Cyclofem and Mesigyna are safe and effective products for fertility regulation, which can be added to the existing range of contraceptive methods[4].

Pharmacology

Cyclofem and Mesigyna contain short-acting estradiol esters (cypionate and valerate, respectively), which yield elevated estradiol serum levels for no more than 15 days, followed by a rapid decline which induces an estrogen withdrawal bleeding 2–3 weeks after the injection. It was showed by Oriowo and colleagues[5], that estradiol cypionate gives lower peak levels of estradiol and estrone than estradiol valerate and benzoate, but the duration of estrogen rise is shorter in the valerate group (7–8 days) than in the cypionate group (11 days). On the other hand, detectable amounts of the progestational component of Cyclofem and Mesigyna are observed over the entire cycle of treatment, but at lower concentrations than those observed in users of progestin-only injectables[6]. However, their effect dominates the second phase of the treatment cycle, as is reflected in some metabolic changes. DMPA and NET-EN safety has been extensively studied and confirmed. The long-lasting concerns and controversies that still existed on the safety of DMPA finally came to an end on October 29, 1992, when the US Food and Drug Administration (FDA) officially approved it for contraceptive use in the United States.

Mechanism of action

The main contraceptive mechanism of monthly injectables relies on their ability to inhibit ovulation, although some additional actions exerted by the progestin component on the endometrium, tubes and cervical mucus, contribute to the overall effect. Ovulation inhibition is consistently observed during the first 30 days following the injectable administration, but a rapid recovery occurs after its discontinuation. Indeed, several studies have shown the presence of follicular activity within the first month post-treatment with Cyclofem and Mesigyna[7], and a complete luteal activity some weeks later (59–87 days after discontinuation). However, the possibility of ovulating during the first month post-treatment does exist, and therefore it is of the utmost importance to repeat the injectable administration within an interval of 30 ± 3 days.

Contraceptive efficacy

As was mentioned, all monthly injectables are highly effective in preventing pregnancy. Five phase III clinical trials have been conducted in several countries, to assess effectiveness and safety of Cyclofem and Mesigyna. Three of them were comparative trials, and the remaining two referred only to Mesigyna. In total, such studies include information on 4234 Cyclofem users (41 226 woman-months of use) and 5559 Mesigyna users (60 832 woman-months of use)[8]. The highest 1-year life-table pregnancy rate observed for Cyclofem was 0.2% and 0.4% for Mesigyna. This is similar to that observed with the use of progestin-only injectables (DMPA: 0.3%; NET-EN: 0.4%), subdermal implants (0.4%), and permanent methods ($< 1\%$).

Side-effects

Cyclofem and Mesigyna are safe formulations. The side-effects reported on the five phase III clinical trials were few, and mostly related to the irregularities of bleeding patterns. Even though these are less than those observed with the use of DMPA or NET-EN alone, they still represent a problem since they are the major method-related cause for discontinuation.

Bleeding irregularities observed are variable. After the first injection most women experience an anticipated bleeding (10–12 days after the injection), which corresponds to estradiol withdrawal. In general it is followed by fairly regular menstrual-like periods, but a number of women continue exhibiting prolonged and irregular bleeding episodes during the first 3 months of use. Nonetheless, by the end of the 1st year of

Table 2 Percentage of women with clinically acceptable bleeding patterns in the World Health Organization phase III trial

Days	Cyclofem	Mesigyna
1–90	43	47.2
91–180	63.8	62.8
181–270	61.3	63.3
271–360	70	68.4

Table 3 Cumulative 12-month life-table discontinuation rates for amenorrhea

	Cyclofem	Mesigyna
Phase III Clinical studies		
World Health Organization	2.1	1.6
Egyptian Fertility Care Society	2.7	1.4
Chinese study	5.2	0.8
Introductory trials		
Indonesia	1.4	—
Jamaica	1.2	—
Mexico	5.2	—
Thailand	5.0	—
Tunisia	13.2	—

use 70% and 68.4% of Cyclofem and Mesigyna users have clinically acceptable bleeding patterns (Table 2). Amenorrhea is also observed in monthly injectable users, and constitutes a potential logistic problem since the possibility of pregnancy needs to be ruled out whenever its duration exceeds 45 days. Table 3 summarizes data on amenorrhea as a reason for discontinuation in clinical and introductory studies.

Current information on the metabolic effects of Cyclofem and Mesigyna is favorable. Multicentric and standardized studies on coagulation and lipid metabolism, supported by WHO/HRP, have shown no increased production of procoagulant factors with either formulation. Only mild and transient changes, without clinical significance, have been observed in the metabolism of lipids, lipoproteins and apolipoproteins[4].

Introduction of combined injectable preparations as a new method

When the clinical assessment of Cyclofem and Mesigyna was satisfactorily completed, the WHO/HRP Task Force on Research on the Introduction and Transfer of Technologies for Fertility Regulation, initiated a systematic program to introduce Cyclofem into the national family planning programs of several countries. The first set of introductory trials has been completed in five countries: Mexico, Thailand, Indonesia, Jamaica and Tunisia[9]. A second set of studies is ongoing in Chile, Brazil, Peru and Colombia.

These studies, undertaken under more realistic conditions of service provision, have confirmed the high efficacy of Cyclofem. They have also disclosed a series of logistic and cultural situations related to the introduction of the new method, which could be a source of problems affecting the quality of health delivery services. It prompted WHO/HRP to reconsider the strategy for the introduction of new methods, as has been described elsewhere[10].

Acknowledgments

This work was undertaken with the support of the Special Programme of Research, Development and Research Training in Human Reproduction, World Health Organization, Geneva, Switzerland. The author thanks Ms. Mariana Olvera for her assistance in preparing this manuscript.

References

1. Siegel, I. (1963). Contraception control by long-acting progestogen: preliminary report. *Obstet. Gynecol.*, **21**, 666–8
2. Koetsawang, S. (1994). Once-a-month injectable contraceptives: efficacy and reasons for discontinuation. *Contraception*, **49**, 387–92
3. Gual, C., Pérez-Palacios, G., Pérez, A. E., Ruiz, M. R., Solis, J., Cervantes, A., Iramain, C. and Schreiber, E. C. (1993). Metabolic fate of a long-acting injectable estrogen-progestogen contraceptive. *Contraception*, **7**, 271–87
4. World Health Organization (1993). Facts about once-a-month injectable contraceptives: memorandum from a WHO meeting. *WHO Bulletin OMS*, **71**, 677–89
5. Oriowo, M. A., Landgren, B. M., Stenström, B. and Diczfalusy, E. (1980). A comparison of the pharmacokinetic properties of three estradiol esters. *Contraception*, **21**, 415–24
6. World Health Organization Task Force on Long-acting Systemic Agents for Fertility Regulation, Special Programme of Research, Development and Research Training in Human Reproduction (1987). A multicentred pharmacokinetic, pharmacodynamic study of once-a-month injectable contraceptives. I. Different doses of HRP 112 and Depoprovera. *Contraception*, **36**, 441–57
7. Bassol, S. and Garza-Flores, J. (1994). Review of ovulation return upon discontinuation of once-a-month injectable contraceptives. *Contraception*, **49**, 441–53
8. Newton, J. R., d'Arcangues, C. and Hall, P. E. (1994). Once-a-month combined injectable contraceptives. *J. Obstet. Gynecol.*, **14** (Suppl. 1), S1-34
9. Hall, P. E. (1994). The introduction of Cyclofem into national family planning programmes: experience from studies in Indonesia, Jamaica, Mexico, Thailand and Tunisia. *Contraception*, **49**, 489–507
10. Cravioto, M. C. and Hall, P. E. (1994). The introduction of new methods: combined monthly injectables. In Popkin, D. R. and Peddle, L. J. (eds.) *Women's Health Today, Proceedings of XIVth World Congress of Gynecology and Obstetrics*, pp. 405–9. (Carnforth, UK: Parthenon Publishing)

Vaginal rings for contraception 7

I. S. Fraser

Introduction

It has been known for some time that the vaginal wall is an excellent surface for absorption of steroids[1], and that any substance absorbed from the vagina also avoids the first-pass effect through the liver. Vaginal rings and pessaries made from a variety of materials have been used for the management of uterine prolapse for many years, and they are usually well retained in the vagina without any discomfort. Retention is excellent even with relatively small rings. When these features are combined with the principle of using the ring as a reservoir for steroids, with an outer sheath made of a polymer which acts as a rate-controlling membrane, the whole device becomes an excellent means of delivering contraceptive steroids at a constant rate.

The vaginal ring approach has now become well recognized amongst some community groups, and the concept has wide appeal in many countries. These systems can provide easy insertion and removal that is controlled by the woman herself as well as different rates of release, different steroid combinations, constant or cyclical use and a high efficacy and acceptability[2,3]. Vaginal rings are but one approach to the concept of long-acting and low-dose hormonal contraception[4], which is already exemplified by the widely available, subdermal, levonorgestrel-releasing implants (Norplant®; Leiras, Finland) and the levonorgestrel-releasing intrauterine system (Levonova®, Mirena®; Leiras, Finland). The vaginal rings have the major advantage of great flexibility in steroid combinations, dosage and patterns of use.

History and development

Use of the first contraceptive vaginal ring releasing medroxyprogesterone acetate was reported in 1970[5]. Although 25 years have passed since this first report, there is still no contraceptive vaginal ring system marketed anywhere in the world. This is partly an indication of how long it takes to bring a new contraceptive concept to full fruition, but is also an indication of the complexity of the new developments in technology and clinical usage which have needed resolving.

Several progestogen-only contraceptive rings have been well studied, and have shown the potential to become highly successful methods[6,7]. These include systems releasing levonorgestrel (20 µg/day) or norethisterone, megestrol and nestorone at varying doses. There are also several systems releasing progesterone (2.4–4.8 mg/day) which have the possibility of becoming very useful options for breastfeeding women[8]. Several successful combination rings are also under development. The first combined ring contained natural estradiol with levonorgestrel[9], but this combination did not give a good balance and has been discontinued. All current combinations utilize ethinylestradiol, and the two systems most advanced in development contain norethisterone acetate or 3-ketodesogestrel as the progestogens[10,11].

Most of the rings utilize a design where the steroids are dispersed in the polysiloxane rods making up the core, which are then surrounded by two precisely extruded half-shells of an exact thickness to provide release at the desired constant rate. This approach can provide release at a near-zero-order rate over periods from 3 to 12 months. Most progestogen-only rings are designed for continuous use while combination rings are designed for cyclical use to mimic the combined oral contraceptive pill. The combination rings are designed to effectively block ovulation while most progestogen-only rings only sometimes block ovulation and therefore rely heavily on other contraceptive mechanisms such as luteal, endometrial and cervical mucus suppression.

Considerable *in vitro* testing of all rings is required after manufacture to ensure that release rates for each batch are within specifications. This type of testing usually gives a good indication of likely pharmacological performance *in vivo*. One of the problems of ring development is the technology and expense required for upgrading of manufacture from a laboratory scale to commercial production.

Clinical performance

Efficacy has been well tested in several of the progestogen-only rings. The levonorgestrel ring gave pregnancy rates of the order of 3–4/100 woman-years in use in phase III trials, which is equivalent to or slightly less than the rates recorded with progestogen-only minipills in the same populations[3]. This suggests that the dosage of 20 µg/day of levonorgestrel is slightly below the optimum dosage required for modern contraceptive performance. More recent progestogen-only rings have aimed at achieving much lower pregnancy rates, but adequate phase III data are not yet available to confirm this. Combination rings will almost certainly have very high efficacy if they are used correctly, and phase II data appear to confirm this. Nevertheless, large-scale phase III data are essential to give a clear idea of ring performance. These data should become available within the next 2–3 years.

The major concern about clinical performance of most long-acting methods has been the almost invariable change in the menstrual cycle which accompanies use of progestogen-only methods[2,3]. This concerns progestogen-only rings, but is not an issue with combination rings. Clinical data to date indicate that combination rings under current development give regular bleeding patterns as good as, if not better than, correctly-used oral contraceptives. However, removal of the combination ring, for example during sexual intercourse, and failure to re-insert it within 2–3 h may lead to a fall in blood hormone levels sufficient to increase the risk of breakthrough bleeding. It is not recommended that rings should be removed during intercourse, since very few partners find that they interfere (only 1–2% in most studies). Some women may wish to remove them for cleaning because of concerns about hygiene, and this is appropriate, especially with the longer duration devices. A simple soapy solution can be used for removal of any secretions, and then the ring should be well rinsed and immediately reinserted. Although progestogen-only rings increase the unpredictability of bleeding episodes and slightly increase the number of bleeding days, they do significantly reduce the total blood loss and increase hemoglobin levels[12].

Increased vaginal secretions and reports of some vaginal discharge are not uncommon (up to 23% compared with 14.5% of pill users[13]), and are probably related to mechanical effects of the ring. Clinical infection is reported at low rates in all studies and is probably coincidental[2]. Such infections can be treated with the ring still in place. It is unusual for any of these symptoms to lead to discontinuation of the ring. Spontaneous expulsions, minor discomfort and odor are sometimes reported and can lead to discontinuation. Other side-effects are uncommon, although some combination rings may cause nausea for 1–2 days after the first insertion due to an accumulation of ethinylestradiol at the ring surface during storage[10].

Ectocervical and vaginal wall changes have been a potential concern ever since the ring concept was proposed. However, only one study has found evidence of ulcerations in the posterior vaginal fornices of a small number of long-term users of a levonorgestrel-releasing device[14]. Extensive subsequent colposcopic inspections of vaginal and cervical changes with several combination and progestogen-only ring types have not yet demonstrated evidence of significant changes.

Acceptability investigations have demonstrated a high level of popularity for all systems studied[15-17]. This is even the case in some cultures where women do not traditionally accept handling their own external genitalia. There is anecdotal evidence to indicate that many women are prepared to change their cultural beliefs when the method offers them significant advantages over available alternatives.

Several studies have examined the metabolic changes occurring with different devices[2,3,10], and the changes found are generally within the range expected with the use of low-dose combination or progestogen-only oral contraceptives. None of the studies have demonstrated worrying findings concerning lipids, carbohydrates, thyroid function, hepatic function or blood coagulation changes.

The future

The concept of vaginal delivery of therapeutic hormones will undoubtedly continue to be actively developed, and it is likely that this route will be explored by a number of agencies and pharmaceutical companies with interests in hormonal therapy. It is also conceivable that this route will be explored for the delivery of other drugs which may be used for long-term treatment of any condition in women. The immediate applications include postmenopausal hormone replacement therapy and endometriosis. Refinements in the contraceptive field will continue with more devices designed for use during lactation, and almost certainly with combination devices designed for tricyclic or continuous use.

References

1. Dziuk, P. J. and Cook, B. (1966). Passage of steroids through silicone rubber. *Endocrinology*, **78**, 208–11
2. Mishell, D. R. (1993). Vaginal contraceptive rings. *Ann. Med.*, **25**, 191–7
3. Diczfalusy, E. and Landgren, B. M. (1981). New delivery systems: vaginal devices. In Fenn, C. C., Griffin, D. and Woolman, A. (eds.) *Recent Advances in Fertility Regulation*, pp. 43–69. (Geneva: Atar S.A.)
4. Fraser, I. S. and Odlind, V. (1992). Long-acting hormonal methods: the answer for fertility control: In Sitruk-Ware, R. and Bardin, C. W. (eds.) *Contraception: Newer Pharmacological Agents, Devices and Delivery Systems*, pp. 1–22. (New York: Marcel Dekker)
5. Mishell, D. R., Talas, M., Parlow, A. F. and Moyer, D. L. (1970). Contraception by means of a silastic vaginal ring impregnated with medroxyprogesterone acetate. *Am. J. Obstet. Gynecol.*, **107**, 100–7
6. Mishell, D. R., Lumkin, M. E. and Jackanicz, T. (1975). Initial clinical studies of intravaginal rings containing norethindrone and norgestrel. *Contraception*, **12**, 253–60
7. Landgren, B. M., Johannisson, E., Masironi, B. and Diczfalusy, E. (1982). Pharmacokinetic and pharmacodynamic investigations with vaginal devices releasing levonorgestrel at constant near zero-order rate. *Contraception*, **26**, 567–85
8. Diaz, S., Jackanicz, T. M., Herreros, C. and Croxatto, H. (1985). Fertility regulation in nursing women VIII. Progesterone-releasing vaginal ring. *Contraception*, **32**, 603–22
9. Sivin, I., Mishell, D. R. and Victor, A. (1981). A multicenter study of levonorgestrel–estradiol contraceptive vaginal rings. 1. Use-effectiveness; an international comparative study. *Contraception*, **24**, 341–58
10. Balogh, S., Mishell, D. R., Lacarra, M., Shoupe, D., Jackanicz, T. M. and Eggena, P. (1994). A contraceptive vaginal ring releasing norethindrone acetate and ethinyl estradiol. *Contraception*, **50**, 517–33
11. Olsson, S. E. and Odlind, V. (1990). Contraception with a vaginal ring releasing 3-keto desogestrel and ethinyl estradiol. *Contraception*, **42**, 563–72
12. Ji, G., Jong-zhu, S., Gui-ying, S. and Li-yuan, M. (1986). Clinical investigation of a low-dose levonorgestrel-releasing vaginal ring. *Fertil. Steril.*, **46**, 626–30
13. Sivin, I., Mishell, D. R. and Victor, A. (1981). A multicenter study of levonorgestrel–estradiol re-

leasing contraceptive vaginal rings. 2. Subjective and objective measures of effects: an international comparative trial. *Contraception*, **24**, 359–76

14. Bounds, W., Szarewski, A., Lowe, D. and Guillebaud, J. (1993). Preliminary report of unexpected local reactions to a progestogen-releasing contraceptive vaginal ring. *Eur. J. Obstet. Gynecol. Reprod. Biol.*, **48**, 123–5

15. Faundes, A., Hardy, E., Reyes, Q., Pastene, L. and Portes-Carasco, R. (1981). Acceptability of the contraceptive vaginal ring by rural and urban populations in two Latin American countries. *Contraception*, **24**, 393–414

16. Elder, M. G., Lawson, J. P., Elstein, M. and Nuttal, I. D. (1991). The efficacy and acceptability of a low-dose levonorgestrel intravaginal ring for contraception in a U.K. cohort. *Contraception*, **43**, 129–37

17. Weisberg, E., Fraser, I. S., Mishell, D. R., Lacarra, M. and Bardin, C. W. (1995). Acceptability of a combined oestrogen–progestogen contraceptive vaginal ring. *Contraception*, **51**, 39–44

2

Infertility

New concepts on the etiology of endometriosis

8

J. L. H. Evers, G. A. J. Dunselman, P. J. Q. v. d. Linden and J. A. Land

Introduction

The clinical case of the woman with severe pelvic pain and only minimal endometriosis is about as common as the woman without any complaint who is accidentally found to have severe endometriosis at an infertility laparoscopy. Do we really know anything about this mysterious disease? In this contribution we want to explore the facts that exist in evidence of the etiology and pathogenesis of endometriosis.

Apart from a few subhuman primates, some bats and the elephant shrew, the human female is the only menstruating mammal. In normal, cycling endometrium, glandular epithelium undergoes rapid growth and remodeling during the follicular phase of the cycle. Growth ceases during the luteal phase and, in the absence of the continued progesterone-dominated environment of pregnancy, patches of tissue separate from the basal layer of the endometrium. Metalloproteinases of the stromelysin family, collagenase and the extracellular matrix degrading enzyme matrilysin are expressed in endometrium and likely play a role in endometrial growth, remodeling, breakdown and possibly in the establishment of ectopic endometriotic tissue and in determining its invasive properties.

Few people, even few medical doctors, recognize that menstruation is a rare event in the animal kingdom. Finn, in a beautifully written monograph, has recently reviewed our knowledge of the phenomenon of menstruation and concluded that the decidual cell reaction in the uterine stroma in a human species-specific adaptation of the endometrial inflammatory response that allows the implanting blastocyst to develop safely inside the uterine tissues, where usually this inflammatory response would have been directed at removal and destruction of the invading foreign object. The premenstrual condition in women whereby the uterus is prepared in advance so as to be able to withstand the invasion of the blastocyst is considered by Finn to represent the latest stage in the evolution of implantation, with menstruation being the price to pay for the fact that, during the menstrual cycle, the human endometrium goes a stage further in the preparation of the stroma for implantation than does the uterus of non-menstruating species. The decidual reaction of the endometrial stroma cells represents a stage of differentiation which does not allow them to return to their former undifferentiated state again. If cells cannot be maintained, they must be discarded. As a result, in order for our species to survive, monthly menstruation troubles its female members.

The reflux implantation theory of Sampson

Sampson, in 1927, was the first to note blood escaping from the fimbrial end of the Fallopian tubes when surgery was performed during the menstrual period[1]. Whether the refluxed endometrium implants on the peritoneal lining of the pelvic organs (reflux implantation theory) or whether it induces a local metaplastic response in the peritoneum, leading to the neogenesis of endometrial tissue by mesothelial metaplasia at the ectopic site (induction theory), is still an unsolved problem and a matter of arduous debate among distinguished endometriologists[2,3]. Most students of endometriosis, however, are favoring the implantation theory nowadays as the most important explanation for the pathogenesis of endometriosis, although not all aspects of the disease may be explained by this theory.

The reflux implantation theory of Sampson is supported by the topographic distribution of lesions in the abdominal cavity[4]; by the demonstration of the viability of shed menstrual endometrium in tissue culture[5]; by the immunohistochemical characteristics of retrogradely shed endometrium and by its similarities to *in situ* endometrium, antegradely shed endometrium and endometriosis lesions in the peritoneal cavity[6]; by the capacity for adhesion and proliferation of peritoneal cells obtained from the peritoneal fluid during the early follicular phase of the cycle; by the high prevalence of endometriosis in girls with congenital menstrual outflow tract obstruction; and by animal experiments in which endometriosis was induced by the creation of uteropelvic fistulas. The reflux implantation theory is based on the assumption that retrograde menstruation takes place, and that viable endometrial cells reach the abdominal cavity, attach to the peritoneal lining, and implant. We may conclude from many studies in the literature that viable endometrial cells reach the abdominal cavity via the Fallopian tubes during the menstrual period in most, if not all, women with patent tubes. Whether the sheer volume or also the tissue properties of the regurgitated menstrual debris determines that endometriosis will develop in some patients and not in others, and whether differences in their peritoneal defense system contribute to the problem, still remains to be elucidated.

Peritoneal defense system

In women with endometriosis, a local, sterile inflammation occurs in the peritoneal cavity. On theoretical grounds this inflammation may be a response to menstrual debris, either regurgitated through the Fallopian tubes or shed locally by the endometriotic implants. Haney and co-workers[7] have shown the latter mechanism to be the least likely one. Elicitation of a reactive inflammatory response may be considered the body's first line of defense against the development of endometriosis. If the defense mechanism fails or if the aggression is too voluminous or too strong, viable endometrial cells will implant and develop into clinical endometriosis. The association between the sterile inflammation of the peritoneal fluid and infertility remains to be elucidated.

The peritoneal response to the invasion of regurgitated menstrual debris is directed at incapacitation, destruction and removal of these cells. This should prevent the adhesion of viable endometrial cells to the peritoneal lining, and their subsequent development into endometriotic lesions. An inadequate response of this defense mechanism has been suggested as a facilitating factor for the development of endometriosis. Immunological factors have been the subject of many studies in this respect, although it should be stressed that no increased occurrence of immunological disorders has been found in endometriosis patients.

Drake and co-workers[8] have reported increased volumes of peritoneal fluid in women with endometriosis, and have interpreted this as a sign of inflammation. Macrophages are involved in phagocytosis and have been implicated, through their secretory products, in inflammatory reactions. They constitute the dominant cell type in the peritoneal fluid cell population. Macrophages are involved in the initiation of the inflammatory response as antigen-presenting cells and in the active phase as tumoricidal and microbicidal cells. Upon stimulation, resident peritoneal macrophages produce factors that stimulate proliferation of monocytes in the bone marrow. These monocytes travel to the site of violation of homeostasis (i.e. the peritoneal cavity) to take part, as activated macrophages, in the inflammatory response and defense reaction[7]. In this respect they may be considered the garbage collection and disposal system of the peritoneal cavity. Halme and co-workers[9] found increased activation of peritoneal macrophages in infertile women with mild endometriosis. Proteolytic enzymes, lysozyme, γ-interferon, interleukins-1 and -2, tumor necrosis factor (TNF) and growth factors are amongst the secretory products of activated macrophages.

Also, the other major cell types of the immune system, T lymphocytes, B lymphocytes and natural killer (NK) cells, have been studied in the peritoneal fluid of endometriosis patients. All cells have the capacity to produce cytokines, and cytokines in turn activate T cells, B cells, NK cells and macrophages. Of particular interest in this regard is the finding by Dunselman and co-workers[10] that, although activated macrophages show increased *in vitro* phagocytosis of sheep red blood cells, their capability to show chemiluminescence after ingestion of zymosan is decreased. This suggests that, in endometriosis patients, macrophages may lack, even when activated in other respects, sufficient capacity to clear the pelvic cavity of regurgitated menstrual debris, i.e. of viable endometrial cells. This is in accordance with an immunological basis for the development of endometriosis, as suggested by Steele and co-workers[11] who found reduced cell-mediated cytotoxicity towards autologous endometrial cells. More recently, Oosterlynck and co-workers[12] reported defective NK-cell activity in endometriosis patients, also resulting in decreased cellular immunity.

From the isolated reports on defense mechanisms in the peritoneal cavity published so far, one may conclude that a highly reactive peritoneal inflammatory response exists in endometriosis patients, which may lower cycle fecundity through interference with intra-abdominal and intratubal reproductive processes. On the other hand, indications exist that isolated defects in these activated immunocompetent cells may explain why endometrial cells may implant and develop into endometriotic lesions. Furthermore, the adhesion of viable endometrial cells may even be facilitated by secretory products of the activated macrophages, e.g. fibronectin, and their outgrowth stimulated by inflammatory cell-derived growth factors, e.g. epidermal growth factors (EGF), transforming growth factors α and β (TGF-α and TGF-β) and insulin-like growth factor-1 (IGF-1). Human breast cancer research has revealed that reduction of E-cadherin expression may play an important role in invasion and metastasis of neoplasms. E-cadherin usually is strongly expressed on the cell–cell boundaries of normal, non-neoplastic tissue. Oka and co-workers[13] showed that the expression of EGF receptor tended to be positive in E-cadherin-positive breast cancers. Zhang and co-workers[14] tested macrophage-conditioned media on an endometrial cancer cell line, ECC-1. They found that the media of six stage III/IV endometriosis patients demonstrated a mitogenic effect, which was blocked by an antibody to EGF. Most macrophage-conditioned media from stage I/II endometriosis patients lacked this effect. When purified cytokines were tested in the tritium-thymidine uptake assay, only EGF and TGF-α were mitogenic on ECC-1, whereas TNF, interleukin-1 (IL-1) and platelet-derived growth factor (PDGF) had no effect.

Malignant tumor research has shown that, after separation of individual or groups of tumor cells from the primary tumor, the three crucial steps of invasion are: adherence of the tumor cells to the host tissue cells; local proteolysis associated with break-down of the extracellular matrix; and migration into the colonized tissue[15]. Regurgitated endometrial cells possess the capacity to attach to the peritoneal lining, as shown by van der Linden and co-workers[6]. These authors concluded from their work that the expression pattern of cell adhesion molecules indicates that the loss of cell adhesion properties may play a role in the shedding of endometrial tissue during menstruation, and that integrins, and perhaps cadherins, may also be operative in attachment of endometrial tissue fragments to the peritoneum. The demonstration of the expression of cell adhesion molecules by cells in menstrual effluent, endometrium, peritoneal fluid, as well as in endometriosis lesions, is no strict evidence that endometriosis originates from endometrium by retrograde shedding of viable tissue fragments. However, all cells potentially involved in the pathogenesis of endometriosis possess the property to express integrin and cadherin cell adhesion molecules during the menstrual phase of the cycle. Although the exact mechanism by which endometrial cells might attach to the peritoneal serosa is still not clear, and although the first endometrial cell making contact with the first serosal cell still has to be sighted, it has been established that early endometriosis invades the peritoneal extracellular matrix: products of local proteolysis, e.g. the amino-terminal propeptide of type III collagen, accumulate in the peritoneal fluid of patients with endometriosis, especially those with early, active lesions. Van der Linden and co-workers[6] showed E-cadherin to be expressed in *in situ* endometrial epithelial cells of 16 of 16 women, but in only one of 16 endometrial cells retrieved from their peritoneal fluids during the menstrual period. Similarity with the loss of E-cadherin expression in invasive breast cancer would suggest a potential role for cadherins in invasive endometriosis. After cell division is resumed, the new endometrial implant will soon reach a critical tissue volume. From then onwards it will have to rely on new vessel ingrowth for support of its further outgrowth and development. In an elegant series of experiments, Oosterlynck and co-workers[16] investigated the presence of angiogenic factors in peritoneal fluid from 24 endometriosis patients and compared the results to those in 24 controls. Angiogenesis was assayed by placing glass fiber filters impregnated with peritoneal fluid on the exposed chorioallantoic membrane of chicken embryos. The peritoneal fluid of endometriosis patients appeared to contain more angiogenic activity than the peritoneal fluid of controls. The reaction remained after charcoal treatment of the peritoneal fluid. TGF-α, TGF-β, TNF-α and EGF all have angiogenic properties and these factors can be produced by activated macrophages. They may, however, also be secreted by endometrial cells, or by immunocompetent cells amidst them. Haining and co-workers[17], in an immunocytochemical study, have shown one of the angiogenic growth factors, EGF, to be produced in eutopic and ectopic endometrium. EGF

receptors are present in endometrium as well as in endometriosis.

Spontaneous resolution

In 1987, David Redwine[17] drew our attention to the age-related evolution in color appearance of endometriosis[18]. He found the mean age of endometriosis patients to increase from 21.5 years, for those with clear papules only, via 26.3 years, for those with red lesions, and 29.5 years, for those with white lesions, to 31.9 years, for those with black lesions. The age range of patients with clear papules only was 17–26 years, the age range of patients with black plus any other lesions was 17–43 and of patients with black lesions only 20–52 years. No patient over the age of 31 was still found to present clear lesions. These findings suggest that endometriosis in many patients is a self-limiting disease. The early, non-pigmented papules (with invasive activity into the extracellular matrix of the host tissue) evolve into well-vascularized, hyperemic, red lesions, and finally will be subdued by the peritoneal defense system and will develop into the familiar black and blue powder-burn lesions, poorly vascularized, quiescent and surrounded by white fibrotic tissue. One wonders what the age range will have been of those (rare) patients that have been described in the literature who showed invisible, i.e. microscopic, lesions only.

The concept of spontaneous resolution of endometriosis is corroborated by the composition of the patient groups usually described in treatment studies. Typically, patients with American Fertility Society (AFS) stage I and II disease constitute the majority of cases, whereas the group of patients belonging to stage III and IV is usually much smaller, irrespective of whether only surgical or also medical treatment studies are considered.

Implications for treatment

Although several studies have suggested that medical treatment of endometriosis is effective in inhibiting progression of endometriosis, other investigations have cast doubt upon this conclusion. If a second look laparoscopy is performed during medical suppression of endometriosis and the findings are compared to the findings at first look laparoscopy (when the pelvic environment was moist, active, with productive endometriotic foci and their inherent hyperemia, hemorrhage, secretion and inflammatory reaction) one may erroneously conclude that the less active, and therefore less visible, foci in the dry, inactive pelvis reflect regression or even resolution of endometriosis[19]. After suppression has been discontinued, however, the foci will become reactivated and the disease will return to its original path of development. The final answer to the question of whether endometriosis is a progressive disease will have to come from long-term prospective investigations studying spontaneous evolution of peritoneal lesions without therapeutic interference. This will require performing a second look laparoscopy in a patient who has not received any treatment in the interval since her first laparoscopy. It is obvious that such groups will be difficult to collect. We may already learn something, however, from the evolution of the disease as detailed in the no-treatment or placebo groups of the few randomized controlled studies published so far. Thomas and Cooke[20] showed, in 17 placebo-treated patients who underwent a laparoscopy before and after 6 months of placebo treatment, unchanged or even diminished endometriosis in 53%, but an increment in 47%. Similar figures were obtained by other investigators. Many other studies give indirect evidence that endometriosis is progressive. D'Hooghe and co-workers[21] studied the spontaneous evolution of endometriosis in baboons and reported a numerical increase in the number of lesions at relaparoscopy at 10 months. The new lesions were mainly subtle, atypical (67%) and localized on the uterine peritoneum. Progression of endometriosis did not, however, go beyond the revised AFS stage I. Repeat laparoscopies in ten baboons with an initially normal pelvis showed endometriosis to be present in seven after 10–12 months. They conclude that endometriosis is moderately progressive in the baboon, but never beyond the borders of revised stage I. Remodeling of endometriosis lesions within stage I took place within a period of several months.

In conclusion

From all the published evidence, we may conclude that endometriosis appears to be a dynamic disease, especially in the early phase, with subtle, atypical lesions emerging and vanishing again. In the end, however, the peritoneal defense system will prevail and the disease will be subdued in the majority of patients.

References

1. Sampson, J. A. (1927). Peritoneal endometriosis due to menstrual dissemination of endometrial tissue into the peritoneal cavity. *Am. J. Obstet. Gynecol.*, **14**, 422–69
2. Meyer, R. (1919). Ueber den Stand der Frage der Adenomyositis und Adenomyome in algemeinen und insbesondere ueber adenomyositis seroepithelialis und Adenomyometritis sarcomatosa. *Zbl. F. Gynaekol.*, **43**, 745–50
3. Dunselman, G. A. J. (1988). *Endometriosis, Clinical and Experimental Aspects*, pp. 8–68. (Maastricht, The Netherlands: Fertility Foundation Publishing Group)
4. Jenkins, S., Olive, D. L. and Haney, A. F. (1986). Endometriosis: pathogenetic implications of the anatomic distribution. *Obstet. Gynecol.*, **67**, 335–8
5. Te Linde, R. W. and Scott, R. B. (1950). Experimental endometriosis. *Am. J. Obstet. Gynecol.*, **60**, 1147–73
6. Van der Linden, P. J. Q., de Goeij, A. F. P. M., Dunselman, G. A. J., van der Linden, E. P. M., Ramaekers, F. C. S. and Evers, J. L. H. (1994). Expression of integrins and E-cadherin in cells from menstrual effluent, endometrium, peritoneal fluid, peritoneum, and endometriosis. *Fertil. Steril.*, **61**, 85–90

7. Haney, A. F., Muscato, J. J. and Weinberg, J. B. (1981). Peritoneal fluid cell populations in infertility patients. *Fertil. Steril.*, **35**, 696–8

8. Drake, T. S., Metz, S. A., Grunert, G. M. and O'Brien, W. F. (1980). Peritoneal fluid volume in endometriosis. *Fertil. Steril.*, **34**, 27–31

9. Halme, J., Becker, S., Hammond, M. G., Raj, M. H. and Raj, S. (1983). Increased activation of pelvic macrophages in infertile women with mild endometriosis. *Am. J. Obstet. Gynecol.*, **145**, 333–7

10. Dunselman, G. A. J., Hendrix, M. G., Bouckaert, P. X. J. M. and Evers, J. L. (1988). Functional aspects of peritoneal macrophages in endometriosis of women. *J. Reprod. Fertil.*, **82**, 707–10

11. Steele, R. W., Dmowski, W. P. and Marmer, D. J. (1984). Immunologic aspects of human endometriosis. *Am. J. Reprod. Immunol.*, **6**, 33–6

12. Oosterlynck, D. J., Meuleman, C., Waer, M., Vandeputte, M. and Koninckx, P. R. (1992). The natural killer activity of peritoneal fluid lymphocytes is decreased in women with endometriosis. *Fertil. Steril.*, **58**, 290–5

13. Oka, H., Shiozaki, H., Kobayashi, K., Inoue, M., Tahara, H., Kobayashi, T. *et al.* (1993). Expression of E-cadherin cell adhesion molecules in human breast cancer tissues and its relationship to metastasis. *Cancer Res.*, **53**, 1696–701

14. Zhang, R. J., Wild, R. A., Medders, D. and Gunupudi, S. R. (1991). Effects of peritoneal macrophages from patients with endometriosis on the proliferation of endometrial carcinoma cell line ECC-1. *Am. J. Obstet. Gynecol.*, **165**, 1842–6

15. Liotta, L. A. (1992). Cancer cell invasion and metastasis. *Sci. Am.*, **266**, 54–9, 62–3

16. Oosterlynck, D. J., Meuleman, C., Sobis. H., Vandeputte, M. and Koninckx, P. R. (1993). Angiogenic activity of peritoneal fluid from women with endometriosis. *Fertil. Steril.*, **59**, 778–82

17. Haining, R. E., Cameron, I. T., van Papendorp, C., Davenport, A. P., Prentice, A., Thomas, E. J. *et al.* (1991). Epidermal growth factor in human endometrium: proliferative effects in culture and immunocytochemical localization in normal and endometriotic tissues. *Hum. Reprod.*, **6**, 1200–5

18. Redwine, D. B. (1987). Age-related evolution in color appearance of endometriosis. *Fertil. Steril.*, **48**, 1062–3

19. Evers, J. L. H. (1987). The second-look laparoscopy for evaluation of the result of medical treatment of endometriosis should not be performed during ovarian suppression. *Fertil. Steril.*, **47**, 502–4

20. Thomas, E. J. and Cooke, I. D. (1987). Impact of gestrinone on the course of asymptomatic endometriosis. *Br. Med. J. Clin. Res. Ed.*, **294**, 272–4

21. D'Hooghe, T. M., Bambra, C. S., Isahakia, M. and Koninckx, P. R. (1992). Evolution of spontaneous endometriosis in the baboon (*Papio anubis, Papio cynocephalus*) over a 12-month period. *Fertil. Steril.*, **58**, 409–12

Medical treatment of endometriosis

9

A. A. Acosta

Introduction

Endometriosis, a very common disease in reproductive medicine, provides a unique clinical and scientific challenge to the gynecologist. Despite being one of the most frequently encountered gynecological diseases requiring medical or surgical treatment, its etiology, pathophysiology and relation to infertility still remains controversial. Considerable research has been carried out in this area in recent years, answering many questions, yet the understanding of endometriosis remains incomplete, restricting the development of effective preventive measures and successful medical treatment modalities. Despite these uncertainties, clinicians have attempted to formulate specific treatments for this very poorly understood disease. There is no drug available to prevent ectopic endometrial implantation or selectively to eradicate ectopic endometrium. Most drugs used in the treatment of endometriosis act indirectly, with different degrees of efficiency, inducing ovarian suppression that should result in atrophy of the hormonally dependent ectopic tissues. The extent of endometriosis regression during such treatment is related to the length of ovarian suppression and may be individually variable.

Although resolution of endometriosis is the main purpose of medical treatment, the ultimate goal for most patients is restoration of fertility. Thus, the effectiveness of different medical treatments in infertile patients with endometriosis has been judged not only by the degree of symptomatic or clinical improvement, regression of the lesions and low rates of recurrence, but primarily by the post-treatment pregnancy rates.

Although danazol was the most commonly used drug in the treatment of endometriosis in the past, and lately the luteinizing hormone releasing hormone (LHRH) analogs, numerous other medications have been used, most altering cyclic ovulation in order to improve or delay the onset of the disease process. Thus, estrogen and a progestogen are used to mimic pregnancy (pseudopregnancy) and gonadotropin releasing hormone (GnRH) analogs or progestogens alone are used to crate sex steroid patterns seen in menopausal women.

The purpose of this presentation is to describe the place of the different drugs in the treatment of endometriosis, describing their mechanism of action, dosage and schedule, and evaluating their efficacy in terms of regression of the lesions, amelioration of symptoms and restoration of fertility.

Combination of estrogens and progestogens: induced pseudopregnancy

Although there is conflicting evidence about the theory, it has long been considered that pregnancy improves endometriosis. A similar hormonal pattern may be achieved with continuous administration of estrogens and progestogens in high doses. Such treatment that simulated pregnancy, aptly called pseudopregnancy, was introduced by Kistner[1], in 1958.

Estrogen/progestogen preparations used for induction of pseudopregnancy are the main components of combination-type oral contraceptives. The estrogens are either 17α-ethinylestradiol or mestranol.

There are a number of synthetic progestogens, each characteristic of the specific oral contraceptive. Some progestogens are related to testosterone C-19 nor configuration (nortestosterone, norethisterone, norgestrel, norethynodrel, lynestrol). Others, such as medroxyprogesterone acetate, megestrol acetate, chlormadinone acetate, dydrogesterone, are related to progesterone (C-21 configuration).

Estrogen–progestogen preparations suppress hypothalamic GnRH and pituitary follicle stimulating hormone (FSH) and LH secretion, resulting in the suppression of ovarian function and decidual endometrial changes. The dose should be individually adjusted, preferably beginning with a low dose, which should be increased if breakthrough bleeding occurs. Pseudopregnancy should be continued for 9 months or longer. The beneficial effect of these preparations depends on their continuous, uninterrupted administration and their predominantly progestational properties.

Side-effects are frequent and many patients tolerate this regime poorly. Most side-effects occur early in treatment and are similar to the signs and symptoms of pregnancy[2].

The efficacy of this regime is questionable. Most reports are based on older, uncontrolled, subjective clinical studies.

The symptomatic response has been reported to be as low as 'a few per cent' or as high as 93%. The corrected pregnancy rates have ranged between 14 and 54%[3]. Annual recurrence rates have ranged between less than 10% and 23%.

There would appear to be virtually no place for a combination of estrogen and progestogen for the treatment of endometriosis in modern practice, mainly because of the unacceptable risks of high doses of estrogen. Perhaps a pseudopregnancy regime may be recommended in selected patients when other therapy is not available or not affordable.

Progestogens

The use of progestational agents alone gained in popularity in the late 1970s. A large number of progestogens have been used, but few of them are currently available for prescription. The main progestogens used in the past were medroxyprogesterone acetate, lynestrol, norethynodrel, dydrogesterone and norethisterone.

The proposed mechanism of action of progestogens consists in decidual transformation of endometrial tissue and eventual atrophy. This action can only take place if progesterone receptors are present, and these receptors are induced through estrogen exposure. Although progestogens have this effect on eutopic endometrium, there is limited information on the histological effect upon ectopic endometrium.

Telimaa and colleagues[4], in the only randomized controlled human trial to date, utilizing high doses of medroxyprogesterone for 6 months, produced total resolution of implants in 50% of patients, and a partial resolution in 13%, whereas corresponding figures for placebo were 12% and 6%, respectively. Most patients in this study had minimal endometriosis.

Three recent studies have shown the efficacy of medroxyprogesterone acetate in the treatment of endometriosis. Moghissi and Boyce[5] treated 35 patients with 30 mg of medroxyprogesterone acetate daily for 90 days. There was subjective and objective improvement in all patients and recurrence was reported in only three cases. Roland and associates[6] had the same result using the same dose in 24 patients. Recently, in patients who underwent laparoscopy pre- and post-treatment, Luciano and co-workers[7], utilizing 50 mg of medroxyprogesterone acetate, found that the score dropped from 18 to 6 with the treatment.

Telimaa and colleagues[4], in a comparative trial with danazol, showed medroxyprogesterone acetate to have equal efficacy.

Hull and co-workers[8] reported a controlled, comparative study using oral medroxyprogesterone acetate, danazol and expectant management in women with early stages of endometriosis. Cumulative pregnancy rates at 30 months were 71%, 46% and 55%, respectively, with no significant differences noted among the groups. Although this study was not a randomized protocol, it suggested that progestational therapy is as efficacious as danazol for treatment of infertility, and that neither is superior to expectant management.

Progestogens may be administered according to a variety of protocols. They have the advantage of oral administration, and withdrawal of the drug will lead to rapid reversibility of side-effects when they occur, or if the patient desires to become pregnant.

The duration of treatment depends on whether the patient wants to conceive or whether the treatment was initiated due to symptoms. In the first case, the treatment should continue for 6 months, and a second-look laparoscopy should be performed after the treatment has ended. If treatment is initiated due to symptoms, the duration of the treatment can be extended much longer.

Side-effects include breakthrough bleeding (38–47%), nausea (0–80%), fluid retention (50%), breast tenderness (5%) and depression (6%)[9].

Progestogens may affect serum lipoprotein levels. The 19-nortestosterone derivatives significantly decrease high-density lipoprotein (HDL), increasing the risks of coronary disease[10]. Data on this effect of medroxyprogesterone acetate are not clear[11].

It is felt that progestogens are an effective treatment for endometriosis, and although they cause side-effects, these are comparable to those of currently available medication.

Gestrinone

Gestrinone (r-2323, ethylnorgestrione) is a triecnic steroid with an ethyl group in position 13, that exhibits anti-estrogenic action, low androgenic activity and marked antiprogestogenic action. In the human, it is probable that gestrinone exerts its effect through a number of mechanisms. It is an androgen, a progestogen and an antiprogestagen. It alters plasma testosterone, plasma LH and plasma estradiol concentrations. Gestrinone produces an important reduction of sex hormone binding globulin (SHBG) in plasma, thus lowering the total plasma concentration but causing an increase in free plasma testosterone[12,13].

Brosens and colleagues[14] showed that gestrinone induced cellular activation and degeneration of endometriotic implants, as well as involuntionary changes in endometriotic implants that resembled a progesterone-withdrawal effect. Gestrinone also inhibits ovarian steroidogenesis. A 50% decrease in serum estradiol levels has been noted after administration[15].

The recommended dose has been 2.5 mg orally twice a week. Hornstein and co-workers[16] reported equal clinical efficacy with a dose of 1.25 mg twice a week.

Its main side-effects are androgenic, probably as a result of raising the concentration of free plasma testosterone levels: seborrhea, acne, breast hypotrophy, hirsutism and hair loss. Mettler and Semm[17] found that 50% of patients treated with gestrinone complained of androgenic side-effects.

Relief of pain with the use of this medication has proven to be excellent. Azadian-Boulanger and associates[18] noted complete relief of pain in 97.4%. Coutinho and co-workers[19], utilizing 5 mg twice a week for 6–8 months, reported pain relief in 19 of 20 patients.

A subsequent study by the same author revealed a complete resolution of pain in 55% and partial improvement in 91% (45 women studied). In these studies, recurrence of pain symptoms was found in 15.8 and 31.1%, respectively, 1 year after the treatment was ended.

Pregnancy rates following gestrinone treatment have been reported by several authors. Coutinho and colleagues[19] reported a 57% pregnancy rate within 1 year, following a dose of 2.5 mg twice weekly for 8 months, and a 56% pregnancy rate in patients treated for 6–8 months with 5 mg twice a week.

Our personal experience, utilizing 2.5 mg twice a week in 200 patients with an early stage of endometriosis, showed a 59% pregnancy rate within 2 years of the treatment[20].

Results indicate that gestrinone is as effective and safe a treatment for endometriosis as are other forms of medical therapy.

Danazol

Danazol, an isoxazole derivative of 17-ethinyl testosterone, exerts diverse effects on the female reproductive system, inhibiting multiple steroidogenic enzymes in the ovary and adrenal gland. Most of these effects are through the creation of a high androgen–low estrogen environment that is detrimental to endometrial growth. Danazol decreases SHBG production and displaces testosterone from SHBG, thus increasing free testosterone concentrations in plasma. Danazol binds to androgen receptors in the central nervous system, ovaries and peripheral tissues, including the endometrium. It may also bind to glucocorticoid and progesterone receptors, but not to estrogen receptors[21].

Danazol suppresses hypothalamic pituitary function, appears to decrease the frequency of GnRH pulses, inhibits midcycle FSH and LH levels and lowers basal FSH and LH levels[22,23].

In the absence of FSH and LH stimulation, ovarian steroidogenesis is abolished. This effect is further potentiated by the direct inhibitory action of danazol on the enzymes of ovarian steroidogenesis. Estradiol and progesterone concentrations are low during the treatment, and ovarian follicular growth and ovulation are suppressed.

It has been demonstrated that danazol binds to endometrial androgen and progesterone receptors. Such an effect in endometriotic implants may result in suppression of cell proliferation and atrophy of the endometriosis. Also, free testosterone may interact with the endometriotic androgen receptor, causing atrophy of the lesions[24,25].

Danazol has immunosuppressive properties and has been shown to inhibit lymphocyte proliferation *in vitro* and to suppress autoantibody production. The immunosuppressive properties of danazol are very attractive if one considers endometriosis to be an autoimmune disease[26,27].

Pseudomenopause is induced with danazol administered at a dose of 400–800 mg daily for a period of approximately 6 months. Treatment is usually begun on the 1st day of the cycle, and after the onset of amenorrhea, depending on the side-effects, the dose may be lowered, keeping in mind that lower dose regimens may result in an incomplete suppression of ovarian function and less clinical improvement.

The well-known side-effects of danazol are due primarily to its androgenic properties. The most common side-effects are androgenic and anabolic manifestations. Weight gain, voice changes, acne, hirsutism and increased appetite are common. Hot flushes, decreased breast size, insomnia, irritability and atrophic vaginitis reflect the hypoestrogenic effect of danazol[28,29]. Breakthrough bleeding, myalgia, edema, nausea, indigestion, alteration in liver function and in lipoprotein metabolism are also general side-effects.

Women with endometriosis typically present with one of two problems: pelvic pain, or infertility. Barbieri and associates[30] examined the effects of 8000 mg daily in 100 women with endometriosis. In these women, 75% had complete relief of dysmenorrhea, 62% had complete relief of dyspareunia and 59% relief of pain not associated with menses.

Laparoscopic resolution has been observed in 70–94% of cases[31]. Reported post-treatment pregnancy rates vary from 38 to 76%, and annual recurrence rates approximate 10%[32].

GnRH analogs

The most recent advance in the medical treatment of endometriosis is the use of GnRH analogs, derived from the natural hormone GnRH. They differ from the original molecule by the substitution of one or more amino acids. Continuous administration of GnRH results in a down-regulation of the gonadotrope, suppression of FSH and LH secretion and a fall in estradiol levels, resulting in a medical oophorectomy that causes a marked regression of endometrial implants and improvement of symptoms[33–37].

The use of GnRH analogs results in more profound hypoestrogenia than occurs with other drugs used in the treatment of endometriosis, and consequently menopausal side-effects are more common with this treatment. However, the androgenic effects and the serum lipid alterations observed in other types of treatment are not found with GnRH analogs[38]. The effect of GnRH analogs on serum gonadotropin levels is rapid: FSH decreases within 2 days of administration and remains low during the treatment. LH is completely suppressed by 4 weeks after the initiation of treatment, and serum estradiol decreases to castration levels in 3–6 weeks[34].

Numerous side-effects of GnRH analogs are reported, most of them related to hypoestrogenia: vaginal bleeding, hot flushes, vaginal dryness, decreased libido, breast tenderness, insomnia, depression, irritability, fatigue and headache. Side-effects due to increased androgen activity, as seen with other medications, are not seen during GnRH treatment[33,39].

Serum electrolyte balance, liver enzymes, lipid metabolism and blood clotting do not change during GnRH analog therapy.

One other significant effect of the analogs is bone resorption and bone loss, well documented in a number of studies[40–44]. These studies have shown that there is a variable amount of bone loss during 6 months of therapy, but studies have also shown that within 6–12 months after finishing treatment, the recovery of this bone loss is back into the normal range. To prevent this temporary bone loss, a group in Scandinavia recently published a report on the combination of GnRH analogs with norethindrone at 1.2 mg/day, which resulted in no significant changes in bone mass during treatment, compared to baseline studies at 6 and 12 months[45].

The effect of GnRH analogs on endometriotic implants has been studied by several authors[46,47]. Atrophic glands and stroma are the rule among biopsied implants post-treatment, but Lemay and co-workers[34] have pointed out that although these implants appear to be inactive, they are capable of growth later. Reductions in the American Fertility Society score classification have been noted by many authors[48].

Pelvic pain has been studied extensively. Dyspareunia, dysmenorrhea and non-cyclic pain were reduced in 80–100% of women treated[34,39,49].

Pregnancy rates have been reported by several authors. Clinical trials have produced pregnancy rates ranging from 10 to 57%[33,34,37,39,50].

Role of hormone therapy in the treatment of endometriosis

Hormone therapy for the treatment of endometriosis has been used for decades in a large number of patients with endometriosis. However, considering that until recent years the objectives of most studies were to report crude pregnancy rates regardless of the extension or severity of the disease, the lack of randomized prospective trials, the lack of controls and the wide choice of treatment modalities available today (both medical and surgical), a re-evaluation of the role of these drugs seems reasonable.

In patients with endometriosis, in whom the chief complaint is pain, a compelling choice for initial therapy would appear to be the fulguration of peritoneal implants at the time of diagnostic laparoscopy. Medical treatment would appear to be indicated in those cases in whom laparoscopic ablation of the implants is incomplete. It would also seem to be indicated in women in whom the primary treatment failed to obtain relief of pain, or in cases of recurrence of pain, when the patient does not desire a second-look laparoscopy.

The role of medical hormonal treatment in promoting fertility is not very clear: the early stages of endometriosis should be clearly differentiated from the advanced stages of endometriosis, in order to make a rational approach. Early stages of endometriosis, if treated, should be treated with laparoscopic fulguration of endometriotic implants at the time of the diagnostic procedure. Perhaps in countries where operative instruments are not available and the laparoscopic ablation cannot be performed, medical treatment could be installed.

Advanced stages of endometriosis are also primarily treated by surgery: laparoscopy or laparotomy. The value of medical therapy as an adjunct to surgical treatment, pre- or postoperatively, is still open[51], although it has been shown in the past that preoperative medical treatment in these cases has improved pregnancy rates as compared to those cases in which the only treatment was surgical removal[28].

To date, there is no clear evidence that medical treatment alone can increase pregnancy rates in infertile patients with endometriosis, and the treatment should be reserved for those cases in which all other treatment modalities are exhausted.

In the patient diagnosed and treated for endometriosis who does not want to become pregnant in the near future, medical treatment could be indicated possibly to delay the recurrence of the disease. The value of prophylactic treatment in young women complaining of pelvic pain and with a strong family history of endometriosis is questionable.

In conclusion, several medical treatments have been shown to be effective in decreasing the size of endometrial implants and relieving pain in patients with associated endometriosis. To date, there is no evidence that medical treatment alone improves fertility in women with endometriosis. Finally, controlled, prospective studies comparing different modalities of treatment and placebo-controlled pain-relief studies are mandatory, and more work is needed to determine the true value of the commonly used medications[52].

References

1. Kistner, R. W. (1958). The use of newer progestins in the treatment of endometriosis. *Am. J. Obstet. Gynecol.*, **75**, 264
2. Noble, A. D. and Letchworth, A. T. (1980). Treatment of endometriosis: a study of medical management. *Br. J. Obstet. Gynaecol.*, **87**, 726
3. Kourides, I. A. and Kistner, R. W. (1968). Three new synthetic progestins in the treatment of endometriosis. *Obstet. Gynecol.*, **31**, 821
4. Telimaa, S., Poolakka, J., Ronnberg, I. and Kaulica, A. (1987). Placebo-controlled comparison of danazol and high-dose medroxyprogesterone acetate in the treatment of endometriosis. *Gynecol. Endocrinol.*, **1**, 13
5. Moghisi, K. S. and Boyce, C. R. K. (1976). Management of endometriosis with oral medroxyprogesterone acetate. *Obstet. Gynecol.*, **47**, 265
6. Roland, M., Leisten, D. and Kane, R. (1976). Endometriosis therapy with medroxyprogesterone acetate. *J. Reprod. Med.*, **17**, 249
7. Luciano, A. A., Turksoy, R. N. and Carleo, J. L. (1988). Evaluation of oral medroxyprogesterone acetate in the treatment of endometriosis. *Obstet. Gynecol.*, **72**, 323–7
8. Hull, M. E., Moghissi, K. S., Magyar, D. F. and Hayes, M. F. (1987). Comparison of different treatment modalities of endometriosis in infertile patients. *Fertil. Steril.*, **47**, 40
9. Luciano, A. A., Turksoy, R. N. and Carleo, J. L. (1985). Clinical and endocrine evaluation of oral medroxyprogesterone acetate in the treatment of endometriosis. *41st Annual Meeting of the American Fertility Society*
10. Hamblen, E. C. (1957). Androgen treatment of women. *South. Med. J.*, **50**, 743
11. Fahraeus, L., Sysdjo, A. and Wallentin, L. (1986). Lipoprotein changes during treatment of pelvic endometriosis with medroxyprogesterone acetate. *Fertil. Steril.*, **45**, 503
12. Moguelewsky, M. and Philibert, D. (1984). Dynamics of the receptor interactions of danazol and gestrinone in the rat. In Raynaud, J. P., Ojasoo, T. and Martini, L. (eds.) *Medical Management of Endometriosis*, p. 163. (New York: Raven Press)
13. Cornillie, F., Brosens, I. A., Vazquez, G. and Riphagen, I. (1986). Histologic and ultrastructural changes in the human endometriotic implants treated with the antiprogesterone steroid gestrinone during 2 months. *Int. J. Gynecol. Pathol.*, **5**, 95
14. Brosens, I. A., Verleyen, A. and Cornillie, F. (1987). The morphologic effect of short-term medical therapy of endometriosis. *Am. J. Obstet. Gynecol.*, **157**, 1215
15. Robyn, C., Delogne-Desnoeck, J., Bordoux, P. and Copinschi, G. (1984). Endocrine effects of

gestrinone. In Raynaud, J. P., Ojasoo, T. and Martini, L. (eds.) *Medical Management of Endometriosis*, p. 207. (New York: Raven Press)

16. Hornstein, M. D., Gleason, R. E. and Barbieri, R. L. (1990). A randomized double blind prospective trial of two doses of gestrinone in the treatment of endometriosis. *Fertil. Steril.*, **533**, 237

17. Mettler, L. and Semm, K. (1984). 3-Step therapy of genital endometriosis in cases of human infertility with lynestrol, danazol and gestrinone administration with the 2nd step. In Raynaud, J. P., Ojasoo, T. and Martini, L. (eds.) *Medical Management of Endometriosis*, p. 23. (New York: Raven Press)

18. Azadian-Boulanger, G., Secchi, J., Tournemine, C., Sakis, E. *et al.* (1984). Hormonal activity profiles of drugs for endometriosis therapy. In Raynaud, J. P., Ojasoo, T. and Martini, L. (eds.) *Medical Management of Endometriosis*, p. 125. (New York: Raven Press)

19. Coutinho, E., Husson, J. M. and Azadien-Boulanger, G. (1984). Treatment of endometriosis with gestrinone – five years experience. In Raynaud, J. P., Ojasoo, T. and Martini, L. (eds.) *Medical Management of Endometriosis*, (New York: Raven Press)

20. Acosta, A. A. (1993). Medical treatment of endometriosis with gestrinone: the Latin American experience. *Revista Latinoam. Esterilidad*, **15**, 132

21. Dmowski, W. P. (1979). Endocrine properties and clinical applications of danazol. *Fertil. Steril.*, **31**, 237

22. Dmowski, W. P., Headly, S. and Radwanska, E. T. (1983). Effects of danazol on pulsatile gonadotropin patterns and on serum estradiol levels in normal cycling women. *Fertil. Steril.*, **39**, 49

23. Wood, G. P., Wu, C. H., Flickinger, G. L. and Mikhail, G. (1975). Hormonal changes associated with danazol therapy. *Obstet. Gynecol.*, **45**, 320

24. Jenkin, G., Cookson, S. I. and Thorburn, G. D. (1983). The interaction of human endometrial and myometrial steroid receptors with danazol. *Clin. Endocrinol.*, **19**, 377

25. Tamaya, T., Wada, K., and Fujimoto, J. (1984). Danazol binding to steroid receptor in human uterine endometrium. *Fertil. Steril.*, **41**, 732

26. Hill, J., Barbieri, R. L. and Anderson, D. J. (1987). Immunosuppressive effects of danazol *in vitro. Fertil. Steril.*, **48**, 414

27. El-Toeiy, A., Dmowski, W. P., Gleicher, N. and Radwanska, E. (1988). Danazol but not gonadotropin-releasing hormone agonist suppresses autoantibodies in endometriosis. *Fertil. Steril.*, **50**, 864

28. Buttram, V. C. Jr, Belue, J. B. and Reiter, R. (1982). Interim report of a study of danazol for the treatment of endometriosis. *Fertil. Steril.*, **37**, 478

29. Buttram, V. C., Reiter, R. C. and Ward, S. (1985). Treatment of endometriosis with danazol. Report of a 6 years prospective study. *Fertil. Steril.*, **43**, 353

30. Barbieri, R. L., Evans, S. and Kister, R. (1982). Danazol in the treatment of endometriosis. Analysis of 400 cases with a 4 year follow-up. *Fertil. Steril.*, **37**, 737

31. Dmowski, W. P. and Cohen, M. R. (1975). Treatment of endometriosis with an antigonodotropin, danazol: a laparoscopic and histologic evaluation. *Obstet. Gynecol.*, **46**, 147

32. Friedlander, R. L. (1973). The treatment of endometriosis with danazol. *J. Reprod. Med.*, **10**, 197

33. Cirkel, U., Schweppe, K. W., Ochs, H. and Schneider, H. P. G. (1986). Effects of LH-RH agonists therapy in the treatment of endometriosis. In Rolland, R., Chadha, D. R. and Willemsen, W. N. P. (eds.) *Gonadotropin Downregulation in Gynecological Practice*, p. 189. (New York: Alan R. Liss)

34. Lemay, A., Maheux, R., Faure, N. and Jean, C. (1984). Reversible pseudomenopause induced by luteinizing releasing hormone LH-RH agonists (buserelin) as a new therapeutic approach to endometriosis. *Fertil. Steril.*, **41**, 863

35. Lemay, A., Maheu, R., Jean, C. and Faure, N. (1986). Efficacy of different modalities of LH-RH agonists (buserelin administration on the inhibition of the pituitary ovarian axis for the treatment of endometriosis. In Rolland, R., Chadha, D. R. and Willemsen, W. N. P. (eds.) *Gonadotropin Down-Regulation in Gynecological Practice*, p. 157. (New York: Alan R. Liss)

36. Meldrum, D., Tsao, Z., Monroe, S. E. and Braumstein, G. D. (1984). Stimulation of LH fragments with reduced bioactivity following Gn-RH agonists administration in women. *J. Clin. Endocrinol. Metab.*, **58**, 755

37. Minaguchi, H., Uemura, T. and Shirasu, K. (1986). Clinical study on finding optimal dose of a potent LH-RH agonist (buserelin) for the treatment of endometriosis – multicenter trial in Japan. In Rolland, R., Chadha, D. R. and Willemsen, W. N. P. (eds.) *Gonadotropin Downregulation in Gynecological Practice*, p. 211. (New York: Alan R. Liss)

38. Shaw, R. W. (1992). The role of GnRH analogues in the treatment of endometriosis. *Br. J. Obstet. Gynaecol.*, **99** (Suppl. 7), 9–12

39. Franssen, A. M., Kauer, F. M., Rolland, R. and Zijlstra, J. A. (1986). The effect of LHRH ago-

nists therapy in the treatment of endometriosis. In *Gonadotropin Down-regulation in Gynecological Practice*, p. 201. (New York: Alan R. Liss)

40. Steingold, K., Cedars, M., Lu, J. K. H., Randle, D. *et al.* (1987). Treatment of endometriosis with a long acting gonadotropin releasing hormone agonist. *Obstet. Gynecol.*, **69**, 403

41. Lewis, V., Ramos, J. and Dawood, M. J. (1987). Changes in bone mineral content in endometriosis patients treated with GnRH agonists. Presented at *34th Annual Meeting of Gynecological Investigation*, March

42. Rock, J. A., Truglia, J. A., Caplan, R. J. and The Zoladex Endometriosis Study Group (1993). Zoladex (goserelin acetate implant) in the treatment of endometriosis: a randomized comparison with danazol. *Obstet. Gynecol.*, **82**, 198–205

43. Dawood, M. Y., Lewis, V. and Ramos, J. (1989). Cortical and trabecular bone mineral content in women with endometriosis: effect of gonadotropin-releasing hormone agonist and danazol. *Fertil. Steril.*, **52**, 21–6

44. Dodin, S., Lemay, A. Maheux, R., Dumont, M. and Turcot-Lemay, L. (1991). Bone mass in endometriosis patients treated with GnRH agonist implant or danazol. *Obstet. Gynecol.*, **77**, 410–15

45. Riis, B. *et al.* (1990). Is it possible to prevent bone loss in young women treated with GnRH agonists? *J. Clin. Endocrinol. Metab.*, **70**, 920

46. Hahn, D. W., Carraher, R. P., Poldesy, R. G. and McGuire, J. L. (1957). Development of an animal model for quantitatively evaluating effects of drugs on endometriosis. *Fertil. Steril.*, **29**, 651

47. Mann. D. R., Collins, D. C., Smith, M. M. and Kessker, M. J. (1986). Treatment of endometriosis in monkeys. Effectiveness of gonadotropin releasing hormone agonists compared to treatment with a progestational steroid. *J. Clin. Endocrinol. Metab.*, **63**, 1277

48. Wheeler, J. M., Knittle, J. D. and Miller, J. D. (1992). Depot leuprolide versus danazol in treatment of women with symptomatic endometriosis I. Efficacy results. *Am. J. Obstet. Gynecol.*, **167**, 1367–71

49. Fedele, L., Bianchi, S., Bicciolone, L., Di Nola, G. and Franchi, D. (1993). Buserelin acetate in the treatment of pelvic pain associated with minimal and mild endometriosis: a controlled study. *Fertil. Steril.*, **59**, 516–21

50. Shaw, R. W., Fraser, H. M. and Boyle, H. (1983). Intranasal treatment with luteinizing-releasing hormone agonists in women with endometriosis. *Br. Med. J.*, **287**, 1667

51. Thomas, E. J. (1992). Combining medical and surgical treatment for endometriosis: the best of both worlds? *Br. J. Obstet. Gynaecol.*, **99** (Suppl. 7), 5–8

52. Olive, D. L. (1989). Medical treatment: alternatives to danazol. In Schenken, R. S. (ed.) *Endometriosis, Contemporary Concepts in Clinical Management*, pp. 189–211

Diagnosis of polycystic ovarian syndrome

10

R. I. Tozzini and L. Colombero

Introduction and definitions

The identification of polycystic ovarian syndrome (PCOS) presents a number of difficulties to the clinician because PCOS is a heterogeneous entity where the clinical aspects together with the results of complementary investigations do not provide a clear-cut definition, more often because of the frequency of closely related entities that do not meet the description provided in 1935 by Stein and Leventhal[1].

It is fairly easy to characterize two diagnostic extremes. The first bases diagnosis on the hormonal derangement: the hyperandrogenism of ovarian origin and insulin resistance[2-8], with some additional participation of anovulation and gonadotropin disequilibrium[9]. For the second diagnostic extreme, some clinicians require the identification of polycystic ovaries by ultrasound[10-14], magnetic resonance (MR) imaging[15] or laparoscopy[16]. Between these extremes there exist a series of intermediate conditions[17-19].

The observed frequency of PCOS has increased with time as a consequence of increased clinicians' awareness of the syndrome and the progress in diagnostic capabilities. Shortly after the report of Stein and Leventhal[1], PCOS was deemed an infrequent condition. Now, Batrinos and colleagues[20] state that PCOS is the most frequent endocrine disorder in young, sexually mature women.

With due caution, therefore, because of the heterogeneity of the syndrome, the available diagnostic criteria are reviewed in the following sections.

Clinical picture

Disorders of the menstrual cycle

The loss of menstrual rhythm is by far the most frequent (close to 100%)[21] clinical feature[3], and is caused by a profound disorder in follicular development and maturation. Very few clinicians suspect PCOS if menstrual cycles are normal. The set of selection criteria employed by different investigators precludes direct comparison of their results; those clinicians that favour hyperandrogenism and sterility will produce different results than those that use echography as a diagnostic tool[22].

As a rule, menstrual cycle disorders appear after a menarche at an early or normal age. Progressively (or not!) one may find polymenorrhea, oligomenorrhea, dysfunctional metrorrhagia, and finally amenorrhea, of great diagnostic value.

Although follicles may produce low levels of estrogens, their increased number appears to produce plasma levels of estradiol similar to those found in the first phase of the menstrual cycle[23]. This metabolic feature indicates the usefulness of the progesterone test as indicated by Kletsky[24] and others[25]. A positive test is characterized by a menstrual-like bleeding following the injection of 100 mg of progesterone in oil or the intake of medroxyprogesterone (10 mg/day during 7 days). According to Fox and colleagues[5] this test is highly effective in differentiating PCOS from pseudo-PCOS in patients with secondary amenorrhea. The occurrence in young women of dysfunctional metrorrhagia, hyperplasia and carcinoma of the endometrium[26] has been attributed to persistent estrogenic levels without adequate complementary progesterone secretion.

The relationship between ovarian morphology and menstrual disorders was investigated by Takahashi and co-workers[27]: more than 10 subcortical follicles (3–8 mm in diameter) are present in 80% of oligomenorrheic patients[27]. Conversely, Fauser and associates[28] have reported PCOS in over 30% of secondary amenorrhea and 87% of oligomenorrhea cases. Both Polson and colleagues[29] and ourselves[30] have reported similar figures. Ardaens and co-workers[31] report 92% of oligomenorrhea when the polycystic image occurs together with stromal hyperplasia. It should be noted, however, that Polson and colleagues[29] have reported that 7% of women with normal menstrual cycles carry polycystic ovaries.

According to Lobo[32], menstrual cycle disorders and obesity are two of the most important variables that indicate insulin resistance.

Hyperandrogenic effects

Hirsutism is one of the most frequent signs and causes of consultation of patients with PCOS. In the review of Goldzieher[3] approximately 70% of patients showed hirsutism; a lower incidence of acne was also recorded. Similar findings have been reported by other investigators[14].

Hirsutism is usually moderate; it appears after the menarche and shows a slow progression with age. On the other hand, it is rare to find net virilization with clitoromegalia, changes in voice-pitch and a male-like phenotype (which suggest virilizing tumors of the ovary, adrenals or the so-called hypertecosis[33]). Baldness is found in a lower number of cases (8% of patients, according to Conway and associates[34]).

The association of oligomenorrhea, positive progesterone test and hirsutism almost coincide, in incidence, with the echographic finding of polycystic ovaries[35]. A strong positive correlation has been reported between hirsutism and the number of follicles or the echogenicity of ovarian stroma[17].

Obesity

According to Insler and co-workers[36] the association of PCOS with a body mass index (BMI) ≥ 26 defines a subgroup of patients characterized by resistance to insulin and increased plasma levels of this hormone. In another investigation[37], significant differences in the circulating levels of insulin, growth hormone (GH), insulin-like growth factor 1 (IGF-1) and sex-hormone binding globulin (SHBG) have been reported as a function of body weight. Obesity has also been found to be correlated with the degree of hirsutism and plasma levels of testosterone[34].

Barbieri and Ryan[38] called attention to the association of acanthosis nigricans, hyperandrogenism, overweight and insulin resistance (HAIR-AN syndrome).

According to Lefebre and associates[6,39] the body fat distribution shows a particular characteristic in cases of hyperandrogenism (increase in the splanchnic or abdominal area), as indicated by the finding that 15 out of 37 PCOS patients had a waist : hip ratio > 0.8.

Acanthosis nigricans

The presence of this skin disorder is observed associated to several pathologies[40] including hyperinsulinism and insulin resistance. It has been reported in 1–4% of patients with PCOS[14,34,39]. It is localized principally in the nape of the neck, axillas and upper part of the trunk.

Laboratory determinations

Although there is no single specific test for PCOS, laboratory measurements provide the most significant data.

Gonadotropins

The diagnostic value of luteinizing hormone (LH) and follicle stimulating hormone (FSH) levels is under review. Increased plasma levels of LH[41], together with low to normal FSH (LH : FSH ratio > 2 or 3), has been considered by many investigators as a hallmark of PCOS.

However, it has been reported that radioimmunoassays (RIAs) also measure the inactive α-subunits of LH and its correlation with bioassays is poor[42]. The recent introduction of highly specific monoclonal antibodies (immunoradiometric assays (IRMAs)) produced distinctly lower LH values[42,43]. It has been also suggested that bioassays should be preferred to IRMAs in order to differentiate between PCOS and apparently similar syndromes.

With respect to LH, most authors do not report the moment of the cycle when blood was drawn, despite the fact that it is known that LH secretion changes during the menstrual cycle. We measured this hormone between the 3rd and 7th day of the cycle or, in the amenorrheic patient, after bleeding induced by a progesterone test.

In general, LH levels in PCOS are higher than in the general population[17,24,35,44–46]. Variability between individuals is, however, large. Franks[14], Conway[34] and Fox[47], and their respective colleagues, reported that, respectively 51%, 44% and 70% of the patients had increased levels of LH. We have published some data in agreement with this, from 35 oligoamenorrheic PCOS patients (RIA LH levels: 16.1 ± 8.3 mIU/ml) vs. 19 normal controls (LH = 9.1 ± 3.2 mIU/ml), $p < 0.001$[48].

Variability is also present in the increased LH : FSH ratio, ranging between 50%[9] and 68%[22]. At the same time, some authors consider a ratio greater than 2 characteristic of PCOS, and others, greater than 3. Robinson and colleagues[49] reported that the ratio measured is dependent upon the reagents employed: 1.6 (average) with RIA and 0.85 with IRMA. Our data[48] are presented in Tables 1 and 2.

The variance of reported data is so large that some authors[14] have suggested abandoning the measured ratio LH : FSH ≥ 2 for the diagnosis of PCOS. Others, however, consider the LH : FSH ratio as one of the most important features of PCOS[3,20,22,50]. Similar findings have been reported for postpubertal patients by Apter and colleagues[51].

The increase in the ratio of bioactive:immunoactive LH has been pointed out by Lobo

Table 1 LRH test in 35 patients with PCOS[48]

	LH (mIU/ml)	FSH (mIU/ml)
Basal	16.1 ± 8.3	7.7 ± 3.1
30 min	48.1 ± 29.9	14.9 ± 6.7
60 min	53.3 ± 31.7	17.2 ± 10.2

Table 2 Different types of response to the LRH test in 35 patients with PCOS

	Patients	
Type of response	n	%
Androgenic disresponse	22	62.9
Normal response	8	22.9
Hypo-response	2	5.7
Atypical response	3	8.5

and colleagues[52] and Fauser and associates[53] as characteristic of PCOS. Also on this line of research, the report by Imse and co-workers[54] is noteworthy; the levels of LH in PCOS patients were measured by bioassay and five different immunoassays with specific antibodies for different epitopes of the LH molecule. A greater number of LH pulses were determined with RIA than with IRMA, together with differences in the time-course of LH levels when measurements with RIA and bioassays were compared.

The pulsatile nature of LH secretion reduces the diagnostic value of isolated determinations of this hormone. When the average LH concentration was determined during an 8-h interval[14], it was found to be above normal in 82% of PCOS patients. In longitudinal studies it has been reported that PCOS patients show a greater LH pulse amplitude[55,56]. The increased frequency of these LH pulses is a matter of debate[54,56–59]. Abnormal secretion patterns during sleep have been reported by Zumoff and associates[60].

Some researchers have attempted to characterize PCOS by measuring LH and FSH following secretion stimulus with gonadotropin releasing hormone[48] (GnRH). This procedure, however, has been discarded because of the frequency of normal, hypo- or atypical responses (37.1% in this series).

Since the report by Yen and colleagues[41] the FSH levels have been unanimously reported as low to normal. According to Fauser and co-workers[53], normal values were obtained irrespective of the method employed (bioassay, RIA or IRMA). These findings are in agreement with the reports of normal[28] or low[61] levels of plasmatic inhibition. The work of Erickson and colleagues[62], who reported a high concentration of FSH in the follicular fluid, suggests that abnormal follicular development may be due to a defect in the association of the hormone with its receptor, or a defect in the subsequent cascade of events.

Estrogens

Plasma levels of estradiol are similar to those of normal women in the early follicular phase of the menstrual cycle[5]. The low estrone and estradiol secretion per follicle is compensated by the increased number of follicles, as ascertained by measurements of estradiol in the ovaric vein[23]. The estrone levels are higher than normal[63,64], producing an inverted estrone : estradiol ratio. Increased estrone levels reflect the contribution of peripheral aromatization of androstenedione. Estrogen levels are comparable to those of the first week of the menstrual cycle, sustained and without the presence of progesterone. They are presumed responsible for the dysfunctional metrorrhagic episodes, hyperplasia and even for endometrial cancer[65–67].

Progestagens

One of the most important consequences of the lack of follicular maturation is anovulation. Its frequency is estimated as 90%, and is highly dependent upon the criteria employed to select the patients for study: it will be higher in sterile PCOS patients and lower if selection is based on echographic findings. In our PCOS patients assessed by laparoscopy, we have only found 7.4% of recent corpora lutea[68].

Anovulation produces progesterone plasma levels < 4 ng/ml, except in some cases of follicular luteinization or inadequate luteal phases when progesterone levels are similar to low to normal postfollicular values. On the other hand, the secretion of 17α-hydroxyprogesterone of ovarian origin (both basal and gonadotropin-stimulated) is increased[40,69]. Ehrman and colleagues[70] and others[9,71] have developed a test with analogs of gonadotropin releasing hormone (GnRH) combined with dexamethasone and corticotropin to identify what they call 'functional ovarian hyperandrogenism (FOH)'. In this case, the plasma 17α-hydroxyprogesterone response to nafarelin was supranormal (58%)[70]. With a similar approach, Ibañez and co-workers[71] have shown, in 58% of postpubertal girls in early puberty, a striking secretion of 17α-hydroxyprogesterone following leuprolide administration. Polycystic ovaries were present in over half of these girls at echographic assessment.

Androgens

Together with change in gonadotropin pattern, hyperandrogenism is another typical feature of the syndrome. Some authors have equated FOH to PCOS[9,72]. Hirsutism, with or without acne, is a frequent clinical finding.

Testosterone is the most important androgen secreted by the ovaries. In normal subjects the ovaries produce half of the circulating testosterone. Abnormal plasma levels are ≥ 2.7 nmol/l (or > 0.8 ng/ml).

PCOS patients present significantly increased levels of testosterone[5,27,35,46,49,73,74], although there is a considerable overlap with normal values. According to Franks[14], 50% of women with an echographic diagnosis of PCOS showed normal testosterone levels. Conway[34] and associates report testosterone levels < 3 nmol/l in 78% of cases identified as PCOS by ultrasound assessment. When patients are identified on clinical signs, higher than normal testosterone levels are found in a greater proportion: from 70%[49] to 80%[8]. Robinson and colleagues[49] consider that testosterone and androstenedione levels are the most useful hormonal markers to define PCOS. We have found testosterone levels > 2.7 nmol/l in 61.5% of cases.

In sterile patients, Pache and colleagues[17] have observed a significant correlation between testosterone levels and ovarian volume, echogenicity of ovarian stroma or the number of subcortical follicles. The correlation is stronger than that observed with LH.

'Free' (not protein-bound) testosterone is a better measurement than total testosterone, and appears to be a better discriminant of PCOS or hyperandrogenism of ovarian origin in hirsute women[22,25,75]. The mean normal value for free testosterone is approximately 1 pg/ml[19]. Significant correlations have been found between testosterone levels and structural changes of the ovaries[27,76], or obesity[5,25].

The daily production[77] and mean plasma levels[78] of androstenedione are increased in PCOS. Plasma levels greater than 6.2 nmol/l (or > 1.8 ng/ml) are considered abnormal. Most frequently, increased testosterone and androstenedione levels are found in PCOS. Some authors recommend that both measurements are performed, although there is no consensus on this point.

With regard to the adrenal androgens dehydroepiandrosterone (DHEA) and its sulfate (DHEAS), between 30 and 50% of patients with FOH have increased levels of DHEAS and an enhanced response to exogenous adrenocorticotropic hormone (ACTH)[2,79,80]. Whilst no relationship has yet been demonstrated between these phenomena and a determined enzymatic defect in adrenal tissue[81], DHEAS level appears to be an excellent marker of the adrenal participation in PCOS. Abnormal DHEAS levels exceed 3600 ng/ml; values greater than 7000 ng/ml strongly suggest an adrenal tumor. The plasmatic concentration of ACTH is normal, however, and this makes the cause of the DHEAS overproduction unclear.

Some authors[82] consider the secretion of 11β-hydroxyandrostenedione to be a more specific marker of adrenal secretion, and its increase in plasma would indicate the adrenal participation in the hyperandrogenism of ovarian origin. It has not yet been included in the diagnostic routine.

Pugent and colleagues[78] have reported high values of 3α-androstanediol and its glucuronide in 72% of PCOS patients compared with 41% in hirsute women showing no PCOS. This steroid is a metabolite of dihydrotestosterone, a marker of peripheral androgen metabolism and of the activity of 5α-reductase. Some investigators assign an adrenal origin to this steroid[83]. It is not considered an important measurement for the diagnosis of PCOS.

Sex hormone binding globulin (SHBG)

Several authors have indicated that diminished levels of this globulin occur in PCOS[8,73,78,84], independently of body weight (obesity is also associated with low plasma levels of SHBG). The normal mean plasma level is around 110 nmol/l. SHBG binds testosterone and so its low concentration increases the bioavailability of the latter. The free androgen index (FAI) is calculated using the formula: testosterone (T) (nmol/l) × 100/SHBG (nmol/l). An elevated FAI (> 4.5) gives the best results in terms of overall accuracy of PCOS diagnosis (94%), similar to the progestogen test (89%)[25]. Pugeat and colleagues challenge the concept that FAI is the only active fraction, in view of the fact that target cells have receptors for SHBG[78]. Nestler[85] regards SHBG as a sensitive marker of insulin resistance and hyperinsulinism. Plymate and associates[86] have reported that insulin downregulates the secretion of SHBG by the liver.

Hyperinsulinism and insulin resistance

Insulin resistance (abnormally high basal levels of insulin or as a response to glucose challenge) is being considered as an integral part of PCOS (especially in obese subjects) despite some conflicting reports[84,87,88].

The determination of basal insulin levels has a low diagnostic value. According to Panidis and co-workers[74], insulin resistance is strongly dependent upon the degree of obesity. Weber and colleagues[89] resorted to glucagon administration to stimulate insulin secretion and concluded that insulin resistance is related to obesity and it is not an etiological factor for hyperandrogenism.

Insulin resistance, according to Robinson and associates[84] is a feature of oligomenorrheic subjects. Insler and co-workers[36] consider different etiologies for obese and lean PCOS patients: insulin resistance and hyperinsulinism in the former and LH and growth hormone increase in the latter. This conclusion is not accepted by several investigators. Buyalos[90], Anttila[91], Chang[92] and Jialal[93] and their respective co-workers have observed a greater than normal insulin response and/or insulin resistance after glucose load in lean PCOS.

According to Yen and colleagues[94] and Lattikainen[95] the mechanism of insulin resistance in PCOS is independent of obesity. The insulin receptors of adipocytes appear to have a normal number of receptors, some deficiency in the mechanism of autophosphorylation, and a clearly hindered, postreceptor transport of glucose. Total circulating insulin would be increased with normal glycemia. A greater activity of IGF-1 would be expected, because of the reduced levels of its binding protein (IGFBP-1).

A very important contribution is the work of Dunaif and colleagues[96]. Employing the euglycemic clamp technique, these investigators found a net insulin resistance in PCOS patients even though basal levels of glucose and insulin may be normal. In agreement, Sharp and co-workers[97] and Poretsky[87] consider insulin resistance as a characteristic and necessary feature for PCOS diagnosis.

Prolactin

According to Futterweit[98] and Luciano and co-workers[99] 15–20% of PCOS patients have higher than normal levels of prolactin. Prolactin determinations, however, do not contribute to PCOS diagnosis. It should be recalled that *ca.* 50% of hyperprolactinemic amenorrheic patients may have polycystic ovaries.

Contribution of image-producing techniques to PCOS diagnosis

Ultrasound

This method has replaced laparoscopy in the determination of polycystic ovaries. Echography has demonstrated polycystic ovaries in normal young women or those affected with diverse pathologies. The impact of these findings has been so large that the issue under current discussion is whether this technique is a kind of 'gold standard'[12,49] or whether endocrine and metabolic data should be favoured over morphological findings[17–19]. It would be very important to reach a consensus, otherwise, the accurate diagnosis of this syndrome is at stake.

Adams and colleagues[100] and Franks[14] have found polycystic ovaries in 32% of amenorrheic, 87% of oligomenorrheic, and 23% of apparently normal women[29]. Clayton and associates[101] have published similar figures for the general population and Gadir and colleagues[102] report a 16% occurrence of polycystic ovaries in healthy Arab women. We have reported the findings from a series of 90 cases with oligoamenorrhea and chronic anovulation[30]; at laparoscopy 87% had polycystic ovaries but only 39% showed hormonal and clinical features of PCOS. Bridges and co-workers[103] found polycystic ovaries in 6% of 6-year-old girls and in 26% of 15-year-old girls. Such ovaries have been also described associated with hypothroidism[102,104], hyperprolactinemic amenorrheas[101,102], adrenal insufficiency[101,105], Cushing's syndrome and acromegaly[101], androgenic tumors[101], in amenorrheic subjects because of loss of weight[106,107], epileptics under valproate treatment[108] and transsexual women with or without androgenic treatment[109].

Echographic characteristics of polycystic ovaries

A number of features differentiate these ovaries from normal ones. The first descriptions were produced by Swanson and colleagues[110] and Matsunaga and co-workers[111], and later systematized by Adams and associates[100].

Follicular distribution   From ultrasound investigations (abdominal approach) emerged the notion that the presence of at least 10 follicles (2–8 mm diameter) at the periphery of the ovarian cortex is required to define a polycystic ovary[100]. However, there is no agreement about the number of follicles 'required' in this definition – i.e. from 5 to 15 or more[5,34,112].

The vaginal approach proposed by Fox and colleagues in 1987[5] has received almost universal acceptance and, for PCOS diagnosis, 15 is the minimal number of follicles required.

Ovarian volume   In the sexually mature women, ovarian volume is around 6 cm^3, and never exceeds 8 cm^3. According to Pache and associates[113] the average volume of polycystic ovaries was 9.8 cm^3, which was significantly different from the controls (5.9 cm^3, $p < 0.001$). Some authors, however, report greater mean volumes ranging from 13.6 to 15.7 cm^3 [35,46,112]. Although increased ovarian volume is a common finding in all series, Yeh and colleagues[112] have observed that 30% of patients with PCOS exhibit normal ovarian volumes.

Ovarian stroma   The increased interstitial echogenicity is another feature of diagnostic importance. Unfortunately, definition of its degree depends upon the experience of the operator. Histologically, it is related to hyperplasia of the 'tecas' and increased cellularity at the interstices. According to Pache and associates[113] 94% of their series showed this feature (2+: 40%, 3+: 54%), while in normals 90% of subjects were assigned a 1+rating.

For Dewailly and co-workers[7], correlating echographic findings with clinical and endocrine data, the increased echogenicity of stroma and the presence of more than five follicles have a unique diagnostic importance in PCOS. The same conclusion is also supported by others[5,14,17,31].

Multifollicular ovaries   The above-mentioned morphological features allow one to differentiate (by the vaginal approach) cases of PCOS from those with multifollicular ovaries, where a crown of follicles is detected without changes in stromal echogenicity or ovarian volume[114]. This condition can be observed in young girls, in cases of hypothalamic anovulation and amenorrhea due to weight loss. At variance with PCOS, these morphological features disappear with the induction of ovulatory cycles.

Finally, it should be mentioned that not all cases of clinically or biochemically defined PCOS show polycystic ovaries at ultrasound assessment[9], and that the latter method shows an excellent correlation with laparoscopy investigation[7]. Echography, especially by the vaginal route, is an excellent (though incomplete) tool for the diagnosis of PCOS.

Magnetic resonance imaging

To assess ovarian morphology, this method provides greater definition and precision than ultrasound[115]. Maubon and colleagues[116] advanced the following criteria for PCOS diagnosis: main ovarian diameter: > 40 mm; > 10 cysts per ovary; and a thickened ovarial 'wall' of *ca.* 2 mm. We find this method perfectly satisfactory.

Doppler echography on ovarian circulation   Schurz and co-workers[117] studied patients with PCOS during induction of ovulation and observed, in the ovarian arteries, a pulsatile index (4.4) that was considerably greater than in normal controls (1.1; $p < 0.001$), during the ovulatory period. The low impedance in normal women is attributed to the process of neo-vascularization around the dominant follicle.

Conclusions

Polycystic ovarian syndrome is a heterogeneous condition. Several authors have attempted to define subgroups[6,17,34,36,37,118]. Diagnosis is achieved by the use of the largest amount of clinical, morphological and biochemical data.

The clinical data include menstrual cycle modifications, and/or hirsutism and/or obesity and metabolic manifestations of insulin resistance. Biochemical data include increased testosterone, testosterone : SHBG ratio or unbound testosterone (or androstenedione) levels.

The tests that measure the degree of ovarian response (17α-hydroxyprogesterone) to GnRH are of great value to define the origin of hyperandrogenism, though they are not essential for PCOS diagnosis.

Hyperandrogenism may or not be associated with an increase in the LH : FSH ratio (as discussed above) or the demonstration of insulin resistance. Basal insulin or glucose levels are of little value, especially in thin women. More complex studies (euglycemic clamp or adipose tissue biopsies) are limited to investigational purposes.

As regards diagnosis through imaging, echography with a vaginal transducer (or magnetic resonance imaging if available) is considered instrumental in defining the morphology of polycystic ovaries.

To summarize: an adequate clinical examination, the measurement of selected plasma hormone levels and data on ovarian morphology supplied by a series of non-invasive methods are the basis of the diagnosis of this pathology despite its heterogeneity.

References

1. Stein, I. and Leventhal, M. L. (1935). Amenorrhea associated with polycystic ovaries. *J. Obstet. Gynecol.*, **29**, 181–91
2. Yen, S. S. C. (1980). The polycystic ovarian disease. *Clin. Endocrinol.*, **12**, 177–208
3. Goldzieher, J. W. (1981). Polycystic ovarian disease. *Fertil. Steril.*, **35**, 371–94
4. Berga, S. L. (1994). Neuroendocrine regulation in polycystic ovary syndrome. In Schats, R. and Schoemaker, J. (eds.) *Ovarian Endocrinopathies*, pp. 157–68. (Carnforth, UK: Parthenon Publishing)
5. Fox, R., Corrigan, E., Thomas, P. G. and Hull, M. G. (1991). Oestrogen and androgen states in oligo-amenorrhoeic women with polycystic ovaries. *Br. J. Obstet. Gynaecol.*, **98**, 294–9
6. Lefebvre, P., Bringer, J., Boulet, F., Clouet, S., Orsetti, A. and Jaffiol, C. (1994). Body composition and regional fat patterning in polycystic ovary syndrome: impact on the hormonal and the metabolic profiles. In Schats, R. and Schoemaker, J. (eds.) *Ovarian Endocrinopathies*, pp. 151–6. (Carnforth, UK: Parthenon Publishing)
7. Dewailly, D., Duhamel, A., Ardens, R. J., Beauscart, R., Lemaitre, L. and Fossati, P. (1993). Interrelationship between ultrasonography and biology in the diagnosis of polycystic ovary syndrome. *Ann. N.Y. Acad. Sci.*, **687**, 206–15
8. Rodin, A., Thakkar, H., Taylor, N. and Clayton, R. (1994). Hyperandrogenism in polycystic ovary syndrome: evidence of disregulation of 11β-hydroxysteroid dehydrogenase. *N. Engl. J. Med.*, **330**, 460–5
9. Escobar-Morreale, H., Pazos, F., Potau, N., Garcia Robles, R., Sanchez, J. M. and Varela, C. (1994). Ovarian suppression with triptorelin and adrenal stimulation with adrenocorticotropin in functional hyperandrogenism: role of adrenal and ovarian cytochrome P450 c17 alfa. *Fertil. Steril.*, **62**, 521–30
10. Kettel, L. M., Roseff, S. J., Berga, S. L., Mortola, J. F. and Yen, S. S. C. (1993). Hypothalamic pituitary–ovarian response to clomiphene citrate in women with polycystic ovary syndrome. *Fertil. Steril.*, **59**, 532–8
11. Fauser, B. C. J. M. (1990). Classification of chronic hyperandrogenic anovulation. In Coelingh-Bennink, H. J. T., Vemer, H. M. and van Keep, P. A. (eds.) *Chronic Hyperandrogenic Anovulation*, pp. 13–17. (Carnforth, UK: Parthenon)
12. Saxton, D. W., Farquhar, C. M., Real, T. and Beard, R. W., Anderson, M. C. and Wadsworth, J. (1990). Accuracy of ultrasound measurement of female pelvis organs. *Br. J. Obstet. Gynaecol.*, **97**, 695–9
13. Takahashi, K., Eda, Y., Okada, S., Abu-Musa, A., Yoshino, K. and Kitao, M. (1993). Morphological assessment of polycystic ovary using transvaginal ultrasound. *Hum. Reprod.*, **8**, 844–9
14. Franks, S. (1989). Polycystic ovary syndrome: a changing perspective. *Clin. Endocrinol.*, **31**, 87–120
15. Maubon, A., Courtieu, C., Vivens, F., Tailland, M. L., Saucerotte, H., Bringer, J., Mares, P. and Rowaneti, P. (1993). Magnetic resonance imaging of normal and polycystic ovaries. *Ann. N.Y. Acad. Sci.*, **687**, 224–9

16. Eden, J. A., Place, J., Carter, G. D., Jones, J., Alaghband-Zadeh, J. and Pawson, M. E. (1989). The diagnosis of polycystic ovaries in sub-fertile women. *Br. J. Obstet. Gynaecol.*, **96**, 809–15

17. Pache, T. D., de Jong, F. H., Hop, W. C. and Fauser, B. C. J. (1993). Association between ovarian changes assessed by transvaginal sonography and clinical and endocrine signs of the polycystic ovary syndrome. *Fertil. Steril.*, **59**, 544–9

18. Fox, R. (1992). Correspondence. *Br. J. Obstet. Gynecol.*, **99**, 938

19. El Tabbakh, G. H., Lotfy, L., Azab, Y., Rahman, H. A., Southren, A. L. and Aleen, F. A. (1986). Correlation of the ultrasonic appearance of the ovaries in polycystic ovarian disease and the clinical, hormonal and laparoscopic findings. *Am. J. Obstet. Gynecol.*, **154**, 892–5

20. Batrinos, M. L. (1993). Intraovarian regulators and polycystic ovarian syndrome. *Ann. N.Y. Acad. Sci.*, **687**, 230–4

21. Gindoff, P. R. and Jewelewicz, R. (1987). Polycystic ovarian disease. *Obstet. Gynecol. Clin. North Am.*, **14**, 931–53

22. Obhrai, M., Lynch, S. S., Holder, G., Jackson, R., Tang, L. and Butt, W. R. (1990). *Clin. Endocrinol.*, **32**, 467–74

23. Wajchenberg, B. L., Achando, S. S., Marthor, M. M., Czeresnia, C. E., Neto, D. G. and Kirschner, M. A. (1988) The source(s) of estrogen production in hirsute women with polycystic ovarian disease as determined by simultaneous adrenal and ovarian venous catheterization. *Fertil. Steril.*, **49**, 56–61

24. Kletsky, D. A., Dawajan, R. M. and Mishell, J. R. D. R. (1975). Classification of secondary amenorrhoea based on distinct hormonal patterns. *J. Clin. Endocrinol. Metab.*, **41**, 660–8

25. Fox, R., Corrigan, E., Thomas, P. A. and Hull, G. R. (1991). The diagnosis of polycystic ovaries in women with oligo-amenorrhoea: predictive power of endocrine test. *Clin. Endocrinol.*, **34**, 127–31

26. Franks, S., Adams, J., Mason, H. and Polson, D. (1985). Ovulatory disorders in women with polycystic ovary syndrome. *Clin. Obstet. Gynecol.*, **12**, 605–32

27. Takahashi, K., Yoshino, K., Nishigaki, A., Eda, Y. and Kitao, M. (1992). The relationship between endocrine and ovulatory abnormalities and polycystic ovaries as diagnosed by ultrasonography. *Int. J. Fertil.*, **37**, 222–6

28. Fauser, B. C. J. M. and Pache, T. D. (1994). Polycystic ovary syndrome: normal and abnormal follicle development. In Schats, R. and Schoemaker, J. (eds.) *Ovarian Endocrinopathies*, pp. 117–27. (Carnforth, UK: Parthenon Publishing)

29. Polson, D. W., Wadsworth, J., Adams, J. and Franks, S. (1988). Polycystic ovaries. A common finding in normal women. *Lancet*, **1**, 870–2

30. Tozzini, R. I. and Pineda, R. L. (1986). *Ginecologia endoscopia*, pp. 96–102. (Buenos Aires: Medica Panamericana)

31. Ardaens, Y., Robert, Y., Lamaitre, L., Fossatti, P. and Dewailly, D. (1991). Polycystic ovarian disease: contribution of vaginal endosonography and reassessment of ultrasonic diagnosis. *Fertil. Steril.*, **55**, 1062–8

32. Lobo, R. A. (1994). *Year Book of Infertility and Reproductive Endocrinology 1994*, 118–94–1–15. (St. Louis, USA: Mosby Year Book)

33. Fraenkel, L. (1943). Thecoma and hyperthecosis of the ovary. *J. Clin. Endocrinol. Metab.*, **3**, 557–60

34. Conway, G. S., Honour, J. W. ad Jacobs, H. (1989). Heterogeneity of the polycystic ovary syndrome: clinical endocrine and ultrasound features in 556 patients. *Clin. Endocrinol.*, **31**, 87–120

35. Falsetti, L. and Pasinetti, E. (1994). Treatment of moderate and severe hirsutism by gonodotropin releasing hormone agonist in women with polycystic ovary syndrome and idiopathic hirsutism. *Fertil. Steril.*, **61**, 817–20

36. Insler, V., Shoham, Z., Barash, A. *et al.* (1993). Polycystic ovaries in non-obese and obese patients: possible pathophysiological mechanism based on new interpretation of facts and findings. *Hum. Reprod.*, **8**, 379–84

37. Insler V., Barash, A., Shoham, Z., Koistinen, R., Seppala, M., Hen, M., Lunenfeld, B. and Zadek, Z. (1994). Overnight secretion pattern of growth hormone, sex hormone binding globulin, insulin-like growth factor-1 and its binding proteins in obese and non-obese women with polycystic ovarian disease. *Isr. J. Med. Sci.*, **30**, 42–7

38. Barbieri, R. L. and Ryan, K. J. (1983). Hyperandrogenism, insulin-resistance and acanthosis nigricans syndrome: a common endrocrinopathy with distinct patholophysiologic features. *Am. J. Obstet. Gynecol.*, **147**, 90–101

39. Bringer, J., Lefebvre, P., Boulet, F., Grigolet, F., Renard, E., Hedon, B., Orsetti, A. and Jaffiol, C. (1993). Body composition and regional fat distribution in polycystic ovarian syndrome. *Ann. N.Y. Acad. Sci.*, **687**, 115–23

40. Cheung, A. and Chang, R. J. (1991). Polycystic ovaries and other ovarian causes of hyperandrogenism. *Infertility and Reproductive Medicine Clinics of North America*, Vol. 2, No. 3, pp. 465–77

41. Yen, S. S. C., Vela, P. and Rankin, J. (1970). Inappropriate secretion of follicle-stimulating hormone and luteinizing hormone in polycystic ovarian disease. *J. Clin. Endocrinol. Metab.*, **30**, 435–42

42. Bart, C., Fauser, J. M. and De Jong, F. H. (1993). Gonadotropins in polycystic ovarian syndrome. *Ann. N.Y. Acad. Sci.*, **687**, 151–61

43. Berga, S. L., Guzic, D. S. and Winters, S. J. (1993). Increased LH and alfa-subunit secretion in woman with hyperandrogenic anovulation. *J. Clin. Endocrinol. Metab.*, **77**, 895–901

44. Burger, C. W., Hompes, P. G., Korsen, T. J. M. and Schoemaker, J. (1989). Ovulation induction with pulsatile luteinizing hormone-releasing hormone in women with clomiphene citrate-resistant polycystic ovary-like disease: endocrine result. *Fertil. Steril.*, **51**, 20–9

45. Corenthal, L., von Hagen, S., Larkins, D., Ibrahin, J. and Santoro, N. (1994). Benefits of continuous physiological pulsatile gonadotropin-releasing hormone therapy in women with polycystic ovarian syndrome. *Fertil. Steril.*, **61**, 1027–32

46. Gadir, A. A., Khatim, M. S., Mowafi, R. S., Al-naser, H. M. I., Alzard, H. G. N. and Shaw, R. W. (1991). Polycystic ovaries: do these represent a specific endocrinopathy? *Br. J. Gynaecol.*, **98**, 300–5

47. Fox, R. and Hull, M. G. R. (1992). Polycystic ovarian disease: diagnostic methods. *Contemp. Rev. Obstet. Gynaecol.*, **4**, 84–9

48. Tozzini, R. I., Pineda, R. L., Turner, D. and Zacarias, H. (1982). Value of the LRH acute test for the study of the alterations of the reproductive axis. In Muldoon, T. G., Mahesh, V. B. and Perez-Ballester, B. (eds.) *Recent Advances in Infertility Research Part A: Developments in Reproductive Endocrinology*, pp. 275–84. (New York: Alan R. Liss, Inc.)

49. Robinson, S., Rodin, D. A., Deacon, A., Wheeler, M. J. and Clayton, R. N. (1992). Which hormone test for the diagnosis of polycystic ovary syndrome? *Br. J. Obstet. Gynaecol.*, **99**, 232–8

50. Crowley, W. F., Hall, J. E., Martin, K. A., Adams, J. and Taylor, A. E. (1993). An overview of the diagnostic considerations in polycystic ovarian syndrome. *Ann. N.Y. Acad. Sci.*, **687**, 235–41

51. Apter, D., Butzow, T., Laughlin, G. A. and Yen, S. S. C. (1994). Accelerated 24-hour luteinizing hormone pulsatile activity in adolescent girls with ovarian hyperandrogenism: relevance to the developmental phase of polycystic ovarian syndrome. *J. Clin. Endocrinol. Metab.*, **79**, 119–25

52. Lobo, R. A., Kletzky, A., Campean, J. D. and Di Zerega, G. S. (1983). Elevated bioactive LH in women with the polycystic ovarian syndrome. *Fertil. Steril.*, **39**, 674–8

53. Fauser, B. C. J., Pache, T. D., Lamberts, S. W. J., Hop, W. C. J., de Jong, F. H. and Dahl, C. D. (1991). Serum bioactive and immunoreactive luteinizing hormone and follicle stimulating hormone levels in women with cycle abnormalities with or without polycystic ovarian disease. *J. Clin. Endocrinol. Metab.*, **73**, 811–17

54. Imse, V., Holzaplel, G., Hinney, B., Kuhn, W. and Wuttke, W. (1992). Comparison of the luteinizing hormone pulsatility in the serum of women suffering from polycystic ovarian disease, using a bioassay and five different immunoassays. *J. Clin. Endocrinol. Metab.*, **74**, 1053–61

55. Kazer, R. R., Kessel, B. and Yen, S. S. C. (1987). Circulating LH pulse frequency in women with polycystic ovary syndrome. *J. Clin. Endocrinol. Metab.*, **65**, 233–6

56. Waldstreicher, J., Santoro, N. F., Hall, J. A., Filicori, M. and Crowley, W. F. (1987). Hyperfunction of the hypothalamic–pituitary axis in women with polycystic ovarian disease. Indirect evidence for partial gonadotroph desensitization. *J. Clin. Endocrinol. Metab.*, **66**, 165–72

57. Burger, C. W., Korsen, T., v. Kessel, H., v. Dop, P. A., Caron, F. J. M. and Schoemaker, J. (1985). Pulsatile LH patterns in the follicular phase of the menstrual cycle, polycystic ovarian disease (PCOD) and PCOD secondary amenorrhea. *J. Clin. Endocrinol. Metab.*, **61**, 1126–32

58. Dunaif, A., Mandeli, J., Fluhr, H. and Dobrjansky, A. (1988). The impact of the obesity and chronic hyperinsulinemia on gonadotropin release and gonadal steroid secretion in the polycystic ovary syndrome. *J. Clin. Endocrinol. Metab.*, **66**, 131–9

59. Venturoli, S., Porcu, E., Fabbri, R., Magrini, O., Gammi, L., Paradisi, R., Forcacci, M., Bolzani, R. and Flamigni, C. (1988). Episodic pulsatile secretion of FSH, LH, prolactin, oestradiol, oestrone and LH circadian variations in polycystic ovary syndrome. *J. Clin. Endocrinol. Metab.*, **28**, 93–107

60. Zumoff, B., Freeman, R., Coupey, S. *et al.* (1983). A chrononbiologic abnormality in luteinizing hormone secretion in teenaged girls with polycystic ovary syndrome. *N. Engl. J. Med.*, **309**, 1206–9

61. Lambert-Messerlian, G. M., Hall, J. E., Sluss, P. M., Taylor, A. S. E., Martin, K. A., Groome, N. P., Cowley, J. R. W. F. and Schneyer, A. L. (1993). Relatively low levels of dimeric inhibin circulate in men and women with polycystic ovarian syndrome using a specific two-site

enzyme-linked immunosorbent assay. *J. Clin. Endocrinol. Metab.*, **79**, 49–50

62. Erickson, G. F. (1994). Polycystic ovary syndrome: normal and abnormal steroidogenesis. In Schats, R. and Schoemaker, J. (eds.) *Ovarian Endocrinopathies*, pp. 103–115. (Carnforth, UK: Parthenon Publishing)

63. Judd, H. L. (1978). Endocrinology of polycystic ovarian disease. *Clin. Obstet. Gynecol.*, **21**, 99–114

64. Gindoff, P. R. and Jewelewicz, R. (1987). Polycystic ovarian disease. *Obstet. Gynecol. Clin. North Am. 14*, 931–53

65. Jafari, K., Javaheri, G. and Ruiz, G. (1984). Endometrial adenocarcinoma and Stein Leventhal syndrome. *Obstet. Gynecol.*, **51**, 97–101

66. Gallup, D. G. and Stock, R. J. (1984). Adenocarcinoma of the endometrium in women 40 years of age or younger. *Obstet. Gynecol.*, **64**, 417

67. Deaton, J. L. (1991). Hyperandrogenism and uterine bleeding. In Pattaway, D. (ed.) *Hyperandrogenism*, pp. 561–83. (New York: W.B. Saunders Co.)

68. Pineda, R. L., Tozzini, R. I. and Reeves, G. (1980). Laparoscopic biopsy of the ovary. In Tozzini, R. I., Reeves, G. and Pineda, R. L. (eds.) *Endocrine Physiopathology of the Ovary*, pp. 335–42. (Amsterdam: Elsevier/North-Holland Biomedical Press)

69. Barnes, R. B., Rosenfield, R. L., Burstein, S. and Ehrmann, D. A. (1989). Pituitary–ovarian responses to nafarelin testing in polycystic ovary syndrome. *N. Engl. J. Med.*, **320**, 559–65

70. Ehrmann, D. A., Rosenfield, R. L., Barnes, R. B., Brigell, D. F. and Sheikh, Z. (1992). Detection of functional ovarian hyperandrogenism in women with androgen excess. *N. Engl. J. Med.*, **327**, 157–62

71. Ibañez, L., Potau, N., Zampolli, M., Prat, N., Gussinye, M., Saenger, P., Vicents-Calvet, E. and Carrascosa, A. (1994). Source localization of androgen axcess in adolescent girls. *J. Clin. Endocrinol. Metab.*, **79**, 1778–84

72. Rosenfield, R. L., Ehrmann, D. A., Barnes, R. B. and Sheikh, Z. (1993). Gonadotropin-releasing hormone agonist as a probe for the pathogenesis and diagnosis of ovarian hyperandrogenism. *Ann. N.Y. Acad. Sci.*, **687**, 162–81

73. Takahashi, K., Yoskino, K., Eda, Y. and Kitao, M. (1992). Prevalence of polycystic ovaries by transvaginal ultrasound and serum androgens. *Int. J. Fertil.*, **37**, 290–4

74. Panidis, D., Rousso, D., Skiadopoulos, S. and Kalogeropoulos, A. (1994). Basal circulating androgen levels in patients with polycystic ovary syndrome and/or without insulin resistance. In Schats, R. and Schoemaker, J. (eds.) *Ovarian Endocrinopathies*, pp. 189–94. (Carnforth, UK: Parthenon Publishing)

75. Yoshino, K., Takahashi, K., Eda, Y., Okada, S. and Ketao, M. (1993). Plasma androgens and sex hormone binding globulin in women with polycystic ovaries diagnosed by transvaginal ultrasound. *J. Reprod. Med.*, **38**, 858–62

76. Takahashi, K., Eda, Y., Abu-Musa, A., Akada, S., Yoshino, K. and Kitao, M. (1994). Transvaginal ultrasound imaging, histopathology and endocrinopathy in patients with polycystic ovarian syndrome. *Hum. Reprod.*, **9**, 1231–6

77. Bardin, C. W. and Lipsett, M. B. (1967). Testosterone and androstenedione blood production rates in normal women with idiopathic hirsutism and polycystic ovaries. *J. Clin. Invest.*, **46**, 891–902

78. Pugeat, M., Nicolas, M. H., Craves, J. C., Alvarado-Dubost, C., Fimbel, S., Déchaud, H. and Lejeune, H. (1993). Androgens in polycystic ovarian syndrome. *Ann. N.Y. Acad. Sci.*, **687**, 124–35

79. McKenna, T. J. (1988). Pathogenesis and treatment of polycystic ovary syndrome. *N. Engl. J. Med.*, **318**, 558–62

80. Turner, E. I., Watson, M. J., Perry, L. A. and White, M. C. (1992). Investigation of adrenal function in women with oligomenorrhoea and hirsutism (clinical PCOS) from north-east England using adrenal stimulation test. *Clin. Endocrinol.*, **36**, 389–97

81. Faber, K. and Hughes, C. L. (1991). Laboratory evaluation of hyperandrogenic conditions. In Pittaway, D. E. (ed.) *Hyperandrogenism*, pp. 495–509. Infertility and Reproductive Medicine Clinics of North America. (New York: W.B. Saunders Co.)

82. Polson, D. W., Reed, M. J., Franks, S., Scanlon, M. J. and James, H. T. (1988). Serum 11-hydroxyandrostenedione as an indicator of the source of excess androgen production in women with polycystic ovaries. *J. Clin. Metab. Endocrinol.*, **66**, 946–50

83. Thompson, D. L., Horton, N. and Ritmaster, R. S. (1990). Androsterone glucuronide is a maker of adrenal hyperandrogenism in hirsute women. *Clin. Endocrinol.*, **32**, 283–92

84. Robinson, S., Kiddy, D., Gelding, S. V., Willis, D., Niththyananthan, R., Busch, A., Johnston, D. G. and Franks, S. (1993). The relationship of insulin insensitivity to menstrual pattern in women with hyperandrogenism and polycystic ovaries. *Clin. Endocrinol.*, **39**, 351–5

85. Nestler, J. E. (1993). Sex hormone-binding globulin: a marker for hyperinsulinemia and/or insulin resistance? *J. Clin. Endocrinol. Metab.*, **76**, 273–4

86. Plymate, S. R., Matej, L. A., Jones, R. E. and Friedl, K. E. (1988). Inhibition of sex hormone binding globulin production in the human hepatoma (Hep g2) cell line by insulin and prolactin. *J. Clin. Endocrinol. Metab.*, **67**, 460–5

87. Poretsky, L. (1994). Role of insulin resistance in the pathogenesis of polycystic ovary syndrome. In Schats, R. and Schoemaker, J. (eds.) *Ovarian Endocrinopathies*, pp. 169–76. (Carnforth, UK: Parthenon Publishing)

88. Poretsky, L. and Piper, B. (1994). Insulin resistance, hypersecretion of LH, and a dual-defect hypothesis for the pathogenesis of polycystic ovary syndrome. *Obstet. Gynecol.*, **84**, 613–21

89. Weber, R. F., Pache, T. D., Jacobs, M. L., Docter, R., Loriaux, D. L., Fauser, B. C. J. M. and Birkenhäger, J. C. (1993). The relation between clinical manifestations of polycystic ovary syndrome and β cell function. *Clin. Endocrinol.*, **38**, 295–300

90. Buyalos, R. P., Geffner, M. E., Bersch, N., Judd, H. L., Bergman, R. N. and Golde, D. W. (1992). Insulin and insulin-like growth factor irresponsiveness in polycystic ovarian syndrome. *Fertil. Steril.*, **57**, 796–803

91. Anttila, L., Koskinen, P., Jaatinen, T. A., Erkkola, R., Irjala, K. and Ruutiainen, K. (1993). Insulin hypersecretion together with high luteinizing hormone concentration augments androgen secretion in oral glucose tolerance test in women with polycystic ovarian disease. *Hum. Reprod.*, **8**, 1179–83

92. Chang, R. J., Nakamura, R. M., Judd, H. L. and Kaplan, S. A. (1983). Insulin resistance in non-obese patient with polycystic ovarian disease. *J. Clin. Endocrinol. Metab.*, **38**, 1165–74

93. Jialal, I., Marker, P., Reddi, K. *et al.* (1987). Evidence for insulin resistance in non-obese patients with polycystic ovarian disease. *J. Clin. Endocrinol. Metab.*, **64**, 1066–70

94. Yen, S. S. C., Laughlin, G. A. and Morales, A. J. (1993). Interface between extra- and intra-ovarian factors in polycystic ovarian syndrome. *Ann. NY Acad. Sci.*, **687**, 98–110

95. Laatikainen, T. (1993). How IGF-I binding protein can be modulated in polycystic ovarian syndrome. *Ann. NY Acad. Sci.*, **687**, 90–7

96. Dunaif, A. (1993). Insulin resistance in polycystic ovarian syndrome. *Ann. N.Y. Acad. Sci.*, **687**, 60–4

97. Sharp, E. S., Kiddy, D. S., Reed, M. J., Anyaoku, V., Johnston, D. G. and Franks, S. (1991). Correlation of plasma insulin and insulin like growth factor I with indices of androgen transport and metabolism in women with polycystic ovary syndrome. *Clin. Endocrinol.*, **35**, 253–7

98. Futterweit, W. (1984). Pathologic anatomy of polycystic ovarian disease. In Futterweit, W. (ed.) *Polycystic Ovarian Disease.* pp. 41–6. (New York: Springer-Verlag)

99. Luciano, A. A., Chapler, F. K. and Sherman, B. M. (1984). Hyperprolactinemia in polycystic ovary syndrome. *Fertil. Steril.*, **41**, 719–23

100. Adams, J., Polson, D. W. and Franks, S. (1986). Prevalence of polycystic ovaries in women with anovulation and idiopathic hirsutism. *Br. Med. J.*, **293**, 355–9

101. Clayton, R. N., Ogden, V., Hodgkinson, J., Worswick, L., Rodin, D. A., Dyer, S. and Made, T. W. (1992). How common are polycystic ovaries in normal women and what is their significance for the fertility of the population? *J. Clin. Endocrinol. Metab.*, **37**, 127–34

102. Abdel Gadir, A., Khatim, M. S., Mowafi, R. S., Alnaser, H. M., Muharif, N. S. and Shaw, R. W. (1992). Implications of ultrasonically diagnosed polycystic ovaries. I- Correlations with basal hormonal profiles. *Hum. Reprod.*, **4**, 453–7

103. Bridges, M. A., Hindmarsk, P. C., Cooke, A., Brook, C. G. D. and Healy, M. J. R. (1993). Standards for ovarian volume in childhood and puberty. *Fertil. Steril.*, **60**, 456–60

104. Abdel Gadir, A., Khatim, M. S., Mowafi, R. S., Alnaser, H. M., Muharif, N. S. and Shaw, R. W. (1992). Implications of ultrasonically diagnosed polycystic ovaries. II- Studies of dynamic and pulsatile hormonal patterns. *Hum. Reprod.*, **7**, 458–61

105. Scharm, P., Zerah, M., Mani, P., Jewelewicz, R., Jaffe, S. and New, M. I. (1992). Nonclassical 3β-hydroxysteroid dehydrogenase deficiency: a review of our experience with 25 female patients. *Fertil. Steril.*, **58**, 129–36

106. Fox, R. and Hull, M. (1993). Ultrasound diagnosis of polycystic ovaries. In *Intraovarian regulators and polycystic ovarian syndrome. Ann. N.Y. Acad. Sci.*, **687**, 217–23

107. Shohan, Z., Conway, G. S., Patel, A. and Jacobs, H. S. (1992). Polycystic ovaries in patients with hypogonadropic hypogonadism: similarity of ovarian response to gonadotropin stimulation in patients with polycystic ovarian syndrome. *Fertil. Steril.*, **58**, 37–45

108. Isojarvi, J. I. I., Laatikainen, T. J., Pakarinen, A. J., Juntunen, K. T. and Myllyia, V. (1993). Polycystic ovaries and hyperandrogenism in women taking valproate for epilepsy. *N. Engl. J. Med.*, **329**, 1383–8

109. Balen, A. H., Schachter, M. E., Montgomery, D., Reid, R. W. and Jacobs, H. S. (1993). Transsexuals. *J. Clin. Endocrinol. Metab.*, **38**, 325–9

110. Swanson, M., Sauerbrie, E. E. and Cooperberg, P. L. (1981). Medical implications of ultrasoni-

cally detected polycystic ovaries. *J. Clin. Ultrasound*, **9**, 219–22

111. Matsunaga, I., Hata, T. and Kitao, M. (1985). Ultrasonographic identification of polycystic ovary. *Asia-Oceania. J. Obstet. Gynecol.*, **11**, 227–32

112. Yeh, H. C., Futterweit, W. and Thorton, J. C. (1987). Polycystic ovarian disease: US features in 104 patients. *Radiology*, **163**, 111–16

113. Pache, T. D., Wladimeroff, J. W., Hop, W. C. and Fauser, B. C. J. (1992). How to discriminate between normal and polycystic ovaries: transvaginal US study. *Radiology*, **183**, 421–3

114. Adams, J., Polson, D. W., Abdulwahid, N., Morris, D. V., Franks, S., Mason, H. D., Tucker, M., Price, J. and Jacobs, H. S. (1985). Multifollicular ovaries: clinical and endocrine features and response to pulsatile gonadotropin releasing hormone. *Lancet*, **2**, 1375–8

115. Outwater, E. K. and Dunton, C. J. (1995). Imaging of the ovary and adnexa: clinical issues and applications of MR imaging. *Radiology*, **194**, 1–18

116. Maubon, A., Courtieu, C., Vivens, F., Tailland, M. L., Saucerotte, H., Bringer, J., Mares, T. and Rouanet, J. P. (1993). Magnetic resonance imaging of normal and polycystic ovaries. *Ann. N.Y. Acad. Sci.*, **687**, 224–9

117. Schurz, B., Schon, H. J., Wenzl, R., Eppel, W., Huber, J. and Reinold, E. (1993). Endovaginal Doppler flow measurements of the ovarian artery in patients with a normal menstrual cycle and polycystic ovary syndrome during *in vitro* fertilization. *J. Clin. Ultrasound*, **21**, 19–23

118. Norman, R. J., Masters, S. C., Hage, W., Beng, C., Pannall, P. and Wang, J. X. (1995). Metabolic approaches to the subclassification of polycystic ovary syndrome. *Fertil. Steril.*, **63**, 329–35

Polycystic ovary syndrome: medical therapy

11

R. Homburg

Introduction

The detailed basic cause of polycystic ovary syndrome (PCOS) is still unknown. There is, therefore, no single effective treatment regimen but a plethora of protocols that do not address the real cause but aim to break the vicious circle of pathological chain reactions. The treatment schedules outlined here are symptomatic therapy, the choice of which is made according to the principal complaint of the patient.

There is, however, one overriding principle for the treatment of obese women with PCOS, whether the main problem is cosmetically unacceptable signs of hyperandrogenism such as hirsutism or acne, infertility or prevention of long-term sequelae. Loss of 5% or more of total body weight is capable of reversing or severely reducing these symptoms and/or facilitating treatment of infertility[1]. This is apparently achieved by reducing insulin and increasing sex hormone binding globulin (SHBG) and insulin-like growth factor binding protein-1 (IGFBP-1) concentrations with a consequent reduction of ovarian androgen production and circulating free testosterone.

More sophisticated methods of reduction of insulin levels with diazoxide[2], metformin[3] or somatostatin[4] have proved to be effective in improving the endocrine milieu. More investigation is needed to examine the clinical feasibility of this mode of treatment.

Therapy for those not wishing to conceive

For women with PCOS who are not interested in conceiving, the treatment of choice is a combination of cyproterone acetate and ethinylestradiol. Cyproterone acetate is a synthetic progesterone with both antigonadotropic and antiandrogenic effects, giving it the advantage for the treatment of PCOS over the majority of progestins in oral contraceptives. In combination with ethinylestradiol, it has been successful in suppressing hyperandrogenism, resulting in improvement of clinical signs and normalization of the hormonal disturbances that characterize PCOS[5]. The efficacy of this treatment is due to the antiandrogenic activity at androgen receptor level, suppression of serum luteinizing hormone (LH) and ovarian androgen levels, reduction in 5α-reductase levels, increased metabolic clearance of testosterone and increase in SHBG concentration. The effect on acne and seborrhea is usually rapid, but, due to the physiological cycle of the hair follicle, at least 6 months' treatment is required before the reduction of hirsutism becomes clinically evident. As previously mentioned, untreated PCOS may be regarded as a progressive syndrome. It is therefore my opinion that early therapeutic intervention will not only temporarily alleviate symptoms but also place the progress of the syndrome 'on hold'. This would appear to be beneficial for future fertility prospects and the possible delay or prevention of long-term sequelae.

Treatment for anovulation

Clomiphene citrate

The chronic anovulation and infertility associated with PCOS can often be successfully treated with clomiphene citrate. Some 75% of those treated with clomiphene citrate in doses of 50–200 mg/day from day 4 or 5 of the cycle for 5 days will respond by ovulating. However, the overall pregnancy rate is only 30–40%. Several reasons have been put forward to explain this apparent discrepancy. The main action of clomiphene citrate is through the hypothalamus, stimulating gonadotropin releasing hormone (GnRH) secretion and increasing follicle stimulating hormone (FSH) release from the hypophysis. This is often accompanied by a striking increase in serum LH concentrations[6] and this may seriously compromise pregnancy rates in these patients[7]. Pretreatment with progesterone is capable of modulating LH pulsatility, reducing LH levels, inducing more FSH synthesis and storage, so creating a more favorable environment for ovulation induction with clomiphene citrate[8]. This treatment has improved the response to clomiphene citrate and consequent pregnancy rates[8]. An additional causative factor in those ovulating but not conceiving is the antiestrogenic effect of clomiphene citrate on the cervical mucus and, possibly, on the endometrium, hypothetically disturbing normal mechanisms of sperm transport and implantation. In some cases, the addition of ethinylestradiol to clomiphene citrate will enhance the pregnancy rate without interfering with the induction of ovulation.

Monitoring by ultrasound examination of the ovaries of those who fail to ovulate on maximal doses of clomiphene citrate will reveal that the majority of these women will show inadequate follicular development, demanding an 'upgrade' of treatment. However, a minority of the non-ovulators will develop large follicle(s) but have an isolated defect of estrogen-mediated positive feedback and may respond to a well-timed injection of human chorionic gonadotropin (hCG). Finally, the addition of dexamethasone in the few who have high dihydroepiandrosterone sulfate levels has been reported to improve results[9].

In our practice, 'clomiphene failure' is regarded as a failure to ovulate on maximal doses

of clomiphene citrate or a failure to conceive, despite apparent ovulation, in six courses of treatment. In the latter case, male and mechanical factors are re-evaluated. Several treatment modes are now available to women with PCOS who are 'clomiphene failures', most of which are reasonably successful in breaking the vicious circle of chain reactions and inducing ovulation and pregnancy without the ability to attack the unknown source.

Pulsatile GnRH

The administration of native GnRH in a pulsatile fashion, either subcutaneously or intravenously in a suggested dose of 15 µg/pulse every 90 min using a pump apparatus, is apparently capable of superimposing the abnormal pattern of secretion with a more physiological pattern, so producing a more balanced output of gonadotropins. This form of treatment is, however, associated with low ovulation rates (50% per cycle) and pregnancy rates per ovulatory cycle of 29%[10]. It is particularly unsuitable for obese, and hyperandrogenic women and the high LH levels observed during induction present a further obstacle[11]. The advantages of this mode of treatment are that it will yield a monofollicular response in a large proportion of women and therefore ovarian hyperstimulation (OHSS) is not encountered and multiple pregnancies are rarely seen if hCG administration is avoided.

Gonadotropin therapy

Stimulation of the ovaries with exogenous gonadotropins is a more acceptable treatment for clomiphene citrate resistant patients. A conventional 'step-up', individually adjusted dose regimen employing human menopausal gonadotropin (hMG) in our hands[12] yields a cumulative conception rate of 82% after six cycles. However, due to the high sensitivity of the polycystic ovary to gonadotropin stimulation and its propensity to multiple follicular development, this treatment regimen is plagued by a high frequency of multiple pregnancies and

OHSS[13]. The use of human urinary FSH has done little to remedy this situation[14–16].

Following the initial publication of Seibel and colleagues[17], several investigators have examined the utility of a chronic low-dose regimen of FSH in an attempt to reduce the complication rate[18–23]. The basic thinking behind this regimen is the 'threshold theory', which demands the attainment and maintenance of follicular development with exogenous FSH, without exceeding the threshold requirement of the ovary[24] which, with supraphysiological doses of FSH, provokes an initial development of a large cohort, stimulates additional follicles and even rescues those destined for atresia[25]. This is what tends to occur in PCOS with its peculiar hypersensitivity to gonadotropins when levels of FSH well above the threshold are induced during conventional treatment. The principle of the chronic low-dose regimen is, therefore, to employ smaller incremental dose rises (e.g. 37.5 IU or less) at intervals of 7 days until follicular development is initiated. A compilation of reported results using this or similar regimens reveals that 218 patients who completed 471 cycles achieved 83 pregnancies (18% per cycle). This rate compares favorably with that of more conventional regimens, but has the advantage that it was accompanied by a very low prevalence of OHSS (one cycle) and multiple pregnancies (5%). A prospective study from our center[23], comparing conventional with low-dose protocols employing 50 women with clomiphene citrate-resistant PCOS, revealed that the low-dose protocol slightly improved pregnancy rates (40% vs. 24%), while completely avoiding OHSS and multiple pregnancies, which are prevalent (11% and 33%, respectively) using conventional incremental rises of FSH dose. We concluded that this treatment modality has distinct advantages and could well replace conventional gonadotropin therapy for these patients.

GnRH analog

The original report of Fleming and co-workers[26] on co-treatment with GnRH analog (GnRH-a) and hMG for anovulatory PCOS encouraged its use for this indication. While hopes that the state of near hypogonadotropic hypogonadism induced by GnRH-a would produce results with hMG as successful as those of World Health Organization group I cases have not been fulfilled, there is a definite place for the incorporation of GnRH-a into stimulation protocols for women with PCOS. The main contribution is the reduction of LH concentrations throughout the follicular phase of the cycle. This almost completely eliminates the troublesome problem of premature luteinization and the need to abandon cycles for this reason, so increasing treatment efficiency. There is now mounting evidence that the ability of GnRH-a to reduce the inordinately elevated concentrations of LH prevalent in PCOS serves to increase ovulation and pregnancy rates and, most importantly, to reduce the prevalence of early spontaneous miscarriage, for which the rates are notoriously high in PCOS accompanied by raised LH concentrations.

In a retrospective analysis from our center[27], 239 women with PCOS received hMG with or without GnRH-a for ovulation induction or superovulation for *in vitro* fertilization/embryo transfer (IVF/ET). Of pregnancies achieved with GnRH-a, 17.6% miscarried compared with 39.1% of those achieved with gonadotropins alone. Cumulative live birth rates for GnRH-a after four cycles were 64% compared with 26% for gonadotropins only. Others[28] have reported similar results. While a randomized, prospective study is sadly lacking to confirm these data, it is our policy to administer GnRH-a to women with high LH concentrations in the follicular phase, on the basis that there is little point in inducing a pregnancy that has a very high chance of being aborted. A further study from our center[29] looked at the performance of women with PCOS undergoing IVF/ET who had high mean LH concentrations, compared with a control group of normally cycling women with mechanical infertility. Pregnancy rates were similar in the groups, but, whereas GnRH-a reduced the miscarriage rate compared with gonadotropins alone in the PCOS group, its administration to the control group had no such effect.

Administration of GnRH-a to women with PCOS reduces LH and androgen concentrations. It has no effect on insulin resistance and hyperinsulinemia, IGF-1 or IGFBP-1 levels[30,31]. The reduction by GnRH-a of intrafollicular concentrations of androgens which would normally induce atresia may be responsible for the increased number of follicles induced by consequent stimulation by GnRH-a/hMG compared with hMG alone[15]. The increased number of developing follicles induced by co-treatment with GnRH-a/hMG is accompanied by a raised incidence of OHSS and multiple pregnancies[15].

Two interesting attempts have been made to utilize the beneficial effects of GNRH-a, increase its efficiency and reduce its undesired influence on multiple follicular development. Filicori and associates[32] followed pretreatment by GnRH-a with pulsatile GnRH. While seemingly paradoxical, this combination produced good ovulation and acceptable pregnancy rates and no multiple pregnancies, but was limited by the long duration of each cycle and a relatively high incidence of abortion and luteal phase abnormalities. The logical idea of combining GnRH-a with low-dose FSH therapy was studied by Scheele and co-workers[33], but failed to reduce multiple folliculogenesis and its consequences. In the opinion of these investigators, the extreme sensitivity of the follicles to FSH once growth is initiated may be tempered by using even smaller incremental dose rises than those employed.

Surgical treatment

Surgical treatment by bilateral wedge resection, although relatively successful in restoring ovulation, has fallen from grace, due to its propensity to adhesion formation. Laparoscopic ovarian diathermy was introduced by Gjonnaess[34], working on the principle that similar results could be achieved while avoiding the introduction of a mechanical factor. In his small study, and in subsequent larger studies[35–37], ovulation rates of 70–90% and pregnancy rates of 40–70% have been achieved. Postoperative laparoscopy has revealed the presence of intraperitoneal adhesions in about 20% of these cases, but they are reported to be mild and unilateral[37,38] and did not apparently affect the high pregnancy rate[39]. Significant falls of LH, androstendione, dihydroepiandrosterone sulfate (DHEAS) and testosterone have been uniformly noted after ovarian diathermy. Laser photodiathermy may lessen adhesion formation and, following the operation, stimulation with hMG gives an enhanced ovarian response compared with the pre-diathermy response[35,38]. The benefit of ovarian diathermy is limited to approximately 6 months, but it is a promising mode of therapy for resistant patients with large ovaries. The ideal protocol following this procedure to yield optimal results has yet to be firmly established.

In vitro fertilization

For patients with PCOS who have failed to conceive during six ovulatory cycles of gonadotropin therapy, we have found that IVF/ET is a very viable alternative. In a study from our centre[29], 68 such women underwent 208 cycles of IVF/ET with a cumulative conception rate of 82% at six cycles, almost identical to that of a control group of women with a pure mechanical factor undergoing similar treatment. There are two possible explanations for the fact that these results were achieved with IVF/ET but not with gonadotropin therapy. Either an overt mechanical factor was present or, more likely, this procedure allowed a more liberal approach to superovulation rather than concentrating on monofollicular development. A fascinating recent development by Trounson and colleagues[40] reports the successful recovery of immature oocytes from the ovaries of untreated PCOS patients and their maturation, fertilization and development in vitro. If this method is successfully adopted, the problems of ovulation induction may well be bypassed.

Summary

In summarizing the treatment of infertility associated with PCOS, the induction of ovulation may be achieved by boosting FSH stimulation of the ovaries either indirectly with clomiphene or native pulsatile GnRH, or directly with gonadotropin preparations. The selection of treatment could not be guided by basal clinical or endocrine features in a series of 306 treatment cycles whose outcome was reported by Farhi and colleagues[12]. However, there seem to be two main determinants of the success of this treatment in achieving a live birth: the degree of hyperinsulinemia and the concentrations of circulating LH. Either of these, when in excess,

not only make induction of ovulation and conception relatively difficult but are associated with high rates of early miscarriage[41,42]. Their correction, particularly in obstinate cases, should be a major consideration in the attempt to achieve optimal results. With such a range of reasonably successful treatments for the induction of ovulation in PCOS, the emphasis in the selection of therapy should now be placed on minimizing the prevalence of undesired side-effects while retaining acceptable efficiency.

References

1. Kiddy, D. S., Hamilton-Fairley, D., Bush, A., Anyaoku, V., Reed, M. J. and Franks, S. (1992). Improvement in endocrine and ovarian function during dietary treatment of obese women with polycystic ovary syndrome. *Clin. Endocrinol.*, **36**, 105–11
2. Nestler, J. E., Barlascini, C. O., Matt, D. W., Steingold, K. A., Plymate, S. R., Clore, J. N. and Blackard, W. G. (1989). Suppression of serum insulin by diazoxide reduces serum testosterone levels in obese women with polycystic ovary syndrome. *J. Clin. Endocrinol. Metab.*, **68**, 1027–32
3. Velaquez, E. M., Mendoza, S., Hamer, T., Sosa, F. and Glueck, C. J. (1994). Metformin therapy in polycystic ovary syndrome reduces hyperinsulinemia, insulin resistance, hyperandrogenemia and systolic blood pressure while facilitating normal menses and pregnancy. *Metabolism*, **43**, 647–54
4. Prelevic, G. M., Wurzburger, M. I., Balint-Peric, L. and Nesic, J. S. (1990). Inhibitory effect of sandostatin on secretion of luteinising hormone and ovarian steroids in polycystic ovary syndrome. *Lancet*, **336**, 900–3
5. Prelevic, G. M., Wurzburger, M. I. and Balint-Peric, L. (1989). Effects of a low dose estrogen–antiandrogen combination (Diane-35) on clinical signs of androgenization, hormone profile and ovarian size in patients with polycystic ovary syndrome. *Gynecol. Endocrinol.*, **3**, 269–80
6. Van den Berg, G. and Yen, S. S. C. (1973). Effect of anti-estrogenic action of clomiphene during the menstrual cycle: evidence for a change in the feedback sensitivity. *J. Clin. Endocrinol. Metab.*, **37**, 356–65
7. Shoham, Z., Borenstein, R., Lunenfeld, B. and Pariente, C. (1990). Hormonal profiles follow-ing clomiphene citrate therapy in conception and non-conception cycles. *Clin. Endocrinol.*, **33**, 271–8
8. Homburg, R., Weissglass, L. and Goldman, J. (1988). Improved treatment for anovulation in polycystic ovarian disease utilizing the effect of progesterone on the inappropriate gonadotrophin release and clomiphene response. *Hum. Reprod.*, **3**, 285–8
9. Daly, D. C., Walters, C. A., Soto-Albors, C. E., Tohan, N. and Riddick, D. H. (1984). A randomized study of dexamethasone in ovulation induction with clomiphene citrate. *Fertil. Steril.*, **41**, 844–8
10. Shoham, Z., Homburg, R. and Jacobs, H. S. (1990). Induction of ovulation with pulsatile LHRH. *Ballière's Clin. Obstet. Gynecol.*, **4**, 589–608
11. Homburg, R., Eshel, A., Tucker, M., Mason, P., Adams, J., Kilborn, J., Sutherland, I. A. and Jacobs, H. S. (1989). One hundred pregnancies following pulsatile luteinising hormone-releasing hormone therapy for ovulation induction. *Br. Med. J.*, **298**, 809–12
12. Farhi, J., Homburg, R., Lerner, A. and Ben-Rafael, Z. (1993). The choice of treatment for anovulation following failure to conceive with clomiphene. *Hum. Reprod.*, **8**, 1367–71
13. Wang, C. F. and Gemzell, C. (1980). The use of human gonadotropin for the induction of ovulation in women with polycystic ovarian disease. *Fertil. Steril.*, **33**, 479–86
14. Garcea, N., Campo, S., Panetta, V., Venneri, M., Siccardi, P., Dargenio, R. and DeTomasi, F. (1985). Induction of ovulation with purified urinary follicle stimulating hormone in patients with polycystic ovary syndrome. *Am. J. Obstet. Gynecol.*, **151**, 635–40

15. Homburg, R., Eshel, A., Kilborn, J., Adams, J. and Jacobs, H. S. (1990). Combined luteinising hormone-releasing hormone analogue and exogenous gonadotrophins for the treatment of infertility associated with polycystic ovary syndrome. *Hum. Reprod.*, **5**, 32–5

16. McFaul, P. B., Traub, A. I. and Thompson, W. (1990). Treatment of clomiphene citrate resistant polycystic ovary syndrome with pure follicle stimulating hormone or human menopausal gonadotropin. *Fertil. Steril.*, **53**, 792–7

17. Seibel, M. M., Kamrava, M. M., McArdle, C. and Taymor, M. L. (1984). Treatment of polycystic ovarian disease with chronic low dose follicle stimulating hormone: biochemical changes and ultrasound correlation. *Int. J. Fertil.*, **29**, 39–43

18. Polson, D. W., Mason, H. D., Saldahna, M. B. and Franks, S. (1987). Ovulation of a single dominant follicle during treatment with low dose pulsatile follicle stimulating hormone in women with polycystic ovary syndrome. *Clin. Endocrinol.*, **26**, 205–12

19. Hamilton-Fairley, D., Kiddy, D., Watson, H., Sagle, M. and Franks, S. (1991). Low dose gonadotrophin therapy for induction of ovulation in 100 women with polycystic ovary syndrome. *Hum. Reprod.*, **6**, 1095–9

20. Shoham, Z., Patel, A. and Jacobs, H. S. (1991). Polycystic ovary syndrome: safety and effectiveness of stepwise and low dose administration of purified follicle stimulating hormone. *Fertil. Steril.*, **55**, 1051–6

21. Dale, O., Tanbo, T., Lunde, O. and Abyholm, T. (1993). Ovulation induction with low dose follicle stimulating hormone in women with polycystic ovary syndrome. *Acta. Obstet. Gynecol. Scand.*, **72**, 43–6

22. Scheele, F., Hompes, P. G. A., Van der Meer, M., Schoute, E. and Schoemaker, J. (1993). The effects of a gonadotrophin-releasing hormone-agonist on treatment with low dose follicle stimulating hormone in polycystic ovary syndrome. *Hum. Reprod.*, **8**, 699–704

23. Homburg, R., Levy, T. and Ben-Rafael, Z. (1995). A comparative prospective study of conventional regimen with chronic low dose administration of follicle stimulating hormone for anovulation associated with polycystic ovary syndrome. *Fertil. Steril.*, **63**, 729–33

24. Brown, J. B. (1978). Pituitary control of ovarian function – concepts derived from gonadotrophin therapy. *Aust. NZ J. Obstet. Gynaecol.*, **18**, 47–54

25. Insler, V. and Lunenfeld, B. (1991). Pathophysiology of polycystic ovarian disease: new insights. *Hum. Reprod.*, **6**, 1025–9

26. Fleming, R., Haxton, M. J., Hamilton, M. P. R., McCune, G. S., Black, W. P., MacNaughton, M. C. and Coutts, J. R. T. (1985). Successful treatment of infertile women with oligomenorrhoea using a combination of a LHRH agonist and exogenous gonadotrophins. *Br. J. Obstet. Gynaecol.*, **92**, 369–73

27. Homburg, R., Levy, T., Berkovitz, D., Farhi, J., Feldberg, D., Ashkenazi, J. and Ben-Rafael, Z. (1993). Gonadotropin-releasing hormone agonist reduces the miscarriage rate for pregnancies achieved in women with polycystic ovary syndrome. *Fertil. Steril.*, **59**, 527–31

28. Balen, A. H., Tan, S. L., MacDougall, J. and Jacobs, H. S. (1993). Miscarriage rates following *in-vitro* fertilisation are increased in women with polycystic ovaries and are reduced by pituitary desensitization with buserelin. *Hum. Reprod.*, **8**, 959–64

29. Homburg, R., Bekovitz, D., Levy, T., Feldberg, D., Ashkenazi, J. and Ben-Rafael, Z. (1993). *In vitro* fertilization and embryo transfer for the treatment of infertility associated with polycystic ovary syndrome. *Fertil. Steril.*, **60**, 858–63

30. Dale, P. O., Tanbo, T., Djoseland, O., Jervell, J. and Abyholm, T. (1992). Persistance of hyperinsulinemia in polycystic ovary syndrome after ovarian suppression by gonadotropin-releasing hormone agonist. *Acta Endocrinol.*, **126**, 132–6

31. Homburg, R., Levy, T. and Ben-Rafael, Z. (1995). Adjuvant growth hormone for induction of ovulation with gonadotropin releasing-hormone agonist and gonadotropins in polycystic ovary syndrome: a randomized, double-blind, placebo controlled trial. *Hum. Reprod.*, in press

32. Filicori, M., Campaiello, E., Michelacci, L., Pareschi, A., Ferrari, P., Bolelli, G. F. and Flamigni, C. (1988). Gonadotropin-releasing hormone (GnRH) analog suppression to ovulation induction with pulsatile GnRH. *J. Clin. Endocrinol. Metab.*, **66**, 327–33

33. Scheele, F., Hompes, P. G. A., Van der Meer, M., Schoute, E. and Schoemaker, J. (1993). The relationship between FSH dose and FSH level and its relevance for ovulation induction with adjuvant gonadotropin-releasing hormone-agonist treatment. *Fertil. Steril.*, **60**, 620–5

34. Gjonnaess, H. (1984). Polycystic ovarian syndrome treated by ovarian electrocautery through the laparoscope. *Fertil. Steril.*, **41**, 20–5

35. Kovacs, G., Buckler, H., Bangah, M., Outch, K., Burger, H. and Healy, D. (1991). Treatment of anovulation due to polycystic ovarian syndrome by laparoscopic ovarian electrocautery. *Br. J. Obstet. Gynaecol.*, **98**, 30–5

36. Aakvaag, A. (1985). Hormonal response to electrocautery of the ovary in patients with polycystic ovarian disease. *Br. J. Obstet. Gynaecol.*, **92**, 1258–64

37. Naether, O. G., Fischer, R., Weise, H. C., Geiger Kotzler, L., Delfs, T. and Rudolf, K. (1993). Laparoscopic electrocoagulation of the ovarian surface in infertile patients with polycystic ovarian disease. *Fertil. Steril.*, **60**, 88–94

38. Dabirashrafi, H., Mohamad, K., Behjatnia, Y. and Moghadami-Tabrizi, N. (1991). Adhesion formation after ovarian electrocauterization on patients with polycystic ovarian syndrome. *Fertil. Steril.*, **55**, 1200–1

39. Greenblatt, E. M. and Casper, R. F. (1993). Adhesion formation after laparoscopic ovarian cautery for polycystic ovary syndrome – lack of correlation with pregnancy rate. *Fertil. Steril.*, **60**, 766–70

40. Trounson, A., Wood, C. and Kausche, A. (1994). *In vitro* maturation and the fertilization and developmental competence of oocytes recovered from untreated polycystic ovarian patients. *Fertil. Steril.*, **62**, 353–62

41. Homburg, R., Armar, N. A., Eshel, A., Adams, J. and Jacobs, H. S. (1988). Influence of serum luteinizing hormone concentrations on ovulation, conception and early pregnancy loss in polycystic ovary syndrome. *Br. Med. J.*, **297**, 1024–6

42. Hamilton-Fairley, D., Kiddy, D., Watson, H., Paterson, C. and Franks, S. (1992). Association of moderate obesity with a poor pregnancy outcome in women with polycystic ovary syndrome treated with low dose gonadotrophin. *Br. J. Obstet. Gynaecol.*, **99**, 128–31

Doppler ultrasound in fertility

12

S. Campbell and J. Zaidi

Introduction

Transvaginal ultrasonography has now super-seded transabdominal scanning as the method of choice in modern fertility management. The addition of color Doppler imaging allows accurate localization of vessels while high-frequency pulsed Doppler has improved the resolution of flow velocity waveforms. This technique can be used to study vascular changes in the uterine, ovarian stromal and follicular blood vessels. Recently, we have also been able to visualize vessels in the subendometrial region and within the endometrium.

Doppler ultrasound can be used to assess blood flow changes to the uterus and ovaries during the menstrual cycle[1-3]. The technique has also been used to study vascular changes in the developing ovarian follicle during the periovulatory period[4,5]. We have assessed vascular changes to the pelvic organs in normal healthy women and in women with the polycystic ovarian syndrome in a prospective longitudinal study using fixed time points during the spontaneous and clomiphene-induced menstrual cycle. This knowledge will provide a basis for understanding the physiological changes in the normal ovulatory cycle, and will allow us to elucidate whether there are any circadian rhythms and to demonstrate any differences in vascularity between women with normal and dysfunctional conditions such as polycystic ovaries.

Normal menstrual cycles

We have studied six women with normal ovaries and regular menstrual cycles in detailed serial studies using color and pulsed Doppler ultra-sound. Ultrasound scans were performed on day 2 of the cycle, then daily from the expected day of ovulation (EDO) −6 and then 6-hourly from EDO −2 until 6 h after follicular rupture. One further scan was performed in the mid-luteal phase. In the women with normal ovaries, we noticed a circadian rhythm in uterine artery index (PI) and time-averaged maximum velocity. There was a lower uterine artery PI and a higher time-averaged maximum velocity in the early morning (06.00) and a rise in PI during the day with an associated decline in velocity. These changes occurred independently of the periovulatory hormonal changes. V_{max} in the follicular vessels and in the adjacent ovarian stroma rose during the follicular phase, being significantly greater after the onset of the luteinizing hormone (LH) surge. V_{max} in the wall of the corpus luteum and in the ovarian stroma remained constant during the mid-luteal phase. There was no change in pulsatility index (PI) in either the follicular wall or the stroma of the dominant ovary. The changes in V_{max} correlated with the changes in LH (follicular vessels: $r = 0.21$, $p = 0.03$; ovarian stroma of the dominant ovary: $r = 0.25$, $p = 0.009$). There was no significant change in V_{max} of PI in the stroma of the contralateral ovary.

This study demonstrates the presence of a circadian rhythm in uterine artery blood flow during the periovulatory period. We have previously reported the presence of a circadian rhythm in uterine artery blood flow during the follicular phase of the menstrual cycle[6] and suggest that there are complex regulatory mechanisms controlling uterine blood flow independent of follicular and periovulatory hormonal changes.

Polycystic ovarian syndrome

Polycystic ovaries are commonly seen in women presenting for infertility treatment. Their response to exogenous gonadotropins in assisted reproduction is quite different to that seen in women with normal ovaries. Women with polycystic ovaries typically produce more follicles and more oocytes, despite receiving lower doses of gonadotropins, and are at a greater risk of ovarian hyperstimulation syndrome[7,8]. Doppler blood flow studies in women with the polycystic ovarian syndrome have revealed significant differences in Doppler indices compared to women with normal ovaries[9] and it has been suggested that Doppler analysis can be a valuable additional tool for the diagnosis of polycystic ovarian syndrome.

We have also studied six women with polycystic ovarian syndrome in detail using the same methodology as for normal cycling women. In women with polycystic ovarian syndrome, the V_{max} in the ovarian stroma was higher throughout the menstrual cycle than in the group with normal ovaries. There was no difference in PI. The uterine artery PI was significantly higher in women with polycystic ovarian syndrome on day 2 of the cycle and during the mid-follicular phase, while V_{max} was lower compared to that in the women with normal ovaries. The increase in stromal blood flow velocity may help to explain the excessive response to gonadotropin stimulation seen in women with polycystic ovarian syndrome.

IVF–ET cycles

Transvaginal Doppler ultrasound, with or without color Doppler, has also been used in *in vitro* fertilization (IVF) cycles to estimate uterine receptivity[10,11]. We have assessed uterine artery PI and subendometrial velocimetry on the day of human chorionic gonadotropin (hCG) administration in order to predict implantation rates. Although there were no significant differences in uterine artery PI between the pregnant and non-pregnant groups, those patients with uterine artery PI less than 3.0 had significantly improved implantation rates. Furthermore, in those patients undergoing blood flow studies of the endometrium, there were eight patients with absent subendometrial blood flow. Embryo implantation failed to occur in all eight cases. Doppler indices of subendometrial blood flow did not predict pregnancy or implantation rates[12].

Conclusion

In summary, transvaginal ultrasonography with color and pulsed Doppler facilities allows assessment of vascular changes in the pelvic organs. Studies of impedance to uterine artery blood flow and presence or absence of subendometrial blood flow may predict implantation rates in IVF programs. There are significant differences in ovarian stromal and uterine artery blood flow between women with normal and polycystic ovaries.

References

1. Scholtes, M. C. W., Wladimiroff, J. W., van Rijen, H. J. M. and Hop, W. C. J. (1989). Uterine and ovarian flow velocity waveforms in the normal menstrual cycle: a transvaginal Doppler study. *Fertil. Steril.*, **52**, 981–5
2. Steer, C. V., Campbell, S., Pampiglione, J. S., Kingsland, C., Mason, B. A. and Collins, W. P. (1990). Transvaginal colour flow imaging of the uterine arteries during the ovarian and menstrual cycles. *Hum. Reprod.*, **5**, 391–5
3. Sladkevicius, P., Valentin, L. and Marsal, K. (1993). Blood flow velocity in the uterine and ovarian arteries during the normal menstrual cycle. *Ultrasound Obstet. Gynecol.*, **3**, 199–208
4. Collins, W. P., Jurkovic, D., Bourne, T. H., Kurjak, A. and Campbell, S. (1991). Ovarian morphology, endocrine function and intra-follicular

blood flow during the peri-ovulatory period. *Hum. Reprod.*, **6**, 319–24

5. Campbell, S., Bourne, T. H., Waterstone, J., Reynolds, K., Crayford, T. J. B., Jurkovic, D., Okokon, E. and Collins, W. P. (1993). Transvaginal color blood flow imaging of the peri-ovulatory follicle. *Fertil. Steril.*, **60**, 433–8

6. Zaidi, J., Jurkovic, D., Campbell, S., Okokon, E. and Tan, S. L. (1995). Circadian variation in uterine artery blood flow during the follicular phase of the menstrual cycle. *Ultrasound Obstet. Gynecol.*, **5**, 406–10

7. MacDougall, M. J., Tan, S. L. and Jacobs, H. S. (1992). *In-vitro* fertilization and the ovarian hyperstimulation syndrome. *Hum. Reprod.*, **7**, 597–600

8. MacDougall, M. J., Tan, S. L., Balen, A. and Jacobs, H. S. (1993). A controlled study comparing patients with and without polycystic ovaries undergoing *in-vitro* fertilization. *Hum. Reprod.*, **8**, 233–7

9. Battaglia, C., Artini, P. G., D'Ambrogio, G., Genazzani, A. D. and Genazzani, A. R. (1995). The role of color Doppler imaging in the diagnosis of polycystic ovary syndrome. *Am. J. Obstet. Gynecol.*, **172**, 108–13

10. Steer, C. V., Campbell, S., Tan, S. L., Crayford, T., Mills, C., Mason, B. and Campbell, S. (1992). The use of transvaginal color flow imaging after *in vitro* fertilization to identify optimum uterine conditions before embryo transfer. *Fertil. Steril.*, **57**, 372–6

11. Favre, R., Bettahar, K., Grange, G., Ohl, J., Arbogast, E., Moreau, L. and Dellenback, P. (1993). Predictive value of transvaginal uterine Doppler assessment in an *in vitro* fertilization program. *Ultrasound Obstet. Gynecol.*, **3**, 350–3

12. Zaidi, J., Campbell, S., Pittrof, R. and Tan, S. L. (1995). Assessment of endometrial thickness, morphology, subendometrial blood flow and intraendometrial perfusion by transvaginal color Doppler ultrasound in an *in vitro* fertilization program. *Ultrasound Obstet. Gynecol.*, **6**, in press

Falloposcopy: its place in the state-of-the-art spectrum of tubal investigation methods

13

S. Rimbach, D. Wallwiener and G. Bastert

Introduction

Based on the personal experience of more than 120 clinical tubal cannulations and falloposcopies[1–3] as well as experimental work[4,5], and preliminary results of an International Multicenter Study on Falloposcopy inaugurated by the author, the following article discusses technical as well as methodological particularities and controversies of falloposcopy including a review of the current literature.

The concept of falloposcopy

In the year 1561, the Italian anatomist Gabriello Falloppio described the organ, that would later carry his name, as thin and coiled[6]. His concept of a narrow and tortuous tubal anatomy, especially of the intramural part, persisted until recent years[7,8], when it was considered impossible to cannulate the tube without harm[9].

Clinical investigations for tubal disease therefore remained restricted to the inspection of the organ's outer appearance by laparoscopy, grossly testing its patency by chromoperturbation and indirect imaging of the interior by radiological hysterosalpingography using contrast media.

First attempts of endoscopic visualization of the tubal lumen, in order to fill this diagnostic gap, started with the work of Mohri[10], Henry-Suchet[11], Cornier[12] and Brosens[13]. Despite interesting correlations to clinical outcome[14–16], their approach of entering the tube from the fimbrial end did not allow investigations of the proximal third beyond the isthmo-ampullary junction.

In 1990, Kerin and colleagues[17] were the first successfully to describe the endoscopic visualization of the intramural and isthmic segments of the tube. In contrast to current opinions about tubal anatomy, assuming a straight rather than tortuous intramural course[18], they did not try to avoid cannulation of the proximal tube but used a transcervical approach including hysteroscopic guide wire catheterization. Both the industrial development of lowest-diameter microfiberendoscopes and recent experiences in tubal cannulation techniques[19–21] favored this concept. The procedure was named falloposcopy, thus allowing terminologic differentiation from the abdominal approaches including fimbrioscopy[22], ampulloscopy[12] and salpingoscopy[13,23], all subsuming under the general idea of tuboscopy[11].

Technique and complications of transcervical tubal catheterization and falloposcopy

Several modifications have been proposed since Kerin and colleagues[17] first described the procedure. All relate to the technique of tubal catheterization, whereas the visualization process is almost uniform in the different methods.

Access to the uterotubal ostium

Access to the uterotubal ostium may be gained either by hysteroscopy, as in the original description, or using the so-called tactile impression technique[24]. Here, the ostium is located blindly with the help of a pre-shaped introductory uterine catheter, delivering the actual tubal catheter. This method proves rather efficient, the catheter being guided to the ostium by the natural shape of the uterine cavity. Especially when a high endometrium disturbs visualization of the tubal ostium or extreme uterine retroflexio complicates its localization, the hysteroscopic approach might be more difficult. On the other hand, the latter allows permanent visual control of the catheterization process and eventual ostial spasms, that frequently and repeatedly occur and might simulate proximal tubal obstruction.

In order to prevent the tubal catheter from kinking within the uterine cavity when using a hysteroscope, sufficient 'back-up support' is essential. This is achieved by keeping the hysteroscope–ostium distance minimal and the hysteroscope–catheter relation coaxial. Hysteroscopes disposing of a deflectable tip fulfil this requirement better than rigid instruments. Additionally, an articulated arm proved helpful firmly attached to the operating table in order to fix the hysteroscope in its position, thus leaving both hands free for manipulating the tubal catheter.

Tubal cannulation

For actual Fallopian tube cannulation, either coaxial over-the-wire catheter systems (e.g. made by Conceptus, USA; Storz, Germany; Cook, USA), using alternatively a hysteroscopic or blind approach, or so-called linear-everting-balloon catheter system (made by Imagyn) for non-hysteroscopic application[25–27], are available. Both systems originated in angiology and have been adapted for their use in gynecology. Each system has its own particular advantages and disadvantages.

The predominant problem of over-the-wire catheters is their tendency to kink whenever the catheter is firmly pushed against a resistance. This may occur in the uterine cavity as discussed above, or in the tubal lumen, but also outside the patient while preparing and introducing the catheter or withdrawing the guide wire to replace it by the fiberscope. Even if cannulation is not impeded, it will be difficult to introduce the falloposcope, once a catheter is kinked.

Simultaneous advancement of catheter and guide wire prevents the wire from dissecting the tubal wall. Sufficient distension is always essential and achieved by continuous irrigation using an electrical roller pump at 5–15 ml/min. Under optimal circumstances, the fluid acts as a 'front wave' and allows the catheter to 'surf' on it. Thus, tubal wall perforations by either wire or cannula are unlikely if movements are controlled by the tips of the index finger and thumb, allowing any resistance to be felt immediately. Complete perforation or partial dissection occurs in 3–10% and has never been followed by any sequelae or any need for further intervention[42] (and preliminary data from the International Multicenter Study on Falloposcopy).

Whereas the narrowest segment of the tube, the intramural part, rarely represents a problem, it is frequently difficult to negotiate the physiological curve of the ampullary segment. The catheter is advanced and bends, seems almost to perforate the thin tubal wall, and lifts up the proximal half of the tube like an arch. Here, the help of laparoscopic manipulation may be needed. Rather than grasping the delicate organ with an atraumatic forceps, running the risk of kinking the catheter or breaking the fiberscope, it is advisable to touch the catheterized isthmic part laterally and to shift it medially. This allows the catheter to straighten out by its own elasticity and to slide past the fimbrial end.

The linear-everting-balloon catheter has been designed to overcome the inherent problems of a straight catheter in following curved structures. Its body is not pre-shaped, but builds up in response to the space given. The system comprises a longer outer and shorter inner cannula, neither to be introduced into the tube. A balloon membrane connects them from the front orifice to the front orifice. Via an inflation side-port at the outer cannula, controlled hydraulic pressure is applied to the membrane, which therefore everts in the form of a ring-like balloon as soon as it is liberated by advancing the inner cannula. The balloon carries the falloposcope forward like a banana being peeled. Compared to an over-the-wire catheter, the balloon's forward movement is also controlled by cannula advancement, but its direction is determined *only* by the path of lowest resistance. For obvious mechanical reasons, the relative movements of the cannula, the balloon and the scope do not follow a one-to-one ratio, as they do in the less sophisticated over-the-wire setting. The surgeon must therefore continuously control the different components, including the pressure applied to the balloon. This requires subtle technical understanding and sufficient *in vitro* training. Unless the learning curve is completed, the intelligent construction, which allows the negotiation of even the most curved lumina, might suggest the risk of perforation in the case of luminal obstructions stronger than the surrounding wall, or the balloon tip being caught in a syphon-like artificial kink of the tubal wall, e.g. in the ampullary region, as outlined above. However, the pressure-controlled inflation of the balloon, concentrating energy at its tip, does not only contribute to the risk of undesired perforation, but also facilitates direct tuboplasty manoevers in case of obstructive pathology.

Visualization

The tube, being successfully cannulated, is visualized by retracting both catheter and scope. A forward movement is also possible, but intense light reflections, so-called white-out effects, impair vision more frequently than with a constant retrograde movement. However, the white-out effect, whenever the fiberscope tip comes close to, or touches tubal wall structures, represents the predominant problem or falloposcopic endotubal exploration. What is 'the Japanese flag' to the hysteroscopist is 'the white flag' to the falloposcopist. To date, a successful procedure is therefore characterized by interpretable imaging within all tubal segments investigated, but only on some occasions by a continuous visualization of the whole tubal interior.

Insufficient illumination, on the contrary, is rarely a problem, but two other factors also play major roles for the success or failure of visualization: soiled lenses and insufficient lumen distension. Continuous fluid irrigation helps to keep the fiberscope lens clear of debris, especially when sliding it through the introduced catheter, and at the same time distending the tubal lumen in order to open its potential space.

In addition to those technical problems, however, a number of anatomical and pathomorphological conditions sometimes render falloposcopy difficult. The everted fimbrial end of a patent tube is hard to distend and can therefore generally not be visualized except for glimpses of floating mucosal folds. In proximal pathology, especially if obstructive, insufficient distension and floating debris may impair vision. Overdistension and perforation may occur in sactosalpinges, which may cause the catheter to curl within the lumen, especially if internally septated or externally deformed by adhesions, thus rendering orientation difficult.

Acknowledging those technical as well as methodological problems as being responsible for a procedure failure rate of 7–10%, falloposcopy still provides endotubal images suitable for clinical interpretation in a considerable 90–93% of the cases (preliminary data from the International Multicenter Study on Falloposcopy).

Description and interpretation of falloposcopic findings

While retracting catheter and scope, the tube is stepwise visualized from its distal end towards the uterine ostium, allowing the evaluation of the distended endotubal space for eventual obstruction or intraluminal lesions, but also the surrounding epithelium with its folds.

Descriptive parameter

Whereas, for the above discussed reasons, the fimbrial segment frequently escapes observation in patent tubes, its agglutinated remnants in sactosalpinges may be evaluated for their mucosal status at the fusion site. In general, however, only ampullary structures will expose themselves to the falloposcopic examination. Predominant for the visual impression of a normal ampulla are extensively ramified and filigreely vascularized fold structures, freely floating with the distension medium. Although ampullary folds represent the best and possibly only structures for direct evaluation of the mucosal vascularization by falloposcopy, the small vessels will only shine through, if a fold floats translucently within the luminal space. This situation is not always achieved despite normal tubal condition. If, however, folds appear flattened, agglutinated by thin, web-like or solid synechiae, hyper- or hypovascularized, it is most likely that (post-)inflammatory changes have provoked such pathologies. Their prognostic value has been investigated earlier when observed at salpingoscopy[13-15,28], resulting in a classification[29] which differentiates five degrees of severity (I, normal fold pattern; II, separation and flattening of folds; III, focal lesions (small adhesions); IV, adhesive or destructive lesions over the entire ampulla; and V, fibrosis and complete loss of folds).

More accurately than in the wide ampullary segment, tubal obstruction or dilatation can be discerned in the isthmic and intramural parts, where a panoramic view of the entire lumen and the surrounding wall surface is possible. Folds, however, physiologically decrease in height and ramification so their importance for evaluation diminishes. Also, physiological vascularity is hard to observe, anatomically situated under the mucosal surface forming capillary networks. Therefore, description concentrates on patency parameter, intraluminal findings such as synechiae, polyps or debris and mucosa surface pattern. The normal mucosa is low in reflex, smooth, and velvet-like with a whitish-rose to pink color. It has a cloud-like appearance and can also be compared to the impression of virgin snow, as opposed to partial or complete atrophic mucosa resembling, respectively, the rough surface of rock and the mirror-like appearance of ice on a glacier.

Using those guidelines, it appears possible to describe numerous endotubal patterns with ac-

ceptable reproducibility. Interobserver variability analysis confirmed high concordance values with conformity rates of 75–95% (preliminary data from the International Multicenter Study on Falloposcopy). Clinical interpretation, however, should remain careful, not all lesions being incompatible with normal reproductive history[30].

If therefore not a functional, at least a morphological discrimination of normal and pathological appears reasonably certain. The results of an experimental study of 30 patients, comparing histopathological findings and falloposcopic images (unpublished data) suggest that morphologically defined pathology is detected by falloposcopy with a high detection rate of 85%, but the falloposcopist has to take into account that a pathological diagnosis can only be considered true in 69%. The certainty, once the diagnosis of normal is made, appears better with 86%, but in almost 30% of the cases pathologies are falsely described in normal tubes. Similar results were found in a study published by Hershlag[31], comparing salpingoscopy to light- and electronmicroscopy. He found a good correlation for the endoscopic detection of severe pathologies but no significant correlation to subtle changes.

Although clinically important, a group of morphologically defined pathologies are most likely to be missed by falloposcopy if limited to the tubal wall, e.g. endometriosis, fibrotic changes, muscular thickening or inflammation. Performing simultaneous laparoscopy, diaphanoscopic inspection allows a limited idea of the tubal wall condition.

Classification and scoring

A falloposcopic classification and scoring system has been proposed by Kerin[32]. It describes the localization, nature and extent of intraluminal findings. Considered parameters are tubal patency (patent, stenosed, obstructed), status of the epithelium (normal, atrophic, featureless), vascularity (normal, intermediate, poor), adhesion formation (none, thin, thick) and dilatation (none, minimal, hydrosalpinx). One to three points are assigned according to the degree of pathological change. Additionally, other findings, such as mucus plugs, debris, polyps, endometriosis, salpingitis isthmica nodosa, together with inflammatory, infectious or neoplastic conditions or absent tubal segments are categorized as moderate or severe. The findings are noted separately for the different tubal segments. Then a cumulative score is calculated for the status of the entire tube. A score of 20 indicates normal tubal lumen, 20–30 moderate tubal lumen disease and more than 30 severe endotubal disease along with a high risk for ectopic pregnancy.

The results of 66 patients in whom this scoring system was evaluated indicate its useful correlation to clinical outcome. Among the patients having normal tubes (score 20), 21% conceived, among those with moderate disease (score 21–30) only 9% and among those with score higher than 30, indicating severe disease, none became pregnant.

Conclusion

Transcervical falloposcopy is definitely the only current method for direct visual examination of the endosalpinx from the uterotubal ostium to the isthmo-ampullary junction, and, as far as the distal tube is concerned, it is complementary to salpingoscopic methods such as fimbrioscopy and ampulloscopy[33,34]. The procedure can be performed on an outpatient basis and without anesthesia[27,35–38], which may result in particular interest for future modifications of assisted reproduction techniques such as gamete and embryo intrafallopian transfer.

The assessment of tubal factors in infertility patients, however, should always include laparoscopy, otherwise compromising valuable information for the therapeutic management in at least 4–8% of patients regarding the tube itself (preliminary results from the International Multicenter Study on Falloposcopy), and, as we can expect from earlier studies on hysterosalpingography[39–41], in a far higher percentage as far as peritubal pathology is concerned. In our experience, laparoscopy was best performed simultaneously with falloposcopy. It is the only method to assist in difficult falloposcopy procedures (which are more frequent, the higher the degree of tubal pathology). It alone can discover and assess complications of falloposcopy such as perforation. The combination of laparoscopy and fimbrioscopy by abdominal route with hysteroscopy and falloposcopy by transcervical route alone allows a complete one-stage diagnosis in order to optimize patient information and therapy planning.

In this setting, falloposcopy reveals endotubal pathologies not detected by previous hysterosalpingography and laparoscopy with chromoperturbation in some 20–46%[42] (and preliminary results from the International Multicenter Study on Falloposcopy), a number confirming earlier results on salpingoscopy[28]. However, falloposcopy does not only provide diagnostic information but also includes therapeutic purposes. As discussed above, it will possibly play a role for future assisted reproduction techniques. In selected cases of proximal obstruction, falloposcopy-guided balloon tuboplasty has been described as a non-invasive method to restore tubal patency[26,42–44]. Risquez reported in 1992[24] two cases of falloposcopically visualized tubal ectopic pregnancies, thus pointing out the possibility of a future non-incisional falloposcopic treatment.

In conclusion, falloposcopy is not only about to become a widespread procedure but is also on its way to a place in the state-of-the-art spectrum of tubal investigation methods. Yet, clinical experiences are still preliminary to date, and only long-term multicentric follow-up studies can define the prognostic value of falloposcopic diagnoses in order to assure this place.

References

1. Rimbach, S., Wallwiener, D., Rauchholz, M. and Bastert, G. (1994). Neue Aspekte in der Therapie des proximalen Tubenverschlusses: die hysterosckopische proximale Tubenkatheterisierung. *Zentralb. Gynakol.*, **116**, 230–5

2. Rimbach, S., Wallwiener, D. and Bastert, G. (1994). Tuben-Endoskopie – minimal invasive Diagnostik bei gestörter Eileiterfunktion. *Minimal Invasive Medizin*, **5**, 9–12

3. Wallwiener, D., Rimbach, S., Kurek, R., Bastert, G. and Menz, W. (1994). Intraluminale Tubenchirurgie mittels Laser – Realität und Fiktion. *Lasermedizin*, **10**, 67–70

4. Rimbach, S., Wallwiener, D., Rauchholz, M. and Bastert, G. (1994). Experimentelle intratubare Laseranwendung unter mikro-endoskopischer Kontrolle – das erste steuerbare Operations-Falloposkop. *Lasermedizin*, **10**, 190–3

5. Wallwiener, D., Morawski, A., Ebbing, A. and Bastert, G. (1988). Tierexperimentelle und klinische Ansätze zur Tuboskopie. *Ber. Gyn.*, **125**, 660–1

6. Herrlinger, R. and Feiner, E. (1964). Why did Versalius not discover the fallopian tubes? *Med. Hist.*, **8**, 335–41

7. Lisa, J. R., Gioia, J. D. and Loffredo, V. (1954). Observations of the interstitial position of the fallopian tube. *Obstet. Gynecol.*, **99**, 159–60

8. Sweeney, W. J. III (1963). The interstitial portion of the uterine tube – its gross anatomy, course and length. *Obstet. Gynecol.*, **109**, 3–5

9. De Cherney, A. H. (1987). Anything you can do I can do better... or differently! *Fertil. Steril.*, **48**, 374–6

10. Mohri, T., Mohri, C. and Yamadori, F. (1970). Tubaloscope: flexible glass fibre endoscope for intratubal observations. *Endoscopy*, **2**, 226

11. Henry-Suchet, J., Tesquier, L. and Loffredo, V. (1981). Endoscopies tubaires: premiers resultats. *Gynecologie*, **23**, 293–5

12. Cornier, E. (1982). La fibroscopie en gynécologie: la fibrohysteroscopie et la fibrotuboscopie. *Nouv. Presse Med.*, **11**, 2841–3

13. Brosens, I., Boeckx, W., Delattin, P., Puttemans, P. and Vasquez, G. (1987). Salpingoscopy: a new preoperative diagnostic tool in tubal infertility? *Br. J. Obstet. Gynaecol.*, **94**, 722–8

14. Henry-Suchet, J., Loffredo, V., Tesquier, L. and Pez, J. P. (1985). Endoscopy of the tube (= tuboscopy): its prognostic value for tuboplasties. *Acta Eur. Fertil.*, **16**, 139–45

15. Mencaglia, L., Hamou, J., Perino, A. and Cosmi, E. (1986). Transcervical and retrograde salpingoscopy: evaluation of the fallopian tube in infertile patients. In Siegler, A. M. (ed.) *The Fallopian Tube: Basic Studies and Clinical Contributions*, pp. 377–81. (Mount Kisco, New York: Futura Publishing Company)

16. Shapiro, B. S., Diamond, M. P. and DeCherney, A. H. (1988). Salpingoscopy: an adjunctive technique for evaluation of the fallopian tube. *Fertil. Steril.*, **49**, 1076–9

17. Kerin, I., Daykhovsky, L., Segalowitz, J., Surrey, E., Anderson, R., Stein, A., Wade, M. and Grundfest, W. (1990). Falloposcopy: a microendoscopic technique for visual exploration of the human fallopian tube from the uterotubal ostium to the fimbria using a transvaginal approach. *Fertil. Steril.*, **54**, 390–400

18. Corfman, R. S. (1990). Falloposcopy: frontiers realised... a fantastic voyage revisited. *Fertil. Steril.*, **54**, 574–6

19. Confino, E., Friberg, J. and Gleicher, N. (1986). Transcervical balloon tuboplasty. *Fertil. Steril.*, **46**, 963–6

20. Sulak, P. J., Letterie, G. S., Hayslip, C. C., Coddington, C. C. and Klein, T. A. (1987). Hysteroscopic cannulation and lavage in the treatment of proximal tubal occlusion. *Fertil. Steril.*, **48**, 493–5

21. Thurmond, A. S., Novy, M. J., Uchida, B. T. and Rösch, J. (1987). Fallopian tube obstruction: selective salpingography and recanalisation. *Radiology*, **63**, 511–14

22. Nezhat, F., Winer, W. K. and Nezhat, C. (1990). Fimbrioscopy and salpingoscopy in patients with minimal to moderate pelvic endometriosis. *Obstet. Gynecol.*, **75**, 15–17

23. Brosens, I. and Puttemans, P. (1989). Double-optic laparoscopy. In Sutton, C. (ed.) *Balliere's Clinical Obstetrics and Gynaecology*, Vol. 3, pp. 595–608

24. Risquez, F. and Confino, E. (1993). Transcervical tubal cannulation, past, present, and future. *Fertil. Steril.*, **60**, 211–26

25. Pearlstone, A., Surrey, E. and Kerin, J. (1992). The linear everting catheter: a nonhysteroscopic, transvaginal technique for access and micro-endoscopy of the fallopian tube. *Fertil. Steril.*, **58**, 4

26. Kerin, J. and Surrey, E. (1992). Tubal surgery from the inside out: falloposcopy and balloon tuboplasty. *Clin. Obstet. Gynecol.*, **35**, 299–312

27. Bauer, O., Diedrich, K., Bacich, S., Knight, C., Lowery, G., Van der Ven, H., Werner, A. and Krebs, D. (1992). Transcervical access and in-

traluminal imaging of the fallopian tube in the non-anesthetized patient: preliminary results using a new technique for fallopian access. *Hum. Reprod.*, **7**, 7–11

28. Puttemans, P., Brosens, I., Delattin, P., Vasquez, G. and Boeckx, W. (1987). Salpingoscopy versus hysterosalpingography in hydrosalpinges. *Hum. Reprod.*, **2**, 535–40

29. De Bruyne, F., Puttemans, P., Boeckx, W. and Brosens, I. (1989). The clinical value of salpingoscopy in tubal infertility. *Fertil. Steril.*, **51**, 339–40

30. Maguiness, S. and Djahanbakhch, O. (1992). Salpingoscopic findings in women undergoing sterilization. *Hum. Reprod.*, **7**, 269–73

31. Hershlag, A., Seifer, D., Carcangiu, M., Patton, D., Diamond, M. and De Cherney, A. (1991). Salpingoscopy: light microscopic and electron microscopic correlations. *Obstet. Gynecol.*, **77**, 399–405

32. Kerin, J., Williams, D., Roman, G., Pearlstone, A., Grundfest, W. and Surrey, E. (1992). Falloposcopic classification and treatment of fallopian tube lumen disease. *Fertil. Steril.*, **57**, 731–41

33. Kerin, J. (1992). Nonhysteroscopic falloposcopy: a proposed method for visual guidance and verification of tubal cannula placement for endotuboplasty, gamete and embryo transfer procedures. *Fertil. Steril.*, **57**, 1133–5

34. Scudamore, I., Dunphy, B., Bowman, M., Jenkins, J. and Cooke, I. (1994). Comparison of ampullary assessment by falloposcopy and salpingoscopy. *Hum. Reprod.*, **9**, 1516–18

35. Scudamore, I., Dunphy, B. and Cooke, I. (1992). Outpatient falloposcopy: intra-luminal imaging of the fallopian tube by trans-uterine fibre-optic endoscopy as an outpatient procedure. *Br. J. Obstet. Gynaecol.*, **99**

36. Dunphy, B., Taenzer, P., Bultz, B., Ingleson, B., Hartman, D. and Dodd, C. (1994). A comparison of pain experienced during hysterosalpingography and in-office falloposcopy. *Fertil. Steril.*, **62**, 67–70

37. Dunphy, B. and Pattinson, H. A. (1994). Office falloposcopy; a tertiary level assessment for planning the management of infertile women. *Aust. N.Z. J. Obstet. Gynecol.*, **34**, 189–90

38. Lower, A., Maguiness, S., Djahanbakhch, O. and Grudzinskas, J. (1992). Transcervical tubal endoscopy (falloposcopy) – a clinically useful tool? *Gynaecol. Endosc.*, **1**, 155–8

39. Fayez, J., Mutie, G. and Schneider, P. (1988). The diagnostic value of hysterosalpingography and laparoscopy in infertility investigation. *Int. J. Fertil.*, **33**, 98–101

40. Okonofua, F. E., Essen, U. J. and Nimalaraj, T. (1989). Hysterosalpingography versus laparoscopy in tubal infertility: comparison based on findings at laparotomy. *Int. J. Gynecol. Obstet.*, **28**, 143–7

41. World Health Organization (1986). Comparative trial of tubal insufflation, hysterosalpingogram and laparoscopy with dye hydrotubation for assessment of tubal patency. *Fertil. Steril.*, **46**, 1101–2

42. Kerin, J. (1994). Transcervical tubal endoscopy: falloposcopy. In Gruzinskas, J., Chapman, M., Chard, T. and Djahanbakhch, O. (eds.) *The Fallopian Tube, Clinical and Surgical Aspects*, pp. 95–109. (London: Springer)

43. Grow, D., Coddington, C. and Flood, J. (1993). Proximal tubal occlusion by hysterosalpingogram: a role for falloposcopy. *Fertil. Steril.*, **60**, 170–4

44. Kovacs, G., Kerin, J., Scudamore, I. and Wood, C. (1992). Falloposcopy – a non-invasive method of salpingostomy. *Gynaecol. Endosc.*, **1**, 159–60

Sporadic and recurrent abortion

14

P. G. McDonough and S. P. T. Tho

Introduction

There is overwhelming evidence from studies in *Drosophila*, *Xenopus* and the mouse that genetic factors are primarily responsible for all stages of early embryonic development. Studies in *Drosophila* and zebra fish indicate that those genes responsible for early axis formation and embryonic patterning are expressed specifically in the maternal oocyte. Mutations in these oocyte-specific genes are invariably embryonic lethals. In humans the study of oocyte-specific genes and the effect of their maternal protein products is just beginning. It is apparent that knowledge of the developmental biology of the human embryo will shed considerable light on the genetic causes of recurrent human abortion. This short treatise addresses the scope of human fetal wastage, and the current state of our knowledge with respect to causes and treatment.

Scope of fetal wastage

Pregnancy is usually not suspected until 5–6 weeks after the last menstrual period and is confirmed by human chorionic gonadotropin (hCG) assays. Clinically recognized pregnancy losses, as evidenced by products of conception, usually occur at least 8 weeks after the last menses and represent 12–15% of all recognizable conceptions[1]. With the advent of ultrasonography, several studies have shown a fetal loss rate of 2.4–3.2% between 8 and 28 weeks of gestation[2,3]. This suggests that most fetuses have died before 8 weeks' gestation. Many investigators have searched for protein markers that would be specific enough and in sufficient quantity to be detected prior to implantation of the blastocyst. Preimplantation pregnancies were diagnosed by Rolfe, using semiquantitation of the early pregnancy factor (EPF)[4]. This specific protein can be detected in human serum within 2 days of fertilization, persists for the first two trimesters of pregnancy and disappears rapidly following death of the conceptus. Unfortunately, this diagnostic technique has not been consistently reproducible.

Early postimplantation embryonic loss has been diagnosed by serial β-hCG determinations. In 1988 Wilcox and co-investigators used a sensitive and specific immunoradiometric urinary hCG assay to follow first morning urinary hCG in 707 cycles of 221 women who were attempting to conceive[5]. Of the 198 pregnancies defined by an increase of hCG at the expected implantation time, 22% (43/198) were preclinically lost while 31% (63/198) represented the total loss rate. In *in vitro* fertilization (IVF) and embryo transfer programs, the reported high success rate of oocyte recovery and fertilization *in vitro* has been in great disparity with the high rate of conception failure (75–80%), in spite of the uniform practice of transferring multiple embryos. One possible reason for this conception failure is the high frequency of lethal chromosomal abnormalities that prevent embryonic development beyond the preimplantation and postimplantation stages[6].

The extensive loss of preimplantation and postimplantation embryos appears to be in agreement with morphological observations. Hertig and colleagues[7] described their findings on 34 fertilized human ova surgically recovered from the Fallopian tubes, uterine cavities and endometria of women of known fertility and coital history who underwent elective hysterectomy. Among the eight preimplantation embryos, four were morphologically abnormal.

Among the 26 postimplantation embryos, six (23%) were morphologically abnormal. Subsequently, Buster and colleagues[8] described 25 intrauterine embryos recovered by lavage from five fertile surrogates. Surrogates received artificial insemination on the day of or the day after their luteinizing hormone (LH) peak and underwent uterine lavage 5 days after the LH surge. The embryos exhibited a wide range of morphological development, from uncleaved zygotes to mature blastocysts. Only five of the 25 embryos recovered were blastocysts and only three of the five blastocysts resulted in pregnancy[8].

Genetic causes of fetal wastage

Chromosomal abnormalities

It is known that at least 50% of clinically recognized first-trimester pregnancy losses result from chromosomal abnormalities[9–12]. In contrast, aneuploidy accounts only for 5–8% of stillborns and for 0.6% of liveborns. Over the past 15 years, chromosomal heteromorphism, defined as normal cytogenetic variations related to differences in heterochromatin, has served as chromosomal markers to distinguish homologous members of a chromosomal pair. Unfortunately, the incidence of cytogenetic heteromorphism in the general population is low (5–7%). Consequently, only a limited number of chromosomes have distinctive cytogenetic markers and this has posed difficulties in the determination of the parental origin of the extra chromosome in trisomies[13]. In 1984, for the first time, Davies and co-workers[14] used restriction fragment length polymorphisms (RFLPs) to identify the parental source of the extra chromosome 21 in a couple with a Down's syndrome infant. This DNA technique, using differences in restriction enzyme cleavage sites to identify polymorphism between homologous chromosomes, is a powerful method of tracing the parental source of a single extra chromosome in an aneuploidic conceptus. Over the past 10 years there has been a proliferation of DNA markers that can be used to determine the parental origin of the extra chromosome in aneuploidic fetuses and liveborns. These markers generated by polymorphic short copy repeat sequences (trinucleotides, dinucleotides, etc.) are being used by selected investigators to study the origin and pattern of recurrent human aneuploidy in couples with recurrent spontaneous abortions.

Sporadic aneuploidic abortions

(1) Autosomal trisomies Autosomal trisomies are by far the most frequently found cytogenetic abnormality in clinically recognized first-trimester abortions and represent 50% of all chromosomal abnormalities identified in sporadic abortion material[12]. Except for chromosome 1, trisomies of all other autosomes have been reported in spontaneously aborted fetuses. Interestingly, trisomy 1 has been found in an abortion from an IVF pregnancy. There appear to be different rates of non-disjunction for each chromosome pair. Trisomy 16 is the most common. In trisomic abortions, the additional chromosome is almost always maternal in origin, irrespective of maternal age[15]. It uniformly results from an error in meiosis I of maternal germ cells.

(2) Triploidy Triploidy is relatively common in human fetuses and accounts for approximately 15% of clinically recognized sporadic abortions in large reported series[12]. Triploid fetuses are characterized by malformations with mostly neural tube defects, omphaloceles and molar degeneration of the placenta. The most common human triploidies are 69,XXY and 69,XXX. In his review of 268 triploid conceptions, Niebuhr found only nine cases with 69,XYY complements, all in spontaneous abortions[16]. Retention of the second polar body leading to digyny, dispermic fertilization and fertilization by a diploid sperm resulting in diandry are the main causes of triploidy. Retention of the first polar body is less frequent than the other three mechanisms[17].

(3) Classic mole Disorders in sperm–egg interaction also result in complete or classic molar

pregnancy. Classic moles in contrast to partial moles are not associated with fetal parts and are diploid with both haploid complements being of paternal origin. Approximately 90% of classic moles are 46,XX and the remainder are 46,XY. The inheritance of two sets of paternal chromosomes in complete mole causes early embryonic death and confers a growth advantage to the placenta through an abnormality in genomic imprinting[18]. This is in contrast to the triploidy condition in which the persistence of a single maternal chromosome complement ($69X^mX^PY$ or $69X^mX^PX^P$) apparently exerts a morphological and biological dilution effect on the compete molar phenotype[17]. A 7-year cytogenetic survey of 192 molar pregnancies compared 54 complete moles of androgenetic origin and 103 partial moles having triploid constitutions. The triploid conceptuses with molar degeneration consistently had two paternal and one maternal haploid complements. The 30 non-molar triploids all had two maternal and one paternal haploid complements[19].

(4) Tetraploidy Tetraploidy is relatively rare in human fetuses and is usually incompatible with life. All tetraploid conceptuses are either XXYY or XXXX. This indicates that their likely origin is failure of cytokinesis at the first cleavage division. Cumulative data have revealed 75 abortuses with 92,XXXX and 45 with 92,XXYY. Heteromorphic banding studies indicated that the 92,XXXX fetuses had duplication of both maternal and paternal chromosomal complements, suggestive of failure of the first cleavage division of the zygote as the mode of origin[20]. A trispermic origin rather than failure of cytokinesis at the first cleavage division is very rare[20].

(5) Monosomy X Monosomy X is the most common single chromosome abnormality, accounting for 20–25% of chromosomally abnormal abortions[12]. Characteristic anomalies include cystic hygroma and generalized edema. The work of Singh and Carr[21] and of Jirasek[22] on 45,X stillborns indicate that X-chromosome privation may be associated with incomplete enveloping of germ cells by follicular cells. This

may affect meiosis control, leading to excessive follicular atresia and development of streak gonads in early childhood or at puberty in surviving 45,X individuals. On the basis of Xg marker studies, it was found that in 70–75% of individuals with 45,X, the single X was maternal[23]. Recently, Hassold and associates[24], using RFLP for seven marker loci on X, determined the origin of the X chromosome in nine informative 45,X spontaneous abortions. In this small number of spontaneous abortions, the X chromosome was maternally derived in six and paternally derived in three[24].

(6) Mosaicism Misdivision of one or more chromosomes by non-disjunction or anaphase lag will give rise to a mosaic conceptus. Mosaicism is relatively common among trisomic abortions. It is generally accepted that approximately 5% of all trisomies are mosaic, with the normal cell line developing after fertilization[25]. Mosaicism appears to be more common in embryos that are derived through *in vitro* fertilization.

(7) De novo unbalanced structural rearrangements The incidence of unbalanced rearrangements in large series of clinically recognized abortions is approximately 1%. It is concluded that as many as 85% of all unbalanced rearrangements are lost before 28 weeks, since the incidence of unbalanced rearrangements found in liveborns is only 0.03%[12].

(8) Chromosomal abnormalities in IVF A European survey of clinically identified abortions after IVF revealed 21 among 34 (62%) having chromosomal abnormalities[26]. These abnormalities included 14 autosomal trisomies, one double trisomy, one triploidy, one tetraploidy, one unbalanced translocation and three abortuses with 45,X karyotypes. The frequency and spectrum of cytogenetic abnormalities are not much different from those in spontaneous abortion material after natural conception.

Cytogenetic studies on preimplantation embryos have met with technical problems which are related to the small number of cells and the difficulty in obtaining dispersed metaphase chromosomes for identification and yet avoiding random loss[27]. In one of the largest series of successful chromosome analyses on 35 pre-embryos, the overall incidence of chromosome aberrations was found to be 14/35 (40%), with 9% for trisomies, 3% for polyploidies, 3% for hypodiploidies and 26% for structural anomalies[6]. Rudak and co-workers[28] studied the frequency of gamete aneuploidy in IVF by karyotyping nine multipronuclear oocytes before the first cleavage division. Two oocytes were clearly dispermic. Among the 24 informative pronuclei, two contained an extra chromosome while in three, one chromosome was missing and the remaining 19 had a normal haploid complement. These data indicate that 20% of the gametes were chromosomally abnormal and that abnormal gametes did not appear to be selected against[28]. The identification of monosomic pre-embryos and pronuclei missing an autosome suggests that monosomy may be a frequent cytogenetic abnormality in preimplantation loss following *in vitro* and *in vivo* conceptions. Trisomy 1, which has never been identified in liveborns or spontaneous abortion material, was found in one *in vitro* fertilized zygote[29]. Mosaicisms and structural anomalies are relatively frequent in IVF embryos in contrast with *in vivo* conceptions.

Recurrent abortions due to chromosomal abnormalities

(1) Balanced parental chromosomal rearrangements
Since the 1966 Geneva conference[30], numerous reports of independent series have shown that balanced chromosomal rearrangements in a parent may predispose to recurrent fetal wastage[31-34]. These studies have indicated that a parent may be a carrier of a balanced cytogenetic abnormality in approximately 2–14% of couples with recurrent abortion with or without fetal malformations.

A balanced translocation in a parent may be produced as a result of a normal meiotic segregation, unbalanced gametes leading to abortions or defective liveborn children or interval infertility. A balanced translocation may also give rise to a balanced gamete, resulting in a balanced carrier, or it may produce a cytogenetically normal gamete. Figure 1 illustrates the unbalanced karyotype of a male abortus [(46,XY, del(6)(pter → q21))]. Figure 2 demonstrates the karyotype of the mother who is a carrier of the balanced translocation 2/6 [46,XX,t (2;6)(q3;q2)]. In rare instances, the balanced rearrangement may induce non-disjunction of other chromosomes during meiosis, leading to aneuploidic gametes by an interchromosomal effect[35].

A brief review of the meiotic behavior of the human heterozygous reciprocal translocation is important for understanding of the clinical observations. At pachytene, each segment of a pair of rearranged chromosomes will pair with its homologous segment to give a cross-shaped configuration. Only if segregation is alternate or diagonally opposite will the resultant gametes be euploid. In Robertsonian translocation carriers, the rearranged chromosome results from centric fusion of two acrocentric chromosomes. During meiotic segregation, two chromosomes will usually proceed to one pole and one to the other pole, yielding six types of gametes. Only two of these types are euploid: one bearing the untranslocated chromosomes and another carrying the large translocation derivative. Among the unbalanced gametes, only the ones resulting in partial trisomy conceptuses are viable.

Although gamete production in female carriers is unaffected, balanced chromosomal rearrangements in some male carriers may cause complete blockage of the sequence of spermatogenesis, leading to sperm maturation arrest. The incidence of balanced chromosomal translocations in couples with multiple abortions was reported as 0–31%. This wide variation is related to the heterogeneous criteria used for patient selection. Since parents with balanced chromosomal rearrangements and history of only repeated abortions have a significant change with each pregnancy of having a child with normal or balanced karyotype, the usual criteria for investigation include at least two abortions or reproductive losses[31]. There is no evidence from several reported series that increasing the num-

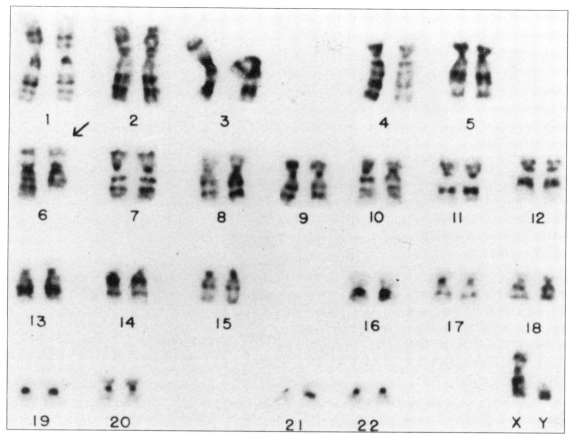

Figure 1   Unbalanced karyotype of a male abortus 46,XY, deleted (6) (pter → q21) with deletion of the long arm of the number 6 chromosome (→). From reference 72, with permission

ber of losses to three or more leads to any change in the yield of chromosomal rearrangements detected[31,32]. From pooled data, it is estimated that the risk of unbalanced offspring derived from parental reciprocal translocations is approximately 12%, whether the carrier is male or female. For Robertsonian translocations, this risk is only for the female carrier and approximates 10%[36–38]. Although there appears to be no risk of unbalanced conception when the male is the carrier, a trisomy 21 child may be born, due to the interchromosomal effect. In the special cases of the homologous 13q13q or 21q21q centric fusion, the rate of pregnancy wastage reaches 100%, because all products of segregation give rise to either monosomic or trisomic zygotes[39].

Another type of chromosomal rearrangement is inversion. A pericentric inversion results when the breaks are on both sides of the centromere. A paracentric inversion involves a single chromosome arm and does not include the centromere. Small paracentric inversions may go undetected even in good-quality preparations. Carriers of chromosome inversions may be phenotypically normal if genes are neither lost, gained nor altered as a result of the breakage and rejoining. However, both types of inversion must form inversion loops to pair with the normal homologs during meiosis. Crossing over within the inversion loop, in case of pericentric inversion, leads to chromosomal duplication or deficiency after segregation, resulting in abortions and abnormal liveborns[40].

109

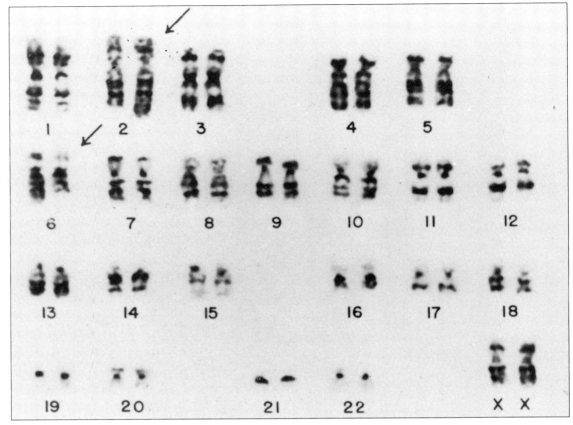

Figure 2 Balanced karyotype of the mother 46,XX, t (2;6) (q3;q2) who produced the abortus in Figure 1. Deleted portion of the long arm of chromosome 6 has been translocated to the long arm of chromosome 2 (→). From reference 72, with permission

Conversely, crossing over within a paracentric inversion loop results in dicentric and acentric segregation products that are both severely unbalanced, leading to early abortions, and rarely, abnormal liveborns[41]. The frequency of unbalanced recombinants detected at amniocentesis in pericentric inversion carriers is 1–2% if ascertained through a history of pure abortions and 10–15% if ascertained through a history of a previous abnormal liveborn child[42].

Finally, in females, X-chromosome mosaicism has been repeatedly reported in association with recurrent abortion histories. Some of these women have also produced liveborn children with Down's syndrome and X-chromosome aneuploidy or mosaicism[43].

It may be concluded that a chromosome analysis using banding techniques and an adequate chromosome count should be performed on couples having a history of recurrent abortion or having a pedigree with one abortion plus one malformed fetus. Parental balanced translocations, pericentric and paracentric inversions, or X-chromosome mosaicism may be uncovered. This detection is important for appropriate counselling and prenatal cytogenetic monitoring.

(1) Recurrent aneuploidy Cumulative cytogenetic data of successive abortions from the same couples indicate a concordance for the normal or abnormal nature of the chromosomal complements. If the karyotype of the first

abortus was normal, about 84% of the second abortuses were also normal. If the karyotype of the first abortus was abnormal, about 66% of the second abortuses were also abnormal, but usually of a different type. When the first abortus was trisomic, 67% of the second abortuses were also trisomic. Triploidic first abortuses were followed by trisomic and triploidic abortuses, 25%[44] and 17%[12] of the time, respectively. In their subsequent study analyzing two consecutive karyotyped abortions in 273 recurrent aborters, Warburton and co-workers found an association between normal karyotypes in successive abortions. However, there was no significant increase in recurrence of trisomy after a previous trisomic abortion when corrections were made for maternal age[45]. Other investigators expressed concern that some undiagnosed trisomic fetuses may potentially survive to term. In a prospective study on a series of 305 young couples with a history of two or more unkaryotyped abortions and normal parental karyotypes, Drugan and associates[46] found five cases (1.6%) of aneuploidy diagnosed at amniocentesis or at birth. Only three aneuploidic conceptions were detected among 979 (0.3%) controls. In this study, the 1.6% frequency of aneuploid conceptions in patients with a history of repeated pregnancy loss in the absence of any other risk factor was roughly similar to the risk for a 40-year-old pregnant woman[46]. Some couples obviously tend to produce aneuploid conceptuses which may abort or survive to term. Aneuploidic conceptions may arise from errors of gametogenesis in the female or male, fertilization, or early cleavage in the zygote.

As regards gametogenesis errors in the female, oocyte aging caused by increased maternal age or secondary to delayed ovulation has been related to gametogenesis or fertilization errors leading to the production of abnormal zygotes. An association between maternal age and aneuploidy has been well documented. However, the mechanism underlying the effect of increased maternal age has not yet been clarified. It has been postulated that the maternal age-dependent trisomies might result from precocious terminalization of chiasmata. This leads to premature disjunction of the bivalents and random segregation of the resulting univalents, a process that should affect chromosomes with the smallest number of chiasmata[47].

Preovulatory gamete aging due to intrafollicular over-ripeness has been shown to contribute to the production of aneuploidic zygotes. Extensive chromosomal aberrations in embryos were described in amphibians by Witschi and Laguens[48] in 1963, in the rat by Butcher and Fugo[49] in 1967 and in *Xenopus*, when ovulation was experimentally delayed, by Mikamo[50] in 1968. Boue and Boue[51] correlated the apparent day of ovulation as suggested by basal body temperature curves with chromosome constitutions of 126 normal, trisomic and polyploid abortuses. More trisomic than normal abortuses were found in cases in which ovulation presumably had occurred after day 18 of the menstrual cycle[51]. The possible underlying mechanism may be spindle degeneration as a result of intrafollicular aging. Errors in the first or second meiotic division that involve an entire haploid genome can give rise to a diploid oocyte leading to a triploid zygote (digyny). Heteromorphic banding techniques have demonstrated that 10% of human triploid conceptuses result from digyny and that the majority of diploid eggs are formed by failure of the second maternal meiotic division[17].

In gametogenesis errors in the male, non-disjunction in the first or second meiotic division can give rise to nullisomic or disomic sperm, leading to monosomic or trisomic conceptions. Errors in meiosis I or meiosis II may involve the entire haploid set of chromosomes, resulting in diploid sperm and triploid conceptions (diandry). Heteromorphic banding studies indicated that 23.6% of triploid fetuses result from fertilization of a haploid ovum by a diploid sperm that is formed by failure of the first meiotic division in the male[17]. Spermatozoan aging in the male tract has been experimentally shown to contribute to increased incidences of reproductive failure in the rabbit by Tesh and Glover[52] in 1966 and in the mouse by Martin-DeLeon and Boice[53] in 1982. The contribution of sperm aging in the female genital tract to abnormal embryonic development was shown in rabbit does by Martin and Shaver[54] in 1972, when sperm were experimentally retained up to 30 h before ovulation. These data indicate that when sperm resided in the male or female tracts for an extended time prior to ovulation, the aging sperm underwent genome alteration prior to losing their capacity for fertilization.

The third cause of aneuploidic conceptions is fertilization errors due to gamete aging. Soon after the fertilizing sperm has bound to the plasma membrane of the oocyte, cortical granule contents are discharged from the egg plasma membrane into the perivitelline space to block fertilization by any other sperm. In all species, eggs that are not fertilized for a given period of time after ovulation lose the mechanism that prevents polyspermy and results in polyploidy[55]. Heteromorphic banding techniques on both parents and their triploid offspring suggest that two-thirds of triploid human conceptuses are formed by fertilization by two sperm (dispermy)[17]. Ill-timed fertilization demonstrated by the analysis of basal body temperature curves with known dates of intercourse has been associated by Boue and associates with an increased frequency of triploidy[36].

Euploidic abortions

On several occasions we have karyotyped 'empty sac', 'blighted ovum' abortions as euploidic 46,XY. Poland and colleagues[56] successfully karyotyped 228 embryos and 59 fetuses among 1126 aborted embryos. Among the 188 embryos with growth disorganization, 79 were cytogenetically normal, as were eight among the 24 (33%) embryos with other phenotypic anomalies and 14 among the 18 (77%) fetuses with abnormal phenotypes. Embryos or fetuses that are phenotypically abnormal but chromosomally normal could have undergone demise from multifactorial conditions, Mendelian disorders or developmental gene mutations.

Multifactorial conditions Some multifactorial conditions may cause early fetal loss and spontaneous abortion[34]. By morphological examina-

tion of 2020 abortuses from 1961 women, Poland and associates[56] found a prevalence of 1.9–3.8% for neural tube defects and 7.9% for cardiovascular system defects. However, neural tube abnormalities noted among pedigrees with multifactorial disorders may represent variants of the Meckel syndrome[57] or be part of chromosomal syndromes such as triploidy or trisomy 18[58]. Cleft lip and cleft palate is another condition which may appear as multifactorial but is truly part of a chromosomal syndrome. Careful examination of external and internal structural abnormalities and tissue karyotyping of defective fetuses are essential for a correct diagnosis and proper counselling. Assuming that the etiologies are similar for the defective fetus and the malformed liveborn, one can give the same recurrence risk whether the defect is identified in an abortus or in a newborn.

Mendelian disorders

(1) Autosomal dominant disorders Such anomalies were rarely identified in the large series of abortuses of Poland and associates[56]. Only one fetus with evidence of osteogenesis imperfecta was found from a couple who had two previous children with this disorder.

(2) Autosomal recessive disorders Alpha-globin gene mutation illustrates an example of these disorders that are lethal in the homozygous state. A human embryo that is homozygous for the deletion of both α-globulin genes does develop normally, but forms imperfect tetrameres of the β-globulin protein and dies prematurely with severe hydrops fetalis. Similarly, the embryonic lethality of a homozygous deletion involving the α-globin gene in mice has been known. A similar DNA deletion in man is associated with fetal hydrops and intrauterine death[59].

(3) X-linked genes mutations X-linked disorders with embryonic lethality in hemizygous males suggest a role for single gene mutations in what otherwise would be euploidic abortion. These pedigrees are characterized by half of the females being affected with the disorder in

question (focal dermal hypoplasia–Goltz syndrome, incontinentia pigmenti, oral–facial–digital I syndrome), male abortuses and phenotypically normal surviving males[60].

Developmental genes mutations

(1) Maternal genes critical for embryonic development Some maternally encoded specific proteins are critical in very early development of the embryo up to the four-cell and eight-cell stage, and others for the first several cleavage divisions of the embryo. Other genes are important for normal body polarity and normal dorsal–ventral asymmetry[61]. These maternal-effect genes appear to be critical in turning on important developmental genes of the embryonic genome. Their mutations may be important in very early embryonic loss. Mutations in such genes provide us with a logical explanation for couples with pure histories of recurrent abortion and no living children.

(2) Homeobox genes Homeobox sequences well studied in *Drosophila* have been highly conserved in a broad array of species, including humans. These genes appear to control the expression of ensembles of genes through transcriptional regulation and to control the developmental determination of groups of cells with respect to their morphogenetic fates[62]. The human homeobox genes Hu-1 and Hu-2 transcripts were shown by Su and co-workers[63] to appear on trophoblast at 4–6 weeks of gestation, to gradually increase in intensity at 8–10 weeks and subsequently to disappear. Embryos with complete disorganization of development or blighted ova should be at high risk for homozygosity for morphogenetic mutants.

(3) Oncogenes The c-*sis* and c-*myc* oncogene transcripts were also found by Su and associates to appear on human trophoblast at 4–12 weeks, gradually to increase in intensity and to disappear thereafter[63]. The expression of these oncogenes appeared to be in a cascading type of sequence, as if one oncogene product might activate the next oncogene in the cascade[64].

This domino effect may even be under the control of other genes similar or identical to homeotic selector genes.

(4) Cell aggregation factors and extracellular matrix genes Cells of the developing human embryo receive regulatory information through cell-to-cell interaction. Cell interactions are modulated by many factors, including the secretion of large aggregation factors that link similar cells together and stabilize the organization of the germ layers. Later in development the plasma membranes of neighboring cells in tissues are linked together at gap junctions to allow ions and small molecules to pass directly from the inside of one cell to the inside of the other[65]. Cells in the multicellular embryo are also in contact with an intricate meshwork of interacting extracellular macromolecules that constitute the extracellular matrix. This holds cells together, and generates and maintains the patterns of cells in tissues and organs during early development. The extracellular matrix contains three major fiber-forming proteins: collagen, elastin and fibronectin. The genes encoding protein products that involve the extracellular matrix are gradually being isolated, cloned and mapped on the human genome.

(5) Collagen type I gene mutation created by insertional mutagenesis Type I collagen is a major component of the extracellular matrix and has an important function in mesenchymal–epithelial interactions during organogenesis. By insertional mutagenesis, a mutation of the collagen type I gene was created and introduced in the germline of mouse embryos that would become adults heterozygous for the mutation. With the use of transgenic animal technology, mouse embryos homozygous for the mutation were produced. The insertion inactivated the collagen type I gene by completely blocking its transcription. Because of the lack of type I collagen in the homozygous embryos, adequate vascular structures were unable to develop as conduits of blood, and vascular rupture caused embryonic death[66].

113

(6) Toxic embryopathy Euploidic embryonic loss may occur through cell toxification. The gene for adenine phosphoribosyl transferase encodes an enzyme that is important in purine metabolism. This enzyme converts xanthine to its degradation products. An increased rate of spontaneous abortions is seen among obligate heterozygote parents. There is growing suspicion that embryos homozygous for the mutation are toxified by the excess of xanthine during early development[67]. Similar types of embryopathy due to a lethal defect in carbohydrate metabolism have been described[68].

Developmental gene mutations involving genes encoding critical structural proteins, homeobox sequences, and proto-oncogenes will no doubt be an integral part of the etiology of euploidic embryonic loss in humans[69]. The precise mutations that are embryonically lethal will have to be characterized, and automated DNA, RNA and protein screening techniques developed[70] and applied to the human euploidic 'blighted embryos'. Molecular analysis in the parents for heterozygosity will ascertain whether the event is sporadic or recurrent. Since some defects may be defects in the translational process, analysis of the protein products of these genes in the abnormal embryos and their comparison with the normal protein profiles will be necessary when molecular screening on the euploidic abortuses is negative.

Counselling

Couples experiencing a *sporadic* abortion should be informed that the frequency of fetal wastage is 12–15% of all clinically recognized pregnancies and that approximately 50% of sporadic abortions are due to chromosomal abnormalities related to sporadic gametogenesis or fertilization errors. A recurrence risk of 25% will be provided in the absence of family history of genetic disorders and advanced maternal age[1]. Couples experiencing two or more abortions or one abortion plus one stillborn or one malformed fetus or liveborn should receive a formal genetic evaluation of *recurrent* fetal wastage.

Evaluation of couples with repetitive reproductive failure

Preparing the history

A complete pedigree analysis is necessary, focusing on the following five key points:

(1) Detection of the history of malformed children or fetuses;

(2) Detection of neural tube abnormality, or other multifactorial defects;

(3) Detection of the history of infertility plus abortion (possible preimplantation wastage);

(4) Detection of clues for recurrent aneuploidy: delayed ovulation or fertilization; and

(5) Detection of the history of male abortuses only.

Laboratory investigations

Cytogenic evaluation of both partners Both partners should have blood leukocyte karyotyping with G and Q banding to identify small rearrangements.

Prenatal diagnosis Couples who are carriers of a heterologous balanced rearrangement should be encouraged to attempt further pregnancies and to have prenatal cytogenetic diagnosis. They may be provided with the cumulative risk figures of unbalanced conceptions according to their type of balanced rearrangements[38,42]. Couples who are carriers of a translocation of two homologous chromosomes should be offered artificial insemination for the male carrier or donor oocyte through IVF for the female carrier.

Couples who have delivered a previous fetus or newborn with a neural tube defect or other multifactorial conditions should attempt further pregnancies with serial targeted ultrasound monitoring. Should abortion occur, a diligent phenotypic examination and karyotyping of the fetus are in order.

The most common couples to manage are those who have a negative history of previous offspring with genetic disorders and an unrevealing complete recurrent fetal wastage evaluation. Future pregnancies may be planned focusing on the two following points:

(1) Basal body temperature curve or urinary LH monitoring should be recorded for several months to ascertain the normal timing of ovulation prior to planning for a future pregnancy. Delayed ovulation should be treated appropriately to avoid intrafollicular ovum over-ripeness. Sperm deposition should be synchronized with ovulation to avoid gamete ageing.

(2) The biochemical diagnosis of pregnancy should be established early and follow-up confirmation and surveillance of a viable pregnancy is best obtained with real-time ultrasonography every 2 weeks from 6–12 weeks' conception. Subsequently, a normal four-chambered heart and normal neural tube will be ascertained. If an unfortunate event occurs and the pregnancy is found arrested early in its course, a transcervical or transabdominal chorionic villus sample should be obtained as soon as possible after embryonic death for a successful karyotype[71]. A careful phenotypic and cytogenetic examination of the abortus is very important.

In brief, transcervical or transabdominal chorionic villus sampling or amniocentesis for fetal fibroblast karyotyping should be offered to individuals with a previous history of cytogenetic or phenotypic abortal abnormalities as well as abnormalities of their own karyotypes. In the absence of this previous history, the data of Drugan and associates[46] may be provided to couples with recurrent abortion in order to select for or against prenatal cytogenetic diagnosis. Ultrasound monitoring should be offered to all couples with a history of fetal wastage. A well-planned pregnancy and appropriate follow-up through early gestation resulted in a successful outcome 62% of the time for couples with a negative pedigree and a negative formal recurrent fetal wastage work-up in our series[34].

Summary
Genetic causes of fetal wastage are overwhelming, as evidenced by the high incidence of chromosomal abnormalities in preimplantation, early postimplantation embryos and first-trimester fetuses. Multifactorial disorders are ten time more prevalent in abortuses than in newborns[32]. Abortion material may be divided into aneuploidic and euploidic conditions. Recurrent aneuploidy due to recurrent gametogenesis or fertilization errors is more common than parental chromosomal rearrangements. Ovulation and fertilization delays may be etiologies of recurrent aneuploidy. Counselling should focus on normalization of ovulation and synchronization of ovulation with sperm deposition through ovulation monitoring. The availability of high-resolution vaginal ultrasonography has provided for close monitoring of fetal viability and improved success of anatomic and cytogenetic analysis in case of aborted development. Euploidic fetal wastage also appears to be of genetic origin, as suggested by the high frequency of severe growth disorganization and phenotypic anomalies in early embryos. The precise genetic causes of euploidic losses in humans have remained a challenge for developmental biologists and interested clinicians.

References
1. Warburton, D. and Fraser, F. C. (1964). Spontaneous abortion risk in man: data from reproductive histories collected in a medical genetics unit. *Am. J. Hum. Genet.*, **16**, 1–25

2. Christiaens, G. C. M. L. and Stoutenbeek, P. (1984). Spontaneous abortion in proven intact pregnancies. *Lancet*, **2**, 571–2
3. Simpson, J. L., Mills, S. L., Holmes, L. B., Ober, C L., Aarons, L. J. and Knopp, R. H. (1987). Low fetal loss rates after ultrasound proved viability in early pregnancy. *J. Am. Med. Assoc.*, **258**, 2555–7
4. Rolfe, B. E. (1982). Detection of fetal wastage. *Fertil. Steril.*, **37**, 655–60
5. Wilcox, A. J., Weinberg, R., O'Conner, J. F., Baird, D. D., Schlatterer, J. P., Canfield, R. E., Armstrong, E. G. and Nisula, B. C. (1988). Incidence of early pregnancy loss. *N. Engl. J. Med.*, **319**, 189–94
6. Papadopoulos, G., Templeton, A. A. and Fisk, N. (1989). The frequency of chromosome anomalies in human preimplantation embryos after *in vitro* fertilization. *Hum. Reprod.*, **4**, 91–8
7. Hertig, A. T., Rock, J., Adams, E. C. and Menkin, M. C. (1959). Thirty-four fertilized human ova, good, bad and indifferent recovered from two hundred and ten women of known fertility: a study of the biological waste in early human pregnancy. *Pediatrics*, **23**, 202–11
8. Buster, J. E., Bustillo, M., Rodi, I. A., Cohen, S. W., Hamilton, M., Simon, J. A., Thorneycroft, I. H. and Marshall, J. R. (1985). Biologic and morphologic development of donated human ova recovered by nonsurgical uterine lavage. *Am. J. Obstet. Gynecol.*, **153**, 211–17
9. Boue, J., Boue, A. and Lazar, P. (1975). Retrospective and prospective epidemiological studies of 1500 karyotyped spontaneous human abortions. *Teratology*, **12**, 11–26
10. Hassold, T. J., Chen, N., Funkhouser, J., Manuel, J. B., Matsuura, J., Matsuyama, A., Wilson, C., Yamane, J. A. and Jacobs, P. A. (1980). A cytogenetic study of 1,000 spontaneous abortions. *Am. J. Hum. Genet.*, **44**, 151–64
11. Kajii, T., Ohama, K., Niikawa, N., Ferrier, A. and Avirachan, S. (1973). Banding analysis of abnormal karyotypes in spontaneous abortion. *Am. J. Hum. Genet.*, **25**, 539–47
12. Warburton, D., Stein, Z., Kline, J. and Susser, M. (1980). Chromosome abnormalities in spontaneous abortion: data from the New York City study. In Porter, I. H. and Hook, E. B. (eds.) *Human Embryonic and Fetal Death*, pp. 261–87. (New York: Academic Press)
13. Jacobs, P. A. and Hassold, T. J. (1980). The origin of chromosome abnormalities in spontaneous abortion. In Porter, I. H. and Hook, E. B. (eds.) *Human Embryonic and Fetal Death*, pp. 289–98. (New York: Academic Pres)
14. Davies, K. E., Harper, K., Bonthron, D., Krumlauf, R., Polkey, A., Pembrey, M. E. and William-son, R. (1984). Use of a chromosome 21 cloned DNA probe for the analysis of non-disjunction in Down syndrome. *Hum. Genet.*, **66**, 54–6
15. Hassold, T. J., Chiu, D. and Yamane, J. A. (1984). Parental origin of autosomal trisomies. *Ann. Hum. Genet.*, **48**, 129–44
16. Niebuhr, E. (1974). Triploidy in man: cytogenetical and clinical aspects. *Hum. Genet.*, **21**, 103–25
17. Jacobs, P. A., Szulman, A. E., Funkhouser, J., Matsuura, J. S. and Wilson, C. C. (1982). Human triploidy: relationship between parental origin of the additional haploid complement and development of partial mole. *Ann. Hum. Genet.*, **46**, 223–31
18. McDonough, P. G. (1991). Cytogenetics in reproductive endocrinology. In Yen, S. S. C. and Jaffe, R. D. (eds.) *Reproductive Endocrinology: Physiology, Pathophysiology and Clinical Management*, 3rd edn., pp. 462–79. (Philadelphia: W.B. Saunders)
19. Hunt, P. A., Jacobs, P. A. and Szulman, A. E. (1983). Molar pregnancies and non-molar triploids: results of 7 year cytogenetic study. Presented at the *34th Annual Meeting of the American Society for Human Genetics*, Abstr. 402, 135A, October, Norfolk, Virginia
20. Sheppard, D. M., Fisher, R. A., Lawler, S. D. and Povey, S. (1982). Tetraploid conceptus with three paternal contributions. *Hum. Genet.*, **62**, 371–4
21. Singh, R. P. and Carr, D. H. (1966). The anatomy and histology of XO embryos and fetuses. *Anat. Rec.*, **155**, 369–83
22. Jirasek, J. E. (1976). Principles of reproductive embryology. In Simpson, J. L. (ed.) *Disorders of Sexual Differentiation: Etiology and Clinical Delineation*, pp. 75–92. (New York: Academic Press)
23. Sanger, R., Tippett, P., Gavin, J., Teesdale, P. and Daniels, G. L. (1977). Xg groups and sex chromosome abnormalities in people of northern European ancestry. An addendum. *J. Med. Genet.*, **14**, 210–11
24. Hassold, T. J., Kumlin, E., Takaesu, N. and Leppert, M. (1985). Determination of parental origin of sex chromosome monosomy using restriction fragment length polymorphism. *Am. J. Hum. Genet.*, **37**, 965–72
25. Hassold, T. J. (1982). Mosaic trisomies in human spontaneous abortions. *Hum. Genet.*, **61**, 31–5
26. Plachot, M. (1989). Chromosome analysis of spontaneous abortions after IVF. A European survey. *Hum. Reprod.*, **4**, 425–9
27. Wramsby, N., Fredga, K. and Liedholm, P. (1987). Chromosome analysis of human oocytes recovered from preovulatory follicles in stimulated cycles. *N. Engl. J. Med.*, **316**, 121–4

28. Rudak, E., Dor, J., Mashiach, S., Nebel, L. and Goldman, B. (1984). Chromosome analysis of multipronuclear human oocytes fertilized *in vitro*. *Fertil. Steril.*, **41**, 538–45

29. Watt, J. L., Templeton, A. A., Messinis, I., Bell, L., Cunningham, P. and Duncan, R. O. (1987). Trisomy 1 in an eight cell human pre-embryo. *J. Med. Genet.*, **24**, 60–4

30. Geneva Conference (1966). Standardization of procedures for chromosome studies in abortion. *Cytogenetics*, **5**, 361–93

31. Husslein, P., Huber, J., Wagenbichler, P. and Schnedl, W. (1982). Chromosome abnormalities in 150 couples with multiple spontaneous abortions. *Fertil. Steril.*, **37**, 379–83

32. Portnoi, M. F., Joye, N., Van Den Akker, J., Morlier, G. and Taillemite, J.-L. (1988). Karyotypes of 1142 couples with recurrent abortion. *Obstet. Gynecol.*, **72**, 31–4

33. Simpson, J. L., Elias, S. and Martin, A. O. (1981). Parental chromosomal rearrangements associated with repetitive spontaneous abortion. *Fertil. Steril.*, **36**, 584–90

34. Tho, S. P. T., Byrd, J. R. and McDonough, P. G. (1979). Etiologies and subsequent reproductive performance of 100 couples with recurrent abortion. *Fertil. Steril.*, **32**, 389–95

35. Lindenbaum, R. H., Hulten, M., McDermott, A. and Seabright, M. (1985). The prevalence of translocations in parents of children with regular trisomy 21: a possible interchromosomal effect? *J. Med. Genet.*, **22**, 24–8

36. Boue, A. and Gallano, P. (1984). A collaborative study of the segregation of inherited chromosome structural arrangements in 1356 prenatal diagnoses. Prenat. Diag., **4**, 45–67

37. Mikkelson, M. (1985). Cytogenetic findings in first trimester chorionic villi biopsies: a collaborative study. In Fraccaro, M., Simoni, G. and Bramati, B. (eds.) *First Trimester Fetal Diagnosis*, pp. 109–20. (Berlin: Springer-Verlag)

38. Simpson, J. L. and Bombard, A. T. (1987). Chromosomal abnormalities in spontaneous abortion: frequency, pathology and genetic counseling. In Bennett, M. J. and Edmonds, D. K. (eds.) *Spontaneous and Recurrent Abortion*, pp. 51–76. (Boston: Blackwell Scientific Publications)

39. Maeda, T., Ohno, M., Takada, M., Matsunobu, A. and Arai, M. (1983). Postzygotic D/D translocation homozygosity associated with recurrent abortions. *Am. J. Med. Genet.*, **15**, 389–92

40. Richter, S., Lockwood, B., Lockwood, D. and Allanson, J. (1989). Abnormal chromosome complement resulting from a familial inversion of chromosome 2. *J. Med. Genet.*, **26**, 725–9

41. Bocian, E., Mazurczak, T. and Stanczak, H. (1990). Paracentric inversion inv (18)

(q21.1q23) in a woman with recurrent spontaneous abortions. *Am. J. Med. Genet.*, **35**, 592–3

42. Daniel, A., Hook, E. B. and Wolf, G. (1989). Risks of unbalanced progeny at amniocentesis to carriers of chromosome rearrangements: data from United States and Canadian laboratories. *Am. J. Med. Genet.*, **31**, 14–53

43. Singh, D. N., Hara, S., Foster, H. W. and Grimes, E. M. (1980). Reproductive performance in women with chromosome mosaicism. *Obstet. Gynecol.*, **55**, 608–11

44. Boue, J. and Boue, A. (1973). Chromosomal analysis of two consecutive abortions in each of 43 women. *Hum. Genet.*, **19**, 275–80

45. Warburton, D., Kline, J., Stein, A., Hutzler, M., Chin, A. and Hassold, T. (1987). Does the karyotype of a spontaneous abortion predict the karyotype of a subsequent abortion? Evidence from 273 women with two karyotyped spontaneous abortions. *Am. J. Med. Genet.*, **41**, 465–83

46. Drugan, A., Koppitch, F. C., Williams, J. C. III, Johnsons, M. P., Moghissi, K. S. and Evans, M. I. (1990). Prenatal genetic diagnosis following recurrent early pregnancy loss. *Obstet. Gynecol.*, **75**, 381–4

47. Hassold, T. J., Jacobs, P., Kline, J., Stein, Z. and Warburton, D. (1980). Effect of maternal age on autosomal trisomies. *Ann. Hum. Genet.*, **44**, 29–36

48. Witschi, E. and Laguens, R. (1963). Chromosomal aberrations in embryos from overripe eggs. *Dev. Biol.*, **7**, 605–16

49. Butcher, R. L. and Fugo, N. W. (1967). Overripeness and the mammalian ova. II. Delayed ovulation and chromosome anomalies. *Fertil. Steril.*, **18**, 297–302

50. Mikamo, K. (1968). Mechanism of non disjunction of meiotic chromosomes and degeneration of maturation spindles in eggs affected by intrafollicular overripeness. *Experientia*, **24**, 75–8

51. Boue, J., Boue, A. and Lazar, P. (1975). The epidemiology of human spontaneous abortions with chromosomal anomalies. In Blandau, R. J. (ed.) *Aging Gametes, Their Biology and Pathology, International Symposium on Aging Gametes*, Seattle, Washington, pp. 330–48. (New York: Karger and Basel)

52. Tesh, J. M. and Glover, T. D. (1966). The influence of aging of rabbit spermatozoa on fertilization and prenatal development. *J. Reprod. Fertil.*, **12**, 414–15

53. Martin-DeLeon, P. A. and Boice, M. L. (1982). Sperm aging in the male and cytogenetic anomalies. An animal model. *Hum. Genet.*, **62**, 70–77

54. Martin, P. A. and Shaver, E. L. (1972). Sperm aging *in utero* and chromosomal anomalies in rabbit blastocysts. *Dev. Biol.*, **28**, 480–6

55. Szolollosi, D. (1975). Mammalian eggs aging in the fallopian tubes. In Blandau, R. J. (ed.) *Aging Gametes, Their Biology and Pathology, International Symposium on Aging Gametes*, Seattle Washington, pp. 98–121. (New York: Karger and Basel)

56. Poland, B J., Miller, J. R., Harris, M. and Livingston, J. (1981). Spontaneous abortion, a study of 1961 women and their conceptuses. *Acta Obstet. Gynecol. Scand.* (Suppl.), **102**, 1–32

57. Lowry, R. B., Hill, R. H. and Tischler, B. (1983). Survival and spectrum of anomalies in the Meckel syndrome. *Am. J. Med. Genet.*, **14**, 417–21

58. Byrne, J. and Warburton, D. (1986). Neural tube defects in spontaneous abortion. *Am. J. Med. Genet.*, **25**, 327–33

59. Gurgey, A., Altay, C., Beksac, M. S., Bhattacharya, R., Kutlar, F. and Huisman, T. H. J. (1989). Hydrops fetalis due to homozygosity for α-thalassemia-1, -(α)-20.5kb: the first observation in a Turkish family. *Acta Haematol.*, **81**, 169–71

60. Wettke-Schafer, R. and Kantner, G. (1983). X-linked dominant inherited diseases with lethality in hemizygous males. *Hum. Genet.*, **64**, 1–23

61. Scott, M. P. and Carroll, S. B. (1987). The segmentation and homeotic gene network in early *Drosophila* development. *Cell*, **51**, 689–98

62. Gehring, W. J. (1985). Homeotic genes, the homeo-box and genetic control of development. *Cold Spring Harbor Symposium on Quantitative Biology*, **50**, 243–51

63. Su, B. C., Strand, D., McDonough, P. G. and McDonald, J. F. (1988). Temporal and constitutive expression of homobox-2 gene (Hu-2), human-heat-shock gene (hsp-70) and oncogenes C-*sis* and N-*myc* in early human trophoblast. *Am. J. Obstet. Gynecol.*, **159**, 1195–9

64. Pfeifer-Ohlsson, S., Rydnert, J., Goustin, A. S., Larsson, E., Betsholtz, C. and Ohlsson, R. (1985). Cell-type specific pattern of *myc* proto-oncogene expression in developing human embryos. *Proc. Natl. Acad. Sci. USA*, **82**, 5050–4

65. Gilula, N. B. (1974). Junctions between cells. In Cox, R. P. (ed.) *Cell Communication*, pp. 1–29. (New York: Wiley)

66. Lohler, J., Timpl, R. and Jaenisch, R. (1984). Embryonic lethal mutation in mouse collagen I gene causes rupture of blood vessels and is associated with erythropoietic and mesenchymal cell death. *Cell*, **38**, 597–607

67. Dush, M. K., Sikela, J. M., Khan, S. A., Tischfield, J. A. and Stambrook, P. J. (1985). Nucleotide sequence and organization of the mouse adenine phosphoribosyl-transferase gene. Presence of a coding region common to animal and bacterial phosphoribosyltransferases that has a variable intron/exon arrangement. *Proc. Natl. Acad. Sci. USA*, **82**, 2731–5

68. Tyson, F. L. and Essien, F. B. (1985). Prenatal expression of a lethal genetic defect in carbohydrate metabolism in mice. *Proc. Natl. Acad. Sci. USA*, **82**, 2101–5

69. McDonough, P. G. (1988). The role of molecular mutation in recurrent euploidic abortion. *Sem. Reprod. Endocrinol.*, **6**, 155–61

70. Covarrubias, L., Nishida, Y. and Mintz, G. (1986). Early postimplantation lethality due to DNA rearrangements in a transgenic mouse strain. *Proc. Natl. Acad. Sci. USA*, **83**, 6020–4

71. Johnson, M. P., Drugan, A., Kopitch, F. C. III, Uhlmann, W. R. and Evans, M. I. (1990). Post-mortem chorionic villus sampling is a better method for cytogenetic evaluation of early fetal loss than culture of abortus material. *Am. J. Obstet. Gynecol.*, **163**, 1505–10

72. McDonough, P. G. and Tho, S. P. T. (1984). Recurrent abortion. In Sciarra, J. J., Speroff, L. and Simpson, J. L. (eds.) *Gynecology and Obstetrics*, 12th edn., Vol. 5, p.2. (Philadelphia, PA: J. B. Lippincott)

Immunological and hematological abnormalities and recurrent pregnancy loss

S. Daya

15

Introduction

Various factors have been suggested to play a role in the etiology of recurrent spontaneous abortion (RSA). Some of these are well established, whereas others are supported only by anecdotal evidence. There remains a substantial proportion of women in whom no obvious cause can be determined. Increasing attention is being drawn towards immunological mechanisms and the treatment of RSA and there is also some information to suggest a role for hematological disorders.

Immunological abnormalities

Alloimmunity and recurrent abortion

The concept of the role of immunology in RSA initially focused on viewing the feto-trophoblast unit as a type of allograft that is rejectable like a kidney graft. Non-specific effector cells, such as macrophages and natural killer (NK) cells, are spontaneously active and can recognize primitive embryonic cells in a non-antigen-specific manner to cause cytolysis and cytostasis. Trophoblast damage and pregnancy loss can occur due to these effector cells. Studies in normal murine and human pregnancy suggest that the action of these effector cells can be prevented by trophoblast cells activating potent, non-T suppressor cells in the decidua[1]. IgG produced in the female against paternal antigens binds to antigens on the trophoblast and also to Fc receptors expressed on the suppressor cells. In this way the suppressor cells are stimulated by

trophoblast to produce molecules which are closely related to transforming growth factor β_2 (TGF-β_2). These molecules have suppressive activity and confer protection to the feto-trophoblast unit by preventing attack by maternal effector cells. It is presumed that in some women with RSA, physiological activation of these cells does not occur or is defective. Thus, when the female is presented with her partner's antigens on the outer surface of the fetal trophoblast at the feto-maternal interface, an adequate protective response does not occur and predisposes her to abortion. The observation that recurrent abortion is partner specific and often does not occur when the female changes her partner supports this notion.

Some of the antigens that are required to activate the protective response in the decidua may be present on the circulating leukocytes of the male partner. Thus, deliberate immunization of the female using large numbers of her partner's leukocytes should induce the required protective response and prevent further miscarriages. Alternatively, passive immunization with intravenous immunoglobulin may be considered.

Active immunization with paternal leukocytes

Attempts to stimulate protective immune responses by immunizing the female with allogeneic leukocytes have resulted in successful pregnancies. The first randomized controlled trial of paternal leukocyte immunization demonstrated significant improvement in the successful pregnancy rate compared to controls[2]. Similar results were also obtained in another smaller randomized controlled study[3]. However, the results in subsequent studies raised doubts about the efficacy of immunization therapy because the difference in outcome between the treated and control groups was not significant. Thus, opinions on the role of allogeneic leukocyte immunization have become polarized with opponents strongly arguing against the use of such therapy.

To try and resolve this controversy, a worldwide collaborative study was commissioned under the auspices of the Ethics Committee of the American Society for Reproductive Immunology. The results demonstrated that the probability of live birth in the group treated with immunization was significantly higher than that in the control group[4,5]. The patient profile associated with a high chance of success was one with unexplained primary RSA, no evidence of pretreatment antipaternal antibody and no autoimmune abnormalities. In such patients, the relative reduction in spontaneous abortion risk is 30%, i.e. the live-birth rate can be improved up to 30% (Figure 1). The challenge that now awaits is to develop better diagnostic tests to identify those patients with alloimmune recognition failure who are likely to derive maximal benefit from this therapeutic approach. The present approach of first excluding other causes of RSA and then offering leukocyte immunization to those with unexplained RSA is not efficient. Long-term follow-up studies are also necessary to identify complications and side effects of this treatment.

Passive immunization with intravenous immunoglobulin Studies in murine models of recurrent abortion have demonstrated that passive transfer of serum from females immunized with paternal antigens is effective in reducing the high rate of fetal resorption. Similar results were also achieved by the use of pooled murine immunoglobulin. These observations suggest that the administration of human polyvalent immunoglobulins prepared from large donor pools might be suitable for the prevention of recurrent abortion in humans.

Several studies on this approach to treatment have been conducted. To date, the results have demonstrated variable outcomes, probably reflecting the variability in patient selection criteria and treatment schedules[6,7]. In general, immunoglobulin is administered intravenously at a dose of approximately 500 mg/kg. Treatment is begun in the follicular phase of the cycle when pregnancy is desired or as soon as pregnancy is confirmed and is continued every 3–4 weeks until delivery or until 28–32 weeks' gestation. The criteria for treatment have included women with two or more abortions, three or more abortions and those with recurrent second trimester losses. Such variability in treatment regimens and patient populations makes it very difficult to compare results from different studies. Nevertheless, there appears to be some evidence from controlled trials to support the role of intravenous immunoglobulin in unexplained RSA.

Autoimmunity and recurrent abortion

The role of autoimmune abnormalities in RSA was initially described in patients with systemic lupus erythematosis and now appears to be generally accepted. Recurrent fetal loss (both miscarriage and intrauterine fetal death) and thrombotic events have been reported in women with autoimmune disease. The antiphospholipid syndrome, which is a milder condition, refers to the presence of antiphospholipid antibodies and RSA, but no history of thrombotic events or autoimmune disease. Although the proposed pathophysiological mechanisms remain unconfirmed, it is believed that the antiphospholipid antibodies cause an alteration in the coagulation pathways by interacting with the platelet-endothelial interface.

Testing for the antiphospholipid syndrome involves the use of a coagulation-based assay to detect the lupus anticoagulant and an enzyme-linked immunosorbent assay to detect anticardiolipin IgG and IgM antibodies. The role of antinuclear antibodies in this disorder is not clear, especially since they are not uncommonly found in women with no history of pregnancy losses.

Several treatment options have been suggested for this syndrome including acetylsalicylic acid (ASA), prednisone and heparin. Although improvement in outcome has been observed in case series, experimental evidence demonstrating efficacy of any of these treatments is lacking. Furthermore, prednisone is associated with significant side effects such as Cushingoid features, pregnancy-induced hypertension, gestational diabetes, poor wound healing, infection, myopathy, osteoporosis, necrosis of the femoral head and intrauterine growth restriction. Until the optimal treatment regimen can be established, women with autoimmune abnormalities and RSA should be treated and monitored in centers with expertise in managing such problems.

Hematological abnormalities

In the last few years, there have been several reports of hematological abnormalities, such as thrombocythemia and impaired fibrinolytic activity (manifested by an imbalance between tissue plasminogen activator and its inhibitor), as risk factors for RSA.

Essential thrombocythemia

Essential thrombocythemia is a relatively uncommon chronic myeloproliferative disorder that is increasingly being observed in asymptomatic patients. Although it presents generally in the 50–70-year age group, it has been reported to be associated with obstetric complications and RSA in younger women[8]. The diagnosis is made by a sustained elevation of the platelet count with values usually greater than $1 \times 10^6/\mu l$. In the peripheral blood smear, the platelets exhibit a wide variation in size and are sometimes seen in aggregates.

Many of the pregnancy complications from this disorder are believed to be due to platelet occlusions that cause recurrent thromboses and placental infarction which lead to placental insufficiency and pregnancy failure. Although

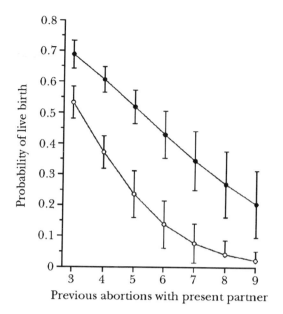

Figure 1 Probability of live birth with allogeneic leukocyte immunization (closed circles) in unexplained primary recurrent spontaneous abortion compared to controls (open circles). Reproduced from reference 5 with permission

ASA administration during pregnancy has been advocated in these patients, the reports of normal outcomes in untreated patients raise doubts about its therapeutic efficacy. Similarly, there is no experimental evidence supporting the other treatment options that have been suggested such as dypyridamol, heparin and plateletpheresis. Thus, recommendations for appropriate management of women with essential thrombocythemia and RSA are difficult to make owing to limited experience in this area.

Impaired fibrinolytic activity

Factor XII (FXII) plays a major role in the initiation of the intrinsic pathway of blood coagulation, fibrinolysis and *in vitro* kinin formation. Deficiency of FXII is an uncommon event that is inherited in an autosomal recessive manner and is associated with vascular thromboses. Although deficiency of factor XII is rare in the general population, it has been reported to be associated with an increased risk of recurrent abortion[9,10]. The reduction in FXII is believed to predispose women to having placental thrombosis because of defects in fibrinolysis activation. The magnitude of FXII deficiency appears to be directly correlated with the number of previous abortions, thereby supporting a possible causal association. Fibrinolytic components are also believed to play a role in trophoblast invasiveness suggesting that RSA may result from limitation of trophoblast growth secondary to impaired fibrinolytic capacity.

Defects in fibrinolysis activation resulting from reduced FXII levels may occur via two possible mechanisms. In the first model, the FXII-dependent generation of kallikreins, which liberate bradykinin, would be reduced thereby causing less stimulation of tissue plasminogen activator. In the second model, the reduction in kallikrein might result in diminished inhibition of plasminogen activator inhibitor 1, which is a major fibrinolysis inhibitor. The finding of higher amounts of plasminogen activator inhibitor activity in women with RSA supports this hypothesis[11]. It has also been observed that activators and inhibitors of the fibrinolytic system are frequently abnormal in women with RSA. Although FXII deficiency may be one predisposing factor for this abnormality, there may be other factors involved.

These interesting observations should prompt further research in the area of hematological abnormalities and RSA so that appropriate diagnostic and treatment recommendations can be made to help these women with RSA have successful pregnancies.

References

1. Daya, S. (1995). Allogeneic leukocyte immunization: treatment for unexplained recurrent miscarriage. In Singal, D. P. (ed.) *Immunological Effects of Blood Transfusion.* (Boca Raton, Fl: CRC Press) (in press)
2. Mowbray, J. F., Gibbings, C., Liddell, H., Reginald, P. W., Underwood, J. and Beard, R. W. (1985). A controlled trial of treatment of recurrent spontaneous abortion by immunization with paternal cells. *Lancet*, i, 941–3
3. Clark, D. A. and Daya, S. (1991). Trials and tribulation in the treatment of recurrent spontaneous abortion. *Am. J. Reprod. Immunol.*, **25**, 18–24
4. The Recurrent Miscarriage Immunotherapy Trialists Group. (1994). Worldwide collaborative observational study and meta-analysis on allogeneic leukocyte immunotherapy for recurrent spontaneous abortion. *Am. J. Reprod. Immunol.*, **32**, 55–72
5. Daya, S., Gunby, J. and The Recurrent Miscarriage Immunotherapy Trialists Group. (1994). The effectiveness of allogeneic leukocyte immunization in unexplained primary recurrent spontaneous abortion. *Am. J. Reprod. Immunol.*, **32**, 294–302
6. Mueller-Eckhardt, G. (1994). Immunotherapy with intravenous immunoglobulin for prevention of recurrent pregnancy loss: European experience. *Am. J. Reprod. Immunol.*, **32**, 281–5
7. Coulam, C. B. (1994). Immunotherapy with intravenous immunoglobulin for treatment of recurrent pregnancy loss: American experience. *Am. J. Reprod. Immunol.*, **32**, 286–9
8. Schafer, A. I. (1991). Essential thrombocythemia. *Progress in Haemostasis and Thrombosis*, **10**, 69–96
9. Schved, J. F., Gris, J. C., Neveu, S., Dupaigne, D. and Mares, P. (1989). Factor XII congenital deficiency and early spontaneous abortion. *Fertil. Steril.*, **52**, 335–6
10. Braulke, I., Pruggmayer, M., Melloh, P., Hinney, B., Kostering, H. and Gunther, E. (1993). Factor XII (Hageman) deficiency in women with habitual abortion: new subpopulation of recurrent aborters? *Fertil. Steril.*, **59**, 98–101
11. Gris, J-C., Neveu, S., Mares, P., Biron, C., Hedon, B. and Schved, J-F. (1993). Plasma fibrinolytic activators and their inhibitors in women suffering from early recurrent abortion of unknown etiology. *J. Lab. Clin. Med.*, **122**, 606–15

Medical care for recurrent pregnancy loss

16

I. Maral and M. Tasdemir

Introduction

Recurrent spontaneous abortion is defined as three or more pregnancy wastages before 20 weeks' gestation with a fetus weighing less than 500 g. Cases with two abortions have also been included recently in the recurrent abortion classification. Recurrent abortion is the cause of childlessness in 2–5% of reproducing couples[1]. The incidence of first-trimester abortion following one loss is 22–25%; after two losses, 26–31%; and after three losses, 32–47%[2]. Primary aborters are sometimes defined as those women who have never had a successful pregnancy, and secondary aborters, as those whose repetitive abortions follow a live birth. The incidence of primary and secondary habitual abortions is 0.7% and 0.2%, respectively, of all pregnancies[3].

Causes of recurrent abortion

Genetic factors

Genetic factors constitute 4–7% of the causes of habitual abortions. For diagnosis, a careful reproductive history including a three-generation pedigree and karyotyping of both parents and any previous aborted material should be obtained. Causes of genetic errors include translocation of paternal chromosomes, chromosomal variation as recombination defects, genetic factors such as biochemical disorders and homozygous dominant inheritance, environmental agents (radiation, chemicals, medications), TORCH infections and delayed fertilization. If the defect is paternal, artificial insemination by donor is the only option available. For a maternal defect, egg donation may be considered.

Anatomical causes

Approximately 12–15% of women with recurrent abortion have various uterine anomalies including septate uterus, cervical incompetence, Müllerian anomalies such as bicornuate or unicornuate uterus, leimyomata, Asherman's syndrome and abnormalities due to diethylstilbestrol exposure *in utero*. Beside hysterosalpingography, the best diagnosis can be achieved by the use of vaginal ultrasonography and magnetic resonance imaging. In treatment, the results of surgery have been very impressive.

Infectious causes

The incidence of infections with *Ureoplasma urealyticum* and *Mycoplasma hominis* has been reported to be significantly higher in patients with recurrent abortions than in a control group[4]. Recently, it has been claimed that *Toxoplasma gondii* may cause sporadic abortion, but not recurrent abortion due to the acquired immunity to this parasite. Other micro-organisms including *Chlamydia trachomatis*[5], herpes simplex, *Treponema pallidum*, *Brucella*, *Listeria monocytogenes* and *Neisseria gonorrhoeae* have been implicated, but their influence has not been substantiated. Antibiotics should be given if infection is confirmed, and appropriate follow-up should be carried out to monitor therapy. It is usually more cost-effective and time-efficient to treat couples empirically with a course of doxycycline (100 mg twice a day for 2 weeks) or erythromycin (250 mg four times a day for 2 weeks) than to pursue sophisticated diagnostic procedures.

Endocrine factors

Hormonal causes of habitual abortion include significant thyroid dysfunction, progesterone insufficiency and uncontrolled diabetes mellitus. It is unlikely that laboratory assessment of thyroid function is worthwhile in relatively healthy women. Although the association between diabetes mellitus and recurrent early pregnancy loss is not clearly established, we generally test patients for this disorder. Luteal phase insufficiency, characterized by deficient ovarian function with inadequate progesterone synthesis, was first defined as the cause of recurrent abortion in the late 1940s. Insufficiency of the corpus luteum is the etiological factor for 23–50% of recurrent abortions[6]. Diagnosis is usually made by serum progesterone measurements at about 3 days before expected menstruation rather than in the midluteal phase[7], by luteal phase endometrial biopsies and by basal body temperature measurements.

Endometrial biopsy has become the standard diagnostic method accepted by most investigators. If repetitive endometrial biopsies indicate a lack in histological development of more than 2 days, or if the basal body chart shows a luteal phase of less than 11 days, the use of progesterone or drugs for induction of ovulation may be indicated accordingly[8].

The most commonly advocated treatment is vaginal suppositories 25 mg twice daily. Successful pregnancy rates of 70–90% have been reported. The risk of producing a missed abortion has limited the use of progesterone[9]. There are controversial reports regarding the use of ovulatory agents such as clomiphene, bromocriptine and gonadotropins[10].

Environmental factors

Environmental factors including various drugs, radiation, alcohol and heavy coffee consumption are associated with an increased risk of recurrent abortion[11]. An increase in risk is proportional to the number of cigarettes smoked[10,12].

Immunological factors

Although mechanisms that prevent rejection of the conceptus are incompletely understood, recent evidence suggests that maternal immunological aberrations may cause repeated abortions. Current methods of detection find no recognized cause in 30–50% of all patients with recurrent abortion. This group of patients may have immunological causes. There are two mechanisms under investigation[13]: first, autoimmune mechanisms; and, second, alloimmune mechanisms.

Autoimmunity Antiphospholipid syndrome is characterized by recurrent pregnancy wastages, vascular thrombosis, thrombocytopenia and the presence of antiphospholipid antibodies. The lupus anticoagulant and anticardiolipin antibodies are antiphospholipid antibodies and are detected in 10–16% of women with recurrent abortions. The antiphospholipid antibodies are directed against platelets and the vascular endothelium, and cause thrombosis, spontaneous abortion and fetal wastage. These antibodies block prostacyclin formation, which results in unbalanced thromboxane activity, leading to vasoconstriction and thrombosis. It is suggested that the maternal vascular and placental lesions are due to thromboxane dominance, which in turn predisposes to vasoconstriction, platelet aggregation and intravascular thrombosis. Clinical features, other than recurrent abortion, associated with antiphospholipid antibodies include thrombotic episodes, thrombocytopenia, chorea gravidarum and a postpartum syndrome consisting of fever, pneumonitis, pleural effusions and myocarditis. The antiphospholipid antibodies prolong the prothrombin time and the partial thromboplastin time. Measurement of the activated partial thromboplastin time is a relatively sensitive screening test. Women with recurrent abortions should be screened for activated partial thromboplastin time, kaolin clotting time and anticardiolipin antibodies[14].

In a recent case–control study, we determined that activated partial thromboplastin time is a valuable screening test for autoimmune causes of recurrent abortion when it is used together with a test for anticardiolipin antibodies. For these women, in an effort to inhibit autoantibody synthesis and to interfere with antigen–antibody interaction, a combination of prednisone (40–60 mg/day) and aspirin (75–80 mg/day) has been recommended as the treatment of choice. Aspirin is added to restore a normal prostacyclin–thromboxane balance and inhibit platelet aggregation. Therapy should be initiated as soon as pregnancy is confirmed. Monitoring of the treatment is by measurement of serum activated partial thromboplastin time. The dose of prednisone is titrated to normalize the activated partial thromboplastin time. After 3–4 weeks, the level returns to normal and the dose of prednisone is tapered off.

With this regimen, successful live-birth rates of 70–75% have been reported. Treatment failure due to insufficient suppression of the abnormal coagulation times may occur. Although neither prednisone nor aspirin is teratogenic, the use of prednisone bears the risk of intrauterine growth retardation and pregnancy-induced hypertension. There is also a high incidence of preterm delivery, fluid retention, acne, gastrointestinal ulceration and immune suppression. Aspirin can cause gastrointestinal upset and ulceration. The efficacy of steroid use remains contentious. Maternal morbidity may increase, due to systemic steroid use, which may cause oropharyngeal candidiasis, acne, facial abscess, tendency for opportunistic infections, pneumonia, cushingoid appearance, delay in wound healing, osteoporosis, gestational diabetes and postprandial adrenal insufficiency[15].

Because of the maternal side-effects of corticosteroids and fetal loss, heparin treatment has been tried[16]. Heparin increases the effect of antithrombin III, which is the inhibitor of factor X and thrombin. The treatment is initiated just after the diagnosis of pregnancy and ceases 24–48 h before the estimated time of delivery. Rosove and co-workers[16] reported 93% success with heparin treatment. Cowchoch and associates (submitted) found no significant difference between steroid and heparin treatments.

Branch and colleagues[17] achieved pregnancy in all of the eight patients treated with heparin and aspirin. Successful results with the use of heparin have been reported in patients with antiphospholipid antibodies[16,18]. Treatment is monitored by coagulation time, adjusted to 1.5–2 times normal. If the activated partial thromboplastin time is long, monitoring is achieved by measurement of thrombin time, adjusted to 100 s. Long-term heparin use may cause bone demineralization of the mother[16]. Heparin should not be used together with corticosteroids, because each drug may potentiate the other's osteoporotic effect. Rarely, thrombocytopenia, thromboemboli, disseminated intravascular coagulation and death are seen[19]. The number of studies about heparin use is limited, and the role of heparin treatment in recurrent abortion is a debatable issue. Further studies are needed to verify its effectiveness and to determine its side-effects. Although there is limited information, success with azathioprine and plasmapheresis has been reported[20,21].

Some investigators have reported successful outcome with close pregnancy follow-up in the treatment of women with recurrent abortion. Trudenger and associates[22] reported live birth in all of the six women who received close clinical follow-up and Doppler examinations. However, close clinical follow-up and Doppler measurements are not helpful in pregnancy loss before 20 weeks of gestation. For this reason, treatment should be initiated as soon as pregnancy is confirmed.

Alloimmunity In general, the alloimmunity involves an abnormal maternal response to antigens on placental or fetal tissues. The mechanism of alloimmune rejection involves presentation of an antigen to the host immune system, which causes the production of antibodies and cytotoxic lymphocytes that return via the bloodstream to destroy the fetoplacental tissue. In normal pregnancy, blocking factors prevent the rejection of the fetus. Couples with recurrent abortions have increased sharing of human leukocyte antigens (HLA), most prominently at the DR locus. This clinical condition is usually associated with lack of blocking factors. On the other hand, many investigators have failed to confirm increased HLA sharing in couples with recurrent abortion. Immunotherapy to achieve a favorable maternal immune response to protect the developing embryo may be indicated. Production of maternal lymphocytotoxic antibodies in response to paternal human lymphocyte antigens has long been recognized. These leukocytotoxic antibodies are found in 12–23% of women with recurrent abortions. Appropriate recognition of fetoplacental antigens by the maternal immune system is needed for implantation and survival of the embryo. Suppressor T cells, present in the endometrium, modulate and suppress the local immune response to the implanting embryo.

Treatment for recurrent abortion

Immunotherapy

Immunization can be divided into two, according to whether it is active or passive.

Active immunization   In this type of immunization, the aim is to initiate the development of blocking and leukocytotoxic antibodies, by, first, immunization with paternal leukocytes, or, second, immunization with third-party (donor) leukocytes.

Although the hypothesis that the immunogenetic compatibility between the mother and fetus is responsible for reproductive problems is debatable, in HLA sharing with absence of blocking antibodies and leukocytotoxic antibodies, paternal leukocyte injection can be employed to induce a beneficial maternal immune response. Several investigators have reported a 70–80% success rate with immunization by paternal and third-party leukocytes[23–25]. In another controlled study, live-birth rates of 78% and 51% have been reported in groups that received partner's leukocytes and isotonic saline solution (control), respectively[26]. The only potential risk is the erythrocyte antigen sensitization from incompatible red cells.

The other type of immunotherapy involves the injection of third-party (donor) leukocytes. Although there is no case reported, in donor immunization maternal infection by HIV, hepatitis virus and cytomegalovirus is a potential risk. For this reason, immunization with frozen donor lymphocytes, trophoblast membrane antigens and vaginal suppositories containing seminal plasma antigens is under investigation.

The success of immunization depends on the development of blocking factors and leukocytotoxic antibodies. Gatenby and colleagues[27] reported a 55% success rate by paternal leukocyte infusion, and claimed that this success was closely related to the early leukocyte antibody development. Carp and co-workers[28] verified this finding with a success rate of 75% following antibody development. If the maternal response of the development of blocking factors and leukocytotoxic antibodies does not occur, the pregnancy usually results in spontaneous abortion. If immunization with paternal leukocytes fails, reimmunization with donor leukocytes is not helpful, either. Unander and associates[29] claimed that the presence of antiphospholipid antibodies may be a predictor for the success of the treatment, but the presence of a high titer of antibodies should warn the clinician of the possibility of coexisting autoimmune diseases such as systemic lupus erythematosus.

Passive immunization   Passive immunization is the intravenous immunoglobulin treatment of pregnant patients with recurrent pregnancy loss caused by antiphospholipid antibodies. Its mechanism of action is unclear, but one possibility is that IgG molecules compete for and bind to receptors on the surface of macrophages, thereby reducing access to pathogenic cells. Immunoglobulins block Fc receptors, leading to their internalization and decreasing the ability of the effector cells to remove platelets. Intravenous immunoglobulin therapy has the ability to hinder the immune response by masking the recognition of the class II major histocompatibility complex[30]. Success rates of 70–80% by passive immunization have been reported[31–33].

The advantages of passive immunization when compared with leukocyte immunotherapy are: (1) the protective effect starts right after the immunization; (2) it is a good alternative for patients who did not respond to leukocyte immunization; and (3) after treatment with leukocytes, HLA immunization occurs, which is potentially hazardous during future blood transfusions and organ transplantation. This is not a problem after passive immunization.

Allergic reactions after intravenous immunoglobulin administration usually occur in IgA-deficient individuals. The anticomplement effects of aggregates of immunoglobulin can produce vasomotor symptoms such as chills, nausea and flushing. Although no case has been reported, there is a potential risk of HIV and hepatitis virus infection with intravenous immunoglobulin treatment, because it is prepared from a large number of donors.

Human chorionic gonadotropin treatment

Human chorionic gonadotropin (hCG) is a placental glycoprotein, produced exclusively by trophoblastic tissue. Its synthesis is suggested to be under the control of placental gonadotropin releasing hormone. Its glycoprotein structure consists of two chains, α and β. Although the α subunit is shared in common with thyroid stimulating hormone and LH, the β subunit determines the unique biological and immunological properties of hCG. hCG in maternal sera can be measured directly after implantation, 8–9 days after the LH surge. It has a crucial role in the maintenance of early pregnancy.

The level of hCG changes during pregnancy. Harrison and co-workers[34] have studied the hCG levels in 20 patients between 4 and 16 weeks of gestation and measured the hCG levels twice weekly. In 14 of these with normal pregnancy, after an initial rise, a plateau at 7–9 weeks of gestation was demonstrated, followed by a further rise, which reached a maximum at the 11th week of gestation. The level of hCG then decreased until the 16th week of pregnancy. If the hCG level does not increase three-fold

weekly, the pregnancy usually results in abortion. hCG is a natural endocrine product of the fetoplacental unit. It does not carry any potential risk when given exogenously. It not only stimulates steroid synthesis exogenously, but also is an alternative to other supporting treatments. In corpus luteum insufficiency, several researchers such as Blumenfeld and Nahhas[35] recommended the administration of hCG to stimulate synthesis of factors and hormones rather than exogenous administration of their supplement. *In vitro*, hCG stimulates steroidogenesis. *In vivo*, it supports the corpus luteum and has a placentatropic effect.

Patient selection and treatment   In patients with no detectable etiology or treatable hormone deficiency, hCG treatment should be considered. In investigating the etiology of recurrent abortion, genetic, anatomical, infectious, endocrine, environmental and immunological causes should be evaluated. The presence of systemic diseases suspected to cause abortion, such as chronic renal insufficiency, should be evaluated.

Treatment should be initiated as soon as the fetal viability is confirmed by ultrasonography. The first clinical report about hCG use in recurrent aborters was in 1953 by Holund[36] who used 6000 IU intramuscularly per day for 5 days and achieved a 72% fetal salvage rate. Sandler and Baillie[37] used hCG 10 000 IU intramuscularly three times a week as a prophylactic treatment for recurrent aborters and achieved a 85% success rate.

Harrison[38] established a cost-effective regimen with a 93% success rate. In a placebo-controlled prospective study[39], we employed this regimen to investigate the effect of hCG in 40 pregnant women with recurrent abortion of unexplained etiology. Patients were randomly allocated into hCG treatment and control groups. Both of the groups consisted of ten ovulation-induced (human menopausal gonadotropin/hCG and clomiphene citrate/hCG) pregnancies and ten spontaneous pregnancies. For the hCG (Pregnyl®, Organon) treatment group, after the initial dose of

Table 1 Pregnancy wastage in pregnancies (generated by ovulation-inducing drugs or spontaneous), treated by human chorionic gonadotropin (hCG) or placebo

	Ovulation induction	Spontaneous pregnancy	Total
hCG			
n	10	10	20
abortions	0	0	0
wastage (%)	0	0	0
Placebo			
n	10	10	20
abortions	8	6	14
wastage (%)	80	60	70
Statistics	$p < 0.05$	$p < 0.05$	$p < 0.05$

10 000 IU, 5000 IU was given twice weekly until the 12th week. Treatment was continued at 5000 IU once a week until the 16th week. Ampules containing equal quantities but no active substance (0.9% NaCl) were used for the control group. As is shown in Table 1, while no abortion was seen in 20 pregnancies treated by hCG, 14 (eight in the ovulation-induced and six in the spontaneous pregnancies) miscarriages occurred in the placebo group. This difference between groups was statistically significant ($p < 0.05$).

We concluded that empirical treatment with repetitive hCG administration between early gestation and the 16th week of gestation is highly effective in decreasing pregnancy wastage in cases with recurrent abortion.

Diagnosing the etiology of recurrent abortion has prime importance for its treatment. A meticulous approach for diagnosis is needed. The treatment should be initiated as soon as the diagnosis is reached. Besides organic causes, the incidence of sociopsychological problems is relatively high in couples with recurrent abortion. The anxiety of abortion is replaced by depression after the loss of pregnancy. For these reasons, while treating these women, psychological support may also be needed.

References

1. Roman, F. (1984). Fetal loss rates and their relation to pregnancy order. *J. Epidemiol. Community Health.*, **38**, 29–35
2. Poland, B. J., Miller, J. R., Jones, D. C. and Trimble, B. K. (1977). Reproductive counseling in patients who have had a spontaneous abortion. *Am. J. Obstet. Gynecol.*, **127**, 685–91
3. McIntyre, J. A., Faulk, W. P., Nichols-Johnson, V. R. and Taylor, C. F. (1986). Immunological testing and immunotherapy in recurrent spontaneous abortion. *Obstet. Gynecol.*, **67**, 169–75
4. Lomey, J. R., Foy, H. M. and Kenny, G. F. (1974). Infection with *Mycoplasma hominis* and T-strains in the female genital tract. *Obstet. Gynecol.*, **44**, 703–8
5. Witkin, S. S. and Leger, W. J. (1992). Antibodies to *Chlamydia trachomatis* in sera of women with recurrent spontaneous abortions. *Am. J. Obstet. Gynecol.*, **167**, 135–9
6. Hargar, J. H., Archer, D. F., Marchese, S. G., Muracca-Clemens, M. and Garver, K. L. (1983). Etiology of recurrent pregnancy losses and outcome of subsequent pregnancies. *Obstet. Gynecol.*, **62**, 574–81
7. Daya, S. (1989). Optimal time in the menstrual cycle for serum progesterone measurement to diagnose luteal phase defects. *Am. J. Obstet. Gynecol.*, **161**, 1009–11
8. Wentz, A. C., Herbert, C. M., Maxson, W. S. and Garner, C. H. (1984). Outcome of progesterone treatment of luteal phase inadequacy. *Fertil. Steril.*, **41**, 856–62
9. Scott, J. R. (1990). Spontaneous abortion. In Scott, J. R., Di Sala, T. J., Hammond, C. B. and Spellacy, W. N. (eds.) *Danforth's Obstetrics and Gynecology*, pp. 215–17. (Philadelphia: Lippincott)
10. Stirrad, G. M. (1990). Recurrent miscarriage II: Clinical associations, causes and management. *Lancet*, **336**, 728–33
11. Regan, L. (1992). Recurrent early pregnancy failure. *Curr. Opin. Obstet. Gynecol.*, **4**, 220–8
12. Harger, J. H., Archer, D. F. and Marchese, S. G. (1983). Etiology of recurrent pregnancy losses

and outcome of subsequent pregnancies. *Obstet. Gynecol.*, **62**, 574–81

13. Carp, H. J. A., Toder, V., Mashiach, S., Nebel, L. and Serr, D. M. (1990). Recurrent miscarriage: a review of current concepts, immune mechanisms and results of treatment. *Obstet. Gynecol. Surv.*, **45**, 657–69

14. Lockwood, C. J., Romero, R., Feinberg, R. F., Clyne, L. P., Coster, B. and Hobbins, J. C. (1989). The prevalence and biologic significance of lupus anticoagulant and anticardiolipin antibodies in a general obstetric population. *Am. J. Obstet. Gynecol.*, **161**, 369–73

15. Hughes, G. R. V. (1983). Thrombosis, abortion, cerebral disease and the lupus anticoagulant. *Br. Med. J.*, **287**, 1088–9

16. Rosove, M. H., Tabsh, K. and Wasserstrum, N. (1990). Heparin therapy for pregnant women with lupus anticoagulant or anticardiolipin antibodies. *Obstet. Gynecol.*, **75**, 630–4

17. Branch, D. W., Blackwell, J. and Dudley, D. J. (1990). Antiphospholipid antibody syndrome (APAS): treated pregnancy outcome and medical follow up. Presented at the *37th Annual Meeting of the Society for Gynecologic Investigation*, p. 285 (abstr.)

18. Scott, J. R., Rote, N. S. and Branch, D. W. (1987). Immunologic aspects of recurrent abortion and fetal death. *Obstet. Gynecol.*, **70**, 645–56

19. Klein, H. G. and Bell, W. R. (1974). Disseminated intravascular coagulation during heparin therapy. *Ann. Intern. Med.*, **80**, 477–81

20. Exner, T., Rickard, K. A. and Kronenberg, H. (1978). A sensitive test demonstrating lupus anticoagulant and its behavioral patterns. *Br. J. Haematol.*, **40**, 143–51

21. Gregorini, G., Setti, G. and Remuzzi, G. (1986). Recurrent abortion with lupus anticoagulant and preeclampsia: a common final pathway for two different diseases? Case report. *Br. J. Obstet. Gynaecol.*, **93**, 194–6

22. Trudenger, B. H., Steward, G. J. and Cook, C. M. (1988). Monitoring lupus anticoagulant positive pregnancies with umbilical artery waveforms. *Obstet. Gynecol.*, **72**, 215–18

23. Mowbray, J. F., Gibbings, J., Liddell, H., Reginald, P. W., Underwood, J. L. and Beard, R. W. (1985). Controlled trial of treatment of recurrent spontaneous abortion by immunization with paternal cells. *Lancet*, **1**, 941

24. McIntyre, J. A., McConnachie, P. R., Taylor, C. G. and Faulk, W. P. (1984). Clinical immunologic and genetic definitions of primary and secondary recurrent spontaneous abortion. *Fertil. Steril.*, **42**, 849–55

25. Unander, A. M. and Lindholm, A. (1986). Transfusions of leukocyte-rich erythrocytes: a successful treatment in selected cases of habitual abortion. *Am. J. Obstet. Gynecol.*, **154**, 516–20

26. Scott, J. R., Rote, N. S. and Branch, D. W. (1987). Immunologic aspects of recurrent abortion and fetal death. *Obstet. Gynecol.*, **70**, 645–56

27. Gatenby, P. A., Moore, H., Cameron, K., Doran, T. J. and Adelstein, S. (1989). Treatment of recurrent spontaneous abortion by immunization with paternal lymphocytes with outcome. *Am. J. Reprod. Immunol.*, **19**, 21–7

28. Carp, H. J., Toder, V. and Gazit, E. (1990). Selection of patients with habitual abortion for paternal leukocyte immunization. *Arch. Gynecol. Obstet.*, **248**, 93–101

29. Unander, A. M. and Lindholm, A. (1986). Transfusions of leukocyte rich erythrocyte concentrates. A successful treatment in selected cases of habitual abortion. *Am. J. Obstet. Gynecol.*, **154**, 516–20

30. Oriveto, R., Achiron, A., Rafael, Z. B. and Achiron, R. (1991). Intravenous immunoglobulin treatment for recurrent abortions caused by antiphospholipid antibodies. *Fertil. Steril.*, **56**, 1013–20

31. Perino, A., Barba, G. and Climino, C. (1989). New perspectives of the therapeutic management of recurrent immunological abortion. *Acta Eur. Fertil.*, **20**, 359–62

32. Mueller-Eckhardt, G. M., Heine, O., Neppert, J., Kunze, W. and Mueller-Eckhardt, C. (1989). Prevention of recurrent spontaneous abortion by intravenous immunoglobulin. *Vox Sang.*, **56**, 151–4

33. Reece, E. A., Gabrielli, S., Cullen, M. T., Zheng, X. Z., Hobbins, J. C. and Harris, E. N. (1990). Recurrent adverse pregnancy outcome and antiphospholipid antibodies. *Am. J. Obstet. Gynecol.*, **163**, 162–9

34. Harrison, R. F., Omoore, R. R. and McSweeney, J. (1980). Maternal plasma β-hCG in early human pregnancy. *Br. J. Obstet. Gynaecol.*, **87**, 705–11

35. Blumenfeld, Z. and Nahhas, G. (1988). Luteal dysfunction in ovulation induction: the role of repetitive human chorionic gonadotropin supplementation during the luteal phase. *Fertil. Steril.*, **50**, 403–7

36. Holund, T. (1953). The use of human chorionic gonadotrophin in threatened abortion. *Acta Endocrinol.*, **12**, 61

37. Sandler, S. W. and Baillie, P. (1979). The use of human chorionic gonadotrophin in recurrent abortion. *S. Afr. Med. J.*, **55**, 832

38. Harrison, R. F. (1985). Treatment of habitual abortion with human chorionic gonadotropin: results of open and placebo controlled studies. *Eur. J. Obstet. Gynecol. Reprod. Biol.*, **20**, 159–68

39. Maral, I., Sozen, U., Balik, E., Kurt, S. and Buyuktosun, C. (1992). Human chorionic gonadotropin in the treatment of recurrent abortion. In Rodríguez-Armas, O., Baumgartner, W. and Burgos-Briceño, L. (eds.) *Fertility and Sterility. Progress in Research and Practice*, pp. 495–502. (Carnforth, UK: Parthenon Publishing)

Management of uterine congenital malformations: diagnosis

17

O. Rodriguez-Armas, O. Rousseau and P. Mares

Congenital anomalies of the female reproductive tract can be caused by a genetic error or by a teratologic event during embryonic development. Some of the abnormalities are major and may lead to severe impairment of menstrual and reproductive functions. (Most of the subprimate mammal species have double uteri. This normal anatomical finding retains the general characteristics of primitive oviducts, but is adapted to varying gestational functions.)

Whatever the embryopathological mechanism, pubertal symptoms, menstrual disorders or pregnancy complications may suggest uterine congenital malformations, sometimes related to urogenital abnormalities.

Many types of examination are available (hysterosalpingography, hysterophlebography, transvaginal ultrasonography, hysteroscopy, and, at times, magnetic resonance imaging and laparoscopy), but their own role has to be determined according to the suspected malformations.

Causes of uterine congenital malformations

Three different mechanisms can lead to uterine congenital malformations.

(1) Bilateral Müllerian agenesis is associated with vaginal aplasia and uterine aplasia. The more frequent and characteristic pathological entity is represented by Rokitansky–Küster–Hauser syndrome. It must be distinguished from Morris syndrome which results from gonadal androgen insensitivity, and is associated with an XY chromosomal constitution but a female phenotype. Urinary tract abnormalities and normal pubal pilosity are usually associated with Rokitansky–Küster–Hauser syndrome.

Unicornuate uterus is related to unilateral Müllerian agenesis. Pseudo-unicornuate uterus is ten times more frequent than the true unicornuate uterus. Frequently, these abnormalities are not associated with other genital tract abnormalities. However, urinary tract malformations, such as a missing or an ectopic kidney, are frequent.

(2) Müllerian fusion defects after 9 weeks' gestation are related to bicornuate uteri. Complete or incomplete duplication of the vagina and the cervix may be associated and are asymptomatic.

(3) Müllerian septum resorption defects lead to septate uteri or cervix atresia.

Detection

There are three types of situations which can lead to detection of uterine congenital malformations – problems with the menstrual cycle and/or sexual activity, obstetric complications and, lastly, fertility problems.

Primary amenorrhea, isolated and generally painless, is the usual means by which bilateral Müllerian agenesis is revealed, and whose diagnosis is suggested by vaginal aplasia. This revealing manifestation is often associated with dyspareunia or with apareunia.

Dysmenorrhea should lead one to suspect a pseudo-unicornuate uterus, or, exceptionally, a pseudo-unicornuate uterus with canaliculated rudimentary cornu, or sometimes asymmetric partitioned uteri (Robert's uterus), or, lastly and more rarely, cervico-isthmic atresia. The malformative origin of dysmenorrhea is revealed by the fact that primary dysmenorrhea increases progressively, is resistant to analgesic treatment and is recurrent after childbirth.

Obstetric complications include late, sometimes repetitive, spontaneous abortion (partitioned and bicornuate uterus), prematurity (unicornuate uterus, 15–25%), more rarely, delayed intrauterine growth and, lastly, podalic presentations. The incidence of uterine malformations in obstetric history is difficult to estimate, especially for late spontaneous abortions, but would seem to be around 15–30% (bicornuate, unicornuate and partitioned uteri combined).

Lastly, hypofertility and its evaluation are important ways of detecting congenital uterine anomalies. Whether it is primary or secondary, anamnesis (exposure to diethylstilbestrol), obstetric antecedents, surgery and the morphological and etiological evaluation (hysterosalpingography, hysteroscopy, coelioscopy) enable one to suspect, to detect and then to make an accurate diagnosis, although the impact on fertility is as yet not easily proven. The incidence of malformation in hypofertility may be estimated to be between 1.5 and 3%.

Diagnosis

While the clinical examination plays a vital part in the evaluation and detection of a bilateral Müllerian agenesis, it is of little effect in the diagnosis of bicornuate, partitioned or unicornuate uteri, if it does not occur in conjunction with a cervico-vaginal anomaly.

In the same way, a clinical examination of the uterus too rarely reveals the presence of a partition or a spur in the fundus uteri and is not a substitute for hysterographic examination.

Very often, the clinical examination also allows the differentiation between a 46,XY and a Rokitansky–Küster–Hauser syndrome by urethral position, the development of the labia minora and the axillo-pubic pilosity. The karyotype examination remains the basic reference

and prior urological explorations (intravenous urography, ultrasonography) enable etiological and therapeutic orientations to be detected and channelled.

Superpubic ultrasonography mostly confirms the absence of a uterine cavity and the presence of two sterile 'buds'. Coelioscopy usually only operates as a means of evaluating the upper genital apparatus and possibly for carrying out a surgical cure of vaginal aplasia using the modified Vecchietti technique.

Imaging acquires great importance in the diagnosis of unilateral agenesis and fusion and resorption defects.

At present, hysterography is the most widely used diagnosing method – a *posteriori* for certain obstetric complications and a *priori* for hypofertility evaluations looking for problems of tubal patency, where the detection of a malformed uterus is generally fortuitous. However, it is not always easy to differentiate between a bicornuate uterus and a partitioned one (angulation). It may show a communication between the two cavities. But when the two cavities are totally independent, it cannot detect the presence and the type of cavity which has not been canuled (unicornuate uterus, or pseudo-unicornuate).

By contrast, ultrasonography seems very sensitive where diagnoses of bicornuate and partitioned uteri are concerned, but very deficient with regard to unicornuate or pseudo-unicornuate uteri, all studies showing that the latter malformations are the most difficult to detect by ultrasonography. It cannot be a substitute for coelioscopy and/or hysterography and should supplement them for evaluating the characteristics of a rudimentary cornu. Ultrasound has an obvious contribution to make in the case of bicornuate uteri by making visible the intercornual vesical 'angle' (or the V) and may make possible some prophylactic treatment where detection occurs early in pregnancy.

The role of magnetic resonance imaging remains to be determined. Its sensitivity in the diagnosis of partitioned or bicornuate, and even pseudo-unicornuate uteri seems interesting. Its cost, which is still high, could be an obstacle.

If the improvement in imaging techniques, and especially ultrasonography, means that uterine malformation can be suspected or even diagnosed, it cannot at present replace the following diagnostic hierarchy: hysterography, and/or hysterophlebography, coelioscopy and hysteroscopy. This is especially true in the evaluation of hypofertility and late spontaneous abortions.

The tubal passage, examination of the fundus uterus, the communication between the two cavities, the inferior edge of a partition and the differentiation between certain corporic bicornuate uteri and partitioned uteri amount to a number of arguments in favor of this diagnostic strategy, all the more because coelioscopy and hysteroscopy allow for a concomitant therapeutic application.

Further reading

Fedele, I., Dorta, M., Vercellini, P., Brioschi, D. and Candiani, G. B. (1987). Reproductive performance of women with unicornuate uterus. *Fertil. Steril.*, **47**, 416–19

Nicolini, U., Bellotti, M., Bonazzi, B., Zamberietti, D. and Canadiani, G. B. (1987). Can ultrasound be used to scan uterine malformation? *Fertil. Steril.*, **47**, 89–93

Randolph, J. R., Kong Ying, Yu, Maier, D. B., Schmidt, C. L. and Riddick, D. H. (1986). Companion of real time ultrasonography, hystero-salpingography and laparosocpy/hysteroscopy in the evaluation of uterine abnormalities and tubal patency. *Fertil. Steril.*, **46**, 828–32

Management of uterine congenital malformations: evaluation of outcome

18

T. Makino

Introduction

The process of human reproduction is complex and inefficient[1,2]. According to recent reports, it has been suggested that approximately 10–20% of known conceptions terminate in spontaneous abortion. In our early report[3], hysterosalpingography revealed that about 14.6% of infertile women with a history of recurrent reproductive wastage have some congenital uterine anomalies, suggesting that this anomaly may have an influence on ovum implantation and early fetal development, and could consequently be involved in the etiology of spontaneous abortion.

In this study, we investigated (1) the exact incidence of congenital uterine malformation among infertile women, (2) the mechanism of induction of wastage, (3) the presurgical examination of suture threads for metroplasty, (4) the modification of metroplastic surgery for improvement of clinical prognosis in terms of the successful maintenance of pregnancy, (5) the post-operative management of patients, and (6) a control study.

These comprehensive studies could improve the outcome of pregnancy in women with a congenital uterine anomaly.

Subjects and methods

A total of 1838 couples were registered for this study by the end of 1993. The ages of female partners were distributed between 19- and 48-years-old, with a mean age of 31.43 ± 4.2 years (mean ± SD). The mean number of spontaneous abortions was 2.67 ± 1.0. As one of the routine examinations for habitual abortion 1666 hysterosalpingographies were performed in these patients.

Basic studies

Histology of the uterine septum The removed tissue specimen during metroplastic surgery was studied for the distribution of uterine arteries by a computerized tissue analyzing system[4].

Examination of surgical threads Several absorbable threads, which were utilized for metroplastic surgery, were implanted into goat uterine muscles for 2–13 weeks and the period required until complete absorption was histologically examined.

Effect of surgical threads on embryonic implantation Several absorbable threads were implanted into the rat uterus as an intrauterine device (IUD), then it was observed how soon fertility function for ovum implantation could be recovered.

Clinical studies

Diagnosis on hysterosalpingography To investigate the exact diagnosis and the incidence of uterine anomaly, uterine cavity deformity was evaluated by X/M ratio on hysterosalpingography; a method in which the longitudinal length of the uterine cavity (M) is compared with the dent of the uterine cavity (X)[2,4].

Metroplastic surgery A modified metroplasty was performed on the uterine anomalies using absorbable threads and by inserting an IUD to prevent postoperative adhesion of the reconstructed cavity. Eighty-two patients of those operated on were investigated for their subsequent pregnancy.

Study of postoperative management Contraceptive periods, time for IUD removal and management of child delivery were studied by collecting clinical opinions from 33 other institutes.

Results

Our study on the removed uterine septum revealed that these tissues from patients with congenital uterine anomaly have an inadequate blood supply[4]. In another basic study using goat uteri, it was observed that synthetic monofilamental absorbable thread was less reactive to the uterine muscles as compared to conventional catgut thread in terms of inflammatory changes and scar granulation formation. When this synthetic absorbable thread was inserted into the rat uterus as an IUD, the infertile effect lasted for the next 8 weeks inhibiting ovum implantation, but such an antifertility effect completely diminished 10 weeks after IUD insertion, showing a comparable number of the embryo implantations compared to those in the control horns.

A total of 227 congenital uterine anomalies (13.6%) were detected in the 1666 hysterosalpingographies, by applying the X/M ratio. Table 1 summarizes the incidence of each anomaly and Table 2 indicates the number of spontaneous abortions in these groups. The data show that the major group of anomalies was the $0 < X/M < 1/3$ (arcuate group), with an incidence of 61.2%, but an equal number of spontaneous abortions was detected in each group. A modified metroplasty based on our basic study performed on these 82 patients, 74 of whom had become pregnant by the time we summarized this report. Table 3 indicates that more than 81% of postoperative pregnancies were successfully terminated in two major (arcuate and partial septate) groups.

We surveyed clinical opinions on the postoperative management from 33 other institutes

Table 1 Classifications of congenital uterine anomalies by the X/M ratio using hysterosalpingography ($n = 227$). X, dent of uterine cavity; M, longitudinal length of uterine cavity

Group	Number of patients (%)
$0 < X/M < 1/3$ (arcuate)	139 (61.2)
$1/3 \leq X/M < 1$ (partial septate)	73 (32.2)
$X/M = 1$ (complete septate)	3 (1.3)
Unicornuate	6 (2.6)
T-shape	6 (2.6)
Total	227 (100)

Table 2 Grade of uterine cavity deformity and number of spontaneous abortions in 227 patients

Group	n	Total pregnancies	Spontaneous abortions	%
Arcuate	139	383	371	96.9
Partial septate	73	225	224	99.6
Complete septate	3	8	8	100
Unicornuate	6	15	15	100
T-shape	6	17	17	100

Table 3 Pregnancy outcome in 82 patients after metroplasty

	n	Full-term (%)	Spontaneous abortions	Not pregnant
Arcuate	37	28 (75.7)	4	5
Partial septate	45	39 (86.7)	3	3

where metroplastic surgery was being performed, for the treatment of habitual abortion, and this survey indicated that a minimum of three menstrual cycles after metroplasty was recommended as a contraceptive period and all pregnant cases were indicated for Cesarean section at term.

Discussion

Embryologically, fusion of the Müllerian ducts, which develop into a single uterine cavity in the human, is repeated three times at different embryonic periods. Consequently, uterine malformation can be induced at any of these stages. Among the general population, congenital uterine anomaly is not frequent, with an estimated incidence of 0.5–2.0%. However, the incidence is considerably higher among patients with a history of recurrent spontaneous abortion. In the present study, 227 congenital uterine anomalies were detected from 1666 hysterosalpingographies, showing an incidence of 13.6%. Since the incidence of reproductive wastage in the lowest grade of uterine cavity deformity (arcuate group) was as high as that revealed in groups with more severe anomalies, any congenital uterine anomaly could constitute a major cause of reproductive wastage. We designed a method of ideal surgical resection and reconstitution on the ischemic part of the uterine cavity, based on our histological findings, in the removed tissue specimen, and basic study for the selection of ideal absorbable threads for the surgery. After these metroplasties, more than 81% of subsequent pregnancies were successfully maintained, whereas more than 96% of presurgical gestations were not carried to full-term labor. The data are comparable with the reports by others[5,6]. These results should be evaluated with an appropriate control study and our previous control study[7] demonstrated that more than 94.4% of total pregnancies in 47 patients who had uterine anomalies but did not receive metroplasty terminated in spontaneous abortion.

Metroplastic surgery, for the patients with a history of recurrent fetal loss, is only a part of the total management for congenital uterine malformation. Generous information on clinical management of the postsurgical period was supplied from 33 institutes and surveyed to obtain an appropriate and ideal management, including contraceptive period and method of child delivery.

All these data indicate that congenital uterine malformation with an etiology for reproductive wastage is curable by the treatment based on both basic and clinical investigations, and outcome of treatment also totally depends on not only surgical manipulation, but on comprehensive therapeutic planning including preoperative diagnosis and postoperative management before pregnancy.

References

1. Makino, T. (1989). Reproductive wastage. In Bantaleb, Y. and Gzouli, A. (eds.) *New Concepts in Reproduction, Proceedings of the XIIIth World Congress of Fertility and Sterility*, pp. 85–92. (Carnforth, UK: Parthenon Publishing)
2. Makino, T., Hara, T., Oka, C., Toyoshima, K., Sugi, T., Iwasaki, K., Umeuchi, M. and Iizuka, R. (1992). Survey of 1120 Japanese women with a history of recurrent spontaneous abortions. *Eur. J. Obstet. Gynecol. Reprod. Biol.*, **44**, 123–30
3. Makino, T., Sakai, A., Sugi, T., Toyoshima, K., Iwasaki, K., Maruyama, T., Saito, S., Umeuchi, M. and Iizuka, T. (1991). Current comprehensive therapy of habitual abortion. *Ann. NY Acad. Sci.*, **626**, 597–604
4. Nakada, K., Makino, T., Tabuchi, T. and Iizuka, R. (1989). Analysis of congenital uterine anomalies in habitual abortions, evaluation of metroplasty. *Jpn. J. Fertil. Steril.*, **34**, 842–7
5. Querleu, D., Brasme, T. L. and Parmentier, D. (1990). Ultrasound-guided transcervical metroplasty. *Fertil. Steril.*, **54**, 995–8
6. Rock, J. A. and Zacur, H. A. (1983). The clinical management of repeated early pregnancy wastage. *Fertil. Steril.*, **39**, 123–40
7. Makino, T., Umeuchi, M., Nakada, K., Nozawa, S. and Iizuka, R. (1992). Incidence of congenital uterine anomalies in repeated reproductive wastage and prognosis for pregnancy after metroplasty. *Int. J. Fertil.*, **37**, 167–70

Environment and reproduction

19

S. Tabacova

Introduction and general considerations

Reproduction is a complex biological social and behavioral process, strongly dependent on both intrinsic factors (e.g. genetics, health background) and extrinsic (environmental) factors. This progressive process, beginning with gametogenesis, gamete interaction and implantation, proceeding through embryonic development, growth, parturition, and postnatal adaptation[1] is shaped by the genotype and modified by a constantly changing internal and external biological, physical and social environment. As Barton Childs has put it, 'In this personal evolution, the genes set the limits of homeostatic capacity: the genes propose, the environments dispose, and if these limits are exceeded the result is illness or death'[2].

In a broad context, reproductive health has been defined as 'a state in which the reproductive process is accomplished in a state of complete physical, mental and social well-being, and not merely in the absence of disease or disorders in the reproductive system'[3]. The indexes of reproductive health, therefore, 'need to be defined both in terms of the ability to reproduce and also with regard to the successful outcome of the reproductive process which includes infant and child survival, growth and healthy development'[4]. The ascertainment of the impact of environmental agents on reproductive health, therefore, must be within the scope of these considerations.

The word 'environment' has been defined in the *Oxford English Dictionary* as 'the sum total of influences which modify and determine the development of life and character'. Environmental influences are exercised from both social factors (emerging from interrelationships within and among population groups) and environmental agents of a chemical, physical or biological nature that can be of either manmade or natural origin. There are no 'reproductive toxins' *per se*; there are levels (thresholds) above which agents may become capable of affecting reproduction. Except for genotoxicants, it is the dose that makes an agent a reproductive toxicant. On the other hand, a deficiency of a specific agent could be no less important than its excess. The long list of elements essential for reproduction includes micro-elements, such as zinc, copper, selenium, cobalt, nickel; macroelements, such as calcium, magnesium, iron; and a host of vitamins and essential organic compounds. Natural deficiencies of bioessential elements in endemic areas have been associated with reproductive and developmental disorders, a classic example being iodine deficiency in many parts of the world[5]. From the viewpoint of environmental toxicology, bioessential elements are important not only with regard to their essentiality in the physiological processes of reproduction, but also with regard to their ability to counteract reproductive toxicants by various mechanisms, thereby preventing or diminishing their harmful effect. A protective effect of zinc and selenium against the developmental toxicity of lead, arsenic and cadmium has been documented[6–8]. The interplay between 'toxic' and 'essential' chemicals in the environment has been found to be an important determinant of human reproductive health parameters[9].

Having in mind that reproduction is a continuum of mutually linked and interdependent biological events, starting with gametogenesis and extending into adult life up to the cessation of reproductive function, it is clear that the temporal scope of exogenously induced effects on reproduction extends from preconception to senescence. The manifestation of the effect induced by a given agent will depend on the time of the insult, therefore the effect is time-specific. Thus, prepregnancy exposures might be expected to affect fertility in the male and female; first-trimester exposures would potentially affect fetal viability or produce birth defects; second- or third-trimester exposures might affect complications of pregnancy, fetal growth, or timing of delivery[10].

Pathways of induction of reproductive damage vary widely among different agents. Vulnerable sites for injury by environmental toxicants include the hypothalamus, anterior pituitary, male and female gonads and accessory organs, the processes of fertilization, implantation, intrauterine development and maturation. Yet the outcomes resulting from these various insults are few: namely, failure to achieve pregnancy, pregnancy loss and developmental disorders in prenatal and/or postnatal life. Therefore the endpoint measured does not necessarily provide an insight into the etiology and pathogenesis of a given reproductive disorder. Although at present a number of environmental agents have been identified as harmful to reproduction, the role of environmental factors in the etiology of reproductive disturbances and their impact on reproduction are largely unknown. After the known causes of birth defects, such as chromosomal damage, heredity, genetic origin, maternal disease, drugs and chemicals are accounted for, about 60% of malformations in humans remain of unknown etiology[11]. Of the estimated 60 000 chemicals currently used in the world, a small fraction has been assessed for reproductive and developmental toxicity in animal models; even less are the agents known as human reproductive hazards[12]. This accentuates the necessity of further efforts for assessment of human reproductive risks.

The reproductive risk of a given agent clearly depends on its potency to induce reproductive and developmental disturbances, which in turn is a function of its toxicokinetics and toxicodynamics. However, the impact of the risk from a specific agent would depend on a number of other factors, such as:

(1) The endpoint affected. If the outcome is of a rare background occurrence, such as that of most birth defects, even a high risk posed by a teratogen may not result in an identifiable impact. For example, valproic acid increases 200-fold the risk for neural tube defects, yet its impact on the overall risk for a major malformation is less than 0.5%[13]. In contrast, if the affected endpoint is of common occurrence, e.g. pregnancy loss, the impact would be greater even in the case of a lower risk.

(2) The availability of the agent in the environment – accessibility to the population. The more common the occurrence of a given reproductive risk factor, the greater the impact. Obvious illustrations are smoking and alcohol abuse.

(3) The persistence of the agent in the environment (e.g. DDT), or environmental transformations to more toxic products (e.g. ultraviolet light-catalyzed transformations of motor vehicle exhaust).

(4) The number of the population at risk, as illustrated by the disastrous effects of pandemics, major accidents and nutritional deficiencies.

Environmental factors

Classification and characteristics

As a biological entity, humans owe their existence to Nature and rely for subsistence on Earth's natural ecosystems, of which they are an integral part. As social beings, they are dependent for survival on the social and man-made environment. Therefore, they are subjected to extrinsic factors of natural, social and man-made origins, which are mutually interdependent (Figure 1).

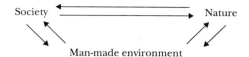

Figure 1 The extrinsic factors affecting humans

Thus, human civilisations and societies have been shaped by natural factors; in turn, social and man-made factors have been influencing the natural resources of the Earth, to culminate in global contemporary changes, such as the greenhouse-related climate change, thinning of stratospheric ozone, land degradation and top-soil loss, depletion of groundwater, reduction in genetic and ecosystem diversity and acidification of waterways and soils[14]. Examples of the above three groups of factors, relevant to reproduction, are: natural geochemical deficiencies or excesses of bioactive elements; man-made pollution of ambient, occupational and household environments by chemical, physical, or biological agents; and social factors, such as the socioeconomic state that determines nutrition, housing, lifestyle, education, health care availability, etc. All three groups of extrinsic factors can affect reproduction directly or indirectly, e.g. through influencing intrinsic factors important for reproduction, such as genetic material and health background. In turn, the reproduction of species can influence natural resources, the man-made human environment and societal characteristics (Figure 2).

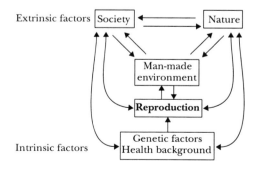

Figure 2 Reproduction of the species can influence natural resources

The relative impact of each group of factors on reproduction across countries depends on socioeconomic development and geographical location. In affluent industrial economies, man-made pollution is of higher priority than natural and socioeconomic factors, while in less developed economies, the socioeconomic and natural factors would play a role superior to that of man-made pollution. On a global scale, social factors are the leading extrinsic determinant of reproductive health. Social factors can modify both the level and impact of other extrinsic factors. For example, a resourceful society would have the economic means to prevent or abate environmental pollution, to provide supplementation for natural deficiencies and to ensure public health care for primary, secondary and tertiary prevention of reproductive health.

Social factors include: demographic characteristics (e.g. density, age and sex structure of the population); cultural factors; socioeconomic factors (e.g. income), family status, education, housing, lifestyles, psychosocial factors (e.g. stress), health care, etc.

Natural factors include: geographic, topographic, climatic, geochemical, physical and biological factors that constitute the natural background of a population.

Man-made factors are, according to their nature, subdivided into chemical, physical, or biological agents that are introduced into the environment by human activity.

Environmental pollution by chemical, physical or biological agents may arise from either man-made or natural sources, such as industry, agricultural practices, community sources, accidents, natural processes or disasters. Exposures can take place in the household, occupational, or ambient environment, via different media (ambient or indoor air, drinking water, foodstuffs) and by different routes (inhalation, ingestion, dermal absorption, etc.). In addition, use of some therapeutic or non-therapeutic drugs may constitute a reproductive risk. Further discussion will concentrate on major environmental factors and agents that are known at present as human reproductive hazards.

141

Social factors

Effects of social factors on reproduction are best perceived from a world perspective. In this review, based on the World Development Report of the World Bank, 1993[15], data on maternal, perinatal and child mortality and morbidity world-wide are used as indicators of reproductive health.

Across countries, more than 75% of the difference in health is associated with income differences. Poverty is a major determinant of poor health due to maternal and perinatal causes: in the developing countries, these causes are the top contributors to the overall burden of disease. Table 1 lists the six conditions that make the largest contribution in developing and industrial countries to the overall burden of disease, expressed as disability-adjusted life year loss (DALY), a measure that combines healthy life years lost because of premature mortality with those lost as a result of disability. In the developing countries of Asia, Africa and Latin America, perinatal and maternal causes constitute more than 10% of the total burden of disease, compared to less than 3% in the industrialized countries.

Infant mortality rate in low-income economies is nine times, and in middle-income economies, five times that of high-income economies; the same applies to child mortality under 5 years of age (Table 2).

In 1991, the number of maternal deaths in the developing group of countries was 428 000 against 3000 in the established market economies and former socialist economies. The leading causes of maternal death in the developing

Table 1 Main contributors to the global burden of disease in developing and industrialized countries[15]

	Associated DALY (millions)	
	Demographically developing countries	*Industrial countries*
Perinatal and maternal causes	125	4
Respiratory infections	119	4
Diarrheal diseases	99	< 0.5
Cardiovascular diseases	58	27
Childhood cluster (diphtheria, polio, pertussis, measles, tetanus)	67	< 0.5
Tuberculosis	46	1
All conditions	1210	152

DALY, disability-adjusted life year loss, a measure that combines healthy life years lost because of premature mortality with those lost as a result of disability[15]

Table 2 Maternal, infant and child mortality per 1000 live births by income of economies world-wide[15]

	Low income economies	*Middle income economies*	*High income economies*
GNP *per capita*, 1991 (US$)	350	2480	21 050
Maternal mortality	3.1	1.1	NR
Infant mortality	71	38	8
Under age 5 mortality	200	98	17
Population per physician	6760	2060	420
Adult illiteracy (%)	40	21	4
Malnutrition under age 5 (%)	14–60	2–38	NR

GNP, gross national product; NR, not registered

Table 3 Deaths by cause and demographic group, 1990 (thousands)[15]

	Demographically developing group	Established market economies and former socialist economies
Maternal (total)	428	3
hemorrhage	130	—
sepsis	79	—
eclampsia	45	—
hypertension	31	—
obstructed labor	40	—
abortion	60	1
Perinatal	2402	89
Congenital anomalies	595	61
Other		
protein/energy malnutrition	207	6
iodine deficiency	19	—
vitamin A deficiency	35	—
alcohol dependence	31	22
drug dependence	14	3

countries were hemorrhage, sepsis, abortion, eclampsia, obstructed labor and hypertension. Except for abortion, no maternal deaths due to these causes were registered in industrial countries. Dramatic differences were also present in the number of perinatal deaths and deaths from congenital malformations (Table 3).

The total impact of income on reproductive health, as illustrated in Tables 2 and 3, includes effects that work directly through income (such as food consumption), as well as those that work indirectly through factors that are mainly dependent on income, such as availability of physicians, access to safe water and sanitation, or abatement of diseases that constitute a reproductive hazard (e.g. rubella, malaria, hepatitis, endocrine and cardiovascular diseases or deficiency states). In a sample of 51 developing countries, a 10% increase in income *per capita*, all else being equal, reduced infant and child mortality rates by between 2 and 3.5%. Within one and the same country and city, there are large differences in child survival between rich and poor neighborhoods. Income growth has more impact in poor populations, because additional resources buy basic necessities, particularly food and shelter, that yield especially large health benefits.

It is not just income *per capita* that is relevant; the distribution of income and the number of people in poverty matter as well. In Sri Lanka, an increase in *per capita* public spending on health was 22 times more effective in reducing infant mortality than was the same increase in average income. The distribution of income within households is also important. Increasing women's access to income can be especially beneficial. In Guatemala, for example, it takes 15 times more spending to achieve a given improvement in child nutrition when income is earned by the father than when it is earned by the mother; in Brazil, income in the hands of the mother has a bigger effect on family health than income controlled by the father.

Throughout the 20th century, life expectancy, which is greatly dependent on infant and child mortality, has been strongly associated at the national level with income *per capita*. According to the World Bank, the factors that have been important along with income growth for the dramatic mortality declines of the past 100 years, and particularly in the developing countries since World War II, are improvements in medical technology, education, and public health programs combined with the spread of knowledge about health. The introduction of

143

public health measures – particularly clean water, sanitation and food regulation – certainly contributed to the decline of infant and child mortality in the early 20th century. The geographic distribution of mortality declines suggests, however, that until people began to understand the sources of poor health, such public health measures were responsible for only a small part of the progress made. World Bank data for 13 African countries between 1975 and 1985 show that a 10% increase in female literacy reduced child mortality by 10% whereas changes in male literacy made little difference. The beneficial effect of maternal education on infant and child health is exercised through many ways, such as age of marriage, family planning, birth spacing, avoidance of unsafe abortion, greater use of prenatal care, better domestic hygiene, wiser use of medical services, etc. Thus, in Brazil, child health benefits from a father's education mostly through his income, while almost all the effect of maternal education comes from learning about health through newspapers, television and radio. Maternal education works also through improved family lifestyles: for example, in Cote d-Ivoire, a doubling of household income under women's control reduced the share of alcohol in the family budget by 26% and the share of cigarettes by 14%. Educated mothers are also less likely to condone abuse and ethnic practices detrimental to female reproductive health.

Thus, on a global, regional, national and household level, reproductive health is strongly dependent on socioeconomic factors that determine conditions closely relevant to reproduction, such as nutrition, availability of health care and prophylactics, family planning, public health measures, parental education, healthier lifestyles, greater occupational and environmental safety and improvements in medical technology.

Lifestyle factors (smoking, alcohol and drug abuse)

Smoking Parental and particularly maternal smoking has been linked to many adverse effects on reproduction. Known or suspected effects include a delay in time to conception, placental pathology, low birth weight, prematurity, increased perinatal mortality and postnatal morbidity, and interference with growth and development[16,17]. Such toxicity can be attributed to the many constituents of cigarette smoke: carbon monoxide, hydrogen cyanide, nitrogen oxides, heavy metals, nicotine and carcinogens such as polycyclic aromatic hydrocarbons, dimethylnitrosoamine, β-naphtylamine and formaldehyde[18]. According to the World Bank[15], *per capita* consumption of tobacco is decreasing in industrial countries and has remained relatively unchanged in the formerly socialist economies; in contrast, it is rising in many developing countries among both men and women and is expected to increase by about 12% between 1990 and 2000.

Smoking before pregnancy interferes with conception: it was found that the fertility of smokers was approximately 72% of that of non-smokers, and that this effect was dose-dependent in that heavy smokers (> 20 cigarettes/day) experienced lower fertility than did smokers of less than 20 cigarettes/day, respectively 57% and 75% of the pregnancy rate of non-smokers[19]. Long-term maternal smoking has been linked in a dose-dependent manner with increased rates of placental pathology, e.g. placenta previa, abruptio placentae, placental infarcts and microscopic placental changes indicative of underperfusion resulting from vasoconstriction[20]. A 92% increase in the rate of placenta previa, and a 86% increase of abruptio placentae were reported in smokers of one or more packs per day in comparison to non-smokers[21]. It has been suggested that the fetal hypoxia ensuing from the vasoconstrictive effect of nicotine[22] and from carbon monoxide-induced limitation in oxygen availability[23] may be the reason for retarded fetal growth and increased fetal wastage. A 1.2–1.8-fold increase in the spontaneous abortion rate among smokers over non-smokers has been reported[17], along with a 30–35% increase in late fetal deaths (independent of the decrease in birth weight) in smokers of one or more packs per day[21,24].

One of the most constant findings has been the reduced birth weight. Many recent epidemiological studies, reviewed by Campbell and Landrigan[16], have shown that babies of smoking mothers are on the average 150–250 g lighter than non-smokers' babies, and that, among smoking women, there is a doubling of the proportion of newborn infants weighing less than 2500 g. Because this reduction occurs mainly during the last half of pregnancy, mothers who quit smoking by the 4th month of pregnancy have babies whose mean birth weight does not differ from those of non-smoking mothers[16]. Paternal smoking during pregnancy was found to reduce birth weight by 120 g per pack of cigarettes per day[25], and 'passive smoking' of women exposed to sidestream smoke for at least 2 h/day during pregnancy was associated with a two-fold increased risk of a low birth weight newborn[26]. A statistically significant decrease in body length at birth has also been noted[27]. A study of patterns of growth retardation in term infants born to smoking mothers has shown that smokers are more likely to have infants with symmetrical growth retardation (short body length for dates), which was felt to represent a general cessation of fetal growth long before birth that resulted in proportional deficits in body weight and length[28]. It has been suggested that smoking-related nutritional factors could contribute to intrauterine growth retardation and fetal survival. Such factors include the appetite-suppressing effect of smoking that could lead to decreased maternal weight gain in pregnancy, and depletion of vitamins, essential for growth[27]. Increased risk of preterm birth by 26–38% was associated with maternal smoking in several studies[21]; smoking of one or more packs per day increased this risk to 50%. Additionally, it was found that 13–14% of all preterm births could be attributed to smoking[21]. At present, no consistent data are available to support a relationship between maternal smoking and congenital malformations[16,17].

Concern over maternal smoking during pregnancy recently has expanded to the postnatal and postneonatal periods. Nicotine is secreted into the breast milk of smoking women;

it has been detected in the milk of women who smoked as few as one cigarette per day[29]. A 26% increase in neonatal death rate of offspring from smoking mothers was reported[24]; termination of smoking prior to the 4th month of pregnancy lowered the mortality risk. Increased respiratory morbidity of bronchitis, pneumonia and virus infection, proportional to the amount of parental smoking and most evident in a child's first 2 years of life, has been observed[18]. Physical developmental delays, most expressed at the age of 1 year, but seen in one study even at the age of 7 years, have been reported[16].

Smoking has also been shown to render the maternal organism more vulnerable to the effects of low-level environmental pollution by metals[30].

Alcohol At present, alcohol is the most prevalent drug or chemical developmental toxicant in humans; it is estimated that 'fetal alcohol effects' may be seen in one in 100 livebirths[17]. It is also the most prevalent chemical human teratogen: an estimated 5% of all congenital malformations is considered to be due to prenatal alcohol exposure; in addition, fetal alcohol syndrome appears to be the leading known cause of mental retardation[31]. Fetal alcohol syndrome, described by Jones and colleagues in 1973[32], is characterized by intrauterine growth retardation, microcephaly, characteristic facial dysmorphism (short palpebral fissures, flat philtrum, maxillary hypoplasia, thin upper lip, micrognathia or retrognathia), and other somatic structural defects (e.g. cardiac abnormalities). The most devastating effect of fetal alcohol syndrome is mental retardation, which occurs in about 85% of children identified as having this condition[33].

Major morphological effects are associated with exposures during 2–8 weeks of gestation; 'binge drinking' early in pregnancy has been suggested to be associated with neural tube defects[31]. Chronic consumption of large amounts of alcohol in pregnancy (6 ounces, or about 160 ml of absolute alcohol daily) constitutes a high risk of full-blown fetal alcohol syndrome[31]; consumption of lesser amounts of alcohol may give rise to 'fetal alcohol effect' manifestations that may vary in severity[17]. Because subtle effects may go unrecognized, no absolutely safe level of alcohol consumption during pregnancy has been established[17]. Reduction of alcohol consumption at any time in pregnancy reduces the severity of fetal alcohol syndrome, but may not significantly reduce the risk of physical or behavioral impairment[31].

The central nervous system (CNS) dysfunction in the newborn period is demonstrated by irritability, poor sucking, inconsolable crying, hypertonia and, sometimes, tonic–clonic seizures in neonates undergoing 'alcohol withdrawal'[34]. In childhood, hyperreactivity, varying degrees of reduced IQ, speech-related and hearing problems, and abnormal patterns of growth are found[17]. Growth catch-up is generally restricted to children only mildly affected. The social impact of alcohol abuse is evident from the lifetime neurobehavioral handicaps of children with fetal alcohol syndrome or fetal alcohol effects[35].

Drug abuse The problem of drug abuse and drug dependence is a major problem confronting contemporary society. In the past decade the production and use of illicit drugs, especially cocaine, appear to have increased considerably worldwide; users typically fall in the age group 15–44, although most are in their mid-20s[15]. Drugs of abuse that may affect the fetus and the newborn encompass a variety of pharmacological agents, including major opioids (e.g. morphine, heroin), stimulants (cocaine, amphetamines), hallucinogens (cannabis, LSD), opioid analgesics (codeine, morphine), and non-opioid CNS depressants (barbiturates, benzodiazepines)[17]. Drug usage patterns vary over time; the most recent drug 'epidemics' in the 1980s involved the widespread use of cocaine. Many abused drugs produce similar manifestations of maternal, fetal and perinatal toxicity; the contribution of individual drugs is difficult to assess, because the frequency of multiple drug abuse is high, end effects are confounded by the high incidence of infections and sexually transmitted diseases, neglect of nutrition and

health care, and by the concomitant use of legal products such as tobacco and alcohol among drug abusers[17,31]. Despite these difficulties, it has been established beyond doubt that drugs of abuse can affect pregnancy and directly affect fetal growth and development, since they cross the placenta easily[17]. Of the different drugs, heroine, methadone and cocaine have been most extensively studied.

Pregnancy complications (abruptio placentae, placental insufficiency, premature onset of labor), fetal wastage and intrauterine growth retardation have been linked with abuse of heroin, cocaine, marijuana, benzodiazepines, barbiturates and toluene[31]. However, with the exception of cocaine, there does not appear to be a significant increase in teratogenic risk associated with the abuse of these drugs. Cocaine has teratogenic potential associated with various types of vascular disruption produced by the sympathomimetic effects of this drug[31]. Placental vasoconstriction, increased uterine contractility and a reduction in uterine blood flow that may cause hypoxia and infarction in the developing fetus have been reported in pregnant women using cocaine[36,37]. The reported fetal effects all appear to be various types of vascular disruptive phenomena: congenital limb amputations, cerebral infarctions, and certain types of visceral and urinary tract malformations. The risk of major malformation from cocaine is low, but the malformations may be severe[31].

Important perinatal and early postnatal risks in drug abusers are associated with the neonatal abstinence syndrome encompassing the CNS, gastrointestinal, respiratory and autonomic nervous system signs that may cause serious morbidity and mortality of 34–93% when abstinence is unrecognized or improperly treated[38]. Reports of long-lasting neurobehavioral effects have currently been rare, but intrauterine exposure to narcotics may predispose susceptible infants to sudden infant death syndrome (SIDS) during infancy. Narcotics are known to reduce brainstem responsiveness to carbon dioxide and to depress the pontine and medullar centers which control respiration[17]. The incidence of SIDS in drug-addicted infants has been found to be 7–20 times higher than in the general population[39–41].

Hormonal regulation of the reproductive system can be altered at different levels of function of the hypothalamic–pituitary–gonadal axis. Anesthetics, analgesics, sedatives and tranquillizers have been associated with reversible alterations in female fertility[42]. In particular, marijuana is disruptive to normal reproductive functions by inhibiting the secretion of both luteinizing hormone (LH) and follicle stimulating hormone (FSH). In the male, centrally acting neuropharmacological agents can also impair reproductive function by affecting the control of gonadotropin release and, as a potential secondary effect, steroid synthesis and release[43]. Marijuana, narcotics and alcohol may also act in this capacity[42].

Environmental chemicals

Heavy metals (lead, mercury, cadmium)

(1) *Lead* Excessive exposures to lead can result from a variety of sources, both occupational (e.g. metal smelting, lead storage battery manufacturing, soldering, stained glass and lead crystal production, printing) and environmental (e.g. leaded gasoline use in motor vehicles, industrial pollution of ambient air, water and soil, leaded paint and cosmetics).

Contemporary evidence suggests that lead, in environmentally relevant concentrations, is associated with impaired spermatogenesis, adverse birth outcomes and postnatal neurodevelopmental disorders[16,44]. Increased frequency of abnormalities in spermatogenesis, including asthenospermia, hypospermia and teratospermia, has been found in workers exposed to lead[45,46]. Such changes seem to occur among males with exposures resulting in blood lead levels higher than 40–50 µg/dl[44]. Although a limited number of epidemiological studies of paternal exposure and reproductive outcome has been reported, the available data show that significantly increased odds of spontaneous abortion were associated with paternal blood lead levels greater than 30 µg/dl, measured within 1 year of the presumed period of spermatogenesis[47], and that paternal exposures in the year prior to the child's birth were associated with elevated risk of death in the perinatal period[48]. There have been more studies linking maternal exposures to adverse birth outcomes. During pregnancy, lead has been found to cross the placenta[49,50] and reach levels in fetal tissues similar to those in maternal ones[51]. It has been estimated that lead transfer first begins at about 14 weeks' gestation and increases throughout pregnancy[51]; concern has been raised about the possibility that during pregnancy lead is mobilized from maternal stores acquired prior to conception[52]. Pregnant women may also be at increased risk for lead absorption as a consequence of calcium and iron deficiencies that occur commonly in pregnancy and enhance lead absorption from the gastrointestinal tract[16]. In pregnancies ending with spontaneous abortion and early neonatal death, a pronounced increase of lead in maternal blood and placenta was found[53,54]. Two times greater risk of stillbirth was associated with maternal exposure to lead via drinking water at levels greater than 0.08 mg/l[55]. Increased risk of preterm delivery was associated with maternal blood levels at or above 25 µg/dl[56], and even with lower levels, such as 8–14 µg/dl[57]; in another study, length of gestation decreased by 0.46 weeks per unit increase in maternal blood lead in the range of 1–27 µg/dl[58]. Lead at high doses has been shown to be teratogenic in experimental animal models[59]; however, data on the ability of lead to produce birth defects in humans have been inconclusive and no specific syndrome of anomalies has been identified[44]. In summary, epidemiological studies have shown limited evidence for an association of low-dose prenatal lead exposure with birth weight, gestational age at birth and congenital defects[44].

In contrast, much more consistent information has emerged with regard to postnatal neurodevelopmental disorders induced by prenatal lead exposures in humans. Several case studies have supported the adverse impact of maternal lead poisoning on the early neurobehavioral development of offspring[60,61]. Low-level prenatal lead exposures have been repeatedly associated with significantly slower mental development in infancy[58,62]. Although this effect appeared to be transient and was no longer detected at school age, it has been suggested that even transient effects could have long-lasting cognitive or behavioral sequelae to which traditional psychometric tests are not sensitive[44]. At relatively higher lead exposures (e.g. mean cord blood lead level of 22.4 μg/dl), an enduring association between prenatal exposure and development was found at the age of 4 years[63]; deficiencies in central auditory processing at the age of 5 years and in fine motor function at 6 years were also associated with elevated neonatal blood lead levels[64,65]. Most of the studies point consistently to an inverse relationship between general intellectual function and neonatal blood lead levels. No threshold for this association has been identified[66]. On the basis of meta-analysis of these studies, the World Health Organization has estimated that, within the 0–25 μg/dl range, each 10 μg/dl increase in lifetime mean blood lead level is associated with a 1–3-point decline in IQ[44]. Recent data suggest that a negative relationship with IQ is detectable even within a range of blood lead as low as 0–10 μg/dl[67].

(2) *Mercury* Methylmercury appears to be the most toxic of the mercurial compounds for the fetus and can have devastating effects, particularly on the developing nervous system. It penetrates the placental barrier more easily than do inorganic or arylmercurial compounds[68], resulting in approximately equal concentrations in maternal and fetal blood in exposed human populations[69,70]. A significant burden of methylmercury can be transferred from a mother to her infant via breast milk[71]. Since methylmercury is lipid soluble, it diffuses across cell membranes, and up to 10–20% of the total body methylmercury content can accumulate in the brain[82]. In general, both prenatal and postnatal effects of methylmercury in humans result from interference with the normal processes of

development and maturation of the CNS[16]. The neurotoxic and teratogenic effects of methylmercury on the developing human first became known through an outbreak of methylmercury poisoning by consumption of fish and shellfish contaminated through discharge of inorganic and organic mercury effluent from an acetaldehyde and vinylchloride plant into Minamata Bay, Japan[73]. The poisoning resulted in a syndrome of functional and morphological congenital neurological manifestations in the prenatally exposed infants, now known as congenital Minamata disease. It was clinically manifested by microcephaly (in 60% of the cases) and/or postnatal neurological deficits, such as cerebral palsy, mental retardation, cerebellar signs, movement disorders (chorea, athetosis), strabismus, visual defects and pyramidal symptoms, on the background of either lacking, or minor, maternal toxicity[74]. Pathological findings included diffuse neuronal disintegration with gliosis, particularly in the granular layer of the cerebellar hemispheres, and degeneration of neurons in the cerebellar cortex[75]. Similar changes were found in subsequent episodes of poisoning in Iraq, Guatemala and Pakistan during the 1970s, from the ingestion of flour and wheat seed treated with methyl- and ethylmercury compounds[76].

Although the information on the reproductive effects of exposures to inorganic mercury compounds is limited, in a case–control study on adverse pregnancy outcomes in dentists and dental assistants exposed to mercury as an amalgam, a positive association was found between maternal hair mercury levels and occurrence of reproductive failures, including spontaneous abortions, congenital malformations (predominantly spina bifida) and stillbirths[77]. Ovarian functional disturbances, associated with urinary mercury levels, were found in a study of women of reproductive age, occupationally exposed to inorganic mercury vapors at a plant for production of luminescent lamps[78]. Anovulatory cycles and menstrual disturbances (oligo- and hypomenorrhea) were observed after only 1 year of employment. The mean urinary mercury level was significantly higher among the women who had abnormal cycles (3.9 μg/dl) in comparison to controls (1.1 μg/dl).

(3) *Cadmium* Cadmium is an occupational and environmental pollutant that has raised great concern during the last decades. Its industrial production started at the beginning of this century, and since then it has almost doubled every 10 years, at least up to 1970[79]. For the general population, the two main sources of exposure are the diet (from contaminated water and crops grown on polluted soil) and tobacco smoking. An important toxicological feature of cadmium is its exceptionally long biological half-life in the human organism (10–30 years)[79]; it mainly accumulates in the kidney[80]. Since the beginning of this century, environmental cadmium pollution in Europe may have caused a 50-fold rise in the concentration of metal in the human renal cortex[81].

Japan is, to date, the only known location where cadmium exposure was high enough to affect significant groups of the regional population in areas of cadmium pollution. In the Japanese experience with cadmium, the clinical extreme of which is renal osteomalacia and osteoporosis known as Itai-Itai disease, the individuals found to be most vulnerable to the effects of cadmium were postmenopausal women with a history of multiple childbirths as well as calcium and vitamin D deficiency. This suggests that women in general are possibly at special risk and it also points to nutritional status as being an important determinant of the adverse health effects of cadmium[82].

Even low-level exposures to cadmium result in prolonged retention in the body, especially in the kidney and liver, but also in the placenta. Cadmium is the only agent to date well documented as a placental toxin in multiple species, including humans[83]. The placenta concentrates cadmium highly; placentae from cigarette smokers concentrate cadmium to higher levels than placentae from non-smokers[84]. While limiting the passage of cadmium into the fetal circulation, the retention of cadmium in the placenta produces direct cellular damage, manifested by

placental necrosis, stromal edema and a decrease in uteroplacental blood flow. Ultrastructural and biochemical changes in the trophoblast, leading to a decrease in content and release of human chorionic gonadotropin and reduction of zinc transfer into the fetal circulation, occur much earlier, beginning at 4 h of initial exposure to cadmium, with a tissue burden of 45 nmol/g[83]. Currently, a no-effect level for cadmium has not been established for the human placental perfusion model. In rodent experiments, placental necrosis and fetal death occur at doses that do not produce renal toxicity, pointing to the fact that the placenta is the main target site of cadmium toxicity[85]. These observations have been the basis for considering the placenta as a possible critical organ in cadmium exposure for the general population[72]. Although few data are available to assess the effect of cadmium on human reproduction, there is suggestive evidence linking cadmium with intrauterine growth retardation[86,87]. Significantly reduced birth weights and increased rate of stillbirth were found in women in the former USSR occupationally exposed to cadmium oxide, although the course of pregnancy and delivery was normal[86]. These findings, supported by the evidence from animal studies, argue for pregnant women being a special group at risk from cadmium by virtue of potential deleterious effects on the fetus. However, insufficient information currently exists for quantification of a dose–effect and dose–response relationships.

Extensive experimental evidence documents the effects of cadmium on the gonads, especially the testes, in animal models as reviewed by the United States Environmental Protection Agency[82]. Severe testicular necrosis has been established as being a consequence of high-level cadmium exposure; the necrosis has been shown to involve endocrine cells within the testes as well as testicular vasculature and germinal epithelium. Leydig cell tumors were repeatedly observed after systemic injections of cadmium to different animal species. However, these have not been found when cadmium was administered orally at lower dose levels. The environmental relevance of these findings is questionable[82]. In humans, occupational exposure to cadmium (primarily as oxide) has been associated with increased risk of prostatic cancer[88]. Cadmium has been classified by the International Agency for Research on Cancer as a possible human carcinogen (group 2A), based on sufficient evidence of carcinogenicity in experimental animals and limited evidence in humans[88].

Environmental and dietary estrogens Humans are exposed to both natural and industrial chemicals that are capable of disrupting the endocrine system. These chemicals mimic or interfere with endogenously produced hormones, neurotransmitters, growth factors and inhibiting substances. Examples include different structural classes of industrial chemicals, such as organochlorine pesticides (*o,p'*-DDT, *p,p'*-methoxychlor, endosulphan, toxaphene, dieldrin), commercial PCB mixtures, and alkylphenols used as components of detergents, which have been reported by several research groups to have estrogenic activities, as well as antiestrogenic compounds that inhibit estrogen-induced responses, such as the aryl hydrocarbon receptor (AhR) agonist 2,3,7,8-tetrachlorodibenzo-*p*-dioxin (TCDD) and related halogenated aromatics, including polychlorinated dibenzo-*p*-dioxins (PCDDs), dibenzofurans (PCDFs) and PCBs[89]. Other AhR agonists, such as polynuclear aromatic hydrocarbons, also exhibit antiestrogenic activities, but their relative potency as antiestrogens is 1000 times smaller in comparison to TCDD[89]. Environmental exposure to estrogenic chemicals is not confined to industrial compounds. Naturally occurring estrogens have been identified, such as plant bioflavonoids and various mycotoxins, including zearalenone and related compounds. In addition, a number of plant foodstuffs contain 17β-estradiol and estrone[90]. A mass balance of dietary levels of industrial and natural estrogens, coupled with their estimated estrogenic potencies, has indicated that the contribution of estrogenic industrial compounds is 0.0000025% of the daily intake of estrogenic flavonoids in the diet, thus suggesting that the overall contribution of industrial estrogenic chemicals to human reproductive risks would be negligible in comparison to naturally occurring estrogens[89]. However, the extreme persistence in the environment of some industrial estrogenic chemicals (such as DDT and PCBs), their high bioaccumulation, placental transfer, passage to breastmilk and their ability to induce adverse reproductive effects should not be disregarded.

A number of laboratory studies suggest that fertility among populations exposed to estrogenic chemicals may be at risk[91]. The motility of sperm from men experiencing fertility problems (< 20 million sperm/ml) was inversely proportional to the concentration of three PCB congeners in their semen[92]. It has been hypothesized that increased environmental estrogen exposure may be responsible for falling sperm counts[93] by over 40% during the past 50 years[94]. It was during this period that humans were first exposed to synthetic estrogenic chemicals. This hypothesis has been challenged on the grounds that the observed decline in sperm counts was an artifact due to the changed reference range of 'normal' over time[95], and that there was a lack of corresponding decrease during the time in which environmental levels of organochlorine compounds were maximal[89,96].

Accidental epidemic exposures to halogenated hydrocarbons have shown that adverse effects on the fetus and developing infant can occur. In Japan in 1968, and subsequently in Taiwan in 1979, PCB-contaminated cooking oil was consumed by the population and resulted in congenital PCB poisoning, demonstrated by a syndrome of congenital abnormalities, including hyperpygmentation ('cola-colored babies') and alterations of the gums, teeth, nails, skin and hair generally consistent with an acquired neuroectodermal dysplasia[97], as well as perinatal and infant mortality, and neurological developmental delay[16]. The parents of children in the Japanese rice oil incident were exposed to PCB at 63 μg/kg body weight per day for 3 months[91]. Much lower maternal exposures (0.093 μg/kg body weight per day) from PCB-contaminated fish in Michigan were associated with a lower birth weight and smaller head circumference[98] and with impaired visual recognition memory at 7 months and short-term memory problems at 4 years[99]. Even in cases of no known exposure, a prospective birth cohort study of approximately 900 subjects in North Carolina found almost universal contamination of human milk[100].

Methylisocyanate Methylisocyanate (MIC) is one of the more recent additions to the list of chemicals that have been involved in major environmental disasters[101]. The hazards associated with exposure to MIC were tragically demonstrated during a release from a pesticide manufacturing plant in Bhopal, India[102]. In this incident, an estimated 30–40 tons of methylisocyanate and other MIC hydrolysis reaction products was accidentally released into the atmosphere over Bhopal during a 2–3-h period on the night of December 2/3, 1984, resulting in deaths and injuries on a 'scale unprecedented in modern industrial history'[101]. Out of the more than 200 000 exposed, the estimated number of deaths was between 2500 and 5000, and the number of seriously injured as high as 60 000[103].

In a survey of 3270 families living close to the source of the MIC release, 43% of 865 observed pregnancies did not result in the birth of a live infant[104]. Of 486 live births, 14.2% of infants died within the first month of life. Compared to the expected rates of 6–10% for abortions and 2.6–3% for neonatal mortality usually seen in these or similar areas[104], these data show substantial increases in spontaneous abortions and neonatal deaths. The results of subsequent animal studies[105] were in concordance with these observations. Malformations were not reported, and no teratogenic and adverse effects of fertility were observed in experimental studies[104,105]. Whether these effects on pre- and postnatal mortality represent a direct fetotoxicity of MIC or reflect maternal toxicity remains to be determined[101]. Among the survivors, long-lasting effects other than persistent lung damage have not been registered. A cause of concern are the

results of genetic toxicity assessments, which suggest that MIC might disrupt the integrity of eukaryotic chromosomes through interaction with nuclear proteins, and gave grounds to conclude that MIC should be considered weakly genotoxic[106]. However, their implications for the survivors in Bhopal are not yet clear[101].

Physical factors

Ionizing radiation Sources of human exposure to radiation include background radiation (from cosmic and terrestrial radiation and radionuclides deposited within the body), occupational and accidental exposure from the production and use of nuclear energy and weapons, occupational and medical exposure from the use of X-irradiation and radiopharmaceuticals, and other miscellaneous sources[107].

Ionizing radiation affects living tissues by disrupting the atomic structure of biological molecules through dislodging electrons from atoms and producing ionization. The resulting deleterious effects are of a stochastic and/or non-stochastic nature. The harm that follows from a single, random modification in a cell component, which might have resulted from a single ionization event, is termed a 'stochastic' effect. Stochastic effects, such as carcinogenicity and mutagenicity resulting from mutations induced in somatic or germ cells, may not have a threshold dose below which no adverse effects occur. Non-stochastic effects are produced by numerous or repeated damage resulting in cell death; such effects have a threshold dose that defines the smallest dose that induces detectable harm[108]. Examples are radiation-induced infertility and embryonic death. Prenatal irradiation may induce either stochastic or non-stochastic effects in the conceptus, depending on the developmental stage at the time of insult.

Specific doses of ionizing radiation are capable of affecting fertility by selectively killing germ cells, without producing gross tissue damage. Testicular doses of 15 or more rad (rad is defined as the amount of energy absorbed per unit mass of tissue; 1 rad = 100 ergs/g) have led to oligospermia, and doses above 50 rad to aspermia, resulting from deleterious effects on spermatogonia[109,110]. With higher doses, later stages of spermatogenesis, such as spermatids, are affected. There is a ten-fold difference between the radiosensitivity of spermatogonia and spermatocytes[111]. Recovery of normal sperm concentrations after doses between 100 and 600 rad takes between 9 months and more than 5 years[110]. The repopulating of germinal cells becomes less and less efficient as radiation exposures increase. The ovary is most sensitive to ionizing radiation in the prenatal period, since radiation sensitivity is highest in oogonia undergoing mitosis, which degenerate shortly after birth. It has been estimated that acute doses above 25 rad absorbed by the fetus during gestation are likely to result in sterility in the human female[112]. In sexually mature women, acute exposure of the ovary to 300–400 rad, depending on age at exposure, can result in impairment of fertility[107]; a fractionated dose of 2000 rad over 5–6 weeks is considered likely to produce complete sterility in 95% of young women[113]. While the early stages of gametogenesis are sensitive to the killing effect of radiation, the late stages (meiotic and postmeiotic) are selectively sensitive to its mutagenic effect. The Committee on the Biological Effects of Ionizing Radiation of the US National Academy of Sciences has estimated that 50–250 rem (1 rem = 1 rad plus a correction factor to equalize biological effects for different types of radiation) would be the dose of radiation sufficient to double the natural human mutation rate[107]. However, follow-up studies of the children of Japanese atomic bomb survivors have not given indications for radiation-induced mutations[114].

Ionizing radiation has a direct effect on the developing embryo that depends on the absorbed dose, the dose rate and the stage of gestation at the time of exposure[115]. As shown by experimental studies in mammals, exposures during the preimplantation period can lead to death of the conceptus, but the surviving conceptuses appear not to be impaired. After implantation, during the period of major organogenesis (from the 2nd to the 9th week of gestation in humans), the embryo is extremely sensitive to induction of major malformations. Birth defects reported in humans after intrauterine irradiation greater than 100 rad during this period involve the CNS (microcephaly, hydrocephaly, spina bifida, mental retardation), the eye (microphthalmos, retinal degeneration, cataracts, coloboma, chorioretinitis, optic atrophy), cleft palate, skeletal defects (skull malformations, clubfeet, syndactyly), genital deformities, effects on germ cell populations and growth retardation[107,116,117]. Exposures during the early fetal stage are characterized by less sensitivity to teratogenic effects, with the exception of the still developing CNS[16]. Effects of later exposures include hypoplastic organs, neoplasia, functional alterations and shortening of life span[115]. Since the developing human CNS is sensitive to radiation throughout gestation and into the neonatal period, the most prominent among the radiation effects observed in humans are microcephaly and mental retardation, which, along with growth retardation, are the cardinal manifestations of intrauterine effects in the human. Microcephaly was seen in the atomic bomb survivors exposed *in utero* to 10–19 rad of mixed neutron and gamma radiation[118], with a 28% incidence rate for exposures during 4–13 weeks' gestation and a 7% incidence rate for exposures at other times during gestation[107]. Growth retardation was associated with an estimated average dose of 25 rad[107]. Studies of children prenatally exposed at Hiroshima and Nagasaki have shown that the highest risk of forebrain damage occurs at 8–15 weeks' gestational age[119], which corresponds to the period of maximum neuronal proliferation and migration[120]. During this period, the dose–response model did not indicate the existence of a threshold dose that would not impair the brain growth, and the probability of increasing the incidence of mental retardation was 0.40% per rad of radiation (four additional cases of mental retardation for each 1000 births). The sensitivity of the CNS decreases from 16 through 24 weeks of gestation, although the CNS is still vulnerable during this period. The estimated decrease in intelligence test scores caused by *in utero* irradiation during these two gestational periods of vulnerability is a 20-point loss in IQ tests for each additional mrad of exposure[121,122]. Radiation exposures before the 8th week and after the 25th week of gestation were not associated with any increased risk of mental retardation.

Although an association between prenatal X-ray exposure and leukemia in children has been reported[123], no excess of deaths from malignant disease in childhood was demonstrated, even among the highest risk group of Japanese atomic bomb survivors, who received 0.5 Gy (50 rad) or more of irradiation *in utero*, according to the UNSCEAR report, 1988[124]. At present, there is no indication that radiodiagnostic doses of ionizing radiation (< 5 rad) during gestation significantly increase the incidence of malformations or genetic mutations in the human population. Such doses, however, may increase the incidence of neoplastic disease in children by 100–240 cases per million persons per rad[108].

(1) *The Chernobyl accident: contamination* T h e accident on 26 April 1986 at the fourth unit of the Chernobyl nuclear power station in Ukraine has been the most serious non-military nuclear accident to date. Damage to the reactor containment and core structures led to the release of large amounts of radioactive materials from the plant. The release did not occur in a single massive event. Only 25% of the materials released escaped during the 1st day of the accident; the rest escaped over a 9-day period. Only two earlier reactor accidents caused significant releases of radionuclides: the one at Windscale (Sellafield, UK) in October 1957, and the other at Three Mile Island (USA) in March 1979. It has been estimated that the Windscale accident released twice the amount of noble gases that were released at Chernobyl, but 2000 times less ^{131}I and ^{137}Cs. The Three Mile Island accident released approximately 2% as much noble gases and 0.00002% as much ^{131}I as the Chernobyl accident.

The released radioactive material affected mainly the western part of the USSR (Byelo-russia, Ukraine and Russia) and the countries of Europe. Long-range atmospheric transport spread the released activity throughout the northern hemisphere. In the southern hemisphere, no airborne activity from Chernobyl has been reported. In Europe, the highest effective dose equivalents in the 1st year were 760 µSv in Bulgaria, 670 µSv in Austria, 590 µSv in Greece and 570 µSv in Romania, followed by those of other countries of northern, eastern and southeastern Europe. For reference, the average annual effective dose equivalents from natural sources is 2400 µSv. The doses in the countries farther to the west of Europe and in Asia, Africa and North and South America were much less. The main pathways and nucleotides contributing to doses were external irradiation from deposited radioactive materials (primarily ^{137}Cs in the longer term) and the dietary ingestion of radionuclides (^{131}I during the first month and, after that, ^{134}Cs and ^{137}Cs). The pathways of cloud gamma-exposure and inhalation of radionuclides were effective only for the short period before the airborne material had been deposited. Transfers along the two primary pathways have been continuing for a length of time that depends on the half-lives of the radionuclides, e.g. some tens of days for ^{131}I, and some tens of years for ^{137}Cs. Initially, 80% of the total radioactivity registered was due to ^{131}I, which characterized the accident as an 'iodine major disaster'. Contributions to the 1st-year committed effective dose equivalents were dominated by ^{131}I, ^{134}Cs and ^{137}Cs. In most countries, ^{134}Cs and ^{137}Cs together contributed over 50% of the dose from ingestion. For the committed 1st-year thyroid dose equivalent, ^{131}I contributed over 90%. The easy absorption of iodine and its accumulation in the thyroid gland, along with the endemic iodine deficiency in a number of heavily contaminated areas, have raised concerns about the related health consequences, particularly in infants and children. Doses of ^{131}I in the environment are generally higher to infants than to adults, because the main pathway is through milk consumption and also because infants are characterized by greater ^{131}I uptake and smaller thyroid mass. Infant thyroid dose equivalents in Europe generally ranged from 1 to 20 mSv, but there were higher doses in some parts of Bulgaria, Greece, Romania, Switzerland and the former USSR.

(2) *The Chernobyl accident: health effects* During 1990–91, the International Chernobyl Project (ICP) was carried out by several international organizations[125] in order to assess radiological and health situations in areas of the former USSR affected by the Chernobyl accident. Based on an evaluation of the estimated doses of irradiation to the population in these areas, possible health effects were expected to be of a stochastic nature (e.g. carcinogenic and mutagenic). Since blood neoplastic diseases are considered to be one of the earliest manifestations of radiation-induced carcinogenicity (with a latency period of 5–7 years, but sometimes as short as 2 years), studies have been performed to assess their incidence in irradiated territories. Increased rates of hemoblastoses in 1989/90 were registered in some of the contaminated areas in the former USSR, e.g. in Bryansk and Rovno[126], but the results were confounded by flaws in medical registers. In one of the most heavily polluted regions of Byelorussia, the Gomel region, a sharp increase in thyroid cancer among children under 15 years of age was reported in 1990/91. In 1991 only, 38 cases of papillary thyroid carcinoma were diagnosed in Gomel[127]. A considerable increase in chromosomal and chromatid aberrations in comparison to the spontaneous background rate was found in a study of 200 children born in Ukraine after the accident and exposed prenatally to 'low' radiation doses[128]. Increased rates of chromosomal structural aberrations in blood cells were seen in Donbass children evacuated from the Chernobyl high-pollution zone. The number of aberrations tended to increase proportionally with the length of time of residence in the zone before evacuation; it was also higher in children whose parents had been employed as 'liquidators' in the zone of high radiation[129].

Outside the former USSR, no other countries have reported an increase in malignancies, including leukemia and thyroid cancer, in children after the accident. The European Childhood Leukaemia–Lymphoma Incidence Study[130] did not find any increase in the incidence of childhood leukoses in many European countries, including Byelorussia, Russia, Estonia, Lithuania, former Czechoslovakia, Hungary, Poland, Slovenia and Bulgaria in 1987/88. No data indicative of increased germ-cell mutations (e.g. specific malformations and genetic diseases) have been reported after the accident in any of the European countries, including the most heavily contaminated regions in Ukraine, Byelorussia and Russia[125].

However, a number of studies performed after the accident in heavily exposed areas in Ukraine and Byelorussia point to adverse effects on pregnancy, intrauterine development, and infant and child health. A survey of 688 mother–infant pairs and 7000 birth histories from two districts (the Chechersky district in Byelorussia and the Polessky district in Ukraine) encompassed a period of 3 years before and 5 years after the accident[131]. Fifty-three per cent of the Ukrainian and 20% of the Byelorussian patients resided in areas of high radioactive soil contamination ($> 740 \times 10^6$ Bq/m^2). The birth rates after the accident decreased from a pre-accident level of 17% to 11% in the more heavily exposed Polessky, and to 14.2% in the Chechersky district; the lowest rate was recorded in 1987. The drop in the birth rates was attributed to the increased number of induced abortions, wider use of contraception, and population evacuation from the polluted territories. Over two-fold increase in the rates of spontaneous abortion and pre-eclampsia was noted along with a rise in extragenital pathology during pregnancy (anemia, arterial hypertension, renal disorders). Maternal thyroid hyperplasia, attributed to exposure to radioisotopes and lack of prophylactic measures, was found in 57.5% of the Ukrainian pregnancies in 1990. The highest level of perinatal mortality (37.4%) was recorded in 1987 in the Ukrainian district; stillbirth and early neonatal mortality rates were 20.6% and 16.8%, respectively. There was a two-fold increase in the incidence of birth defects after the accident; congenital heart disease was the most common finding, and it often coexisted with hydrocephaly, anencephaly and multiple malformations. There were no changes in the average birth weight. Clinical laboratory analyses in pregnancy showed declining maternal thyroid function (decreased serum levels of triiodothyronine, thyroxine and thyroxine-binding globulin), impaired immune function (decreased immunoglobulins, increased C-reactive protein), hormonal imbalance and peripheral blood changes. Placental abnormalities, such as increased placental size and weight, increased dystrophic changes, high (45%) prevalence of basal deciduitis and/or chorioamnionitis, hemodynamic disturbances causing hemorrhage, placental infarctions and decreased synthesis of specific proteins (trophoblastic β-2-globulin, α-2-microglobulin), were found in up to 75% of the women. In infants, a pronounced leukopenia (average cell counts 60% lower than normal), signs of destruction in the lymphocytes, erythropenia with anisocytosis and poikilocytosis were found on the first day of life and progressively in the early neonatal period. These findings pointed to defective compensatory and adaptive, maternal and fetoplacental mechanisms that resulted in increased neonatal morbidity rates[131]. Increased rates of maternal and perinatal pathologies were also reported from other areas in Ukraine. In Donetzk, the incidence of EPH gestosis (pre-eclampsia) increased by nearly 30% during the year after the accident in comparison to the preceding year. The increase was associated with a radiation-induced excessive peroxidation in maternal blood and placenta[132]. In Kiev, the overall incidence of congenital malformations during a 6-year period after the accident was elevated by 43% in comparison to pre-accident levels[133].

Postnatal effects were also reported by a number of studies. A follow-up of 509 infants, prenatally exposed in the evacuation zone and the nearby town of Pripyat (thyroid irradiation dose range from 18 to 120 sGy), during their 1st year of life showed higher rates of thyroid hyperplasia, neurovegetative disturbances indicative of a sympathetic/parasympathetic imbalance, suppression of T cells of immunity, immuno-

globulin imbalance, increased free-radical oxidation processes, and delays in neurobehavioral and mental development in comparison to less severely exposed children[134]. A study of 136 children aged 1–15, who had been living in Kiev at the time of the accident, showed a high prevalence of thyroid hyperplasia (in 19%), immunological disorders (dys-immunoglobulinemia, T-lymphocyte decrease), and high morbidity of cholangiopathies (in 44%), neurological disorders (in 23%), and upper respiratory tract infections[135]. Persistent changes in immune competence, manifested by suppression of the T system of immunity (e.g. decreased T lymphocytes and T suppressor cells), increase and functional changes in B lymphocytes, and decreased immunoglobulin (IgA and IgM) levels, along with elevated morbidity rates were reported in children of preschool age who had been exposed both prenatally and postnatally to radiation in the towns of Kiev and Korosten[136]. Six years after the accident, persisting significant decreases in blood immunoglobulin content were found in children aged 9–15, who had been exposed to low radiation levels[137]. The most frequent causes of increased post-Chernobyl morbidity during 1988–90 among child populations of heavily irradiated villages within the evacuation zone in Ukraine were chronic inflammatory diseases (tonsillitis, lymphadenitis, respiratory infections), thyroid pathology and allergic diseases that affected predominantly the younger age groups (under 7 years). Sixty-eight per cent of the children in these villages had been diagnosed with one or more of the above conditions during their 1st year of life, and 13.5% had a history of perinatal pathology. The infant and neonatal morbidity rates in these heavily exposed areas were three times as high as those in control areas[138]. Along with radiation, other unfavorable environmental factors were also at play, such as protein deficiency (diet protein content being only 24–35% of that recommended), vitamin deficits (up to 60% for thiamine, 34% for niacin, 33% for riboflavin and 21% for ascorbic acid), as well as high content of pesticides, nitrates and heavy metals in locally produced foodstuffs[139].

Most of the studies on the occurrence of developmental and birth defects in Europe after Chernobyl have reported negative results. However, in Denmark, an excess of spina bifida cases has been reported[140]. In Finland, an increased number of malformed infants with low gestational age was seen[141], and studies in Turkey indicated an association between neural tube defects and Chernobyl fallout in areas with a high background occurrence of these defects[142,143]. In Germany, a deviation from a generally falling trend in perinatal and early neonatal mortality was seen in high-dose areas after the Chernobyl accident[144]; in Hungary, an increased number of premature births was registered during the first 2 months after the accident[145]. In Norway, a positive association was found for hydrocephaly and total radiation dose (external and food-based), received in the second month of gestation[146]; however, no associations were found for conditions, expected to be associated with radiation, such as small head circumference, low birth weight and spina bifida. Studies in Croatia and Hungary have not found any increase in 'marker' malformations and malformative syndromes indicative of genetic damage[147]. Therefore, except for the most heavily irradiated territories in the former Soviet Union, where the observed maternal and child problems followed a distinct pattern (thyroid hyperplasia, impaired immune function, late pregnancy complications and non-specific perinatal and postnatal morbidity increase), no consistent changes in reproductive health parameters attributable to Chernobyl have been found in Europe.

References

1. Mattison, D. (1985). The mechanisms of action of reproductive toxins. *Am. J. Ind. Med.*, **4**, 65–79
2. Childs, B. (1980). Genetic factors in human disease. In Kabak, M. (ed.) *Genetic Issues in Pediatric and Obstetric Practice*, pp. 3–16. (Chicago: Year Book)
3. Fathalla, M. F. (1988). Promotion of research in human reproduction: global needs and perspectives. *Hum. Reprod.*, **3**, 7–10
4. Bajaj, J. S., Mistra, A., Rajalakshmi, M. and Madan, R. (1993). Environmental release of chemicals and reproductive ecology. *Environ. Health Perspect.*, **101** (Suppl. 2), 125–30
5. Levin, H. M., Pollit, E., Galloway, R. and McGuire, J. (1991). *Micronutrient Deficiency Disorders*, pp. 5–8. (Washington: The World Bank)
6. US Environmental Protection Agency (1987). *Summary Review on the Health Effects Associated with Zinc and Zinc Exposure*, p. 24. (Washington: US EPA)
7. Holmberg, R. E. and Ferm, V. H. (1969). Interrelationships of selenium, cadmium, and arsenic in mammalian teratogenesis. *Arch. Environ. Health.*, **18**, 873–7
8. Ferm, V. H. and Carpenter, S. J. (1968). The relationship of cadmium and zinc in experimental mammalian teratogenesis. *Lab. Invest.*, **18**, 429–32
9. Tabacova, S. and Vukov, M. (1992). Issues of human exposure to agents causing developmental toxicity. *Cong. Anom.*, **32** (Suppl.), 21–30
10. Savitz, D. and Harlow, D. (1991). Selection of reproductive health endpoints for environmental risk assessment. *Environ. Health Perspect.*, **90**, 159–64
11. Kalter, H. and Warkany, J. (1983). Congenital malformations. Etiologic factors and their role in prevention (First of two parts). *N. Engl. J. Med.*, **308**, 424–31
12. Mattison, D. (1993). Sites of female reproductive vulnerability: implications for testing and risk assessment. *Reprod. Toxicol.*, **7**, 53–62
13. Fabro, S., Brown, N. A. and Scialli, A. R. (1983). Valproic acid and birth defects. *Reprod. Toxicol.*, **2**, 9–11
14. McMichael, A. J. (1993). Global environmental change and human population health: a conceptual and scientific challenge for epidemiology. *Intern. J. Epidemiol.*, **22**, 1–8
15. The World Bank (1993). *World Development Report*, pp. 17–106. (New York: Oxford University Press)
16. Campbell, C. C. and Landrigan, P. J. (1991). Chemical and physical agents. In Sweet, A. Y. and Brown, E. G. (eds.) *Fetal and Neonatal Effects*

of Maternal Disease, pp. 414–47. (St Louis: Mosby Year Book)

17. Kandall, S. R. (1991). Drug abuse. In Sweet, A. Y. and Brown, E. G. (eds.) *Fetal and Neonatal Effects of Maternal Disease*, pp. 401–14. (St Louis: Mosby Year Book)

18. American Academy of Pediatrics Committee on Environmental Hazards (1986). Involuntary smoking – a hazard for children. *Pediatrics*, **77**, 755–7

19. Baird, D. D., Wilcox, A. J. and Weinberg, C. R. (1986). Use of time to pregnancy to study environmental exposures. *Am. J. Epidemiol.*, **124**, 470–80

20. Naeye, R. L. (1979). The duration of maternal cigarette smoking, fetal and placental disorders. *Early Hum. Dev.*, **3**, 229–37

21. Meyer, M. B., Jonas, B. S. and Tonascia, J. A. (1976). Perinatal events associated with maternal smoking during pregnancy. *Am. J. Epidemiol.*, **103**, 464–76

22. Mochizuki, M., Maruo, T. and Masuko, K. (1984). Effects of smoking on fetoplacental-maternal system during pregnancy. *Am. J. Obstet. Gynecol.*, **149**, 413–20

23. Kelly, J., Mathews, K. A. and O'Connor, M. (1984). Smoking in pregnancy: effects on mother and fetus. *Br. J. Obstet. Gynaecol.*, **91**, 111–17

24. Butler, N. R., Goldstein, H. and Ross, E. M. (1972). Cigarette smoking in pregnancy: its influence on birth weight and perinatal mortality. *Br. Med. J.*, **2**, 127–30

25. Rubin, D. H., Leventhal, J. M. and Krasilnikoff, P. A. (1986). Effect of passive smoking on birthweight. *Lancet*, **2**, 415–17

26. Martin, T. R. and Bracken, M. B. (1986). Association of low birthweight with passive smoke exposure in pregnancy. *Am. J. Epidemiol.*, **124**, 633–42

27. Holsclaw, D. S. and Topham, A. L. (1978). The effects of smoking on fetal, neonatal, and children development. *Pediatr. Ann.*, **7**, 105–36

28. Miller, H. C., Hassanein, K. and Hensleigh, P. A. (1976). Fetal growth retardation in relation to maternal smoking and weight gain in pregnancy. *Am. J. Obstet. Gynecol.*, **125**, 55–60

29. Wolff, M. S. (1983). Occupationally derived chemicals in breast milk. *Am. J. Ind. Med.*, **4**, 259–81

30. Tabacova, S., Baird, D. D., Balabaeva, L., Lolova, D. and Petrov, I. (1994). Placental arsenic and cadmium in relation to lipid peroxides and glutathione levels in maternal–infant pairs from a copper smelter area. *Placenta*, **15**, 873–81

31. Beckman, D. A. and Brent, R. L. (1990). Teratogenesis: alcohol, angiotensin-converting-enzyme inhibitors, and cocaine. *Curr. Opin. Obstet. Gynecol.*, **2**, 236–45

32. Jones *et al.* (1973), as cited by Beckman, D. A. and Brent, R. L. (1990). Teratogenesis: alcohol, angiotensin-converting-enzyme inhibitors, and cocaine. *Curr. Opin. Obstet. Gynecol.*, **2**, 236–45

33. Streissguth, A. P., Herman, C. S. and Smith, D. W. (1978). Intelligence, behavior, and dysmorphogenesis in the fetal alcohol syndrome: a report on 20 patients. *J. Pediatr.*, **92**, 363–7

34. Pierog, S., Chandavasu, O. and Wexler, I. (1977). Withdrawal symptoms in infants with the fetal alcohol syndrome. *J. Pediatr.*, **90**, 630–3

35. Day, N. L., Jasperse, D., Richardson, G., Robles, N., Sambamoorthi, U., Taylor, P., Scher, M., Stoffer, D. and Cornelius, M. (1989). Prenatal exposure to alcohol: effect on infant growth and morphologic characteristics. *Pediatrics*, **84**, 536–41

36. Chasnoff, I. J., Bussey, M. E. and Savich, R. (1986). Perinatal cerebral infarction and maternal cocaine use. *J. Pediatr.*, **108**, 456–9

37. Chasnoff, I. J. and Griffith, D. R. (1989). Cocaine: clinical studies of pregnancy and the newborn. *Ann. NY Acad. Sci.*, **562**, 260–6

38. Kandall, S. R., Albin, S. and Gartner, L. M. (1977). The narcotic-dependent mother: fetal and neonatal consequences. *Early Hum. Dev.*, **1**, 159–69

39. Rajegowda, B. K., Kandall, S. R. and Falciglia, H. (1978). Sudden unexpected death in infants of narcotic-dependent mothers. *Early Hum. Dev.*, **2**, 219–25

40. Chavez, C. J., Ostrea, E. M. and Stryker, J. C. (1979). Sudden infant death syndrome among infants of drug-dependent mothers. *J. Pediatr.*, **95**, 407–9

41. Finnegan, L. P. (1979). *In utero* opiate dependence and sudden infant death syndrome. *Clin. Perinatol.*, **6**, 163–80

42. Smith, C. G. (1983). Reproductive toxicity: hypothalamic–pituitary mechanisms. *Am. J. Ind. Med.*, **4**, 107–12

43. Smith, C. G. (1982). Drug effects on male sexual function. *Clin. Obstet. Gynecol.*, **25**, 525–31

44. Bellinger, D. (1994). Teratogen update: lead. *Teratology*, **50**, 367–73

45. Cullen, M. R., Kayne, R. D. and Robins, J. M. (1984). Endocrine and reproductive dysfunction in men associated with occupational inorganic lead intoxication. *Arch. Environ. Health.*, **39**, 431–40

46. Assennato, G., Paci, C. and Baser, M. E. (1986). Sperm count suppression without endocrine

dysfunction in lead-exposed men. *Arch. Environ. Health*, **41**, 387–90

47. Lindbohm, M.-L., Sallmen, M., Anttila, A., Taskinen, H. and Hemminki, K. (1991). Paternal occupational lead exposure and spontaneous abortion. *Scand. J. Work Environ. Health.*, **17**, 95–103

48. Kristensen, P., Irgens, L., Dalveit, A. and Andersen, A. (1993). Perinatal outcome among children of men exposed to lead and organic solvents in printing industry. *Am. J. Epidemiol.*, **137**, 134–44

49. Needleman, H. L., Rabinowitz, M., Leviton, A., Linn, S. and Schoenbaum, S. (1984). The relationship between prenatal exposure to lead and congenital anomalies. *J. Am. Med. Assoc.*, **251**, 2956–9

50. Gershanic, J., Brooks, G. and Little, J. (1974). Blood lead values in pregnant women and their offspring. *Am. J. Obstet. Gynecol.*, **119**, 508–11

51. Barltrop, D. (1969). *Mineral Metabolism in Pediatrics: A Glaxo Symposium.*, pp. 135–51. (Oxford: Blackwell Scientific Publications)

52. Silbergeld, E. K. (1986). Maternally mediated exposure of the fetus: *in utero* exposure to lead and other toxins. *Neurotoxicology*, **7**, 557–68

53. Rom, W. N. (1976). Effects of lead on the female and reproduction: a review. *Mt Sinai J. Med.*, **43**, 542–52

54. Wibberley, D. G., Khera, A. K. and Edwards, J. H. (1977). Lead levels in human placetae from normal and malformed births. *J. Med. Genet.*, **14**, 339–45

55. Aschengrau, A., Zierler, S. and Cohen, A. (1993). Quality of community drinking water and the occurrence of late adverse pregnancy outcomes. *Arch. Environ. Health*, **48**, 105–13

56. Fahim, M. S., Fahim, Z. and Hall, D. G. (1976). Effects of subtoxic lead levels on pregnant women in the state of Missouri. *Res. Commun. Chem. Pathol. Pharmacol.*, **13**, 309–31

57. McMichael, A. J., Vimpani, G. V. and Robertson, E. F. (1986). The Port Pirie cohort study: maternal blood lead and pregnancy outcome. *J. Epidemiol. Community Health*, **40**, 18–25

58. Dietrich, K., Krafft, K., Bornschein, R., Hammond, P., Berger, O., Succop, P. and Bier, M. (1987). Low-level fetal lead exposure effect on neurobehavioral development in early infancy. *Pediatrics*, **80**, 721–50

59. Kimmel, C. A. (1984). Critical periods of exposure and developmental effects of lead. In Kacew, S. and Reasor, M. J. (eds.) *Toxicology and the Newborn*, pp. 219–35. (Amsterdam: Elsevier Science Publishers)

60. Bellinger, D. and Needleman, H. (1985). Prenatal and early postnatal exposure to lead: developmental effects, correlates, and implications. *Int. J. Mental Health*, **14**, 78–111

61. Hu, H. (1991). Knowledge of diagnosis and reproductive history among survivors of childhood plumbism. *Am. J. Public Health.*, **81**, 1070–2

62. Bellinger, D., Leviton, A., Waternaux, C., Needleman, H. and Rabinowitz, M. (1987). Longitudinal analyses of prenatal and postnatal lead exposure and early congnitive development. *N. Engl. J. Med.*, **316**, 1037–43

63. Wasserman, G., Graziano, J., Factor-Litvak, P., Popovac, D., Morina, N., Musabegovic, A., Vrenezi, N., Capuni-Paracka, S., Lekic, V., Preteni-Redjepi, E., Hadjialjjevic, S., Slavkovich, V., Kline, J., Shrout, P. and Stein, Z. (1994). Consequences of lead exposure and iron supplementation on childhood development at age 4 years. *Neurotoxicol. Teratol.*, **16**, 233–40

64. Dietrich, K., Succop, P., Berger, O. and Keith, R. (1992). Lead exposure and the central auditory processing abilities and cognitive development in urban children: the Cincinnati Lead Study cohort at age 5 years. *Neurotoxicol. Teratol.*, **14**, 51–6

65. Dietrich, K., Berger, O. and Succop, P. (1993). Lead exposure and the motor developmental status of urban six-year-old-children in the Cincinnati Prospective Study. *Pediatrics*, **91**, 301–7

66. Schwartz, J. (1994). Low-level lead exposure and children's IQ: a meta-analysis and search for a threshold. *Environ. Res.*, **65**, 42–55

67. Bellinger, D., Stiles, K. and Needleman, H. (1992). Low-level lead exposure, intelligence and academic achievement: a long-term follow-up study. *Pediatrics*, **90**, 855–61

68. Leonard, A., Jacquet, P. and Lauwerys, R. R. (1983). Mutagenicity and teratogenicity of mercury compounds. *Mutat. Res.*, **114**, 1–18

69. Koos, B. J. and Longo, L. D. (1976). Mercury toxicity in the pregnant woman, fetus, and newborn infant. *Am. J. Obstet. Gynecol.*, **126**, 390–409

70. Tsuchiya, H., Mitani, H. and Kodama, K. (1984). Placental transfer of heavy metals in normal pregnant Japanese women. *Arch. Environ. Health.*, **39**, 11–17

71. Elhassani, S. B. (1982). The many faces of methylmercury poisoning. *J. Toxicol. Clin. Toxicol.*, **19**, 875–906

72. Clarkson, T. W., Nordberg, G. F. and Sager, P. R. (1985). Reproductive and developmental toxicity of metals. *Scand. J. Work. Environ. Health.*, **11**, 145–54

73. Chisolm, J. J. (1980). Poisoning from heavy metals (mercury, lead, and cadmium). *Pediatr. Ann.*, **9**, 458–68

74. Harada, M. (1978). Congenital Minamata disease: intrauterine methylmercury poisoning. *Teratology*, **18**, 285–8

75. Matsumoto, H., Koya, G. and Takeuchi, T. (1964). Minamata disease. A neuropathological study of two cases of intrauterine intoxication by a methylmercury compound. *J. Neuropathol. Exp. Neurol.*, **24**, 563–74

76. Amin-Zaki, L., Elhassani, S. and Majeed, M. A. (1976). Perinatal methylmercury poisoning in Iraq. *Am. J. Dis. Child.*, **130**, 1070–6

77. Sikorski, R., Juszkiewicz, T. and Paszkowski, T. (1987). Women in dental surgeries: reproductive hazards in occupational exposure to metallic mercury. *Int. Arch. Occup. Environ. Health*, **59**, 551–7

78. Panova, Z. (1988). *Occupational Obstetric Gynaecological Pathology*, pp. 33–7 (in Bulgarian). (Sofia: Medicina i Fizkultura State Publishing House)

79. Lauwerys, R., Amery, A., Bernard, A., Bruaux, A., Buchet, J.-P., Claeys, F., De Plaen, P., Ducoffre, G., Fagard, R., Lijnen, P., Nick, L., Roels, H., Rondia, D., Saint-Remy, A., Sator, F. and Staessen, J. (1990). Health effects of environmental exposure to cadmium: objectives, design and organization of the Cadmibel Study: a cross-sectional morbidity study carried out in Belgium from 1985 to 1989. *Environ. Health Perspect.*, **87**, 283–9

80. Bernard, A. and Lauwerys, R. (1986). Effects of cadmium exposure in humans. In Foulkes, E. C. (ed.) *Handbook of Experimental Pharmacology*, pp. 135–77. (Heidelberg: Springer-Verlag)

81. Drasch, G. A. (1983). An increase in cadmium body burden for this century. An investigation on human tissues. *Sci. Total Environ.*, **26**, 111–19

82. United States Environmental Protection Agency (1981). *Health Assessment Document for Cadmium*, pp. 4–61. (Research Triangle Park, NC: Environmental Criteria and Assessment Office)

83. Wier, P. J., Miller, R. K., Maulik, D. and di Sant' Agnese, P. A. (1990). Toxicity of cadmium in the perfused human placenta. *Toxicol. Appl. Pharmacol.*, **105**, 156–71

84. Miller, R. K., Ng, W. W. and Levin, A. A. (1983). The placenta: relevance to toxicology. In Clarkson, T., Nordberg, G. and Sager, P. (eds.) *Reproductive and Developmental Toxicity of Metals*, pp. 569–605. (New York: Plenum Press)

85. Levin, A. A., Miller, R. K. and di Sant' Agnese, P. A. (1983). Heavy metal alterations of placental function: a mechanism for the induction of fetal toxicity with cadmium in the rat. In Clarkson, T., Nordberg, G. and Sager, P. (eds.) *Repro-* *ductive and Developmental Toxicity of Metals*, pp. 633–54. (New York: Plenum Press)

86. Tsvetkova, R. P. (1970). Influence of cadmium compounds on the generative function (in Russian). *Gig. Tr. Prof. Zabol.*, **14**, 31–3

87. Huel, G., Boudene, C. and Ibrahim, M. A. (1981). Cadmium and lead content of maternal and newborn hair. Relationship to parity, birth weight and hypertension. *Arch. Environ. Health.*, **36**, 221–7

88. International Agency for Research on Cancer (1987). *IARC Monographs on the Evaluation of the Carcinogenic Risks to Humans*, Suppl. 7, pp. 139–41. (Lyon: World Health Organization)

89. Safe, S. H. (1994). Environmental and dietary estrogens and human health: is there a problem? *Environ. Health Perspect.*, **103**, 346–51

90. Verdeal, K. and Ryan, D. S. (1979). Naturally-occurring estrogens in plant foodstuffs – a review. *J. Food Protection*, **42**, 577–83

91. Colborn, T. (1994). The wildlife/human connection: modernizing risk decisions. *Environ. Health Perspect.*, **102** (Suppl. 12), 55–9

92. Bush, B., Snow, J. and Koblintz, R. (1986). Polychlorinated (PCB) congeners, p,p′-DDE, and sperm function in humans. *Arch. Environ. Contam. Toxicol.*, **15**, 333–41

93. Sharpe, R. M. and Skakkebaek, N. F. (1993). Are oestrogens involved in falling sperm counts and disorders of the male reproductive tract. *Lancet*, **341**, 1391–5

94. Carlsen, E., Giwercman, A., Keiding, N. and Skakkebaek, N. (1992). Evidence for the decreasing quality of semen during the past 50 years. *Br. Med. J.*, **305,** 609–12

95. Bromwich, P., Cohen, J., Stewart, I. and Walker, A. (1994). Decline in sperm counts: an artefact of changed reference range of normal. *Br. Med. J.*, **309**, 19–22

96. Ramilow, M. (1994). As cited by Safe, S. (1994). Environmental and dietary estrogens and human health: is there a problem? *Environ. Health Perspect.*, **103**, 346–51

97. Rogan, W. J., Gladen, B. C. and Hung, K. (1988). Congenital poisoning by polychlorinated biphenyls and their contaminants in Taiwan. *Science*, **241**, 334–6

98. Fein, G. G., Jacobson, J. L. and Jacobson, S. W. (1984). Prenatal exposure to polychlorinated biphenyls: effect on birth size and gestational age. *J. Pediatr.*, **105**, 315–20

99. Tilson, H. A., Jacobson, J. L. and Rogan, W. J. (1990). Polychlorinated biphenyls and the developing nervous system: cross-species comparison. *Neurotoxicol. Teratol.*, **12**, 239–48

100. Rogan, W. J. and Gladen, B. C. (1985). Study of human lactation for effects of environmental

contaminants: The North Carolina Breast Milk and Formula Project and some other ideas. *Environ. Health Perspect.*, **60**, 215–21

101. Bucher, J. R. (1987). Methylisocyanate: a review of health effects research since Bhopal. *Fund. Appl. Toxicol.*, **9**, 367–79

102. Heylin, M. (1985). Bhopal. *Chem. Eng. News*, Feb. 11, 14–15

103. Lepkowski, W. (1985). Bhopal. Indian city begins to heal but conflicts remain. *Chem. Eng. News*, Dec 2, 18–32

104. Varma, D. R. (1987). Epidemiological and environmental studies on the effects of methylisocyanate on the course of pregnancy. *Environ. Health Perspect.*, **72**, 151–5

105. Schwetz, B. A., Adkins, B. Jr, Harris, M., Moorman, M. and Sloan, R. (1987). Methylisocyanate: reproductive and developmental toxicology studies in Swiss mice. *Environ. Health Perspect.*, **72**, 147–50

106. Shelby, M. D., Allen, J. W., Caspary, W. J., Haworth, S., Ivett, J., Klingerman, A., Luke, C. A., Mason, J. M., Myhr, B., Tice, R. R., Valencia, R. and Zeiger, R. (1987). Results of *in vitro* and *in vivo* genetic toxicity tests of methylisocyanate. *Environ. Health Perspect.*, **72**, 181–5

107. Committee on the Biological Effects of Ionizing Radiations, Division of Medical Sciences, Assembly of Life Sciences, National Research Council (1980). *The Effects on Populations of Exposure to Low Levels of Ionizing Radiation (BEIR III)*. (Washington, DC: National Academy of Sciences)

108. Lione, A. (1987). Ionizing radiation and human reproduction. *Reprod. Toxicol.*, **1**, 3–16

109. Heller, C. G. (1967). Effects on the germinal epithelium. In Langham, W. H. (ed.) *Radiological Factors in Manned Space Flight*, NRC Publication 1487, pp. 124–33. (Washington DC: National Academy of Sciences, National Research Council)

110. Rowley, M. J., Leach, D. R. and Warner, G. A. (1974). Effect of graded doses of ionizing radiation on the human testis. *Radiat. Res.*, **59**, 665–78

111. Lushbauch, C. C. and Ricks, R. C. (1972). Some cytokinetic and histopathologic considerations of irradiated male and female gonadal tissues. *Front. Radiat. Ther. Oncol.*, **6**, 229–48

112. Brent, R. L. (1977). Radiations and other physical agents. In Wilson, J. G. and Frazer, F. C. (eds.) *Handbook of Teratology*, Vol. 1, pp. 153–223. (New York: Plenum Press)

113. Lushbaugh, C. C. and Casarett, G. W. (1976). The effects of gonadal irradiation in clinical radiation therapy: a review. *Cancer*, **37**, 1111–20

114. Schull, W. J., Otake, M. and Neel, J. W. (1981). Hiroshima and Nagasaki: a reassessment of the mutagenic effect of exposure to inoizing radiation. In *Population and Biological Aspects of Human Mutation*, pp. 277–303. (New York: Academic Press)

115. Jensh, R. P. (1985). Ionizing radiation and the conceptus: neurophysiologic effects of prenatal x-irradiation on offspring. *Ann. Clin. Lab. Sci.*, **15**, 185–94

116. Brent, R. L. (1980). Radiation teratogenesis. *Teratology*, **21**, 281–98

117. Russel, L. B. and Russel, W. L. (1952). Radiation hazards to the embryo and fetus. *Radiology*, **58**, 369–76

118. Beebe, G. W. (1981). The atomic bomb survivors and the problem of low-dose radiation effects. *Am. J. Epidemiol.*, **114**, 761–83

119. Otake, M. and Schull, W. J. (1984). *In utero* exposure to A-bomb radiation and mental retardation: a reassessment. *Br. J. Radiol.*, **57**, 409–14

120. Dobbing, J. and Sands, J. (1973). Quantitative growth and development of human brain. *Arch. Dis. Child.*, **48**, 757–67

121. Mettler, F. A. and Moseley, R. D. (1985). *Medical Effects of Ionizing Radiation*, p. 288. (New York: Grune & Stratton)

122. International Commission on Radiological Protection (1986). *Developmental Effects of Irradiation on the Brain of the Embryo and Fetus*, Annals of the ICRP, 16(4), p. 43 (Oxford, New York: Pergamon Press)

123. Stewart, A., Webb, J. and Hewitt, D. (1958). A survey of childhood malignancies. *Br. Med. J.*, **1**, 1495–508

124. United States Scientific Committee on the Effects of Atomic Radiation (UNSCEAR) (1988). *Sources, Effects, and Risks of Ionizing Radiation: 1988 Report to the General Assembly, with Annexes.* (New York: United Nations)

125. International Atomic Energy Association (1991). *The International Chernobyl Project. Report by an International Advisory Committee.* (Vienna: IAEA)

126. Vygovskaya, Y., Kachorovsky, B. and Mazurok. A. (1992). Cases of hemoblastosis in regions of the Rovno province contaminated with radionuclides in the result of the Chernobyl accident (in Russian). Presented at the *3rd Scientific Conference on Scientific–Practical Aspects of Preserving of Health in Persons Exposed to Radiation Impact in the Result of the Chernobyl Accident*, April, Gomel, Minsk

127. Baverstock, K., Egloff, B., Pinchers, A., Ruchti, C. and Williams, D. (1992). Thyroid cancer after Chernobyl. *Nature (London)*, **359**, 21–2

128. Vanyurikhina, K. A. (1993). Evaluation of genetic sequelae of prenatal exposure to low doses of ionizing radiation (in Russian). Presented at the *International Scientific–Practical Conference on Radiational, Ecological and Medical Aspects of the Accident at the Chernobyl Atomic Electric Station*, June, Kiev

129. Barilyak, I. G., Frolov, V. N. and Peresadin, N. A. (1993). Chromosomal characteristics of peripheral blood cells in children under the influence of low-intensity radiation in an ecologically unfavourable region in Ukraine (in Russian). Presented at the *International Scientific–Practical Conference on Radiational, Ecological and Medical Aspects of the Accident at the Chernobyl Atomic Electric Station*, June, Kiev

130. Parkin, D., Gardis, E., Masuyer, E., Friedl, H., Hansluwka, H., Bobev, D., Ivanov, E., Sinnaeva, J., Agustin, J., Plesko, I. and Storm, H. (1993). European Childhood Leukaemia–Lymphoma Incidence Study. *Eur. J. Cancer*, **29A**, 87–95

131. Kulakov, V. I., Sokur, T. N., Volobuev, A. I., Tzibulskaya, I. S., Malisheva, V. A., Zikin, B. I., Ezova, L. C., Belyaeva, L. A., Bonartzev, L. B. and Orlova, N. S. (1993). Female reproductive function in areas affected by radiation after the Chernobyl power station accident. *Environ. Health Perspect.*, **101** (Suppl. 2), 117–24

132. Tchayka, V. K., Kvashchenko, V. P., Akimova, I. K. and Zolotukhin, N. S. (1993). Epidemiological aspects of the effect of pre-morbid doses of radiation on the course of pregnancy and birth in Donbass (in Russian). Presented at the *International Scientific–Practical Conference on Radiational, Ecological and Medical Aspects of the Accident at the Chernobyl Atomic Electric Station*, June, Kiev

133. Golota, V. Ya., Mikhasyuk, S. E. and Makarenko, G. I. (1993). Obstetric–gynecological pathology in the town of Kiev in 1986–1992 (trends, problems) (in Russian). Presented at the *International Scientific–Practical Conference on Radiational, Ecological and Medical Aspects of the Accident at the Chernobyl Atomic Electric Station*, June, Kiev

134. Stepanova, E. I., Kondrashova, V. G., Galichanskaya, T. Ya., Kolesnikov, Yu, A. and Vdovenko, V. Yu. (1993). Children irradiation *in utero*. (Clinical aspects) (in Russian). Presented at the *International Scientific–Practical Conference on Radiational, Ecological and Medical Aspects of the Accident at the Chernobyl Atomic Electric Station*, June, Kiev

135. Tyazhkaya, A. V., Androshchuk, A. A., Lutai, T. I., Pomytkina, L. R., Antoshkima, A. N., Kazakova, L. N., Vasyukova, M. M., Kazmirchuk, V. E., Daletskaya, L. P., Martynova, L. E. and Aleksinskaya, I. M. (1993). Some health indicators of children and their parents permanently residing in the town of Kiev (in Russian). Presented at the *International Scientific–Practical Conference on Radiational, Ecological and Medical Aspects of the Accident at the Chernobyl Atomic Electric Station*, June, Kiev

136. Androshchuk, A. A., Tyazhkaya, A. V., Antoshkina, A. N., Daletskaya, L. P., Makarchak, N. M., Kruglikova, A. A., Pomytkina, L. R., Aleksinskaya, I. M., Lutai, T. I. and Kazakova, L. N. (1993). Status of the immune system and nonspecific factors of resistance in children residing in zones with different levels of radiation contamination (in Russian). Presented at the *International Scientific–Practical Conference on Radiational, Ecological and Medical Aspects of the Accident at the Chernobyl Atomic Electric Station*, June, Kiev

137. Kaminskaya, T. A., Gulyaev, G. K. and Luzin, A. V. (1993). On some aspects of the assessment of health status in children who arrived in Evpatoria spa from zones of radionuclide contamination (in Russian). Presented at the *International Scientific–Practical Conference on Radiational, Ecological and Medical Aspects of the Accident at the Chernobyl Atomic Electric Station*, June, Kiev

138. Zvinyatskovskii, Ya, I., Serykh, L. V., Berdnik, O. V., Zaykovskaya, V. Yu. and Stoyan, E. F. (1993). Health status of children populations residing in rural areas with different radiation situation (in Russian). Presented at the *International Scientific–Practical Conference on Radiational, Ecological and Medical Aspects of the Accident at the Chernobyl Atomic Electric Station*, June, Kiev

139. Salii, N. S., Matasar, I. T. and Dzyuba, M. G. (1993). Ecological situation, nutrition, and general population health in the controlled districts in Ukraine (in Russian). Presented at the *International Scientific–Practical Conference on Radiational, Ecological and Medical Aspects of the Accident at the Chernobyl Atomic Electric Station*, June, Kiev

140. EUROCAT Working Group (1988). Preliminary evaluation of the impact of the Chernobyl radiological contamination on the frequency of central nervous system malformations in 18 regions in Europe. *Paediatr. Perinat. Epidemiol.*, **2**, 253–64

141. Harjulehto, T., Aro, T. and Rita, H. (1989). The accident at Chernobyl and outcome of pregnancy in Finland. *Br. Med. J.*, **298**, 995–7

142. Guvenc, H., Uslu, M. A. and Okten, A. (1989). Incidence of anencephaly in Elazig, eastern Turkey. *Paediatr. Perinat. Epidemiol.*, **3**, 230–2

143. Mocan, H., Bozkaya, H. and Mocan, M. Z. (1990). Changing incidence of anencephaly in eastern Black Sea region of Turkey and Chernobyl. *Paediatr. Perinat. Epidemiol.*, **4**, 264–8

144. Lining, G., Schmidt, M. and Scheer, J. (1989). Early infant mortality in West Germany before and after Chernobyl. *Lancet*, **334**, 1081–3

145. Czeizel, A. and Billege, B. (1988). Teratological evaluation of Hungarian pregnancy outcomes after the accident in the nuclear power station of Chernobyl (in Hungarian). *Orvosi Hertilap*, **129**, 457–62

146. Lie, R. T., Irgens, L. M., Skjaerven, R., Reitan, J. B., Strand, P. and Strand, T. (1992). Birth defects in Norway by levels of external and food-based exposure to radiation from Chernobyl. *Am. J. Epidemiol.*, **136**, 377–88

147. Czeizel, A., Elek, C. and Susanszky, E. (1991). The evaluation of the germinal mutagenic impact of Chernobyl radiological contamination in Hungary. *Mutagenesis*, **6**, 285–8

Influences of nutrition on the menstrual cycle and fertility in women

20

J. Bringer, E. Renard, P. Lefebvre, B. Hedon and C. Jaffiol

Introduction

The impact of unbalanced nutrition on humans has been largely investigated in women where it clearly induces overt abnormalities of the menstrual cycle. The greater frequency of dysovulation in obese women is associated with various alterations in hormone secretion, transport and metabolism. The abdominal android fat distribution is positively correlated to menstrual irregularities[1], whereas it is negatively correlated with conception rate[2]. Being overweight reduces the effectiveness of follicular stimulating agents and, in this condition, ovulatory function is improved by a significant weight loss[3,4]. Food deprivation and excessive thinness inhibit ovulation and cause infertility both in animals[5,6] and in women[7,8]. The basal gonadotropin levels and response of luteinizing hormone (LH) to gonadotropin releasing hormone (GnRH) are related to weight and tightly correlated to basal metabolism[9], which is a marker of energy balance. Taken together, these data suggest that weight, body composition, fat distribution and food intake greatly influence the fertility of women. Therefore, the evaluation of these nutritional parameters represents an essential step in assessing every woman with infertility or menstrual dysfunction.

Obesity, ovulatory disorders and infertility

A higher incidence of *obesity* was found in amenorrheic women (45%) when compared to populations of normal cycling controls (9.5 and 13%)[10]. It has been suggested that amenorrhea in such women develops shortly after a period of rapid weight gain[11]. Successful weight loss in women could have a salutary effect in restoring normal menstrual function[11–13]. Moreover, weight reduction in obese anovulatory and hyperandrogenic women resulted in a marked fall in plasma levels of androgens[3,4] and LH[4], which coincided with the return of ovulatory function[4].

The fact that most obese women have normal ovulatory menstrual cycles and remain fertile suggest that obesity *per se* is not the only mechanism able to explain the disorders of ovulation and fertility seen in some obese women[12].

The quantity of fat is not the main factor influencing reproduction in obese women but the body location of the excess fat is a determining factor[14]. Independently of the weight, the *abdominal distribution of fat* seems to have a deleterious effect on female fecundity. The waist-to-hip ratio (WHR), assessed in 12 000 women aged between 20 and 39 years, is positively correlated to the prevalence of oligomenorrhea[1]. WHR is negatively correlated to the conception rate of women submitted to an insemination by donor semen[2]. This negative correlation remains after adjustment for age, parity, weight, duration of cycles and tobacco consumption[2]. Therefore, the endocrine metabolic alterations observed in women with abdominal obesity may be involved in their oligo-ovulation and relative infertility. Women with excess fat in the glutofemoral region usually do not have such disturbances and rarely have abnormal menstrual cycles[14].

The coexistence of upper body obesity, hyperandrogenism and *polycystic ovarian syndrome*

(PCOS) raises the possibility that obesity, frequently associated with PCOS[15], is able to reveal or reinforce the hormonal and ovulatory disorders accompanying this condition. The higher levels of non-cyclic estrogen (estrone) produced in fat[16] could induce an abnormal secretory pattern, with predominance of LH over follicle stimulating hormone (FSH) that stimulates ovarian androgen synthesis, follicular dysfunction and polycystic ovaries[4]. Changes in peripheral aromatization of androgens to estrogens[17] and inappropriate gonadotropin secretion are associated with other hormonal features involving a decrease in sex hormone binding globulin (SHBG) and an increase in adrenal and ovarian androgen production[12].

The possibility that obesity may entirely cause PCOS in some women remains controversial, although it is obvious that a rapid increase of weight sometimes reveals a previous masked syndrome. There is evidence that weight, body composition, fat distribution and eating habits are able to modulate the following (Figure 1 and Table 1):

(1) Clinical and biological phenotypes and, therefore, the severity of the hormonal and metabolic abnormalities seen in PCOS, as well as their long-term vascular consequences;

(2) The prognosis of infertility and response to follicle stimulating agents;

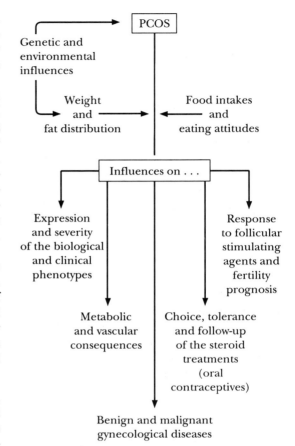

Figure 1 Influences of weight and nutrition on clinical aspects of polycystic ovarian syndrome (PCOS)

Table 1 Polycystic ovarian syndrome: main phenotypes and their clinical consequences

	Normal* weight	Overweight and/or abdominal fat location
Body mass index (kg/m^2)	≤ 25	> 25
Waist-to-hip ratio	≤ 0.80	> 0.80
% of women with PCOS	45	55
Higher risk for		
metabolic disorders (X syndrome)	no	yes
vascular disease	no	yes
endometrial cancer	?	++
Higher tendency to increase weight and abdominal fat with age	no	yes
Tolerance of treatment (oral contraceptives) to restore regular cycles and prevent gynecological consequences	usually excellent	various (weight increase, metabolic etc.)
Ovarian response to follicular stimulating agents	easy (hyperstimulation)	lower

*Women with acanthosis nigricans are excluded: PCOS, polycystic ovarian syndrome

(3) Morbidity in pregnancy and especially the risk of gestational diabetes[18];

(4) Choice, tolerance and follow-up of the sex steroid compounds regulating the menstrual cycle, treating hyperandrogenic symptoms and preventing endometrial hyperplasia;

(5) Risks of benign or malignant gynecological diseases such as uterine fibroids[19], endometrial carcinoma[20] and, to a lesser extent, breast carcinoma[21,22].

This paper reviews advances in the first three issues related to fertility.

The influence of nutrition on PCOS phenotypes (Figure 1 and Table 1)

Fifty per cent of PCOS women are obese[15,23], and most of them have a waist-to-hip ratio with a predominant upper body fat patterning. Lean PCOS patients differed significantly from obese PCOS in LH, SHBG, free testosterone and insulinemia[23,24]. Weight positively correlated to free testosterone, whereas weight and fat negatively correlated to SHBG[15,23]. Many reports have shown that women with PCOS may be insulin-resistant[25,26]. It has been suggested that insulin resistance and the subsequent hyperinsulinemia is a feature of PCOS independent of weight[25,26]. Studies in lean patients with PCOS are conflicting. Data using the glucose clamp technique, intravenous or oral glucose tolerance test and insulin tolerance test have suggested insulin resistance. However, few studies have taken into account the impact of the fat distribution, and none have quantified visceral fat or evaluated lifestyle and eating pattern, factors largely involved in insulin sensitivity. Patients with PCOS show a significant increase of abnormal eating patterns and are two times more likely to have subclinical bulimia, as demonstrated by a bulimia investigation test[27]. Overweight, hirsutism and acne frequently seen in PCOS are in direct conflict with socially normal views of femininity, explaining the high levels of anxiety and misacceptance of their self-

evaluated body shape, resulting in bulimia. Such alterations in food intake, and particularly binge eating, may modulate insulin secretion and sensitivity in individuals submitted to rapid changes in visceral fat.

Other studies, employing an insulin test with a low physiological dose during a glucose clamp, found no evidence of impaired insulin sensitivity in lean PCOS patients with androgen levels 2–3-fold higher than normal, compared to that in control subjects which were well matched for body mass index, WHR and free fat mass[28]. Moreover, with an extensive methodological approach, the insulin sensitivity was found to be normal in muscle, liver and adipose tissue[28].

Finally, it appears clearly that the majority of European studies do not detect hyperinsulinemia and insulin resistance in PCO women of normal weight[15,24,28–30], whereas most of the studies in the USA do[25,26,31]. An initial explanation for these controversial results may be that US patients tend to be heavier[26,31] than those included in the European studies where moderately overweight women and not solely obese subjects were excluded from the data[15,24,28–30]. Moreover, it is obvious that food customs in the USA differ qualitatively from those in European. Differences in body fat distribution, and therefore insulin sensitivity and secretion, could result from these discrepancies in 'food culture' between the two continents.

Another explanation for the conflicting results observed between studies on PCOS may be the exclusion[15,28,29], or not, of the particular subgroup with clinical acanthosis nigricans and extreme insulin resistance, so-called HAIR-AN syndrome (hyperandrogenism, insulin resistance, acanthosis nigricans). In this rare syndrome, occurring in less than 10% of PCOS patients, the marked hyperinsulinemia usually reveals a gene defect located on subunit α or β of the insulin receptor[15].

Taken together, the results of these studies suggest that the great majority of lean hyperandrogenic women with PCOS and without acanthosis nigricans are normosensitive to insulin and have similar insulin levels, serum lipoprotein lipid profile (including plasma free fatty acid) to control subjects[15,24,28–30]. Finally, except for the HAIR-AN phenotype, lack of sensitivity to insulin and atherogenic disturbances of lipids in PCOS patients could be related to their abdominal fat distribution without a significant difference between patients with PCOS and their visceral fat-matched controls[15,24,28,29]. The origin of the insulin resistance is at the post-receptor level and involves a defect in the insulin signal transduction chain[31] between the receptor kinase and glucose transport. Therefore, the increased prevalence of diabetes, hypertension and myocardial infarction seen in PCOS women aged 45–60 years[32] could be related to the X syndrome commonly associated with abdominal-visceral obesity.

Prognosis of infertility and response to follicular stimulating agents

Weight is positively correlated with the dosage of clomiphene citrate required to achieve ovulation, although once ovulation has occurred obesity does not appear to affect the ability to conceive[33]. There is also a direct relationship between weight and the amount of human menopausal gonadotropin (hMG) needed to induce follicular development, ovulation and/or pregnancy[34].

GnRH pulsatile treatment gives a lower rate of ovulations and pregnancies in overweight women with eugonadotropic chronic anovulation[35,36]. Weight loss induces a decrease in LH, total and free testosterone and has a beneficial effect on ovulation and fertility in obese women[4].

On the other hand, lean women with PCOS have a higher rate of hyperstimulation with hMG and human chorionic gonadotropin procedures. The recommendations for the induction of ovulation in overweight women point out the necessity of achieving a significant weight loss before stimulation (Figure 2).

Obesity and pregnancy outcome

Being overweight alters the course and outcome of pregnancy. The prevalences of hypertension,

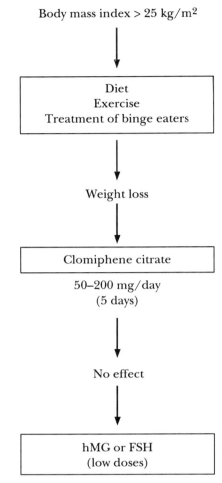

Figure 2 Management of induction of ovulation in overweight women with polycystic ovarian syndrome

toxemia, gestational diabetes and fetal macrosomia are related to maternal body weight[18]. Cesarean section is more frequently performed in overweight women[18]. Management and strict follow-up of the pregnancy and infant risks result in a significant extra cost in obese women[18].

Negative energy balance and infertility

Pubertal delay, menstrual cycle abnormalities, ovarian dysfunction and infertility among women are associated with excessive weight loss, low body fat content, and intensive exercise[12,37,38]. Oliogmenorrheic women reported a higher intake of crude fiber, dietary fiber and a lower intake of saturated and total fats relative to their classmates with similar weight and eumenorrhea[7,8,37–49]. Consistent with this finding, a significant increase in menstrual cycle length was experienced by women shifting from a high-fat (40% of calories) to a low-fat (20% of calories) diet. Many features of exercise-associated amenorrhea overlap with those of anorectic or restricted vegetarian patients who have a selective low-fat food intake. Excessive weight loss, depleting fat reserves, and abnormal eating patterns occur in women with a high self-consciousness concerning body and body image. Psychological stress has been implicated as the cause of an occasional missed period. However, a number of studies have established that emotional upsets do not contribute to prolonged amenorrhea of several months' duration[50,51]. It seems, therefore, more likely that metabolic or nutritional stress is an essential determining factor, although psychological stress is a permissive factor.

A negative energy balance may be the common link between amenorrheic states in athletes, dancers, patients with eating disorders, recreational joggers and hyperactive dieters who experience only moderate weight loss[42,43,46,52,53]. Although critical body weight and fat mass may be one prerequisite for normal reproduction, factors other than body weight and composition are clearly involved.

Low body fat is not invariably associated with menstrual irregularity in humans, as seen in constitutionally low-weight women with normal cycles. Mild caloric restriction may cause anovulatory cycles and luteal phase defect in the majority of young women of normal weight, even when their body weight does not fall below 100% of the ideal body weight[46]. A vegetarian diet affects the cycle more than a non-vegetarian diet, when both induce the same weight loss[7].

Most of animal studies found no evidence to support the exclusive body fat hypothesis[5,6,54]. Ovulation is regulated somehow in relation to whole-body energy balance and the amount of energy stored in adipose tissue is an important component of energy balance.

Changes in reproductive status may be related to the general availability of metabolic fuels rather than to the direct causal action of the fat reserve[5,6,53]. If not fat, what are the mechanisms that alter the activity of the GnRH pulse generator, and subsequent secretion of gonadotropins? Several candidates are receiving attention: thermogenesis, the availability of metabolic fuels as free fatty acids or glucose, and insulin.

To investigate the hypothesis that *thermogenesis* could be involved as a regulator of the gonadotropin secretion, we evaluated, in 21 women with anorexia nervosa aged 14–38 years, the relationship between plasma LH and FSH levels and the resting metabolic rate (RMR) assessed by indirect calorimetry[9]. Before refeeding, average LH concentrations were markedly reduced, whereas FSH levels were altered less. During renutrition, a multivariate analysis showed that the RMR appeared to be the closest factor related to LH response to the GnRH test ($r = 0.616$; $p < 0.0001$)[9] (Figure 3).

As shown in Figure 4, refeeding of a woman with severe anorexia nervosa restores the resting metabolic rate and the physiological response of LH to GnRH, in spite of the patient being persistently underweight[53]. This supports the possible role of a lack of thermogenesis in neuroendocrine–metabolic alterations (Figure 5).

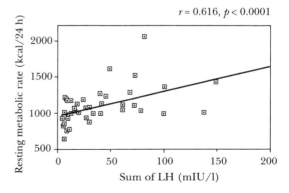

Figure 3 During refeeding of anorexia nervosa patients, the resting metabolic rate is correlated to LH response (sum of LH) to GnRH test

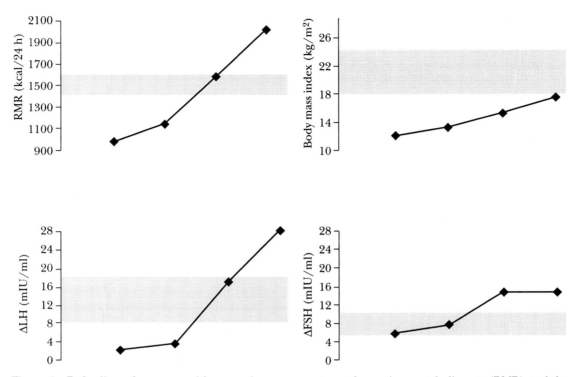

Figure 4 Refeeding of a woman with anorexia nervosa restores the resting metabolic rate (RMR) and the physiological response of LH to the GnRH test in spite of the patient being persistently underweight

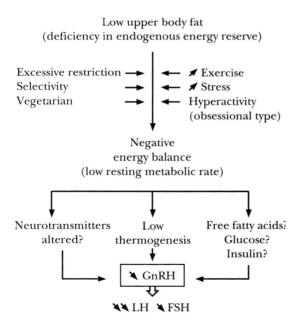

Figure 5 Psychonutritional hypothalamic amenorrhea

In regard to the *metabolic fuels*, it is becoming clear in animal models that ovulation is dependent upon the availability of oxidizable metabolic fuels – *glucose* and *fatty acids*[5,6]. Acute starvation blocks the estrous cycle of the Syrian hamster, an effect that can be countered by adding glucose to the drinking water[54]. Concerning the role of body fat, lean hamsters were more susceptible to starvation-induced anestrus than fat hamsters[6]. Simultaneous pharmacological block of both fatty acid oxidation and glycolysis inhibited reproduction, but, as long as one of these metabolic pathways could be used, estrous cycles continued[6]. Possibly related to this mechanism is the observation that food-restricted female rats exhibit high-amplitude LH pulses a few hours after eating their one daily meal, but not at any other time[5].

The suggestion that *insulin* may influence GnRH pulse generator in altering glucose, fatty acids and amino acid substrates is controversial.

Supporting this idea are the observations that availability of amino acids by insulin is necessary for the synthesis of norepinephrine and serotonin, both influencing the GnRH pulse generator[5]. The infusion of insulin, glucose and a mixture of amino acids is able to increase LH levels in animals[55].

On the other hand, cerebroventricular infusion of insulin was without effect on LH secretion in underfed lambs, and decreased LH pulsing in fed females[56].

In rhesus monkeys, stimulation of LH secretion by food intake does not appear to be mediated by insulin, as shown by the persistence of LH food-induced pulses after suppression of insulin secretion by diazoxide[57].

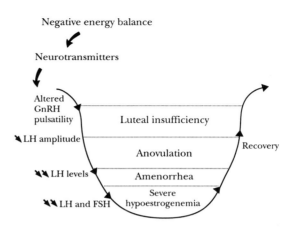

Figure 6 Influences of energy balance on menstrual cycle

Management of infertile women with negative energy balance

Careful evaluation of eating attitude, food intake and exercise is the main step in investigating the possible causal factors involved in ovulatory disorders responsible for infertility. The data presented above suggest that the hypothalamic–pituitary–ovarian axis is extremely sensitive to relatively mild restrictions of caloric intake, inducing a negative energy balance.

Alterations of diet composition may contribute to disturbances of gonadal function. Rapidity of weight loss is another co-factor. Many women submitted to heavy exercise experience relative eating insufficiency disorders. Clinical and experimental data give support to the role of reduction in resting energy expenditure as a common signal for the suppression of pulsatile GnRH and LH secretions (Figure 5). The hormonal profile of these 'psychonutritional' hypoestrogenic anovulations shows a dissociation between markedly low LH and normal (or moderately low) FSH levels (Figure 6). A further decrease in FSH levels occurs in severe weight loss (Figure 6). Food intake has to be monitored along with the woman's feelings and beliefs about eating, and the woman is gradually encouraged to reach the desired caloric level and food composition. Physicians

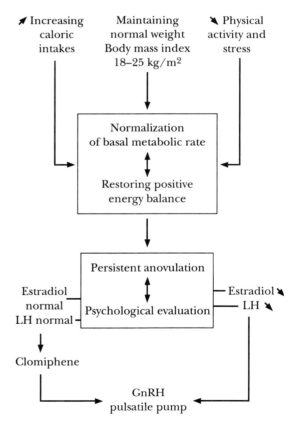

Figure 7 Induction of ovulation in women with low resting metabolic rate

must accept that dietary intake does not always conform to prescribed eating plans.

Weight regain has to be accomplished by applying behavioral techniques to reinforce eating. Modification of the nutritional attitude often justifies cognitive behavioral therapy and treatment dealing with body image disturbances and irrational beliefs about food. Follicular stimulation and induction of ovulation may be useful when intervention on nutrition does not succeed in restoring cycles (Figure 7). GnRH pulsatile administration by pumps[36] is usually the most convenient means to induce ovulation.

References

1. Hartz, A. J., Rupley, D. C. and Rimm, A. A. (1984). The association of girth measurements with disease in 32856 women. *Am. J. Epidemiol.*, **119**, 71–80

2. Zaadstra, B. M., Seidell, J. C., Van Noord, P. A. H. *et al.* (1993). Fat and female fecundity: prospective study of effect of body fat distribution on conception rates. *Br. Med. J.*, **306**, 484–7

3. Bates, G. W. and Whitworth, N. S. (1992). Effect of body weight reduction on plasma androgens in obese infertile women. *Fertil. Steril.*, **38**, 406

4. Pascali, R., Antenucci, D., Casimirri, F., Venturoli, S., Paradisi, R., Fabbri, R., Balestra, V., Melchionda, N. and Barbara, L. (1989). Clinical and hormonal characteristics of obese amenorrheic hyperandrogenic women before and after weight loss. *J. Clin. Endocrinol. Metab.*, **68**, 173–9

5. Bronson, F. H. and Manning, J. M. (1991). The energetic regulation of ovulation: a realistic role for body fat. *Biol. Reprod.*, **44**, 945–50

6. Schneider, J. E. and Wade, G. N. (1989). Availability of metabolic fuels controls estrous cyclicity of Syrian hamsters. *Science*, **244**, 1326–8

7. Pirke, K. M., Schweiger, U., Laessle, R., Dickhaut, D., Scweigger, M. and Waechtler, M. (1986). Dieting influences the menstrual cycle: vegetarian versus non vegetarian diet. *Fertil. Steril.*, **46**, 1083–8

8. Frisch, R. E. (1978). Population, food intake and fertility. *Science*, **199**, 22–30

9. Lefebvre, P., Martinez, T. H., Sultan, C. H., Sabatini, M., Isnard, M., Jaffiol, C., Orsetti, A. and Bringer, J. (1995). Impact of renutrition on gonadotropin in functional hypothalamic amenorrhea. Role of basal metabolic rate. Presented at *The Endocrine Society*, Washington DC, June, abstr. P 3–358

10. Rogers, J. and Mitchell, G. W. (1952). The relation of obesity to menstrual disturbances. *N. Engl. J. Med.*, **247**, 53–5

11. Given, W. P., Gause, R. W. and Douglas, R. G. (1950). Rational therapy for secondary amenorrhea. *N. Engl. J. Med.*, **243**, 357

12. Reid, R. L. and Van Vugt, D. A. (1987). Weight related changes in reproductive function. *Fertil. Steril.*, **48**, 905–13

13. Mitchell, G. W. and Rogers, J. (1953). The influence of weight reduction on amenorrhea in obese women. *N. Engl. J. Med.*, **249**, 835–7

14. Givens, J. R. (1991). Reproductive and hormonal alterations in obesity. In Björntorp, P. and Brodoff, B. N. (eds.) *Obesity*, Vol. 45, pp. 540–9. (Philadelphia: J. B. Lippincott)

15. Bringer, J., Lefebvre, P., Boulet, F., Grigorescu, R., Renard, E., Hedon, B., Orsetti, A. and Jaffiol, C. (1993). Body composition and regional fat patterning in polycystic ovarian syndrome: relationship to hormonal and metabolic profiles. *Ann. NY Acad. Sci.*, **687**, 115–23

16. Zhang, Y. W., Stern, B. and Rebar, R. W. (1984). Endocrine comparison of obese menstruating and amenorrheic women. *J. Clin. Endocrinol. Metab.*, **58**, 1077–83

17. Deslypere, J. P., Verdonck, L. and Vermulen, A. (1985). Fat tissue: a steroid reservoir and site of steroid metabolism. *J. Clin. Endocrinol. Metab.*, **61**, 564–70

18. Galtier Dereure, F., Montpeyroux, F., Boulot, P., Bringer, J. and Jaffiol, C. (1995). Weight excess before pregnancy: complication cost. *Obesity*, in press

19. Shikora, S. A., Niloff, J. M., Bistrian, B. R., Forse, R. A. and Blackburn, G. L. (1991). Relationship between obesity and uterine leiomyomata. *Nutrition*, **7**, 251–5

20. Schapira, D. V., Kumar, N. B., Lyman, G. H. *et al.* (1991). Upper-body fat distribution and endometrial cancer risk. *J. Am. Med. Assoc.*, **266**, 1808–11

21. Schapira, D. V., Kumar, N. B., Lyman, G. H. and Cox, C. E. (1990). Abdominal obesity and breast cancer risk. *Ann. Intern. Med.*, **112**, 182–6

22. Schapira, D. V., Kumar, N. B., Lyman, G. H. and Cox, C. E. (1991). Obesity and body fat distribution and breast cancer prognosis. *Cancer*, **67**, 523–8

23. Holte, J., Bergh, T., Giennarelli, G. and Wide, L. (1994). The independent effects of polycystic ovary syndrome and obesity on serum concentrations of gonadotrophins and sex steroids in premenopausal women. *Clin. Endocrinol.*, **41**, 473–81

24. Holte, J., Bergh, T., Berne, C. and Lithell, H. (1994). Serum lipoprotein lipid profile in women with the polycystic ovary syndrome: relation to anthropometric, endocrine and metabolic variables. *Clin. Endocrinol.*, **41**, 463–71

25. Chang, J. R., Nakamura, R. M., Judd, H. L. and Kaplan, S. A. (1983). Insulin resistance in non-obese patients with polycystic ovarian disease. *J. Clin. Endocrinol. Metab.*, **57**, 356

26. Dunaif, A., Segal, K. R., Futterweit, W. and Dobrjansky, A. (1989). Profound peripheral insulin resistance independent of obesity in polycystic ovary syndrome. *Diabetes*, **38**, 1165–74

27. McCluskey, S., Evans, C., Lacey, J. H. and Pearce, J. M. (1991). Polycystic ovary syndrome and bulimia. *Fertil. Steril.*, **55**, 287–91

28. Ovesen, P., Moller, J., Ingerslev, H. J., Jorgensen, J. O., and Mengel, A. (1993). Normal basal and insulin-stimulated fuel metabolism in lean women with the polycystic ovary syndrome. *J. Clin. Endocrinol. Metab.*, **77**, 1636–40

29. Weber, R. F. A., Pache, T. D., Jacobs, M. L., Docter, R., Lynn Loriaux, D., Fauser, B. C. J. M. and Birkenhäger, J. C. The relation between clinical manifestations of polycystic ovary syndrome and β-cell function. *Clin. Endocrinol.*, **38**, 295–300

30. Rajkhowa, M., Bicknell, J., Jones, M. and Clayton, R. N. (1994). Insulin sensitivity in women with polycystic ovary syndrome: relationship to hyperandrogenemia. *Fertil. Steril.*, **61**, 605–12

31. Ciaraldi, T. P., El-Roeiy, A., Madar, Z., Reichart, D., Olefsky, J. M. and Yen, S. S. C. (1992). Cellular mechanisms of insulin resistance in polycystic ovarian syndrome. *J. Clin. Endocrinol. Metab.*, **75**, 577–83

32. Dahlgren, E., Janson, P. O., Johansson, S., Matthson, L. A. *et al.* (1992). Women with polycystic ovary syndrome wedge resected in 1956 to 1965: a long term follow-up focusing on natural history and circulating hormones. *Fertil. Steril.*, **57**, 505–13

33. Shepard, M. K., Balmaceda, J. P. and Leija, C. G. (1979). Relationship of weight to successful induction of ovulation with clompihene citrate. *Fertil. Steril.*, **32**, 641

34. Chong, A. P., Rafael, R. W. and Forte, C. C. (1986). Influence of weight in the induction of ovulation with human menopausal gonadotropin and human chorionic gonadotropin. *Fertil. Steril.*, **46**, 599–603

35. Bringer, J., Hedon, B., Jaffiol, C. Nicolau, S., Gilbert, F., Cristol, P., Orsetti, A., Viala, J. L. and Mirouze, J. (1985). Influence of the frequency of gonadotropin-releasing hormone (GnRH) administration on ovulatory responses in women with anovulation. *Fertil. Steril.*, **44**, 42–8

36. Bringer, J., Boulet-Gilbert, F., Clouet, S., Hedon, B., Mares, P. and Jaffiol, C. (1989). Administration pulsatile de la LH-RH: applications diagnostiques at thérapeutiques. *J. Steroid. Biochem.*, **33**, 783–8

37. Bringer, J., Hedon, B., Giner, B., Richard, J. L. and Jaffiol, C. (1990). Influence sur la fertilité féminine des anomalies pondérales et des déséquilibres alimentaires. *Presse Med.*, **19**, 1456–9

38. Frisch, R. E. (1988). Fatness and fertility. *Sci. Am.*, **258**, 88–95

39. Scott, E. C. and Johnston, F. E. (1982). Critical fat, menarche, and the maintenance of menstrual cycles. *J. Adol. Health Care*, **2**, 249–60

40. Frisch, R. E., Gotz-Welbergen, A. V., McArthur, J. W., Albright, T., Witschi, J., Bullen, B., Birnholz, J., Reed, R. B. and Hermann, H. (1981). Delayed menarche and amenorrhea of college athletes in relation to age of onset of training. *J. Am. Med. Assoc.*, **246**, 1559–63

41. Frisch, R. E. (1987). Body fat, menarche, fitness and fertility. *Hum. Reprod.*, **2**, 521–33

42. Cumming, D. C. (1987). The reproductive effects of exercise and training. *Curr. Prob. Obstet. Gynecol. Fertil.*, **10**, 225–85

43. Loucks, A. B., Horvath, S. M. (1985). Athletic amenorrhea: a review. *Med. Sci. Sports. Exer.*, **17**, 56–72

44. Sinning, W. E. and Little, K. D. (1987). Body composition and menstrual function in athletes. *Sport Med.*, **4**, 34–45

45. Glass, A. R., Deuster, P. A., Kyle, S. B., Yahiro, J. A., Vigersky, R. A. and Schoomaker, E. D. (1987). Amenorrhea in olympic marathon runners. *Fertil. Steril.*, **48**, 740–5

46. Pirke, K. M., Schweiger, U. and Strowitzki, T. (1989). Dieting causes menstrual irregularities in normal weight young women through impairment of episodic luteinizing hormone secretion. *Fertil. Steril.*, **51**, 263–8

47. Schweiger, U., Laessle, R., Pfister, H., Hoehl, C., Schwingenschloegel, M., Schweiger, M. and Pirke, K. M. (1987). Diet-induced menstrual irregularities: effects of age and weight loss. *Fertil. Steril.*, **48**, 746–51

48. Snow, R. C., Schneider, J. L. and Barbieri, R. L. (1990). High dietary fiber and low saturated fat intake among oligomenorrheic under-graduates. *Fertil. Steril.*, **54**, 632–7

49. Jones, D. Y., Judd, J. T., Taylor, P. R., Campbell, W. S. and Nair, P. P. (1987). Influence of dietary fat on menstrual cycles and menses length. *Hum. Nutr. Clin. Nutr.*, **41c**, 341

50. Schachter, M. and Shoham, Z. (1994). Amenor-rhea during the reproductive years – is it safe? *Fertil. Steril.*, **62**, 1–16

51. Fries, H., Nillius, S. J. and Petersson, F. (1974). Epidemiology of secondary amenorrhea. II. A retrospective evaluation of etiology with special regard to psychogenic factors and weight loss. *Am. J. Obstet. Gynecol.*, **118**, 473–8

52. Luke, A. and Schoeller, D. A. (1992). Basal me-tabolic rate, fat free mass and body cell mass during energy restriction. *Metabolism*, 450–6

53. Bronson, F. H. (1987). Puberty in female rats: relative effects of exercise and food restriction. *Am. J. Physiol.*, **252**, R140–4

54. Morin, L. P. (1986). Environment and hamster reproduction: response to phase-specific starva-tion during estrous cycle. *Am. J. Physiol.*, **251**, R663–9

55. Cameron, J. L. (1989). Influence of nutrition on the hypothalamic–pituitary–gonadal axis in pri-mates. In Pirke, K. M., Wuttke, W. and Schweiger, U. (eds.) *The Menstrual Cycle and Its Disorders*, pp. 66–78. (Heidelberg: Springer Verlag)

56. Schneider, J. E. and Wade, G. N. (1989). Availa-bility of metabolic fuels controls estrous cyclicity of Syrian hamsters. *Science*, **244**, 1326–8

57. Williams, N. I., Lancas, M. J. and Cameron, J. L. Stimulation of luteinizing hormone (LH) secre-tion in male rhesus monkeys by food intake: evidence against a role for insulin. Presented at the *Endocrine Society*, Washington DC, June, abstr. OR22-3

Vaginismus 21

C. M. Harrison

Introduction

Vaginismus is the involuntary spasm of the muscles surrounding the entrance to the vagina, which occurs whenever an attempt is made to introduce any object including a penis into the vagina. Usually the spasm is confined to the vaginal opening but many women also suffer from spasms of the muscles of the thighs, anus, abdomen and buttocks[1].

It is believed that the term 'vaginismus' was first used by the American gynecologist, Sims in the 1860s. He was the first to describe the condition at a meeting of the Obstetrical Society in London in 1861. Further reference is made to vaginismus by Havelock Ellis (1859–1939), a British physician specifically interested in researching sex, relating to a case study in 1896[2].

The earliest known medical reference to vaginismus can be traced back to Quincy's *Lexicon medicum* which was published in London in 1802. At the time, suggested treatments were surgical, as psychotherapy did not exist. Other references can also be found in the homeopathic medical text books of the 1880s. There was no understanding of the influence that the mind can have on the body until the time of Sigmund Freud (1856–1939). Even he, the greatest contributor to the study of sexuality in the early twentieth century, mainly focused on male psychology and sexuality. He introduced the concept of association between mind (psyche) and body (soma), hence psychosomatic. The condition of vaginismus is psychosomatic, induced it is believed often by deep-routed fear and anxiety. Freud discussed the condition with his colleague Karl Abraham in a letter in 1924[3], and his concepts and techniques still influence some of the therapies that are

used today in the treatment of vaginismus. It was not until the late 1950s that the condition of vaginismus became identified as a treatable condition, and this was due to the work of Masters and Johnson[4–5]. They are seen as the pioneers of sex therapy as we know it today.

Vaginismus is not a physical disability or a disease. It is an emotional condition which has psychological causes that manifest themselves in a physical response. It is not so much about sexuality itself but about intimacy, conflicts relating to dependency and issues of trust, and the woman's relationship with her own body. It is an aspect of women's psychological and sexual experience that has remained hidden for centuries. It carries with it a great deal of shame which means that women and their partners often suffer in silence and are very reluctant to address the problem.

We live in a society that equates being sexual with penetrative intercourse and couples find it very difficult to admit that they are not able to do what they imagine everyone else is doing spontaneously. Because vaginismus renders a couple infertile, it is often the desire to have a baby that finally pressurizes them to come forward for treatment. This can be after many years of non-consummation and distress.

It was believed in the past that vaginismus was a rare condition, but, as more and more research is carried out, this is no longer believed to be so. Vaginismus affects an estimated 0.17% of the women in the UK. One doctor specializing in the treatment of sexual problems in Ireland[6], estimated that vaginismus occurs in approximately five out of every 1000 Irish married couples. Another survey in Britain[7] revealed that 16 out of every 100 women consulting one birth-control clinic were suffering from vaginismus. In the United States, approximately 20% of the women seeking help at the Masters and Johnson Institute in St. Louis had a demonstrable degree of vaginismus[8]. Approximately 40% of the women seen at the Center for Human Sexuality, State University of New York Health Science Center, Brooklyn had vaginismus[9].

Overcoming vaginismus is not only about being able to tolerate full penetrative intercourse without severe pain and anxiety. It is also about understanding oneself as a woman and what lies behind the body's resistance to intercourse, why it is saying 'no' and just what saying 'yes' would fully entail.

Because vaginismus can range from mild to severe, because it can be primary (where intercourse has never taken place) or secondary (where the condition occurs when intercourse has been able to take place in the past) and because it can also be situational, only occurring in certain situations, the treatment necessary to overcome it will vary. The shame and embarrassment attached to vaginismus render it a subject that is seldom discussed openly or written about. Therefore, it is not known how many couples resolve the problem themselves or how many accept the condition and learn to live with it. We only know of those where the pressure has become so great that they feel forced to seek help. However, it *is* known that the earlier help is sought the better.

In the past, treatment for vaginismus has included surgical intervention (widening of the introitus and the vagina) and psychotherapy, including, at times, psychoanalytical therapy and sex therapy (the latter is a generic term used to describe any method of treatment that seeks to help a man, woman or couple with a sexual problem).

Psychotherapy which includes sex therapy is the most common method of treatment for vaginismus at the present time in the UK and Ireland, as the prognosis is very positive with high success rates (personal communication). This approach can include psychodynamic and behavioral methods of treatment, varying according to the needs of the client. Where the

history includes sexual abuse or other severe childhood or adolescent traumas, these may need to be addressed first to give the woman more insight into her own psychology. When working with a couple where the relationship is generally not satisfactory and there is conflict between them, it is essential that these issues are addressed and overcome before sex therapy commences. If it is apparent that it is a purely learned or sexual problem, the emphasis will be on the behavioral components of treatment.

Method of treatment

In the Department of Human Assisted Reproduction in the Rotunda Hospital, Dublin all referred couples are initially assessed by a sex and marital therapist, together, or when no partner exists, individually. At this session the problems as seen by the client(s) are explored in detail and, if appropriate, the goals of therapy are established jointly between clients and therapist and a verbal contract agreed upon. Drenth advocates that therapists should not set the goals of therapy, but rather liberate the vaginismic woman to set her own goals in conjunction with her partner[10].

A detailed history of both parties is taken over several sessions, at one of which partners are seen separately in case any confidential information exists which they do not wish to discuss in front of their spouse/partner. Behavioral therapy specifically designed to treat sexual problems then commences together with a more psychodynamic approach addressing issues relating to the problem.

The form of behavioral therapy used was originally developed in the late 1950s by Masters and Johnson[4,5]. It has since been updated considerably and varies to some extent according to the individual therapist's own professional orientation and the clients' needs. With some clients, where their knowledge of sexual function or their own anatomy and physiology is limited, it is necessary to spend some time giving basic information regarding these matters at this stage.

The behavioral program has three main purposes:

(1) It provides a structured approach which allows couples to rebuild their sexual relationship gradually – treatment is broken down into small steps which are tackled one at a time.

(2) It helps the couple and therapist to identify the factors which are contributing to and maintaining the sexual dysfunction, highlighting areas of their sexuality and communication where things are going wrong. Homework tasks are set and how these are tackled gives insight into attitudes and values in this area, leading to more understanding for the couple.

(3) It provides the couple with specific techniques to deal with particular problems.

In the case of vaginismus, treatment very often starts with a self-focus program working only with the woman where she concentrates on her own body and how she feels about it. When she is comfortable with this, treatment progresses to non-genital sensual exercises with her partner. These exercises then become more genitally focused and gradually vaginal containment is introduced, first with the client's own fingers then her partner's and then eventually with her partner's penis without movement and then with movement. Together with these exercises, some work is done on relaxation generally which is an important aspect of treatment (particularly relaxation with thigh and pelvic floor muscles). Occasionally, it may be necessary to introduce vaginal dilators (Amielle®, Owen Mumford, Oxford, UK) at this point in time. The use of fantasy can also be an important aspect of treatment.

Generally couples or individuals are seen fortnightly, but weekly at times especially if a 'block' should occur which they are finding difficult to overcome.

Once penile containment is taking place, the use of contraception is strongly advised even where a pregnancy is desired, as this could impair treatment at this stage. When the goals of treatment have been reached, a 6-week follow-up session always takes place to establish that the desired outcome is long-standing and that no other problems have occurred in the meantime.

Results and analysis

Between August 1989 and December 1994, 32 referrals for vaginismus were seen by the sex and marital therapist in the Department of Assisted Reproduction in the Rotunda Hospital, Dublin – 26 were from within the hospital setting and six were outside referrals from general practitioners and other agencies. Vaginismus was the initial reason for referral in 31 cases and primary impotence was the reason for referral in one case where it became apparent that the female partner also suffered from vaginismus early on in treatment. Of the 32 cases in the study, 28 were seen with partners (they were all married), and four women were seen alone. Two of these had married partners who refused to attend and two of the women were single.

The women ranged in age from 23 to 39 years (mean, 31.67 years), and the men from 27 to 51 years (mean, 33.7 years). Of the 30 married couples, the duration of marriages ranged from 6 months to 15 years with a mean of 5.76 years. Of the two couples living together but not married, one couple had been together 10 years and the other couple, 18 months.

At the commencement of treatment, 27 women suffered from primary vaginismus where penetrative intercourse had never taken place. None were able to use tampons or insert their own fingers into their vagina. A further three women had secondary vaginismus. Two of these had severe marital problems, their partners refused to attend and they did not complete treatment or overcome their problems. One suffered from vaginismus following a miscarriage and she dropped out of treatment after one session. The final two women had occasional vaginismus, one associated with a congenital abnormality of the vagina. All but the two with marital problems were having active sexual lives.

Of the 32 cases presented, 26 completed treatment, 22 successfully (85%). They attended for between two and 23 sessions (mean, 9.5). All these were able to achieve full penetrative intercourse with no discomfort and were still experiencing a full sexual relationship including regular intercourse when followed up 6 weeks after completion of treatment. Eight out of the 22 had received previous treatment elsewhere without success.

The remaining six dropped out before completing treatment. Two found the distance to travel to hospital too far. For two women, their relationship was very poor and their partners refused to attend. The remaining failed to keep their appointments. Seven of the 22 couples who completed treatment successfully have reported a pregnancy since. However, not all wished to become pregnant as pregnancy was not the goal for all these couples. Others would not necessarily have contact us.

Where couples were seen together ($n = 28$), nine male partners also exhibited a sexual dysfunction. Eight of these became apparent for the first time during the course of treatment. Three had some form of erectile dysfunction, four suffered from premature ejaculation and one had inhibited sexual desire. One man was referred for primary impotence (erectile dysfunction) and his partner's vaginismus became apparent during the course of treatment.

Discussion

At the Rotunda Hospital, Dublin, it is apparent that, as young doctors and health-care workers become more aware of the area of human sexuality, more and more women suffering from vaginismus are referred. This is true of clinics in Britain and Ireland[6]. Sadly for some, it is only when they reach the stage of a postcoital test at the infertility clinic in the hospital that they are forced to disclose their dilemma. But many women are now starting to look for help sooner than they did in the past, because they want it for themselves and their partners, and not just to have a baby.

Unfortunately, considerable shame and anxiety is still associated with sexual dysfunction generally, and specifically with vaginismus. Sadly, in the past, lack of training and knowledge on the part of the medical profession, particularly the family practitioner has meant that these problems have sometimes been overlooked and not detected at an early stage. In a study carried out by Ogden and Ward[11] in

Figure 1 One woman's perception of progress through treatment of vaginismus. (a) Confusion, frustration, the problem is so complex I don't know where to start. The original problem has now become engulfed and entangled by anger, frustration, etc. from previous attempts at treatment. (b) After sifting through the complexities and talking through the anger and hurt, I can cut it all back and focus on myself, my body and my mind. (c) As self-focus develops, I come to terms with my body and the next step is to come to terms with my genital area. (d) Close-up of flower head/bud represents genital area, just looking at it. (e,f) Exploration becomes possible, the lips can be parted and accepted but the vagina still firmly closed (bud). (g) Vagina is a sore spiny place where nothing can go in without pain. This is a transverse section of the bud showing the inside – the immature parts of the flower (spiny) which are to grow and come out the bud walls (representing vagina). The inside will eventually develop into anthers and style of flower (sexual parts of flower) and fully function sexually, as will I hopefully. (h) As self-focus develops, a finger can now go in a slight bit, most of the pain has reduced but still remains as more of a discomfort (one spine). (i) One finger can go in with little or no discomfort and inside becomes smooth. (j) Two fingers can go in now and vagina becomes more accessible so bud walls open – not so tight and allow inside develop upwards. (k,l) Sexual parts of flower (anthers and style) develop and expand and bud walls open more. Likewise, the penis can enter a small bit at first and then fully. (m) Whole view of flower head, petals bloom and grow, maturity is reached, the sexual function of the flower can now start. Full penetration is achieved and orgasms for both of us (at different times). But note, although the penis can enter, the walls of the vagina, i.e. bud of flower, have not fully let go, although loads has already been achieved. (n) What I really want to achieve is a fully bloomed flower, no caution, no discomfort, no holding back, where my body can be given freely, not tentatively. The bud walls open wide and expose the sexual parts of the flower. Likewise I want to achieve this in mind and body. Is it possible?

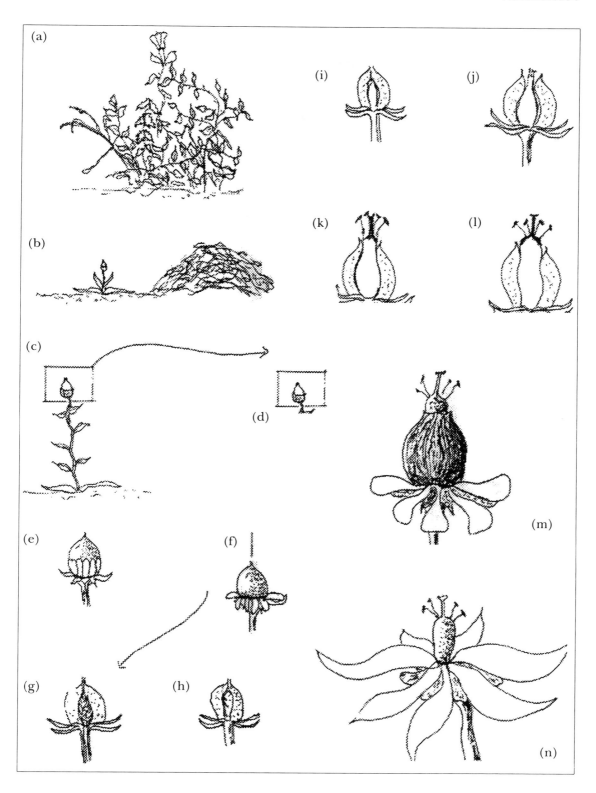

Britain, although the general practitioner was the most frequently sought source of help, the vaginismus sufferers perceived them as being least helpful, with only 22% ($n = 14$) of the subjects who had visited their general practitioner saying that they found this contact helpful.

Of the subjects who had visited a counsellor, 51.8% ($n = 14$) found this helpful, while 55.6% ($n = 15$) of the subjects who had visited a gynecologist, 61.9% ($n = 26$) of those who had visited a sex therapist and 75.8% ($n = 25$) of those who had visited a psychotherapist found these contacts helpful. As medical students receive more training in human sexuality generally and in sexual dysfunction, it is hoped that this will change and that they will recognize if and when it is necessary to refer their patients on to somebody specializing in work in this area, or, if they have the time or inclination, to seek further specialized training themselves.

The majority of couples in this study had good relationships generally. Only two had poor relationships where the male partners refused to attend. For these women, the vaginismus was secondary, one would image as a result of the anger and resentment associated with the poor relationship. The remaining couples were very close and were having an active sexual relationship. Most of the women were experiencing orgasms by clitoral stimulation and enjoying all sexual contact providing this did not lead to sexual intercourse. No woman should be made to feel abnormal if she cannot tolerate intercourse. Couples should feel free to find ways of expressing their sexuality in their own way without necessarily conforming to the rigid norms of our society. However, all the clients seen felt very strongly that they did want to have intercourse. They felt they were missing out on something. Also many wished to have children, although not all had this as their primary goal.

Some general trends became evident as a result of observations made at the Rotunda Hospital. Quite frequently, the relationship between the husband and the wife was close, but paternalistic, with the women dependent in many ways on the man. Often, one would hear comments from the women that they had had fears of intercourse since childhood. These fears were sometimes related to stories told by mothers of sex being something that one has to tolerate or of difficult births, stillbirths or miscarriages. An unusually strong bond or enmeshment among some of the women with their families of origin, especially with their mothers was also observed. This is not to say that the relationship was always a good one, but frequently seemed to be one where the mother had retained a great deal of power and control. It would seem to be that this very strong mother/daughter relationship inhibited in some ways the daughter from becoming fully sexual and 'letting someone else in'. Such women had to address this issue at the start of therapy and only by letting go and stepping back from this relationship in some ways could they allow intercourse to take place with their partners, even though this is what they very much wanted at a conscious level. It is known that there is a high incidence of vaginismus in Ireland[6] and some of these trends could be peculiar to that society.

As can be seen from the results of this study, quite often partners of women with vaginismus developed or exhibited premature ejaculation or erectile dysfunction and these needed to be treated alongside the vaginismus. It is not always clear whether this was a reaction by the man as the woman became able to have intercourse or whether the problem was already present. It does indicate the necessity of treating the couple together rather than the woman in isolation.

When a couple reach their desired goal of therapy, it is an exciting time for them and a rewarding experience for the therapist. It is a privilege to work with couples on such an intimate level, joining in the joy of each successful step and trying to help them to overcome some of the hurdles. All couples who overcame their problem claim that not only had their sexual relationship improved but that they had become closer in other ways.

Figure 1 on the previous page shows the drawings of one woman as she progressed

178

through treatment for vaginismus. They illustrate very clearly how she felt her body was gradually responding to treatment, how she was opening up and becoming receptive to her partner. Her accompanying interpretations clarify this as she takes us through her journey from anger and frustration to a sense of letting go and blooming.

References

1. Orbach, S. (1991). In Valins, L. (ed.) *When a Woman's Body Says No to Sex. Understanding and Overcoming Vaginismus*, pp. ix–xi. (London: Penguin)
2. Ellis, H. (1900). *Studies in the Psychology of Sex*, Vol. 3. (New York: Random House)
3. Freud, S. and Abraham, K. (1965). A psychoanalytic dialogue. In Abraham, H. C. and Freud, E. L. (eds.) *The Letters of Sigmund Freud and Karl Abraham 1907–1926*. (London: Hogarth Press and Institute of Psychoanalysis)
4. Masters, W. H. and Johnson, V. E. (1966). *Human Sexual Response*. (Boston: Little Brown & Co.)
5. Masters, W. H. and Johnson, V. E. (1970). *Human Sexual Inadequacy*. (Boston: Little Brown & Co.)
6. Barnes, J. (1986). Primary vaginismus, Part I, social and clinical features. *Ir. Med. J.*, **79**, 59–62
7. Duddle, M. (1975). The clinical management of sexual dysfunction. *Br. J. Obstet. Gynaecol.*, **82**, 295–6
8. Masters, W. H. (1990). In Valins, L. (ed.) *When a Woman's Body Says No to Sex. Understanding and Overcoming Vaginismus*, p. 23. (London: Penguin) (1992 edition)
9. Dunne, M. E. (1992). In Valins, L. (ed.) *When a Woman's Body Says No to Sex. Understanding and Overcoming Vaginismus*, p. 23. (London: Penguin)
10. Drenth, J. J. (1988). Vaginismus and the desire for a child. *J. Psychosom. Obstet. Gynaecol.*, **9**, 125–37
11. Odgen, J. and Ward, E. (1995). Help – seeking behaviour in sufferers of vaginismus. *Sex. Marital Ther.*, **10**, 23–30

Female age and fecundity

22

M. G. R. Hull

Introduction

Age is often a dominating factor for women wanting to conceive. Some choose to delay childbearing because of their careers. Many infertile couples go through protracted and indefinite investigations and treatment which can cause critical delay. The average age at which women seek specialist help is usually about 30 years, and 35 years by the time they undergo *in vitro* fertilization (IVF). Many reach the required treatment when the chance of success is declining substantially. Natural fecundity (the monthly chance of conception) in the woman declines gradually after the age of 30 years; the decline accelerates some time between 35 and 40 years and fecundity reaches almost zero by 45 years. The review considers the underlying causes and relevant clinical information with a view to their practical importance.

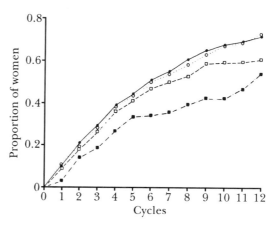

Figure 1 Cumulative conception rates by donor insemination treatment (French national data[1]). Filled circles, ≤ 25 years; open circles, 26–30 years; open squares, 31–35 years, filled squares, ≥ 36 years

Age and infertility treatments

The best clinical evidence of the true decline in female fecundity comes from donor insemination studies, which completely control for coital frequency and the spouse's age[1], as shown in Figure 1. Treatments such as gonadotropin therapy to induce ovulation[2] and gamete intrafallopian transfer (GIFT)[3] should largely control for coital timing, and the results, illustrated in Figures 2 and 3, demonstrate the great importance of the woman's age in determining therapeutic outcome and therefore choices. Figure 3 further emphasizes that the declining chance of pregnancy is compounded by an exponential rise in the risk of miscarriage in reducing the ultimate hope of successfully having a baby. But what are the underlying mechanisms?

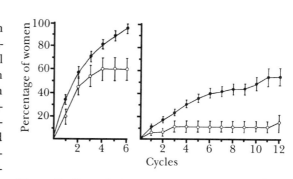

Figure 2 Cumulative pregnancy rates resulting from gonadotropin therapy to induce ovulation according to the cause of ovulation failure and the age of the woman: (left) hypothalamic–pituitary amenorrhea; (right) other disorders, mainly due to polycystic ovaries[2]. Filled circles, < 35 years; open circles, ≥ 35 years

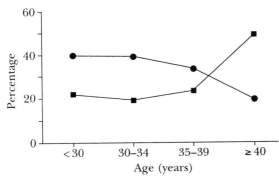

Figure 3 Pregnancy per cycle (●) and miscarriage rates (■) resulting from gamete intrafallopian transfer treatment related to the woman's age[3]

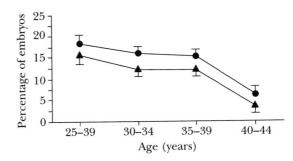

Figure 4 Implantation rates per individual embryo after *in vitro* fertilization treatment related to the woman's age, in ovulatory women with normal uterus and partner with normal sperm (M. G. R. Hull and colleagues, unpublished data). Bars show standard error; circles, pregnancy sacs ($p < 0.02$); triangles, babies ($p < 0.01$)

Underlying mechanisms: evidence from IVF studies

IVF and embryo transfer offer a model for specific study. Every report demonstrates an age-related decline in pregnancy and birth rates, associated with declining numbers of oocytes and consequently embryos to transfer, but oocyte fertilization rates remain normal. Our own specific study controlling for the number of embryos transferred and other confounding factors showed a gradual decline with age, but after 40 years the chance of each embryo implanting was reduced by more than half, and of producing a baby was reduced by more than two-thirds (Hull and colleagues, unpublished data), as illustrated in Figure 4. The remarkable success of egg donation to postmenopausal women[4,5] strongly suggests that oocyte quality is the main factor, which is further supported by a recent controlled study[6]. Furthermore, egg donation studies in women (donors and recipients of all ages) show that the age-related increase in miscarriage is determined largely by oocyte quality[7,8].

Endometrial and uterine receptivity should not be entirely dismissed as causes[9]. There is animal experimental evidence showing declining receptivity with age, but on the other hand enhanced receptivity after prolonged lack of estrogen. That is echoed by enhanced success rates in women receiving donated eggs if they

have postmenopausal amenorrhea rather than if still menstruating[10]. There is also evidence from ultrasonography that endometrial development is frequently impaired in women over 40 years, although in most cases there was also obvious uterine pathology, such as multiple fibroids or severe synechiae[11]. If the uterus appears normal its receptivity seems to remain favorable.

Declining oocyte quality and genetic defectiveness

The decline in fertility potential of the oocyte is accompanied by increasingly frequent chromosomal abnormalities, which occur exponentially and seem to be linked to acceleration in the rate of depletion of oocytes in the ovaries. The acceleration seems to occur when the complement of follicles remaining in each ovary has fallen to about 25 000, at around 37 years of age on average[12].

One possible cause of the accelerated follicular atresia is the emergence of a relative preponderance of genetically defective oocytes, which would also explain the reduced implanting ability and increased risks of miscarriage and congenital abnormalities. The classical explanation is prolonged meiotic arrest of the oocyte, making it vulnerable to ageing and environmental influences. However, a leading current hypothesis is that the defective oocytes are defective from the start, and due to their defectiveness are also less readily recruited for ovulation than healthy oocytes, until the latter have declined in number. This model[13] would explain the exponential rise in genetic abnormalities affecting pregnancies in women over 37. It also implies that women approaching a premature menopause, for whatever reason including sometimes iatrogenic ovarian damage or loss, carry the same risks of declining fertility and increasing risks of miscarriage and congenital anomalies as older premenopausal women. Experimental evidence in mice shows that removal of one ovary leads to shortening of reproductive life and earlier rise in aneuploidy[14].

The need for ovarian conservation

In women, removing an ovary in early adult life would not halve the reproductive span, because oocyte depletion occurs exponentially, but it would be expected that the menopause would be advanced by 7 years[12]. Large-scale reduction of ovarian mass, as can occur in surgical excision of endometriosis, for example, can be disastrous. Ovarian conservation should be a dominating priority of surgery – and if it were possible, of radiotherapy and chemotherapy – in young women. In surgery for ovarian endometriosis, internal ablation of cysts should probably be preferred to attempting excision.

Ovarian responsiveness and FSH levels

The typical gross elevation of follicle stimulating hormone (FSH) and luteinizing hormone (LH) that marks the menopause is preceded by a gradual rise in FSH levels for at least 5–6 years before the menopause, although in LH levels for only about 1 year before, despite continuation of apparently normal ovulatory cycles[15]. The rise in FSH is still within the normal range at first, but in most cases is clearly abnormal 3–4 years before reaching the menopause. The presumed explanation is falling inhibin levels,

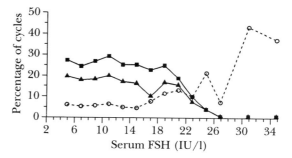

Figure 5   Results of *in vitro* fertilization treatment per cycle started (for the cancellation rate) or attempted egg recovery, related to the basal (day 3) serum concentration of follicle stimulating hormone (FSH) (upper normal limit in this assay, 22 IU/l)[17]. Squares, total pregnancies; triangles, ongoing pregnancies; circles, cancelled cycles

which may be due to diminishing numbers of follicles recruitable for maturation and is associated with reduced production by granulosa cells[16].

As FSH levels rise, in women apparently still ovulating normally, ovarian responsiveness to stimulation declines. This results in progressively fewer oocytes being yielded for IVF treatment, and as Figure 5 shows, increasing cancellations due to inadequate responses and diminishing pregnancy rates[17]. The pregnancy rate dived when the FSH level reached the upper limit of normal (22 IU/l by the assay of Toner and co-workers[17]) and reached zero when it was only slightly higher. The decline seemed to be more sharply related to FSH than to age, but the distinction was not analyzed.

Our own study has demonstrated significant reduction in ovarian responsiveness even when FSH levels have risen into the upper half of the normal range, and of course it was further reduced when FSH was above the normal limit (9 IU/l by our assay). In particular, analysis of variance showed the FSH level to be a more important independent determinant of ovarian responsiveness than age[18]. In other words, biological age of the ovary appears to be more important than chronological age.

The value of FSH measurement has been further refined by dynamic testing, in particular the responsiveness to clomiphene[19]. However, predictiveness is not reliable enough in individual cases and ovarian responsiveness is probably best tested by gonadotropin therapy in (provisional) preparation for ovulation induction or IVF, as required. Even so, what really matters is oocyte quality and whether FSH levels and ovarian responsiveness reflect this[20]. Our own studies have recently shown that in women over 40 years, a raised FSH level provides no significant additional information, but younger women with a raised basal FSH level have substantially reduced implanting ability of the oocytes after fertilization *in vitro*: implantation rates per embryo were reduced from 16% to 4% (C. Fleming and associates, unpublished observations). Those findings are consistent with recent evidence that the FSH response to clomiphene is a good predictor of natural conception rates in young infertile women, but not in those over 40 years[21]. This evidence supports the routine use of basal FSH measurement in the investigation of infertility.

In practice it is important to appreciate the wide variation between FSH assays. Whilst a raised FSH level is a valuable prognostic index, the normal range must be properly determined by each laboratory.

Conclusions

It is important in infertility practice to recognize the major impact of advancing age on the chance of any treatment leading to pregnancy, and furthermore on the chance of any pregnancy reaching a successful conclusion. Women should not delay their attempts at childbearing too long, and doctors should minimize delays in the process of diagnosis and treatment of infertility in women aged 35 years or more. Measurement of basal FSH levels in young infertile women is prognostically valuable. Furthermore, in any young women requiring pelvic surgery, ovarian conservation should be a dominating priority to protect their future fertility.

References

1. Federation CECOS (1982). Female fecundity as a function of age. *N. Engl. J. Med.*, **306**, 404–6
2. Dor, J., Itzkowic, D. J., Mashiach, S., Lunenfeld, B. and Serr, D. M. (1980). Cumulative conception rates following gonadotropin therapy. *Am. J. Obstet. Gynecol.*, **136**, 102–5
3. Craft, I., Ah-Moye, M., Al-Shawaf, T. *et al.* (1988). Analysis of 1071 GIFT procedures – the case for a flexible approach to treatment. *Lancet*, **1**, 1094–8
4. Sauer, M. V., Paulson, R. J. and Lobo, R. A. (1993). Pregnancy after 50: application of oocyte donation to women after natural menopause. *Lancet*, **341**, 321–3
5. Borini, A., Bafaro, G., Violini, F., Bianchi, L., Casadio, V. and Flamigni, C. (1995). Pregnancies in postmenopausal women over 50 years old in an oocyte donation program. *Fertil. Steril.*, **63**, 258–61
6. Navot, D., Drews, M. R., Bergh, P. A., Guzman, I., Karstaedt, A., Scott, R. T., Garrisi, G. J. and Hofmann, G. E. (1994). Age-related decline in female fertility is not due to diminished capacity of the uterus to sustain embryo implantation. *Fertil. Steril.*, **61**, 97–101
7. Abdalla, H. I., Burton, G., Kirkland, A., Johnson, M. R., Leonard, T., Brooks, A. A. and Studd, J. W. W. (1993). Age, pregnancy and miscarriage: uterine ovarian factors. *Hum. Reprod.*, **8**, 1512–17
8. Balmaceda, J. P., Bernardini, L., Ciuffardi, I., Felix, C., Ord, T., Sueldo, C. E. and Asch, R. H. (1994). Oocyte donation in humans: a model to study the effect of age on embryo implantation rate. *Hum. Reprod.*, **9**, 2160–3
9. Meldrum, D. R. (1993). Female reproductive aging – ovarian and uterine factors. *Fertil. Steril.*, **59**, 1–5
10. Edwards, R. G., Morcos, S., Macnamee, M., Balmaceda, J. P. *et al.* (1991). High fecundity of amenorrhoeic women in embryo-transfer programmes. *Lancet*, **338**, 292–4
11. Sher, G., Herbert, C., Maassarani, G. and Jacobs, M. H. (1991). Assessment of the late proliferative phase endometrium by ultrasonography in patients undergoing *in-vitro* fertilization and embryo transfer (IVF/ET). *Hum. Reprod.*, **6**, 232–7
12. Faddy, M. J., Gosden, R. G., Gougeon, A. *et al.* (1992). Accelerated disappearance of ovarian

follicles in mid-life: implications for forecasting menopause. *Hum. Reprod.*, **7**, 1342–6

13. Zheng, C. J. and Byers, B. (1992). Oocyte selection: a new model for the maternal-age dependence of Down syndrome. *Hum. Genet.*, **90**, 1–6

14. Brook, J. D., Gosden, R. G. and Chandley, A. C. (1984). Maternal ageing and aneuploid embryos – evidence from the mouse that biological and not chronological age is the important influence. *Hum. Genet.*, **66**, 41–5

15. Lenton, E. A., Sexton, L., Lee, S. and Cooke, I. D. (1988). Progressive changes in LH and FSH and LH : FSH ratio in women throughout reproductive life. *Maturitas*, **10**, 35–43

16. Pellicer, A., Mari, M., de los Santos, M., Simon, C., Remohi, J. and Tarin, J. J. (1994). Effects of aging on the human ovary: the secretion of immunoreactive α-inhibin and progesterone *Fertil. Steril.*, **61**, 663–8

17. Toner, J. P., Philputt, C. B., Jones, G. S. and Muasher, S. J. (1991). Basal follicle-stimulating hormone level is a better predictor of *in vitro* fertilization performance than age. *Fertil. Steril.*, **55**, 784–91

18. Cahill, D. J., Prosser, C. J., Wardle, P. G., Ford, W. C. L. and Hull, M. G. R. (1994). Relative influence of serum follicle stimulating hormone, age and other factors on ovarian response to gonadotrophin stimulation. *Br. J. Obstet. Gynaecol.*, **101**, 999–1002

19. Scott, R. T. and Hofmann, G. E. (1995). Prognostic assessment of ovarian reserve. *Fertil. Steril.*, **63**, 1–11

20. Wallach, E. E. (1995). Pitfalls in evaluating ovarian reserve. *Fertil. Steril.*, **63**, 12–14

21. Scott, R. T., Opsahl, M. S., Leonardi, M. R., Neal, G. S., Illions, E. H. and Navot, D. (1995). Life table analysis of cumulative pregnancy rates based on the results of ovarian reserve screening and patient age in a general infertility population. *Hum. Reprod.*, **10**, 1706–10

Genetic screening in practice

23

J. L. Simpson

Introduction

Genetic screening implies routine monitoring for the presence or absence of a given condition in apparently normal individuals. Specialists in reproductive medicine who are not primarily obstetricians need to be conversant with standard indications, including screening certain ethnic groups and screening for heterozygote detection. These issues apply to screening gamete donors as well as to screening pregnant women. Overall, about 20% of couples will volunteer some genetic information that needs to be pursued, but relatively few will be at substantive risk[1]. A similar proportion holds for gamete donors[2]. Eventually, invasive prenatal diagnostic procedures may be required and the risks for these procedures must also be appreciated.

Genetic history

One should inquire into the health status of first-degree relatives (siblings, parents, offspring), second-degree relatives (nephews, nieces, aunts, uncles, grandparents), and third-degree relatives (first cousins, especially maternal). Such adverse reproductive outcomes as repetitive spontaneous abortions, stillbirths, and anomalous liveborn infants should be pursued; couples having such histories should undergo chromosomal studies in order to exclude balanced translocations[3]. If a birth defect exists in a second-degree relative (uncle, aunt, grandparent, nephew, niece) or third-degree relative (first cousin), the risk for that anomaly will generally not prove substantially increased over that in the general population. For example, identification of a second- or third-degree relative with an autosomal recessive trait places the couple at little increased risk for an affected offspring, an exception being if the patient and her husband are consanguineous. However, a maternal first cousin with an X-linked recessive disorder would place the couple at increased risk for a similar occurrence.

Advancing maternal age is known to carry increasing risk of chromosomal abnormalities. At age 35 the risk of Down's syndrome is 1/365; at age 40 the risk is 1/109. The risk for all chromosomal abnormalities is about twice the above. Paternal age in the upper fifth and sixth decades increases the risk for fresh mutations, by 1% over background.

Ethnic origin should be recorded to exclude disorders to be described below. This applies for both assisted reproductive technology as well as pregnancies achieved by natural means.

Heterozygote screening

Tay-Sachs disease (deficiency of serum hexosaminidase A), α-thalassemia, β-thalassemia and sickle cell anemia are the only disorders for which it is accepted as standard to screen adults in order to determine whether they are heterozygous. These autosomal recessive disorders are amenable to prenatal diagnosis (Table 1). Jewish individuals should be screened for Tay-Sachs disease. Couples may be uncertain whether they are of Ashkenazic or Sephardic descent; thus, one should probably screen all Jewish couples, and possibly even those in which only one partner is Jewish. Heterozygote detection for β-thalassemia is appropriate in southeast Asians, Chinese and Philippinos. Mean corpuscular volume (MCV) greater than 80% excludes heterozygosity for α- or β-thalassemia. Values less than 80% are more likely to reflect

Table 1 Genetic screening in various ethnic groups. Cystic fibrosis screening is recommended but not considered standard unless the male partner has absence of the vas deferens

Ethnic group	Disorder
Ashkenazi Jews	Tay-Sachs
Black	sickle cell
Mediterranean people	β-thalassemia
Southeast Asians/Chinese	α-thalassemia
Northern European Caucasians	cystic fibrosis

iron deficiency anemia than heterozygosity, but additional confirmatory tests are indicated to exclude the thalassemias. The above genes have been isolated and cloned, but molecular heterogeneity is considerable for all save sickle cell anemia. For this reason, screening still utilizes enzymatic methods, with the possible exceptions of sickle cell anemia and Tay-Sachs disease.

Heterozygote screening may also be appropriate for cystic fibrosis. Here the approach must utilize molecular methods, and again, considerable molecular heterogeneity exists. Deletion of three nucleotides at position 508 (ΔF508) with loss of phenylalanine is the most common mutation. In northern European populations, ΔF508 accounts for 75% of all cystic fibrosis mutations; the next 10–15 mutations account for only an additional 15%. If one screened only for ΔF508, 60% of affected fetuses could be detected[4]. With multiplex polymerase chain reaction for 15 mutations, one would detect only 85–95% of affected fetuses. For this reason universal screening for cystic fibrosis is not an accepted recommendation. Cystic fibrosis screening should be pursued if the pedigree reveals cystic fibrosis, or if the father has absence of the vas deferens. Such men can be homozygous or heterozygous for cystic fibrosis, although not necessarily ΔF508.

Loss rates after invasive procedures

Screening is usually offered routinely for: all individuals of certain ethnic groups (Table 1); all pregnant women to detect elevated maternal serum α-fetoprotein for diagnosing fetal neural tube defects; all pregnant women 35 years of age and above to undergo invasive tests for detecting Down's syndrome; and all pregnant women under the age of 35 years to undergo maternal serum screening for detecting Down's syndrome. Surveillance ultimately requires an invasive procedure. None of these procedures is without risks, principally procedure-related fetal loss of about 0.5%.

Traditional amniocentesis

In 1976 the US National Institute of Child Health and Human Development published the first major prospective study of genetic amniocentesis (1040 subjects and 992 matched controls)[5]. Of all the women who underwent amniocentesis, 3.5% experienced fetal loss between the time of the procedure and delivery compared with 3.2% of controls; the difference was not statistically significant and disappeared completely when corrected for maternal age. The most recent large-scale study was a Danish randomized controlled study of amniocentesis that involved 4606 women aged 25–34 years who were without known risk factors for fetal genetic abnormalities[6]. Amniocentesis was performed under real-time ultrasound guidance with a 20-gauge needle by experienced operators. The spontaneous abortion rate after 16 weeks was 1.7% in the amniocentesis group compared with 0.7% in controls ($p < 0.01$), with a 2.6-fold relative risk of spontaneously aborting if the placenta was traversed. Despite the introduction of ultrasound guidance for amniocentesis in the mid-1980s, the risk of pregnancy loss secondary to traditional amniocentesis was thus not inconsequential. Doubtless, risks are lowest in experienced hands and with good-quality ultrasound.

Early amniocentesis (≤ 14 weeks' gestation)

With the advent of high-resolution ultrasound equipment, physicians began offering amniocentesis before 15 weeks' gestation. No large randomized studies exist; thus, risks are unclear.

In one series of 936 amniocenteses at ≤ 12.8 weeks' gestation, loss rates were 0.7% (7/936) within 2 weeks of amniocentesis, an additional 2.2% before 28 weeks and an additional 0.5% stillbirths or neonatal deaths[7]. Total losses (32/936 or 3.4%) were considered comparable with the 2.1–3.2% in ultrasonographically normal pregnancies not undergoing a procedure; however, no corrections for maternal age and gestational age were made. Henry and Miller[8] also reported favorable results in amniocentesis at 12, 13 and 14 weeks' gestation. Pregnancy losses prior to 28 weeks were 5/193 (2.6%), 5/426 (1.2%), and 18/1172 (1.5%), respectively. This author also believes that amniocentesis at 12–14 weeks' gestation should be relatively safe in experienced hands, but extant data cannot support the claim that early amniocentesis is equal in safety to traditional amniocentesis.

Chorionic villus sampling

Chorionic villus sampling (CVS) offers the attractive option of first-trimester testing. The United States Collaborative Study[9] (1985–87) and the Canadian Collaborative study[10] reported pregnancy loss rates following transcervical CVS to be only slightly higher than following traditional amniocentesis. Neither difference, 0.8% and 0.6%, respectively, was statistically significant. In a later US National Institute of Child Health and Human Development (1988–90) collaborative study[11], 1144 patients were randomized to either transcervical or transabdominal CVS. The loss rates of cytogenetically normal pregnancies during 28 weeks were 2.5% and 2.3%, respectively. The total 1988–90 loss rate (background plus procedure-related) following CVS decreased by 0.8% compared to the earlier (1985–87) period in which only transcervical CVS was available. This decrease probably reflects both increasing operator experience as well as availability of both transcervical and transabdominal approaches.

Multiple gestations

Multiple gestations arise commonly in infertility therapy. Fortunately, invasive diagnostic procedures can usually be performed. In experienced hands, amniocentesis is performed successfully in more than 95% of twin pregnancies[12]. Anderson and Goldberg[13] reported a post-procedure twin-loss rate of 3.57% during 28 weeks, a rate interpreted as not increased over the sum of background twin-loss rate plus the loss rate associated with singleton amniocentesis. Analogous to sampling twins, triplets and other multiple gestations can be tested similarly by sequentially injecting dye into successive sacs. So long as clear fluid is aspirated, one can be reassured that a new amniotic sac has been entered.

Chorionic villus sampling in multiple gestation is less established. In four experienced centers, 99% of fetuses could be sampled[14]. No diagnostic errors occurred among the 126 twin and two triplet gestations. Loss rates appear comparable to CVS for singleton pregnancies. However, XX/XY mixture occurred in six of 256 samples, giving an overall frequency of cell contamination of 4.6%; thus, accuracy is not quite so high as in singleton pregnancies.

References

1. Simpson, J. S., Elias, S., Gatlin, M. and Martin, A. O. (1981). Genetic counseling and genetic services in obstetrics and gynecology. *Am. J. Obstet. Gynecol.*, **140**, 70–7
2. Verp, M. S., Cohen, M. R. and Simpson, J. L. (1983). Necessity of formal genetic screening in artificial insemination by donor. *Obstet. Gynecol.*, **62**, 474–9
3. Simpson, J. L., Meyers, C. M., Martin, A. O., Elias, S. and Ober, C. (1989). Translocations are infrequent among couples having repeated

spontaneous abortions but no other abnormal pregnancies. *Fertil. Steril.*, **51**, 811–14

4. Lemna, W. K., Feldman, G. L., Kerem, B. S., Fernbach, S. D., Zevkovich, E. P., O'Brien, W. E., Riordan, J. R., Collins, F. S., Tsui, L. C. and Beaudet, A. L. (1990). Mutation analysis for heterozygote detection and the prenatal diagnosis of cystic fibrosis. *N. Engl. J. Med.*, **322**, 219–96

5. National Institute of Child Health Development National Registry for Amniocentesis Study Group (1976). Midtrimester amniocentesis for prenatal diagnosis: safety and accuracy. *J. Am. Med. Assoc.*, **236**, 1471–6

6. Tabor, A., Philip, J., Madsen, M. I., Bang, J., Obel, E. and Nørgaard–Pedersen, B. (1986). Randomized controlled trial of genetic amniocentesis in 4,606 low risk women. *Lancet*, **1**, 1287–93

7. Hanson, F. W., Tennant, F., Hune, S. and Brookhyser, K. (1992). Early amniocentesis: outcome, risks, and technical problems at ≤ 12.8 weeks. *Am. J. Obstet. Gynecol.*, **166**, 1707–11

8. Henry, G. P. and Miller, W. A. (1992). Early amniocentesis. *J. Reprod. Med.*, **37**, 396–402

9. Rhoads, G. G., Jackson, L. G., Schlesselman, S. E., de la Cruz, F. F., Desnick, R. J., Golbus, M. S., Ledbetter, D. H., Lubs, H. A., Mahoney, M. J., Pergament, E., Simpson, J. L., Carpenter, R. J., Elias, S., Ginsberg, N. A., Goldberg, J. D., Hobbins, J. C., Lynch, L., Shiono, P. H., Wapner, R. J., Zachary, J. M. and the NICHD (1989). The safety and efficacy of chorionic villus sampling for early prenatal diagnosis of cytogenetic abnormalities. *N. Engl. J. Med.*, **320**, 609–17

10. Canadian Collaborative CVS – Amniocentesis Clinical Trial Group (1991). Multicentre randomized clinical trial of chorionic villus sampling. *Lancet*, **337**, 1491–9

11. Jackson, L. G., Zachary, J. M., Desnick, R. J., Golbus, M. S., Ledbetter, D. H., Mahoney, M. J., Pergament, E., Schulman, J. D., Simpson, J. L., Fowler, S. E. and the NIH CVS and Amniocentesis Study Group (1992). A randomized comparison of transcervical and transabdominal chorionic villus sampling. *N. Engl. J. Med.*, **327**, 594–8

12. Elias, S. and Simpson, J. L. (1992). Amniocentesis. In Milunsky, A. (ed.) *Genetic Disorders and the Fetus*, 3rd edn., pp. 33–57. (New York: Plenum Press)

13. Anderson, R. L. and Goldberg, J. D. (1991). Prenatal diagnosis in multiple gestation: 20 years' experience with amniocentesis. *Prenat. Diagn.*, **11**, 263–70

14. Pregament, E., Schulman, J. D., Copeland, K., Fine, B., Black, S. H., Ginsberg, N. A., Frederiksen, M. C. and Carpenter, R. J. (1992). The risk and efficacy of chorionic villus sampling in multiple gestations. *Prenat. Diagn.*, **12**, 377–84

3

Endocrinology of reproduction

The endometrium and implantation 24

I. D. Cooke

Introduction

The blastocyst makes contact with the uterine luminal epithelium and then penetrates to become interstitial, being completely covered with endometrium by the 12th day of pregnancy. The attachment itself induces differentiation of endometrial stromal cells, which become decidual cells. The segment of the blastocyst containing the inner cell mass makes first contact with the endometrium. It is very difficult to study human implantation and some model systems have been devised. Endometrium has been grown in Matrigel® to achieve a three-dimensional structure. Mouse embryos have been cultured on explanted endometrial strips and the trophoblast/endometrial interface has been studied by culturing blastocysts with extracellular matrix purified from mouse endometrium on day 4 of pregnancy.

Clinical studies of endometrial receptivity

In natural human pregnancy, plasma human chorionic gonadotropin (hCG) rises from days + 6 to + 10 following the luteinizing hormone (LH) surge, inferring that implantation probably began on days LH +5 to + 9. On the other hand, in *in vitro* fertilization, embryo transfer occurs on days LH + 3 or + 4. In women with premature ovarian failure after endometrial development by sequential estradiol and progesterone, embryos transferred on days 3–5 after the start of progesterone administration have the best prospects of successful implantation.

There is evidence that receptivity may be influenced by the quality of the blastocyst and there is much evidence from the practice of *in vitro* fertilization (IVF) that egg and embryo quality may be suboptimal, to account in major part for the 75% loss of embryos. Although it might be thought that the hyperstimulation involved in IVF would cause major endometrial changes, scanning electron microscopy of the endometrium reveals no differences compared to normal endometrium. The higher estradiol/progesterone ratio in the early luteal phase has been suggested as increasing the rate of embryo transport, contributing to implantation failure. Zona hardening may contribute to this failure, but assisted hatching by breaching the zona pellucida may optimize synchronization. Clinical assessment of the endometrium at the time of embryo transfer has suggested that ultrasonic measurement of endometrial thickness may allow prediction of a better outcome, the thickness being variably estimated at greater than 6 mm or greater than 9 mm. A typical triple pattern has been described, although the precise histological association of these patterns is unclear. An alternative way of assessing endometrial preparation is assessment of endometrial vascularity, resistance to blood flow being variously described as a resistance or pulsatility index. More sophisticated imaging such as magnetic resonance has been able to identify implantation sites in rats, using enhancement techniques such as gadolinium, the different resonances being attributed to associated changes such as extracellular fluid volume, vascular permeability or uterine blood flow.

Simpler endometrial assessment has long been carried out using endometrial biopsy. There has been much controversy, but it seems that a midluteal phase sample (directed towards the time of implantation) is more likely to detect retarded development than late biopsies, which are more likely to reflect preparation for menstruation. Premature luteinization, a not uncommon feature of IVF, can cause lack of synchrony of both endometrial glands and stroma and this has been mimicked experimentally by premature progesterone administration in an otherwise standard sequential replacement regime in castrate patients.

Experimental studies of endometrium

Experimental studies have examined whole tissue as well as the constituent parts. Whole tissues possibly reflect more truly the integrated nature of gland and stromal interaction and are not of course subject to the disruption involved in experimental manipulation. The changes demonstrated by the effect of estradiol and progesterone are dependent on the respective receptors being developed at appropriate times. Estradiol and progesterone receptors during the follicular phase are present in both glands and stroma, peaking just prior to midcycle. Again, the premature ovarian failure patient has been used as a model. In the luteal phase there is first an early disappearance of estradiol receptors and only later of the progesterone receptors. They are both present in the same cells, but the rate of disappearance depends on the duration of progesterone administration. On the other hand, the stroma demonstrates progesterone receptors throughout the luteal phase. The progesterone receptor antagonist mifepristone and the anti-estrogen tamoxifen downregulate these receptors.

Platelet activating factor (PAF) was suggested as an early component in implantation when thrombocytopenia was found as the first sign of pregnancy in mice. PAF induces vascular permeability and would be a candidate for producing a transient, virtually avascular zone around the implanting blastocyst. However, a variety of PAF antagonists in rabbits was ineffectual in preventing implantation. PAF could reasonably be associated with major changes in the environment of the implanting blastocyst, as the PAF receptor is functionally linked to inositol lipid hydrolysis, intracellular calcium mobilization and activation of a tyrosine kinase pathway. Interestingly, calcitonin, a peptide hormone involved in calcium homoeostasis is also expressed in gland cells at implantation.

Epidermal growth factor (EGF) may mediate estradiol action in endometrium, and in stromal cells it stimulates DNA and protein synthesis. The EGF receptor has been found in gland cells. In conjunction with leukemia inhibitory factor (LIF), it is postulated[1] as being secreted into the lumen and influencing the implanting blastocyst to secrete matrixmetalloproteases. Plasminogen is activated by urokinase from trophoblast, to create plasmin, activating the matrixmetalloproteases by proteolytic cleavage.

The role of the immunosuppressive placental protein 14(PP14) is unclear. It is, however, secreted in huge amounts from endometrial gland cells and can be leached from the endometrium by flushing, in quantities 1–2 orders of magnitude greater than the serum concentration. The role of PP14 is speculative at present, although it has been shown to be acted upon by the cytokine interleukin (IL)-6, which in turn has been demonstrated to produce T cell growth, differentiation and activation. Interleukin-1 also stimulates its secretion and acts synergistically with IL-6 on T cells and B cells.

Peptide secretion from endometrial samples can be profiled. There is cycle fluctuation and some pathological conditions, such as endometriosis, are associated with different patterns, which may have implications for endometrial function and a reduced probability of implantation.

Studies on isolated glands

Both the classic and alternative pathways of complement activation, known to take part in phagocytosis and immunoregulation, have had components demonstrated in endometrial glandular tissue. The fact that complement receptor type 1 has been found only on stroma cells and type 3 on infiltrating leukocytes suggests that there may be a dialog between these elements.

Of the secreted glycoproteins, keratan sulfate in particular has been better characterized. Its passage through the cell from basal to apical and into the lumen by secretion is driven by progesterone. The process has been postulated as a marker of normal differentiation[2]. It is a lactosaminoglycan of mucin type, but epitope expression is heterogeneous, both from endometrial gland and stroma as in other tissues, multiple types being recognized. Cholesterol sulfate is accumulated in association with a lyophilic proteoglycan and its accumulation is also stimulated by progesterone. One of the mucins, polymorphic epithelial mucin MUC1, which has been cloned and sequenced, is transcriptionally regulated by progesterone in the endometrium. Postovulation mRNA is translated and glycosylation of the polypeptide occurs in the domain containing tandem repeats. A function for MUC1 has been sought and it has been suggested that implantation might comprise initial reactions other than direct blastocyst–luminal epithelium contact. MUC1 might create steric hindrance to direct contact, because the molecule projects further from the luminal epithelium than other potential ligands. The oligosaccharide of MUC1 may bind weakly to the luminal epithelial glycocalyx initially, but an adhesion cascade, similar to that used by neutrophils during extravasation at inflammatory sites, may subsequently lead to more substantial integrin binding of blastocyst and endometrial luminal cells[3].

Studies on isolated stroma

Stromal cell differentiation is known as decidualization, an essential component of implantation. Prostaglandin binding sites have been identified on proliferative phase cells, prostaglandin E_2 stimulation resulting in expression of prolactin. This expression has been used as a marker for decidualization and is promoted by estradiol and progesterone. Transforming growth factor-β (TGF-β) stimulates DNA synthesis in stromal cells but inhibits it in glandular

cells. Insulin like growth factor (IGF) 1 (and 2 in the rat) show structural homology to proinsulin, having effects on cell proliferation, growth, differentiation and metabolism. They occur not only in the endometrium but also in the embryo. IGF1 binds to endometrial IGF receptors that have the same binding affinity as IGF binding protein 1, which is produced by decidualized stroma cells. It may play a role in inhibiting IGF action at the endometrial trophoblastic interface.

Studies on leukocytes

In the rodent, leukocytes/macrophages have been termed large granular leukocytes or, previously, granulated metrial gland cells. They have recently been thought to be presumptive cytolytic natural killer cells or at least an organ-specific subset of these[4]. They produce granulocyte macrophage colony stimulating factor (GM-CSF), which is in turn stimulated by IL-1, IL-2, IL-4, IL-6 and tumor necrosis factor α (TNF α). It enhances the function of macrophages and stimulates endothelial cells, contributing to a modulatory cascade. T cells increase in the endometrium in response to progesterone. T suppressor/cytotoxic, CD8[+] cells are reduced and T helper/inducer, CD4[+] cells are increased in unexplained infertility consistent with deviations found in recurrent abortion.

Studies on vessels

Vessels are important as a probable source of leukocyte transmigration through the epithelial cells into the stroma, which takes place under the effects of chemoattractants. A potent chemoattractant for neutrophils and T lymphocytes is the cytokine IL-8, produced by blood mononuclear cells and epithelial cells. It has recently been immunohistochemically identified perivascularly, but localized to arteriole smooth muscle cells rather than to endothelial cells[5]. It may also play a role in prostaglandin stimulation.

Studies on luminal epithelium

The uterine lumen containing the blastocyst has low oxygen tension, high potassium and low sodium concentrations in luminal fluid. The uterine luminal epithelium can influence these concentrations by a sodium pump, suggesting that it has a major role in generating and maintaining the distinctive ionic composition.

IL-1 acts on its receptor, which is located in the luminal epithelium. Blockade of this receptor by an IL-1 receptor antagonist in the mouse leads to failure of blastocyst attachment and therefore of implantation[6]. There is no detrimental effect on the blastocyst formation, its hatching or its ability to attach to fibronectin, its outgrowth or its trophoblastic migration *in vitro*, so it seems that the IL-1 stimulation of its receptor is crucial to attachment and implantation.

The luminal epithelial glycocalyx is believed to play a role in implantation. Fucose is well represented in complex carbohydrates such as a fucosylated H type 1 carbohydrate, an epitope found on the glycocalyx. The enzyme α (1–2) fucosyltransferase is under distinct endocrine control, peaking at estrus and then falling sharply, reflecting its stimulation by estrogen and strong inhibition by progesterone. This may suggest that the enzyme plays a crucial role in the final step of oligosaccharide synthesis that determines the epitopes presenting for initial binding by the blastocyst.

More potent binding receptors are integrins, heterodimeric molecules comprising dissimilar α and β subunits. The extracellular ligand-binding domains are large and each is connected through a transmembrane region to cytoplasmic domains that bind to the cytoskeleton and trigger second messengers. There are two cycle-dependent integrins, α4β1 and αVβ 3, which span the implantation window and are postulated to play a role in uterine receptivity. They are receptors for cell-matrix adhesion and recognize vitronectin, in particular the amino acid sequence Arg-Gly-Asp (RGD)[7]. When both cells contain these sequences, they may adhere through the RGD binding sites or through a bridging molecule.

Studies on trophoblast endometrial interaction

The urokinase-type plasminogen activator (u-PA) and inhibitors 1 and 2 are localized at the trophoblast surface. The activator converts plasminogen to plasmin, which is hypothesized to activate TGF-β. Invasive trophoblast expresses αV integrins. The control of the extracellular matrix component glycoproteins laminin and fibronectin limits the invasiveness of trophoblastic villi[8]. They bind the integrin receptors expressed on the trophoblast cell membrane. Trophoblast is invasive when the receptors are distributed in a non-polarized way. They do not bind to ligands and secrete matrixmetalloproteases (MMPs), particularly the MMP9 otherwise known as gelatinase B or collagenase IV. Proteases act on the MMP family, which have similar structures. MMP2 lacks the type V collagen-like domain, whereas MMP1, 8, 3 and 10 lack the fibronectin-like gelatin-binding domain. These form the family of stromelysins. Finally, a putative uterine metalloprotease (PUMP-1) lacks any vitronectin-like domain with its major carbohydrate component. All four types bind zinc. When the integrin receptors are clustered on the trophoblast surface, protease secretion is reduced by tissue inhibitors of MMP (TIMPs) and the villi lose their ability to invade.

Apoptosis plays a role in implantation, but it is not clearly defined. Trophoblast invasion initially occurs between the luminal epithelial cells ultimately replacing them, apoptosis seemingly programmed at the interface between the conceptus and maternal tissue. LIF also plays a regulatory role by stimulating TGF-β within the endometrium, which in turn stimulates TIMPs to limit the secretion of metalloproteases, LIF itself being subject to estrogen and progesterone stimulation[1]. Judging by its name, LIF was previously described as a cytokine that inhibited embryonic stem cell differentiation. It may act on decidua at the implantation site either directly or indirectly, by inducing the expression of other cytokines. These regulate both in time and space the proteolytic activity that determines the effectiveness of implantation.

196

At present, implantation seems to be a description of separate events of receptor binding and stimulation. An understanding of the interaction of these events developing into cascades, as has occurred in leukocyte activation, will doubtless show a complex series of proteolytic and immunomodulatory cascades. All elements will participate and, as their interactions clarify the understanding of implantation, its potential control will be clearer. Until then, we must be content with fragmented data and hypotheses. The process of acquiring these data and this understanding will provide much excitement in the forthcoming decade.

References

1. Harvey, M. B., Leco, K. J., Arcellana-Panlilo, N. Y., Zhang, X., Edwards, D. R. and Schultz, G. A. (1995). Roles of growth factors during peri-implantation development. *Mol. Hum. Reprod.*, **10**, 712–18

2. Graham, R. A., Li, T. C., Cooke, I. D. and Aplin, J. D. (1994). Keratan sulphate as a secretory product of human endometrium: cyclic expression in normal women. *Hum. Reprod.*, **9**, 926–30

3. Aplin, J. D. (1994). Models of human embryo implantation and placental morphogenesis. In Ward, R. H. T., Smith, S. K. and Donnai, D. (eds.) *Early Fetal Growth and Development*, pp. 154–69. (London: Royal College of Obstetricians and Gynaecologists)

4. King, A., Wooding, P., Gardner, L. and Yoke, Y. W. (1993). Expression of perforin, granzyme A and TIA-1 by human uterine CD 56$^+$ NK cells implies that they are activated and capable of effector functions. *Hum. Reprod.*, **8**, 2061–7

5. Critchley, H. O. D., Kelly, R. W. and Kooy, J. (1994). Perivascular location of a chemokine interleukin-8 in human endometrium: a preliminary report. *Hum. Reprod.*, **9**, 1406–9

6. Simon, C., Frances, A., Piquette, G. N., el-Danasouri, I., Zurawski, G., Dang, W. and Polan, M. L. (1994). Embryonic implantation in mice is blocked by interleukin-1 receptor antagonist. *Endocrinology*, **134**, 521–8

7. Lessey, B. A., Castelbaum, A. J., Buck, C. A., Lie, Y., Yowell, C. W. and Sun, J. (1994). Further characteristics of endometrial integrins during the menstrual cycle and in pregnancy. *Fertil. Steril.*, **62**, 497–506

8. Bischof, P., Redard, M., Gindre, P., Vassilakos, P. and Campana, A. (1993). Localization of alpha 2, alpha 5, and alpha 6 integrin subunits in human endometrium, decidua and trophoblast. *Eur. J. Obstet. Gynecol. Reprod. Biol.*, **51**, 217–26

Antiprogestins and the implantation process

25

M. Bygdeman, M. L. Swahn and K. Gemzell Danielsson

Introduction

During recent years, a number of antiprogestins have been developed, such as mifepristone (Roussel Uclaf, Paris, France), onapristone and lilopristone (Schering AG, Berlin, Germany) which interact with the progesterone receptor preventing progesterone from expressing its biological effect. Since progesterone is essential for the formation of the secretory endometrium, which is required for nidation of the conceptus, an effect of antiprogestin on implantation is likely.

Effect of antiprogestin during the follicular phase

Administration of antiprogestin in the mid- or late follicular phase delays the luteinizing hormone (LH) surge and postpones ovulation. Estrogen levels fail to increase and follicular development is delayed or arrested. No bleeding is induced and endometrial development does not seem to be influenced[1–5]. After cessation of antiprogestin treatment, there is a resumption of follicular growth or recruitment of a new follicle and the following luteal phase is normal in most women[4]. It seems likely that the inhibitory effect of antiprogestins on ovulation is due to a blocking of the effect of progesterone at the pituitary level[6–8]. There are no data indicating that administration of antiprogestin in the follicular phase has any effect on implantation.

Effect of antiprogestin during the luteal phase

The effect of antiprogestins during the luteal phase is dependent on the time of treatment and the dose of antiprogestin given. Even if a high dose of mifepristone, 200 mg, is administered immediately after ovulation (two days after LH surge, LH + 2) no bleeding is induced except for occasional spotting after 2 to 3 days and the length of the luteal phase and the levels of ovarian steroids are not significantly influenced[9]. Administration of high doses of mifepristone later during the luteal phase results in the shedding of the endometrium and the subsequent bleeding a few days after the initiation of treatment[4,10]. Available evidence strongly suggests that the effect is due to withdrawal of progesterone influence on the endometrium[9,11]. Since no bleeding occurs if antiprogestin is administered during the follicular phase, immediately after ovulation or to anovulatory women[4,8,12] progesterone influence and secretory transformation of the endometrium seems to be a prerequisite for antiprogestin-induced bleeding. The dose of antiprogestin is also of importance since small doses of antiprogestin do not induce any bleeding in spite of an inhibition of endometrial development[13–15].

Administration of antiprogestin early in the luteal phase has profound effects on endometrial development and function. A significantly decrease in glandular diameter and increase in the number of glandular and stromal mitoses have been demonstrated[9,10]. Treatment with mifepristone will significantly inhibit the normal down-regulation of progesterone receptor concentration in the luteal phase[16-18]. The effect of mifepristone on the secretory activity of the endometrium has been evaluated in different ways. The reduction in the amount of uterine fluid at midluteal phase in comparison with at ovulation time is less pronounced and the concentration of prostaglandin ($PGF_{2\alpha}$) in uterine fluid is significantly reduced[19]. The same is true for 17β-hydroxysteroid dehydrogenase which is the major enzyme in the endometrium, metabolizing estradiol into the biologically less active estrogen estrone[17]. The secretory components of the endometrium detected by lectin histochemistry are also significantly reduced[15,18]. The plasma concentration of placental protein 14 (PP14) is another marker of endometrial function. After treatment with mifepristone, the plasma concentration of PP14 at menstruation is significantly lower than in control cycles[15,20] (Table 1).

Effect on implantation

The mechanism of implantation of the human blastocyst in the endometrium is considered to be initiated by a dialog between the embryo and maternal tissue[21]. Studies in animals have shown that the developmental stages of both the blastocyst and the endometrium require a temporal synchronization for implantation to be possible[22]. This permissive stage of the endometrium is sometimes referred to as 'the implantation window'[23]. Human implantation occurs approximately 5–6 days after ovulation, which corresponds to approximately 7–8 days after the LH surge[24]. Studies of women with ovarian failure undergoing embryo transfer have shown that the window of implantation is restricted to 3–4 days[25].

That the inhibition of endometrial development and secretory function following treatment with antiprogestin is sufficient to prevent implantation has been demonstrated in clinical studies. In one study, 21 sexually active women were given 200 mg mifepristone in the very early luteal phase of the menstrual cycle (day LH + 2) as their sole method of contraception. The women used the treatment for periods of 1–12 months. There was only one pregnancy in a total of 157 ovulating cycles. In 124 cycles, at least one act of intercourse occurred in the 3 days around ovulation. The duration of the menstrual cycle and amount and duration of menstruation was not affected[26]. That treatment with mifepristone is sufficient to prevent implantation was also demonstrated in two studies in which 600 mg mifepristone was given within 72 h of unprotected intercourse[27,28]. No pregnancy occurred following mifepristone in either study. Based on the number of days that had elapsed since the last menstruation, a substantial number of women were treated around ovulation when the contraceptive effect of mifepristone must have been due to its inhibitory action on endometrial development and function.

Future development

These three studies strongly suggest that the endometrial effect of mifepristone is sufficient to prevent pregnancy. However, the doses of mifepristone used (200–600 mg) are also so high that the ovulation is inhibited if administered in the follicular phase. Much lower doses of antiprogestin may still influence endometrial function without inhibiting ovulation. Once weekly administration of 5 or 10 mg onapristone to bonnet monkeys did not inhibit ovulation but caused atrophic changes in endometrial glands as well as in the stroma[14]. A recent study from the same group of investigators using the same antiprogestin, also in bonnet monkeys, indicated that this effect on the endometrium is sufficient to prevent implantation[29]. A similar difference in endometrial and ovarian sensitivity to mifepristone seems also to be present in the human. Treatment once weekly with 2.5 or 5 mg mifepristone did not induce bleeding or inhibit ovulation, while a delay in endometrial development, an inhibition of the down-regulation of progesterone receptor concentration, a significant reduction in the secretory activity of the endometrium and in serum concentration of PP14 could be demonstrated[15]. Daily administration of 1.0 mg mifepristone will also only occasionally suppress ovulation but consistently

Table 1 Review of endometrial effects of antiprogestin in the luteal phase

Site of action	Effect
Endometrial development[4,10]	delayed or inhibited
Volume of uterine secretion[19]	increased
Progesterone receptor concentration[15]	inhibition of down-regulation
Concentration of $PGF_{2\alpha}$ in uterine secretion[19]	decreased
DBA-lectin binding[15]	reduced
Placenta protein 14[15,20]	reduced

inhibit endometrial development[6,30]. If these effects on the endometrium are sufficient to prevent implantation remains to be established. However, not only inhibition of endometrial development but also impaired secretory activity of the endometrium has been demonstrated as a cause of infertility[31,32]. It may thus be possible to develop a contraceptive method based on very low doses of antiprogestin, preventing implantation without an effect on ovarian function and the bleeding pattern of the menstrual cycle.

Conclusions

Treatment with antiprogestin will inhibit endometrial development and function. Clinical stu-dies have shown that these effects are highly effective in preventing implantation, at least if high doses of mifepristone are given. The endometrium seems more sensitive to antiprogestin than the ovulatory process, and with small daily or once weekly doses of mifepristone, an effect on the endometrium can be demonstrated without inhibiting ovulation. If these effects on the endometrium are sufficient to prevent implantation remains to be established.

Acknowledgements

These studies were supported by the Knut and Alice Wallenberg Foundation and by the Swedish Medical Research Council (05696).

References

1. Liu, J. H., Garzo, G., Monis Strenkel, C., Ul-mann, A. and Yen, S. C. C. (1987). Disruption of follicular maturation and delay of ovulation after administration of the antiprogestin RU 486. *J. Clin. Endocrinol. Metab.*, **65**, 1135–40

2. Shoupe, D., Mishell, D. R., Page, M. A., Mad-kour, H., Spitz, J. M. and Lobo, R. A. (1987). Effects of the antiprogesterone RU 486 in nor-mal women. *Am. J. Obstet. Gynecol.*, **157** 1421–6

3. Luukainen, T., Heikinheimo, O., Haukkamaa, M. and Lähteenmäki, P. (1988). Inhibition of folliculogenesis and ovulation by the antipro-gesterone RU 486. *Fertil. Steril.*, **49**, 361–3

4. Swahn, M. L., Johannisson, E., Daniore, V., de la Torre, B. and Bygdeman, M. (1988). The effect of RU 486 administered during the proliferative and secretory phase of the cycle on the bleeding pattern, hormonal parameters and the endo-metrium. *Hum. Reprod.*, **3**, 915–21

5. Puri, C. P., Patel, R. K., Elger, A. G., Vadigoppula, A. D. and Pongula, J. M. R. (1989). Gonadal and pituitary responses to pro-gesterone antagonist ZK 98,299 during the follic-ular phase of the menstrual cycle in bonnet monkeys. *Contraception*, **39**, 227–43

6. Batista, M. C., Cartledge, T. P., Zellmar, A. W., Merino, M. J., Axiotis, C., Loriaux, D. L. and Nieman, L. K. (1992). Delayed endometrial maturation induced by daily administration of the antiprogestin RU 486. A potential new con-traceptive strategy. *Am. J. Obstet. Gynecol.*, **167**, 60–5

7. Batista, M. C., Cartledge, T. P., Zellmar, A. W., Nieman, L. K., Merriam, G. R. and Loriaux, D. L. (1992). Evidence for a critical role of pro-gesterone in the regulation of the midcycle gonadotropin surge and ovulation. *J. Clin. En-docrinol. Metab.*, **74**, 565–70

8. Puri, C. P. and Van Look, P. F. A. (1991). Newly developed competitive progesterone antagonists for infertility control. In Agarwal, M. K. (ed.) *Antihormones in Health and Disease. Frontiers of Hormone Research.* Vol. 19, pp. 127–67. (Basel: Karger)

9. Swahn, M. L., Bygdeman, M., Xing, S., Cekan, S., Masironi, B. and Johannisson, E. (1990). The effect of RU 486 administered during the early luteal phase on bleeding pattern, hormonal parameters and endometrium. *Hum. Reprod.*, **5**, 402–8

10. Li, T.-C., Dockery, P., Thomas, P., Rogers, A. W., Lenton, E. A. and Cooke, I. D. (1988). The effects of progesterone blockade in the luteal phase of normal fertile women. *Fertil. Steril.*, **50**, 732–42

11. Croxatto, H. B., Spitz, J. M., Salvatierra, A. M. and Bardin, C. W. (1985). The demonstration of the antiprogestin effects of RU 486 administered to the human during hCG-induced pseudopregnancy. In Baulieu, E. E. and Segal, S. J. (eds.) *The Antiprogestin Steroid RU 486 and Human Fertility Control.* pp. 263–71. (New York: Plenum Press)

12. Schaison, G., George, M., Lestrat, N., Reinberg, A. and Baulieu, E. E. (1985). Effects of the antiprogesterone steroid RU 486 during midluteal phase in normal women. *J. Clin. Endocrinol. Metab.*, **61**, 484–9

13. Greene, K. E., Kettel, L. M. and Yen, S. S. C. (1992). Interruption of endometrial maturation without hormonal changes by an antiprogesterone during the first half of the luteal phase of the menstrual cycle: a contraceptive potential. *Fertil. Steril.*, **58**, 338–43

14. Ishawad, P. C., Katkam, R. R., Hinduja, I. N., Chwalisz, K., Elger, W. and Puri, C. P. (1993). Treatment with a progesterone antagonist ZK 98.299 delays endometrial development without blocking ovulation in bonnet monkeys. *Contraception*, **48**, 57–70

15. Gemzell Danielsson, K., Westlund, P., Johannisson, E., Swahn, M. L., Seppälä, M. and Bygdeman, M. (1995). Effect of low weekly doses of mifepristone on ovarian function and endometrial development. *Hum. Reprod.*, in press

16. Berthois, Y., Salat-Baroux, J., Cornat, J., De Brux, J., Kopps, F. and Maric Martin, P. A. (1991). Multiparametric analysis of endometrial estrogen and progestrone receptors after postovulatory administration of mifepristone. *Fertil. Steril.*, **55**, 547–54

17. Mäentausta, O., Svalander, P., Gemzell-Danielsson, K., Bygdeman, M. and Vihko, R. (1993). The effects of an antiprogesterone, mifepristone, and an antiestrogen, tamoxifen, on endometrial 17β-hydroxysteroid dehydrogenase and pro-

gestin and estrogen receptors during the luteal phase of the menstrual cycle. An immunohistochemical study. *J. Endocrinol. Metab.*, **77**, 913–18

18. Gemzell Danielsson, K., Svalander, P., Swahn, M. L., Johannisson, E. and Bygdeman, M. (1994). Effect of a single postovulatory dose of RU 486 on the endometrial maturation in the implantation phase. *Hum. Reprod.*, **9**, 2398–404

19. Gemzell Danielsson, K. and Hamberg, M. (1994). The effect of antiprogestin (RU 486) and prostaglandin biosynthesis inhibitor (Naproxen) on uterine fluid $PGF_{2\alpha}$ concentrations. *Hum. Reprod.*, **9**, 1626–30

20. Swahn, M. L., Bygdeman, M., Seppälä, M., Johannisson, E. and Cekan, S. (1993). Effect of tamoxifen alone and in combination with RU 486 on the endometrium in the midluteal phase. *Hum. Reprod.*, **8**, 93–200

21. Psychoyos, A. and Martel, D. (1985). Embryo-endometrial interactions at implantation. In Edwards, R. G., Purdy, J. M. and Steptoe, P. C. (eds.) *Implantation of the Human Embryo.* p. 195. (London: Academic Press)

22. Glasser, S. R., Mulholland, J., Mani, S. K., Julian, J., Munir, M. I., Lampelo, S. and Soares, M. J. (1991). Blastocyst-endometrial relationships: reciprocal interaction between uterine epithelial and stromal cells and blastocysts. *Trophoblast Res.*, **5**, 229–80

23. Harper, M. J. K. (1992). The implantation window. In Hamberger, L. and Wikland, M. (eds.) *Baillière's Clinical Obstetrics and Gynaecology*, Vol. 6(2), pp. 351–72. (London: Baillière Tindall)

24. Bergh, P. A. and Navot, D. (1992). The impact of embryonic development and endometrial maturity on the timing of implantation. *Fertil. Steril.*, **58**, 537–42

25. Navot, D., Scott, T. R., Droesch, K., Veeck, L. L., Hung-Ching, L. and Rosenwaks, Z. (1991). The window of embryo transfer and the efficiency of human conception *in vitro*. *Fertil. Steril.*, **55**, 114–18

26. Gemzell Danielsson, K., Swahn, M. L., Svalander, P. and Bygdeman, M. (1993). Early luteal phase treatment with RU 486 for fertility regulation. *Hum. Reprod.*, **8**, 870–3

27. Glasier, A. F., Thong, K. J., Dewar, M., Mackie, M. and Baird, D. T. (1992). Mifepristone (RU 486) compared with high-dose estrogen and progesterone emergency postcoital contraception. *N. Engl. J. Med.*, **327**, 1041–4

28. Webb, A. M. C., Russel, J. and Elstein, M. (1992). Comparison of Yuzpe regimen, danazol and mifepristone (RU 486) in oral postcoital contraception. *Br. Med. J.*, **305**, 927–31

29. Katkam, R. R., Gopalkrishnan, K., Chwalisz, K., Schillinger, E. and Puri, C. P. (1995). Onapri-

stone (ZK 98,299). A potential antiprogestin for endometrial contraception. *Am. J. Obstet. Gynecol.*, in press

30. Croxatto, H. B., Salvatierra, A. M., Croxatto, H. D. and Fuentealba, B. (1993). Effects of continuous treatment with low dose mifepristone throughout one menstrual cycle. *Hum. Reprod.*, 8, 201–7

31. Li, T.-C., Dockery, P., Rogers, A. W. and Cook, I. D. (1990). A quantitative study of endometrial development in the luteal phase: comparison between women with unexplained infertility and normal fertility. *Br. J. Obstet. Gynaecol.*, **97**, 576–82

32. Klentzeris, L. D., Bulmer, J. N., Li, T. C., Morrison, L., Warren, A. and Cooke, I. D. (1991). Lectin binding of endometrium in women with unexplained infertility. *Fertil. Steril.*, **56**, 660–7

Prevention of the ovarian hyperstimulation syndrome

26

B. C. Tarlatzis and G. Grimbizis

Introduction

Ovulatory stimulants have been used successfully in the management of anovulation since the early 1960s, with the introduction of clomiphene citrate (CC) and human menopausal gonadotropin (hMG), and they have also been routinely applied in controlled ovarian hyperstimulation for *in vitro* fertilization since the early 1980s. Despite their efficacy, their administration is accompanied by some complications, the most important and serious being the ovarian hyperstimulation syndrome (OHSS).

Ovarian hyperstimulation syndrome has been reported to occur following treatment with virtually all drugs used for ovarian hyperstimulation[1-4], and the currently available gonadotropin releasing hormone analogs (GnRH-a) seem to be associated with an increased incidence of OHSS[5,6]. The syndrome is associated with a variety of clinical symptoms and signs as well as laboratory findings. The pathophysiological changes observed during its clinical course are thought to result from an acute increase in vascular permeability, leading to third-space shifting of intravascular fluid[2,7].

The existing differences in the severity of clinically apparent OHSS as well as its management create the need for an accurate and useful classification. Since the initial classification proposed by Rubeau and colleagues[8] fits a description of ovarian response rather than OHSS *per se*, a revision based on clinical symptoms and signs was later introduced by Golan and associates[9] which seems to be more appropriate. Thus, according to these authors, OHSS is divided to three categories and five grades:

(1) Mild OHSS

  (a) Grade 1, abdominal distension and discomfort;

  (b) Grade 2, plus nausea, vomiting and/or diarrhea associated with ovarian enlargement of 5–12 cm.

(2) Moderate OHSS

  (a) Grade 3, manifestations of the mild forms plus ultrasonographic evidence of ascites.

(3) Severe OHSS

  (a) Grade 4, features of moderate OHSS plus clinical evidence of ascites and/or hydrothorax or breathing difficulties;

  (b) Grade 5, changes in the blood volume, increased blood viscosity due to hemoconcentration, coagulation abnormalities and impaired renal function with oliguria.

Furthermore, Navot and co-workers[10] proposed a definition of the severest degree of OHSS as 'a critical or life-threatening stage'. Thus, the presence of tense ascites and/or hydrothorax, hematocrit (Hct) ≥ 55%, white blood cells ≥ 25 000 ml, creatinine ≥ 1.6 mg%, creatinine clearance < 50 ml/min, renal failure, thromboembolic phenomena as well as acute respiratory distress syndrome, are thought to be characteristics of this critical stage.

The management of clinically apparent OHSS is mainly based on the knowledge of its pathophysiology. On the other hand, as the syndrome is a potentially life-threatening condition, its prevention seems to be more useful than its treatment.

Prevention

Stimulation protocol

In patients with polycystic ovary syndrome (PCOS), the predisposition for OHSS development is associated with their inherent tendency toward multiple follicular development and their peculiar hypersensitivity to gonadotropins[11-13]. The low-dose step-up protocol was proposed as an alternative to avoid ovarian hyperstimulation. It is based on low-dose gonadotropin administration in order to reach the follicle stimulating hormone (FSH) threshold level and, once ovarian response has been achieved, the lowest effective dose is continued. Thus, multifollicular development associated with conventional regimes is substituted by a mono- or oligofollicular response, producing acceptable ovulation and pregnancy rates[11,12] with elimination of OHSS[11,13].

More recent options in ovulation induction therapy are the step-down regimes. According to these protocols, the FSH threshold is quickly reached by rapid increases in the administered gonadotropin dose and, once adequate ovarian response is achieved, the dose is reduced in order to avoid the continuous recruitment and development of less mature follicles[14]. Preliminary experiences indicate that this protocol is accompanied by satisfactory results, and furthermore severe OHSS appears to be avoided[14].

Another manipulation that has been proposed in order to modify ovarian hyper-responsiveness in PCOS patients is to administer GnRH-a. Although, theoretically, the PCOS hormonal milieu may be altered by GnRH-a administration, it seems that the duration of GnRH-a suppression has to be extremely long (≥ 8 weeks) in order favorably to affect ovarian response[10].

Manipulations with preovulatory human chorionic gonadotropin

Withholding human chorionic gonadotropin (hCG) administration with concomitant discontinuation of ovarian stimulation effectively prevents the occurrence of imminent OHSS but is also accompanied by cycle cancellation[4,10,15]. In patients stimulated with GnRH-a plus gonadotropins, in addition to the aforementioned manipulations, GnRH-a administration may be continued in an attempt further to suppress ovarian activity[6]. However, the value of this practice is doubted by other workers, as endogenous gonadotropin output is thought to be minimal for at least 14 days after GnRH-a discontinuation[15].

Navot and co-workers[10] have proposed the reduction of the hCG dose from the currently used 10 000 IU to 5000 IU, in patients at risk for OHSS with moderate estradiol levels, but the benefits of this practice have not been yet confirmed. Premature hCG administration has also been proposed as an alternative to avoid high estradiol levels on the day of hCG and to rescue the stimulated cycle. However, this is accompanied by ovulation of immature oocytes and poor pregnancy results[4]. Withholding human menopausal gonadotropin (hMG) and administering hCG after a pause of several days has been described as another option to prevent imminent OHSS[4]. However, the conception rates seem to drop in relation to the length of the interval between discontinuation of hMG and hCG injection[4].

Triggering of ovulation with a short-term GnRH-a administration in hMG-stimulated cycles has been reported by several authors[16-19]. The combined luteinizing hormone (LH) and FSH surge which is provoked is thought to provide a more physiological endocrine milieu[16] and potentially protect the patient from imminent OHSS[17]. Although Imoedemhe and co-workers[17] and Shalev and colleagues[19] support that this practice is effective in preventing OHSS development in high-risk patients, van der Meer and co-workers[18] failed to document complete protection in their study population. Induction of ovulation with GnRH-a may also be used in GnRH-a plus gonadotropin-stimulated cycles after previous discontinuation of daily GnRH-a administration for at least 2 days[6]. However, there is no clinical experience to support the effectiveness of this protocol.

Avoidance of endogenous human chorionic gonadotropin production: withholding embryo transfer

One of the benefits of in vitro fertilization (IVF) is the provided capability to dissociate oocyte retrieval and fertilization from subsequent embryo transfer, thus deferring the achievement of pregnancy through cryopreservation of the resulting embryos[10,15]. This procedure lessens the severity of OHSS since pregnancy and luteal hCG supplementation are avoided[15]. Furthermore, the absence of the fear of a subsequent pregnancy allows more liberal and aggressive management of the affected patients[15]. However, the use of this method depends on the availability and the efficacy of the cryopreservation program at the individual IVF center.

In women stimulated with GnRH-a plus gonadotropins, this practice can be associated with prolongation of GnRH-a administration after oocyte retrieval in order to contribute to the patient's improvement[6]. However, the value of this is doubted by others[15] and, therefore, continuation of GnRH-a therapy is indicated only in patients who wish to embark on further treatment without delay[15].

The role of follicular aspiration

Follicular aspiration seems to exert a protective effect on OHSS development. However, OHSS is also observed in IVF cycles, but with higher estradiol levels than in ovulation induction, thus indicating that this protection is incomplete[10]. The reduction of the amount of granulosa cells, the influence of intrafollicular hemorrhage on corpus luteum function as well as the disruption of intraovarian processes which have been implicated in OHSS development (e.g. ovarian

renin–angiotensin system) appear to contribute to the decrease of OHSS incidence and severity[10,20,21].

Hence, conversion of ovulation induction cycles with excessive ovarian response to IVF cycles has been proposed as a protective manipulation against OHSS occurrence and severity with satisfactory results[21]. Additional protection can be achieved by cryopreservation of the resulting embryos, thus avoiding a subsequent pregnancy[21]. As an alternative to follicular aspiration of all the existing follicles in ovulation induction cycles, Belaisch-Allert and co-workers[22] performed selective oocyte retrieval leaving one mature follicle in situ. In this case, the patient may benefit from both natural conception and a subsequent embryo transfer of freeze-thawed embryos. However, the efficacy of this approach has yet to be proved[21].

As an additional preventive measure, Amit and co-workers[20] performed repeated aspiration of early corpus luteum cysts on the day of embryo transfer in IVF cycles when estradiol levels exceeded 3800 pg/ml and more than 20 follicles were observed, and succeeded in decreasing both the incidence and the severity of OHSS.

Luteal phase human chorionic gonadotropin

Luteal phase support can be provided by the administration of hCG or progesterone. Both forms of supplementation are equally effective in hMG-stimulated cycles, increasing significantly the pregnancy rates[23], whereas the use of hCG appears to be more effective than progesterone in GnRH-a plus gonadotropin-stimulated cycles[23]. However, the administration of hCG during the luteal phase is associated with a higher incidence of OHSS development. Furthermore, the severe forms of OHSS are very rare in the absence of hCG supplementation[10,23]. Thus, in high-risk patients progesterone should be routinely used in order to avoid imminent OHSS. In our center, when estradiol levels exceed 1800 pg/ml luteal phase is supplemented only with micronized progesterone[24].

Intravenous administration of human albumin

Asch and co-workers[25] were the first to advocate the prophylactic use of albumin for OHSS prevention because of its two important properties: (1) that of maintaining plasma oncotic pressure and, consequently, intravascular volume, and (2) its role as a carrier protein which acts to bind the elevated active steroid hormones and sequester the vasoactive substances released by the corpora lutea. From the existing data, it seems that intravenous albumin administration can effectively protect against imminent OHSS[25,26]. However, further studies are needed to reach more definite conclusions for its exact role and effectiveness.

References

1. Schenker, J. G. and Weinstein, D. (1978). Ovarian hyperstimulation syndrome: a current survey. *Fertil. Steril.*, **30**, 255–68
2. Editorial (1991). Ovarian hyperstimulation syndrome. *Lancet*, **338**, 1111–12
3. Rizk, B. and Aboulghar, M. (1991). Modern management of ovarian hyperstimulation syndrome (Review). *Hum. Reprod.*, **6**, 1082–7
4. Schenker, J. G. (1993). Prevention and treatment of ovarian hyperstimulation (Review). *Hum. Reprod.*, **8**, 653–9
5. Rizk, B. and Smitz, J. (1992). Ovarian hyperstimulation syndrome after superovulation using GnRH agonists for IVF and related procedures (Review). *Hum. Reprod.*, **7**, 320–7
6. Mordel, N. and Schenker, J. G. (1993). Gonadotrophin-releasing hormone agonist and ovarian hyperstimulation syndrome in assisted reproduction (Review). *Hum. Reprod.*, **8**, 2009–14
7. Bergh, P. A. and Navot, D. (1992). Ovarian hyperstimulation syndrome: a review of pathophysiology. *J. Assist. Reprod. Genet.*, **9**, 429–38
8. Rubeau, E., David, A., Serr, D. M., Mashiach, S. and Lunenfeld, B. (1967). Human menopausal gonadotropins for anovulation and sterility: results of 7 years of treatment. *Am. J. Obstet. Gynecol.*, **98**, 92–8
9. Golan, A., Ron-El, A., Herman, A., Soffer, Y., Weinraub, Z. and Caspi, E. (1989). Ovarian hyperstimulation syndrome: an update review. *Obstet. Gynecol. Surv.*, **44**, 430–40
10. Navot, D., Bergh, P. A. and Laufer, N. (1992). Ovarian hyperstimulation syndrome in novel reproductive technologies: prevention and treatment. *Fertil. Steril.*, **58**, 249–61
11. Schoemaker, J., Van Weissenbruch, M. M., Scheele, F. and Van der Meer, M. (1993). The FSH threshold concept in clinical ovulation induction. *Baillieres Clin. Obstet. Gynaecol.*, **7**, 297–308
12. Ben-Rafael, Z., Levy, T. and Schoemaker, J. (1995). Pharmacokinetic of follicle-stimulating hormone: clinical significance. *Fertil. Steril.*, **63**, 689–700
13. Homburg, R., Levy, T. and Ben-Rafael, Z. (1995). A comparative prospective study of conventional regimen with chronic low-dose administration of follicle-stimulating hormone for anovulation associated with polycystic ovary syndrome. *Fertil. Steril.*, **63**, 729–33
14. Fauser, B. C. J. M., Donderwinkel, P. and Schoot, D. C. (1993). The step-down principle in gonadotrophin treatment and the role of GnRH analogues. *Baillieres Clin. Obstet. Gynaecol.*, **7**, 309–30
15. Wada, I., Macnamee, M. and Brinsden, P. (1993). Prevention and treatment of ovarian hyperstimulation (letter). *Hum. Reprod.*, **8**, 2245–7
16. Emperaire, J.-C. and Ruffie, A. (1991). Triggering ovulation with endogenous luteinizing hormone may prevent the ovarian hyperstimulation syndrome. *Fertil. Steril.*, **65**, 506–10
17. Imoedemhe, D. A. G., Chan, R. C. W., Sigue, A. B., Pacpaco, E. L. A. and Olazo, A. B. (1991). A new approach to the management of patients at risk of ovarian hyperstimulation in an *in-vitro* fertilization programme. *Hum. Reprod.*, **6**, 1088–91
18. van der Meer, S., Gerris, J., Joostens, M. and Tas, B. (1993). Triggering of ovulation using a gonadotrophin-releasing hormone agonist does not prevent ovarian hyperstimulation syndrome. *Hum. Reprod.*, **8**, 1628–31
19. Shalev, E., Geslevich, Y. and Ben-Ami, M. (1994). Induction of pre-ovulatory luteinizing hormone surge by gonadotrophin-releasing hormone agonist for women at risk for developing the ovar-

ian hyperstimulation syndrome. *Hum. Reprod.*, **9**, 417–19

20. Amit, A., Yaron, Y., Yovel, I., Peyser, M. R., David, M. P., Botchan, A. and Lessing, J. B. (1993). Repeated aspiration of ovarian follicles and early corpus luteum cysts in an *in-vitro* fertilization programme reduces the risk of ovarian hyperstimulation syndrome in high responders. *Hum. Reprod.*, **8**, 1184–6

21. Nisker, J., Tummon, I., Daniel, S., Kaplan, B. and Yuzpe, A. (1994). Conversion of cycles involving ovarian hyperstimulation with intra-uterine insemination to *in-vitro* fertilization. *Hum. Reprod.*, **9**, 406–8

22. Belaisch-Allart, J., Belaisch, J., Hazout, A., Testart, J. and Frydman, R. (1988). Selective oocyte retrieval: a new approach to ovarian hyperstimulation. *Fertil. Steril.*, **50**, 654–6

23. Soliman, S., Daya, S., Collins, J. and Hughes, E. G. (1994). The role of luteal phase support in infertility treatment: a meta-analysis of randomized trials. *Fertil. Steril.*, **61**, 1068–76

24. Tarlatzis, B. C. and Grimbizis, G. (1993). Assisted reproduction techniques in polycystic ovarian syndrome. *Ann. NY Acad. Sci.*, **687**, 280–7

25. Asch, R. H., Ivery, G., Goldsman, M., Frederick, J. L., Stone, S. C. and Balmaceda, J. P. (1993). The use of intravenous albumin in patients at high risk for severe ovarian hyperstimulation syndrome (Clinical report). *Hum. Reprod.*, **8**, 1015–20

26. Shoham, Z., Weissman, A., Barasch, A., Borenstein, R., Schachter, M. and Insler, V. (1994). Intravenous albumin for the prevention of severe ovarian hyperstimulation syndrome in an *in vitro* fertilization program: a prospective, randomized, placebo-controlled study. *Fertil. Steril.*, **62**, 137–42

Systemic effects of ovarian hyperstimulation syndrome: implications for the rationale of treatment

27

M. Aboulghar

Introduction

Ovarian hyperstimulation syndrome (OHSS) is the most serious complication of ovulation induction by gonadotropins. The incidence of the severe forms of the syndrome varies from 0.6 to 1.8%. Severe forms are characterized by ovarian enlargement, ascites, hydrothorax, electrolyte imbalance, hypovolemia, oliguria and thromboembolism. The syndrome is a potentially life-threatening condition with serious complications including acute renal insufficiency thromboembolism, adult respiratory distress syndrome and liver dysfunction[1].

Risk factors for the development of OHSS include high serum estradiol and multiple immature and intermediate follicles. Patients with polycystic ovarian disease (PCO) are well known to be predisposed for this syndrome.

Human chorionic gonadotropin (hCG) stimulation triggers the development of OHSS. Pregnancy with its endogenous human chorionic gonadotropin production increases the incidence of OHSS, particularly the severe forms.

The main cause of morbidity and mortality related to this syndrome originates from the acute fluid shift out of the intravascular space, which may result in ascites, hydrothorax and even generalized edema, and is associated with a major electrolyte imbalance, reduced renal perfusion and marked hemoconcentration. Although the pathophysiology of this syndrome has not been completely elucidated, the underlying mechanism appears to be an increase in capillary permeability of mesothelial surfaces.

The pathogenesis of fluid shifting phenomena that cause ascites formation is unclear. Using an experimental rabbit model, it was concluded that the fluid escape is a process which occurs mainly in the ovarian veins; however, recently, this original experiment was challenged and it was found that the fluid is derived from a generalized increase in transudation across serosal surfaces[2]. It was found that, in normal ovulatory women, the volume of peritoneal fluid shows a sudden increase after ovulation which lingers through out the luteal phase. The fluid production was not dependent on the patency or the presence of the Fallopian tubes or uterus. Its origin was felt to be ovarian or peritoneal. One likely mechanism for this cyclic peritoneal fluid change may be related to a marked increase in capillary permeability induced by intraovarian new capillary formation[3].

The ovarian prorenin system may play a crucial role in the normal ovarian physiology and thus may be implicated in the pathophysiology of OHSS. A correlation between the plasma renin level and the severity of OHSS has been found. Treatment with inhibitors of angiotensin converting enzymes has been used. To date, there are no adequately controlled studies to prove its efficiency in prevention of OHSS. These drugs have teratogenic effects on experimental animals, in marked symptomatic hypotension and are contraindicated in renal impairment[4].

Histamine has also been proposed as a possible mediator for OHSS. However, treatment with antihistamines did not improve the outcome[4].

Prostaglandins have been suggested as likely candidates in the pathogenesis of OHSS; however, indomethacin at pharmacological doses failed to prevent ascites and ovarian enlargement in rabbits, despite its ability to suppress ovarian prostaglandin formation. Similarly, human trials of indomethacin for the treatment of OHSS have been disappointing[4].

Recently, there have been numerous reports regarding the cytokine-mediated regulation of ovarian function. It is not unreasonable to anticipate a significant role for this ovarian regulator in the pathophysiology of OHSS. Higher levels of interleukin-2 (IL-2) were demonstrated in patients with OHSS. It is known that IL-2 can cause vascular leak syndrome, which resembles OHSS. These observations, together with the established interaction between the immune and reproductive systems, may suggest a pivotal role of IL-2 in the pathogenesis of OHSS[5].

There are no completely curative therapies for the treatment of OHSS. Therefore, the most effective treatment of OHSS is still prevention. However, complete prevention of OHSS does not seem possible with the currently available means.

Methods of prediction and prevention of OHSS are outside the scope of this paper.

Active management of OHSS

Mild OHSS is usually self-limiting and requires no active therapy other than observation and follow-up.

Severe OHSS requires hospitalization and active monitoring. Since it was realized that the main problem is the shift of fluids from the circulation to the third space which results in hypovolemia, hypoproteinemia, hemoconcentration and electrolyte disturbance, the approach to conservative treatment has changed. Restriction of salt, fluids and the use of diuretics is no longer recommended. Instead, the main line of treatment is to correct the circulatory

volume and the electrolyte imbalance, which will improve the renal perfusion and prevent coagulation problems and possible embolic manifestations. On admission, the woman's general condition is assessed by measuring pulse, temperature, blood pressure, hematocrit, electrolytes, plasma proteins, complete blood count, clotting parameters and creatinine clearance. Abdominal ultrasound is used to measure the diameters of the enlarged ovaries and to identify ascites. Chest X-ray is performed routinely to exclude the presence of undiagnosed hydrothorax. Intravenous fluid therapy should be started immediately. A volume ranging between 4 and 5 l is infused every 24 h in the form of 5% dextrose and lactated Ringer's solution, and a fluid chart is prepared for each patient. Patients with marked reduction of plasma are injected with 5–25 g of human albumen.

Aspiration of the ascitic fluid and pleural effusion in severe OHSS

In a prospective randomized clinical trial, the effects of transvaginal aspiration of ascitic fluid under sonographic guidance in patients with severe OHSS were investigated[6]. The average hospital stay and the period with severe symptoms and disturbed electrolyte balance were much shorter in the group in which aspiration of ascitic fluid was performed when compared with the group that underwent conservative treatment. Aspiration of the ascitic fluid was found to be of paramount importance in relieving symptoms, improving the general condition and increasing urinary output. A marked improvement in symptoms was noted after drainage of as little as 900 ml of ascitic fluid.

There were no adverse hemodynamic effects as a result of the aspiration of large volumes of ascitic fluid. Replacement of the plasma proteins is mandatory because of the high protein content of ascitic fluid (47 ± 22 g/l). This is particularly essential as repeated aspiration was required in 30% of patients. The rate of accumulation of ascitic fluid varied significantly. However, re-collection of a large volume of ascitic fluid sufficient to cause discomfort would require, on average, 3–4 days.

We believe that ultrasonic needle-guided transvaginal aspiration is an effective and safe procedure. Injury to the ovary is avoided by puncture under ultrasonic visualization. No anesthesia is required for the procedure. Better drainage of the ascitic fluid is accomplished because the pouch of Douglas is the most dependent area. In our experience, transvaginal aspiration of ascites in severe forms of OHSS is a fast and effective method of treatment. It is performed routinely in our center, in all severe OHSS cases after our first clinical trial[7].

Autotransfusion of aspirated fluid has also been reported. Both the proteins and electrolytes of the patient were reinfused which may be physiologically advantageous for the treatment of OHSS. To reduce the risk of possible contamination, ultra-filtration could be performed before reinfusion of the ascitic fluid[8].

References

1. Rizk, B. and Aboulghar, M. (1991). Modern management of ovarian hyperstimulation syndrome. *Hum. Reprod.*, **6**, 1082–7
2. Yarali, H., Fleige-Zahradka, B. K., Yuen, B. Y. and McComb, P. F. (1993). The ascites in the ovarian hyperstimulation syndrome does not originate from the ovary. *Fertil. Steril.*, **59**, 657–61
3. Donnez, J., Langerock, S. and Thomas, K. (1982). Peritoneal fluid volume and 17-beta estradiol and progesterone concentrations in ovulatory, anovulatory, and postmenopausal women. *Obstet. Gynecol.*, **59**, 687–92
4. Schenker, J. G. (1993). Prevention and treatment of ovarian hyperstimulation. *Hum. Reprod.*, **8**, 653–9
5. Orvieto, R., Voliovitch, I., Fishman, P. and Ben-Rafael, Z. (1995). Interleukine-2 and ovarian hyperstimulation syndrome: a pilot study. *Hum. Reprod.*, **10**, 24–7
6. Aboulghar, M. A., Mansour, R. T., Serour, G. I. and Amin, Y. (1990). Ultrasonically guided vaginal aspiration of ascites in the treatment of ovarian hyperstimulation syndrome. *Fertil. Steril.*, **53**, 933–5
7. Aboulghar, M. A., Mansour, R. T., Serour, G. I., Sattar, M. Y., Amin, Y. M. and Elattar, I. (1993). Management of severe ovarian hyperstimulation syndrome by ascitic fluid aspiration and intensive intravenous fluid therapy. *Obstet. Gynecol.*, **81**, 108–11
8. Aboulghar, M. A., Mansour, R. T., Serour, G. I., Riad, R. and Ramzi, A. M. (1992). Autotransfusion of the ascitic fluid in the treatment of severe ovarian hyperstimulation syndrome. *Fertil. Steril.*, **58**, 1056–9

Outcome and long-term follow-up after ovarian stimulation

28

R. Ron-El

It is now 34 years since the introduction of clomiphene citrate and 33 years since the first treatment cycle using human menopausal gonadotropin (hMG). Although no worldwide registrations exist of children born after ovulation induction, it is speculated that around 500 000 babies have been born after hMG induction of ovulation. However, there are few reports describing the results of long-term follow-up of these children. A careful search for studies dealing with the outcome and long-term follow-up after ovarian stimulation (Medline) revealed ten papers. Four[1-4] of these papers analyzed series of hMG treatments and six[5-10] dealt with clomiphene citrate-induced ovulations.

Outcome and long-term follow-up of hMG treatment

Out of a total of 527 pregnancies, 128 (24%) were multiple gestations – 88 (17%) were twins, 24 (4.5%) triplets, 13 (2%) quadruplets, one (0.2%) quintuplets and two (0.4%) sextuplets. Of the 527 pregnancies, 141 (26.8%) terminated in early and late abortions. Table 1 shows the modes of delivery of 201 pregnancies which were described in the studies[1,2].

The mean gestational age for singleton births was 271 ± 17.9 days, for twins 247 ± 30.3, for triplets 234 ± 19.4 and for quadruplets 206 ± 59.5 days. Perinatal mortality was 21.5%. There was shown a predominance of girls which was more pronounced in singleton births than in twins and triplets. The male : female sex ratio as 0.64 for singleton births and 0.78 for twin births; whereas the normal male : female sex ratio is 1.06.

Table 1 Mode of delivery of 201 pregnancies following human menopausal gonadotropin therapy

| | Pregnancy type | | |
	Singleton n (%)	Twin n (%)	Triplet or more n (%)
Vaginal delivery*	93 (63)	8 (22)	11 (61)
Cesarean section	54 (37)	28 (78)	7 (39)
Total	147	36	18

*Vaginal delivery includes instrumental and breech deliveries

The congenital malformations of babies born after hMG treatment in comparison with the general population are listed in Table 2. The congenital malformation rate in this cumulative series out of three studies was 4.2% – 10 out of 240 live-born infants. In the fourth study, malformations were not detailed. Nine of the ten malformed babies were singletons and the one with cyclopia (nervous system defect) was the only affected twin. Three of the infants with heart diseases had a ventricular septal defect, one had cyanotic heart disease, another had tricuspid valve atresia and the sixth baby's heart disease was not described. The skeletal malformation was a sacrococcygeal teratoma.

Of the 240 children who were followed up to the age of 4–8 years, all except one had a normal physical and psychomotor development. One child, who was one of a set of triplets, suffered from cerebral palsy, strabismus and mental retardation.

Table 2 Major congenital malformations in babies born after using hMG for ovulation induction

	hMG babies n (%)	General population (%)
Congenital heart disease	6 (2.5)	0.5–1.0
Nervous system defect	1 (0.4)	0.3–0.8
Polycystic kidney/agenesis of kidney	1 (0.4)	0.03
Absence of external auricle	1 (0.4)	0.01
Musculoskeletal defect	1 (0.4)	1.0–2.0

Outcome and long-term follow-up of clomiphene citrate treatment

Out of a total of 2518 reported pregnancies, 191 (7.6%) were multiple gestations. Abortion rate was 16.9% and 1.1% were ectopic pregnancies. Prematurity rate was documented as 9.1% and the perinatal mortality rate of the clomiphene citrate-treated deliveries was 5.9%.

The congenital malformation rate diagnosed in the clomiphene citrate infants was similar to the incidence found in the general population. There were 42 babies out of 1898 (2.2%) born with congenital malformations. Since the malformations are not recorded in the largest series it is impossible to report them here in detail. However, one study mentions developmental disorders in 6% of the children and moderate retardation in psychological tests in 25% of the probands. None of the other studies deals with long-term follow-up.

Discussion

The accumulated data from these studies concerning the outcome and long-term follow-up of children born after ovulation induction show the classic findings already known of the complications involved in such treatment – multiple pregnancy, fetal wastage and a high rate of prematurity and perinatal mortality are the consequences. However, data concerning congenital malformations and long-term follow-up of developmental and psychological disorders are minimal when compared with the vast use of these medications for ovulation induction.

References

1. Hack, M., Brish, M., Serr, D. M., Insler, V. and Lunenfeld, B. (1970). Outcome of pregnancy after induced ovulation. Follow-up of pregnancies and children born after gonadotropin therapy. *J. Am. Med. Assoc.*, **5**, 791–7
2. Caspi, E., Ronen, J., Schreyer, P. and Goldberg, M. D. (1976). The outcome of pregnancy after gonadotrophin therapy. *Br. J. Obstet. Gynaecol.*, **83**, 967–73
3. Seki, K., Seki, M. and Kato, K. (1983). Outcome of pregnancy and follow-up of children conceived by ovulation induction. *Asia Oceania J. Obstet. Gynaecol.*, **9**, 59–69
4. Ben-Rafael, Z., Blankstein, J., Sack, J., Lunenfeld, B., Oelsner, G., Serr, D. M. and Mashiach, S. (1983). Menarche and puberty in daughters of amenorrheic women. *J. Am. Med. Assoc.*, **250**, 3202–4
5. Hack, M., Brish, M., Serr, D. M., Insler, V., Salomy, M. and Lunenfeld, B. (1972). Outcome of pregnancy after induced ovulation. Follow-up of pregnancies and children born after clomiphene therapy. *J. Am. Med. Assoc.*, **10**, 1329–33
6. Gorlitsky, G. A., Kase, N. G. and Speroff, L. (1978). Ovulation and pregnancy rates with clomiphene citrate. *Obstet. Gynecol.*, **51**, 266–9
7. Von Kineses, L., Veres, I., Farkasinszky, T., Wagner, A., Somogyi, I., Szilard, J. and Sas, M. (1981). Nachuntersuchung von kindern aus

induzierten schwangerschaften. *Zentralbl. Gynakol.*, **103**, 502–14

8. Adashi, E., Rock, J. A., Sapp, K. C., Martin, E. J., Wentz, A. and Jones, G. S. (1979). Gestational outcome of clomiphene-related conceptions. *Fertil. Steril.*, **31**, 620–6

9. Macgregor, A. H., Johnson, J. E. and Bunde, C. A. (1968). Further clinical experience with clomiphene citrate. *Fertil. Steril.*, **19**, 616–22

10. Thompson, C. R. and Hansen, L. M. (1970). Pergonal menotropins: a summary of clinical experience in the induction of ovulation and pregnancy. *Fertil. Steril.*, **21**, 844–53

The potential relevance of growth factors to ovarian physiology

29

E. Y. Adashi

The process of ovarian follicular development is a long and arduous one, marked by dramatic proliferation and differentiation of both the somatic and the germ cell elements. To a large extent, this explosive agenda is under the control of conventional endocrine principles, such as pituitary gonadotropins and ovarian steroids. It has become increasingly apparent, however, that several phenomena central to ovarian physiology are not fully accounted for by conventional endocrine principles. As an example, consideration must be given to the process of follicular selection whereby a predetermined number of follicles is recruited, selected, allowed to assert dominance and ultimately ovulate, despite the fact that all follicles are afforded comparable gonadotropic stimulation. These observations have given rise to the suggestion that the regulation of ovarian function may be under the control of yet another group of modulatory principles known under the general term 'putative intraovarian regulators'. It is generally envisioned that the exquisitely timed and highly regionalized expression of these locally derived often peptidergic principles may finally account for those aspects of the ovarian life cycle which at this time defy conventional explanation.

It has been hypothesized that the role of insulin-like growth factor-I (IGF-I) in the context of ovarian physiology is to serve as an amplifier of gonadotropin hormonal action[1]. At this time, significant support for this hypothesis can be documented. More speculative is the notion that IGF-I may take part in intrafollicular inter-compartmental co-ordination, a concept presupposing enhanced follicular development, due to granulosa–theca–interstitial cell cross-talk and improved coupling. It is entirely in the speculative realm that IGF-I may in fact take part in the process of follicular selection – a notion for which relatively limited support can be derived at this time.

General overview of IGF-I

The gene encoding IGF-I does not code for the mature 70 amino acid polypeptide. Rather, a precursor (prepro) form of IGF-I is translated, requiring additional post-translational processing to yield the mature product. Specifically, post-translational modification would be required to clip off the amino terminal signal peptide (pre-domain) as well as the carboxy terminal E peptide, the function of which remains unknown. All told, the IGF-I gene is estimated to span more than 80 kb, incorporating a total of six exons and five introns. Of the six known exons, only two (exons 3 and 4) engage in relatively straightforward coding for the open reading frame. In contrast, exons 5 and 6 engage in alternative RNA processing, yielding two distinct 3' transcripts known as IGF-IE$_a$ and IGF-IE$_b$, respectively. These in turn give rise to two distinct IGF-I proteins, differing both in terms of the size and sequence of the E domain. Similarly, alternatively spliced exons 1 and 2 may give rise to two distinct transcripts, the resultant proteins differing both in the size and sequence of the signal peptide. Current views suggest that the exon 2-coded protein constitutes the endocrine form of IGF-I, the expression of which may be liver-specific and growth hormone-dependent. In contrast, the exon 1-coded version of IGF-I may constitute the autocrine/paracrine form of IGF-I, the expression of which is ubiquitous and growth hormone-independent. Interestingly, it is this latter form of IGF-I that may give rise to the truncated version of the protein (des 1–3) IGF-I, the biological potency of which is substantially enhanced, due to a marked diminution in affinity for circulating binding proteins.

The ovary as a site of IGF-I production

A growing body of information now supports the view that the rat ovary is indeed a *bona fide* site of IGF-I gene expression[2–4]. In one report[5], use was made of total RNA subjected to a liquid hybridization/RNase protection assay using a ^{32}P-labelled riboprobe transcribed from a cDNA designed to highlight exon 1 and exon 2 transcripts. Although both the ovary and the liver are documented as sites of IGF-I gene expression, there is little doubt that the liver is much more active in this regard. Cellular localization studies have clearly established the granulosa cell as the major ovarian cell type concerned with IGF-I gene expression. In contrast, theca–interstitial cells are virtually negative in this regard. These conclusions were confirmed by Oliver and colleagues[6], whose *in situ* hybridization studies clearly localized IGF-I to the membrana granulosa, very little of the signal emanating from the interfollicular theca–interstitial compartment. Note must also be made of the fact that healthy growing follicles proved IGF-I-replete, whereas atretic, poorly growing follicles proved IGF-I-deplete. These observations are viewed as compatible with the notion that IGF-I may play a positive role in the context of follicular development. Immunofluorescent localization has also established the granulosa as the major producer of the IGF-I protein[7].

The ovary as a site of IGF-I reception

Studies by several groups have now clearly established the rat ovary as a site of IGF-I reception[8–12]. Indeed, conventional radioligand receptor assays have documented the presence of specific type I IGF receptors on both granulosa and theca–interstitial cells. Importantly, the binding characteristics of ovarian type I IGF receptors conform to those observed in other tissues so studied. Of greater interest are studies concerned with the regulation of ovarian type I IGF receptors. In particular, special efforts where directed in answering the question of whether or not the granulosa cell complement of type I IGF receptors is on follicle stimulating hormone (FSH). Given the established ability of FSH to induce heterologous receptor systems at the level of the granulosa cell, it is not inconceivable that the acquisition of type I IGF receptors by the cell type may be FSH-dependent. Indeed, both *in vitro* and *in vivo* observations have clearly documented the ability of FSH to effect dose-dependent increments in granulosa cell IGF-I binding. This increase in specific binding was shown to be due to enhanced IGF-I binding capacity rather than to affinity, as attested by the apparent parallelism of the two Scatchard plots[10]. The ability of FSH to induce ovarian type I IGF receptors was further confirmed at the molecular level when the recently cloned cDNA for the rat type I IGF receptor was used. Indeed, treatment of hypophysectomized immature rats with FSH resulted in a substantial increase in the steady state levels of type I IGF receptor transcripts. The systemic provision of diethylstilbestrol proved equally upregulatory. Unlike the ligand, the distribution of which is limited to the granulosa cell, the type I IGF receptor can be found on both granulosa and theca–interstitial cells.

All told, the ovarian type I IGF receptor appears to be expressed in both granulosa and theca–interstitial cells and appears to be dependent of gonadotropin as well as estrogen at the level of the granulosa cell.

The ovary as a site of IGF-I action

A large number of observations have clearly established the rat ovary as a site of IGF-I action[2–4,13–18]. At the level of the murine granulosa cell, IGF-I has been shown to modulate a number of functions either by itself or in concert with pituitary gonadotropins. For the most part, however, IGF-I acted at the level of the granulosa cell to amplify gonadotropin hormonal action. In this respect, the body of information currently available supports the view that intraovarian IGF-I may in fact play a role as an amplifier of gonadotropin hormonal action. Similar statements can be made with respect to the theca–interstitial cell.

Specifically, IGF-I has been shown to promote FSH-supported progestin biosynthesis, estrogen production, induction of the luteinizing hormone (LH) receptor and inhibin biosynthesis. Interestingly, IGF-I has also been shown to promote both the basal and FSH-supported production of proteoglycans by cultured granulosa cells. This observation is particularly intriguing in light of the fact that the very discovery of the somatomedins reflected their so-called 'sulfation factor' activity, i.e. the promotion of incorporation of labelled [^{35}S]sulfate into cartilaginous proteoglycans.

Ovarian IGF binding proteins

IGF binding proteins (IGFBP) constitute a heterogeneous group of at least six distinct proteins capable of binding IGFs (but not insulin), with affinites of 10^{-10}–10^{-9} mol/l. The six known rat IGF binding proteins range in size from 21.5 to 29.6 kDa, as predicted from the non-glycosylated mature protein. It is assumed, although by no means proven, that the IGF binding proteins subserve different functions, thereby justifying the existence of multiple species. Although the exact role of the IGF binding proteins remains a matter of study, general consensus supports a role in the transport of IGFs and in the regulation of their bioavailability.

Mapping studies carried out at the level of the rat ovary combined multiple approaches, including molecular probing, immunoprecipitation and deglycosylation. As a result of these efforts, it would appear that the granulosa cell is a site of IGFBP-4, IGFBP-5 and to some extent IGFBP-6 gene expression. In contrast, the theca–interstitial cell appears to be a site of

IGFBP-2 and IGFBP-3 (possibly IGFBP-4 and IGFBP-6) gene expression. Preliminary regulatory studies at the level of the rat granulosa cell revealed a striking ability of FSH substantially to inhibit the release of otherwise constitutively elaborated IGF binding proteins. These observations are particularly noteworthy for the fact that FSH by its very designation is a follicle stimulating hormone rarely engaged in the inhibition of granulosa cell function. Re-evaluation, however, may suggest that this apparent inhibition may in effect constitute a net stimulatory gain, provided one accepts the hypothesis that granulosa cell-derived IGF binding proteins are inhibitory to IGF hormonal action, the removal of which may well be in the best interest of the granulosa cell. Specifically, diminishing the IGF binding capacity of granulosa cells may enhance the bioavailability of IGFs and hence their potency. Studies are currently under way to evaluate this hypothesis.

Particularly noteworthy are observations made by several groups with respect to the antigonadotropic activity of IGF binding proteins. All told, these findings suggest highly specific antigonadotropic potential, which appears to be dependent on an intact IGF (but not FSH) binding site. These observations suggest that IGF binding proteins may be acting as antigonadotropins, by sequestering endogenously derived IGFs. It is suggested that optimal FSH hormonal action is contingent upon the bioavailability of granulosa cell-derived IGFs and the consequent amplification of the gonadotropic signal. According to this view, intrinsic FSH hormonal action is relatively limited. In contrast, augmented FSH hormonal action, *in vivo* or *in vitro*, consists of a modest intrinsic component complemented by a substantial portion contributed by synergistic interactions between FSH and IGFs. According to this view, FSH requires co-operation from tissue-based regulatory factors to realize its full potential. Preliminary findings suggest that similar statements can be made with respect to LH. Conceivably, this principle may prove generally applicable and perhaps of consequence to the action of other tropic principles, the optimal action of which may depend on interaction with tissue-based modulatory factors.

Summary

A large body of information now supports the existence of an intraovarian IGF system replete with ligands[19,20], receptors and binding proteins. The intraovarian IGF system is most probably concerned with the amplification of gonadotropin hormonal action, other potential regulatory roles remaining speculative at this time. There is every reason to believe that work in this area in the upcoming several years will yield new insight necessary to establish whether or not IGFs are truly indispensable to ovarian function. At this time, this ultimate requirement remains to be demonstrated through selective ablation of ovarian IGF-I gene expression and the examination of the impact of such manipulation on reproductive potential.

Acknowledgement

This study was supported in part by NIH Research Grant HD-19998.

References

1. Adashi, E. Y., Resnick, C. E., D'Ercole, J., Svoboda, M. E. and Van Wyk, J. J. (1985). Insulin-like growth factors as intraovarian regulators of granulosa cell growth and function. *Endocr. Rev.*, **6**, 400–20

2. Adashi, E. Y., Resnick, C. E., Brodie, A. M. H., Svoboda, M. E. and Van Wyk, J. J. (1985). Somatomedin-C-mediated potentiation of follicle-stimulating hormone-induced aromatase activity of cultured rat granulosa cell. *Endocrinology*, **117**, 2313–20

3. Adashi, E. Y., Resnick, C. E., Svoboda, M. E. and Van Wyk, J. J. (1985). Somatomedin-C synergizes with follicle stimulating hormone in the acquisition of progesterone biosynthetic capacity by cultured rat granulosa cells. *Endocrinology*, **116**, 2135–42

4. Adashi, E. Y., Resnick, C. E., Brodie, A. M. H., Svoboda, M. E. and Van Wyk, J. J. (1985). Somatomedin-C enhances induction of luteinizing hormone receptors by follicle-stimulating hormone in cultured rat granulosa cells. *Endocrinology*, **116**, 2369–75

5. Murphy, L. J., Bell, G. I. and Friesen, H. G. (1987). Tissue distribution of insulin-like growth factor I and II messenger ribonucleic acid in the adult rat. *Endocrinology*, **120**, 1279–82

6. Oliver, J. E., Aitman, T. J., Powell, J. F., Wilson, C. A. and Clayton, R. N. (1989). Insulin-like growth factor I gene expression in the rat ovary is confined to the granulosa cells of developing follicles. *Endocrinology*, **124**, 2671–9

7. Hansson, H. A., Nilsson, A., Isgaard, J., Billig, H., Isaksson, O., Skottner, A., Andersson, I. K. and Rozell, B. (1988). Immunohistochemical localization of insulin-like growth factor I in the adult rat. *Histochemistry*, **89**, 403–10

8. Adashi, E. Y., Resnick, C. E., Svoboda, M. E. and Van Wyk, J. J. (1986). Follicle-stimulating hormone enhances somatomedin-C binding to cultured rat granulosa cells: evidence for cAMP-dependence. *J. Biol. Chem.*, **261**, 3923–6

9. Adashi, E. Y., Resnick, C. E., Hernandez, E. R., Svoboda, M. E. and Van Wyk, J. J. (1988). Characterization and regulation of a specific cell membrane receptor for somatomedin-C/insulin-like growth factor I in cultured rat granulosa cells. *Endocrinology*, **122**, 194–201

10. Adashi, E. Y., Resnick, C. E., Svoboda, M. E. and Van Wyk, J. J. (1988). *In vivo* regulation of granulosa cells somatomedin-C/insulin-like growth factor-I receptors. *Endocrinology*, **122**, 1383–9

11. Adashi, E. Y., Resnick, C. E. and Rosenfeld, R. D. (1990). Insulin-like growth factor-I (IGF-1) and IGF-II hormonal action in cultured rat granulosa cells: mediation via I but not II IGF receptors. *Endocrinology*, **126**, 216–22

12. Davoren, J. B., Kasson, B. G., Li, C. H. and Hsueh, A. J. W. (1986). Specific insulin-like growth factor (IGF) I- and II-binding sites on rat granulosa cells: relation to IGF action. *Endocrinology*, **119**, 2155–62

13. Adashi, E. Y., Resnick, C. E., Svoboda, M. E., Van Wyk, J. J., Hascall, V. C. and Yanagishita, M. (1986). Independent and synergistic actions of somatomedin-C in the stimulation of proteoglycan biosynthesis by cultured rat granulosa cells. *Endocrinology*, **118**, 456–8

14. Bicsak, T. A., Tucker, E. M., Cappel, S., Vaughan, J., Rivier, J., Vale, W. and Hsueh, A. J. W. (1986). Hormonal regulation of granulosa cell inhibin biosynthesis. *Endocrinology*, **119**, 2711–19

15. Cara, J. F. and Rosenfeld, R. (1988). Insulin-like growth factor I and insulin potentiate luteinizing hormone-induced androgen synthesis by rat ovarian thecal–interstitial cells. *Endocrinology*, **123**, 733–9

16. Davoren, J. B., Hsueh, A. J. W. and Li, C. H. (1985). Somatomedin C augments FSH-induced differentiation of cultured rat granulosa cells. *Am. J. Physiol.*, **249**, E26–33

17. Magoffin, D. A., Kurtz, K. M. and Erickson, G. F. (1990). Insulin-like growth factor-I selectively stimulates cholesterol side-chain cleavage expression in ovarian theca–interstitial cells. *Mol. Endocrinol.*, **4**, 489–96

18. Zhiwen, Z., Carson, R. S., Herington, A. C., Lee, V. W. K. and Burger, H. G. (1987). Follicle-stimulating hormone and somatomedin-C stimulate inhibin production by rat granulosa cells *in vitro*. *Endocrinology*, **120**, 1633–8

19. Carlsson, B., Carlsson, L. and Billig, H. (1989). Estrus cycle-dependent co-variation of insulin-like growth factor-I (IGF-I) messenger ribonucleic acid and protein in the rat ovary. *Mol. Cell. Endocrinol.*, **64**, 271–5

20. Hernandez, E. R., Roberts, C. H., LeRoith, D. and Adashi, E. Y. (1989). Rat ovarian insulin-like growth factor I (IGF-I) gene expression is granulosa cell-selective: 5'UT mRNA variant representation and hormonal regulation. *Endocrinology*, **125**, 572–4

The potential relevance of insulin-like growth factors and their binding proteins to endometrial physiology

30

M. Seppälä

Introduction

Endometrium undergoes cyclical processes of cell proliferation, differentiation and shedding in response to endocrine stimuli mediated by local autocrine and paracrine mechanisms in which growth factors and cytokines are involved. In this communication, a review is presented of the actions of insulin-like growth factors (IGFs) and their binding proteins as examples of paracrine factors that play a role in endometrial function and endometrial–trophoblast interactions.

The insulin-like growth factor (IGF) system

The IGF system includes IGF-I and IGF-II, their receptors and soluble insulin-like growth factor binding proteins (IGFBPs). IGF-I and IGF-II are peptides which have effects on cell proliferation, growth, differentiation, and metabolism[1]. Most tissues synthesize IGF-I and IGF-II at some phase of pre- and postnatal development. Postnatally, liver is considered to be the major site of IGF-I production. IGF-I production is upregulated by growth hormone (GH) and it mediates the growth-promoting effects of GH in many tissues. In endocrine glands, IGF production is regulated by trophic hormones, and there is feedback from IGF-I to GH[2]. IGF-II is believed to play a key role in fetal development[3]. In rat uterus, estrogen stimulates both IGF-I and IGF-II as well as type I IGF receptor mRNA expression indicating that the proliferative action of estrogen is mediated by the IGFs[4]. In

Table 1 The insulin-like growth factor (IGF) system in the early and late proliferative and secretory phases of human endometrium (abundance of mRNA). Adapted from references 5, 6, 7, 19, 21 and 22

	Proliferative phase		Secretory phase	
	Early	Late	Early	Late
IGF-I mRNA[5]	++	+++	+	+
IGF-II mRNA[5]	++	+	+	+++
Type I IGF receptor[21]	+	+	+	+++
Type II IGF receptor[21]	+	+	+	+++
IGFBP-1[19]	–	–	+	+++
IGFBP-2[6,7]	+	+	++	+++
IGFBP-3[6,7]	+	+	++	++
IGFBP-4[21]	+	+	+	+
IGFBP-5[21]	+	+	+	+
IGFBP-6[22]	++	+	+	++

–, negative; +, ++, +++ = relative abundances of mRNA; IGFBP, insulin-like growth factor binding protein

human endometrium, IGF-I mRNA is abundant in the late proliferative phase and IGF-II mRNA in the early proliferative and secretory phases[5–7] (Table 1). IGF-I and IGF-II mRNAs have been identified in human embryos suggesting that the IGF system plays a role in early embryonic development[8]. Circulating IGFs may also act in an endocrine fashion.

Insulin-like growth factor receptors

Biological effects of the IGFs are mediated through specific receptors on the cell membrane in most tissues including the endometrium[9]. Type I IGF receptor binds IGF-I and IGF-II with high affinity[10]. There are IGF-I and IGF-II receptors in the human placenta[11]. After binding of the ligand, the IGF-I receptor undergoes autophosphorylation, followed by phosphorylation of endogenous substrates within the cell. The same process mediates IGF-I-stimulated glucose uptake, glycogen synthesis and DNA synthesis[10].

Insulin-like growth factor binding proteins

The IGFs are bound to specific binding proteins in serum and extracellular fluids. There are six IGFBPs which differ in structure from each other, and also their tissue distribution, regulation and function are different[12]. Like the IGFs, the IGFBPs are produced by many tissues and cell types.

IGFBP-1

This is the major IGFBP in human endometrium. IGFBP-1 binds IGF-I with an affinity similar to that of the type I IGF receptor[13]. IGFBP-1 is not detectable in proliferative endometrium and it only appears in late secretory phase endometrium[14,15]. Progesterone stimulates IGFBP-1 release from non-pregnant endometrium[16]. IGFBP-1 is abundant in endometrial tissue in women bearing a levonorgestrel-releasing intrauterine contraceptive device[17]. A 1.6-kb IGFBP-1 mRNA is expressed in secretory phase endometrium and decidua in pregnancy, but not in proliferative endometrium[18]. Using *in situ* hybridization histochemistry, Julkunen and colleagues[19] found IGFBP-1 mRNA in predecidualized stromal cells in late secretory phase endometrium and decidual cells. The timing and cellular localization of IGFBP-1 in human endometrium suggest that the protein is functionally related to decidual differentiation of the stroma. Medroxyprogesterone acetate stimulates IGFBP-1 secretion in cultured endometrial stromal cells, and relaxin potentiates this effect[20].

IGFBP-1 as a paracrine marker in epithelial–stromal cell interactions An important paracrine role of endometrial IGFBP-1 is supported by various observations: (1) abundance of IGFBP-1 mRNA compared to other IGFBP mRNAs, (2) a cyclical change in expression of mRNA and protein, (3) tissue-specific regulation by progesterone and relaxin, (4) gene expression in stromal cells which, after implantation, surround the embryo that contains IGF-receptors but does not express IGFBP-1 mRNA, and (5) inhibition of receptor binding of IGF-I by IGFBP-1[9].

Endometrial IGF-I mRNA is stimulated by estrogen and IGFBP-1 is stimulated by progesterone, therefore, the IGF system is likely to be one of the mechanisms through which the biological actions of estrogen and progesterone are mediated. Stromal IGFBP-1 may have an effect on epithelial cells because endometrial epithelium adjacent to decidualized stromal cells (in which IGFBP-1 is abundant) is atrophic during pregnancy and sustained progestogen treatment. The finding that levonorgestrel-releasing intrauterine contraceptive devices induce a strong local decidual reaction with strong IGFBP-1 staining and atrophy in the adjacent epithelium provides indirect evidence that stromal IGFBP-1 may be related to epithelial atrophy[17].

The relative dominance of IGFs over IGFBPs may play a role in uterine neoplasias[21]. Thus, overexpression of the IGFs, or an increase in IGF receptors, or a decrease of IGFBP-1 and possibly of other IGFBPs may lead to enhanced IGF action and contribute to growth stimulation in endometrium. In cystic glandular hyperplasia there is no detectable IGFBP-1 in endometrium. Endometrial carcinoma often develops under conditions in which IGFBP-1 is either reduced or absent[22]. Adenomyosis is characterized by invasion of epithelial and stromal endometrial cells into the myometrium. Again, no IGFBP-1 is found in the invading adenomyotic foci, not even during progestogen treatment which brings about predecidual reaction in the stroma[21].

Role of IGFBP-1 in implantation and early pregnancy In transformed trophoblastic cells (JEG-3), decidual IGFBP-1 prevents receptor binding and biological action of IGF-1[23]. This has also been found in placental membranes suggesting that IGFBP-1 inhibits IGF actions on these sites[24]. Frost and Tseng have shown that IGFBP-1 produced by decidualized endometrial stromal cells is phosphorylated, and the time-course of IGFBP-1 phosphorylation coincides with the growth arrest and decidual differentiation of endometrial stromal cells[25]. Clemmons and co-workers reported that phosphorylated isoforms of IGFBP-1 have higher affinity for IGF-I than does nonphosphorylated IGFBP-1[26], supporting the concept the IGFBP-1 in decidualized endometrial stromal cells has a high affinity for IGFs, and inhibits their actions. According to studies by Koistinen and co-workers, the degree of IGFBP-1 phosphorylation increases from early to late gestation[27].

A few days after implantation, the embryo is surrounded by decidualized endometrial stromal cells. Progesterone-induced local changes are considered to be essential for implantation to take place. Progesterone-stimulated IGFBP-1 release from decidualized stroma is obviously one of these mechanisms. The trophoblast possesses IGF receptors and expresses IGF-II mRNA, but not IGFBP-1 mRNA[7,11,23]. The trophoblast has proliferative capacity but, for an unknown reason, any extensive invasion into the uterine wall is inhibited. If the IGFs stimulate trophoblast proliferation, then it can be postulated that IGFBP-1 may control both proliferation of the trophoblast and its invasion into maternal tissue by inhibiting the receptor binding of IGFs[23,24].

IGFBP-2, -3, -4, -5 and -6 in the endometrium

The roles that IGFBP-2 and IGFBP-3 play in the endometrium are not clear. According to Giudice and co-workers, IGFBP-2 and IGFBP-3 mRNAs are detectable also in the proliferative endometrium, where the proteins are localized to endometrial glands, whereas IGFBP-1 appears in predecidualized/decidualized endometrium only[6,7]. In their studies, progesterone stimulated endometrial IGFBP-2 synthesis, and IGFBP-2 and IGFBP-3 were more abundant in secretory compared to proliferative endometrium. Thus, in addition to IGF-I and type I IGF receptor, there are at least three different IGFBP species synthesized by secretory endometrium during the peri-implantation period, indicating that the actions of IGFs on the endometrium are regulated by a number of binding proteins.

Unlike the expression of IGFBP-1 mRNA in late secretory phase endometrium only, mRNAs for IGFBP-2 and IGFBP-3[7], and IGFBP-4, -5 and -6 are present in endometrium throughout the menstrual cycle[22]. IGFBP-2 and IGFBP-3 mRNAs are differentially expressed in secretory and proliferative endometria, and synthesis of either IGFBP-2 or IGFBP-3 is regulated by estrogen and progesterone[7]. Rutanen and co-workers have shown cyclic variation in IGFBP-6 gene expression in normal endometrium[22]. IGFBP-6 mRNA levels were low or undetectable in midcycle and highest in the early proliferative and late secretory phases (see Table 1). The abundance of other IGFBPs in endometrium is lower compared to IGFBP-1[9,17,21]. Despite the apparent hormone dependence of endometrial IGFBP-1, -2 and -3, their circulating levels show no cyclical change during the menstrual cycle[7,28].

Summary

Endometrium contains all components of the IGF system: the two IGFs, their receptors and six binding proteins. In a simplistic model, the action of IGFs is to stimulate mitoses and that of the binding proteins is to regulate the local actions of these growth factors. Much of this regulation is inhibitory but, except for IGFBP-1, our knowledge on the interplay between the different binding proteins, IGFs and their receptors in the various endometrial cell types is still limited.

Acknowledgements

Original studies reviewed in this communication have been supported by grants from the Academy of Finland, the University of Helsinki, the Nordisk Forsknins Komité, and the Finnish Cancer Foundation.

References

1. Daughaday, W. H. and Rotwein, P. (1989). Insulin-like growth factors I and II. Peptide, messenger ribonucleic acid and gene structure, serum and tissue concentrations. *Endocr. Rev.*, **10**, 68–90

2. Holly, J. M. P. and Wass, J. A. H. (1989). Insulin-like growth factors; autocrine, paracrine or endocrine? New perspectives of the somatomedin hypothesis in the light of recent developments. *J. Endocrinol.*, **122**, 611–18

3. D'Ercole, A. J. (1991). The insulin-like growth factors and fetal growth. In Spencer, E. M. (ed.) *Modern Concepts of Insulin-like Growth Factors*, pp. 9–23. (New York: Elsevier)

4. Murphy, L. J. and Ghahary, A. (1990). Uterine insulin-like growth factor-1: regulation of expression and its role in estrogen-induced uterine proliferation. *Endocr. Rev.*, **11**, 443–53

5. Boehm, K. D., Daimon, M., Gorodeski, I. G., Sheean, L. A., Utian, W. H. and Ilan, J. (1990). Expression of the insulin-like and platelet-derived growth factor genes in human uterine tissues. *Mol. Reprod. Dev.*, **27**, 93–101

6. Giudice, L. C., Lamson, G., Rosenfeld, R. G. and Irwin, J. C. (1991). Insulin-like growth factor-II (IGF-II) and IGF binding proteins in human endometrium. *Ann. NY Acad. Sci.*, **626**, 295–307

7. Giudice, L. C., Milkowski, D. A., Lamson, G., Rosenfeld, R. G. and Irwin, J. C. (1991). Insulin-like growth factor binding proteins in human endometrium: steroid-dependent messenger ribonucleic acid expression and protein synthesis. *J. Clin. Endocrinol. Metab.*, **72**, 779–87

8. Bondy, C. A., Werner, H., Roberts, C. R. Jr and LeRoith, D. (1990). Cellular pattern of insulin-like growth factor-I (IGF-I) and type I IGF receptor gene expression in early organogenesis: comparison with IGF-II gene expression. *Mol. Endocrinol.*, **4**, 1386–98

9. Rutanen, E.-M., Pekonen, F. and Mäkinen, T. (1988). Soluble 34K binding protein inhibits the binding of insulin-like growth factor I to its cell receptors in human secretory phase endometrium: evidence for autocrine/paracrine regulation of growth factor action. *J. Clin. Endocrinol. Metab.*, **66**, 173–80

10. Steele-Perkins, G., Turner, J., Edman, J. C., Hari, J., Pierce, S. B., Stober, C., Rutter, W. J. and Roth, R. A. (1988). Expression and characterization of a functional human insulin-like growth factor I receptor. *J. Biol. Chem.*, **263**, 11486–92

11. Marshall, R. N., Underwood, L. E., Voine, S. J., Fousher, D. B. and Van Wyk, J. J. (1974). Characterization of insulin and somatomedin-C receptors in human placental cell membranes. *J. Clin. Endocrinol. Metab.*, **39**, 283–92

12. Shimasaki, S. and Ling, N. (1991). Identification and molecular characterization of insulin-like growth factor binding proteins (IGFBP-1, -2, -3, -4, -5 and -6). *Prog. Growth Factor Res.*, **3**, 243–66

13. Koistinen, R., Huhtala, M.-L., Stenman, U.-H. and Seppälä, M. (1987). Purification of placental protein PP12 from human amniotic fluid and its comparison with PP12 from placenta by immunological, physicochemical and somatomedin-binding properties. *Clin. Chim. Acta*, **164**, 293–303

14. Rutanen, E.-M., Gonzales, E., Said, J. and Braunstein, G. D. (1991). Immunohistochemical localization of the insulin-like growth factor binding protein-1 in female reproductive tissues by monoclonal antibodies. *Endocrinol. Pathol.*, **2**, 132–8

15. Wahlström, T. and Seppälä, M. (1984). Placental protein 12 (PP12) is induced in the endometrium by progesterone. *Fertil. Steril.*, **41**, 781–4

16. Rutanen, E.-M., Koistinen, R., Sjöberg, J., Julkunen, M., Wahlström, T., Bohn, H. and Seppälä, M. (1986). Synthesis of placental protein 12 by human endometrium. *Endocrinology*, **118**, 1067–71

17. Pekonen, F., Nyman, T., Lähteenmäki, P., Haukkamaa, M. and Rutanen, E.-M. (1992). Intrauterine progestin induces continuous insulin-like growth factor-binding protein-1 production in the human endometrium. *J. Clin. Endocrinol. Metab.*, **75**, 660–4

18. Julkunen, M., Koistinen, R., Aalto-Setälä, K., Seppälä, M., Jänne, O. A. and Kontula, K. (1988). Primary structure of human insulin-like growth factor-binding protein/placental protein 12 and

tissue specific expression of its mRNA. *FEBS Lett.*, **236**, 295–302

19. Julkunen, M., Koistinen, R., Suikkari, A.-M., Seppälä, M. and Jänne, O. A. (1990). Identification by hybridization histochemistry of human endometrial cells expressing mRNAs encoding a uterine β-lactoglobulin homologue and an insulin-like growth factor-binding protein-1. *Mol. Endocrinol.*, **4**, 700–7

20. Bell, S. C., Jackson, J. A., Ashmore, J., Zhu, H. H. and Tseng, L. (1991). Regulation of insulin-like growth factor-binding protein-1 synthesis and secretion by progestin and relaxin in long-term cultures of human endometrial stromal cells. *J. Clin. Endocrinol. Metab.*, **72**, 1014–24

21. Rutanen, E.-M., Pekonen, F., Nyman, T. and Wahlström, T. (1993). Insulin-like growth factors and their binding proteins in benign and malignant uterine diseases. *Growth Regul.*, **3**, 72–5

22. Rutanen, E.-M., Nyman, T., Lehtovirta, P., Ämmälä, M. and Pekonen, F. (1994). Suppressed expression of insulin-like growth factor binding protein-1 mRNA in the endometrium: a molecular mechanism associating endometrial cancer with its risk factors. *Int. J. Cancer*, **59**, 307–12

23. Ritvos, O., Ranta, T., Jalkanen, J., Suikkari, A.-M., Voutilainen, R., Bohn, H. and Rutanen, E.-M. (1988). Insulin-like growth factor (IGF) binding protein from human decidua inhibits the binding and biological action of IGF-I in cultured choriocarcinoma cells. *Endocrinology*, **122**, 2150–7

24. Pekonen, F., Suikkari, A.-M., Mäkinen, T. and Rutanen, E.-M. (1988). Different insulin-like growth factor binding species in human placenta and decidua. *J. Clin. Endocrinol. Metab.*, **67**, 1250–7

25. Frost, R. A. and Tseng, L. (1991). Insulin-like growth factor-binding protein-1 is phosphorylated by cultured human endometrial stromal cells and multiple protein kinases *in vitro*. *J. Biol. Chem.*, **266**, 18082–8

26. Clemmons, D. R., Camacho-Hubner, C., Jones, J. I., McCusker, R. H. and Busby, W. H. Jr (1991). Insulin-like growth factor binding proteins: mechanisms of action at the cellular levels. In Spencer, E. M. (ed.) *Modern Concepts of Insulin-like Growth Factors*, pp. 475–86. (New York: Elsevier)

27. Koistinen, R., Angervo, M., Leinonen, P., Hakala, T. and Seppälä, M. (1993). Phosphorylation of insulin-like growth factor-binding protein-1 from different sources. *Growth Regul.*, **3**, 25–7

28. Rutanen, E.-M. (1992). Insulin-like growth factor binding protein-1. *Sem. Reprod. Endocrinol.*, **10**, 154–63

The potential relevance of inhibin and activin to placental physiology

31

F. Petraglia, M. Lombardo, P. Florio, C. Salvestroni, R. Gallo, P. Scida, M. Stomati, G. D'Ambrogio, P. G. Artini, A. Gallinelli, D. De Vita and A. R. Genazzani

Introduction

Inhibin and activin are two glycoproteins that modulate follicle stimulating hormone (FSH) production and secretion by the anterior pituitary gland[1]. Inhibin exists in two heterodimeric forms, inhibin A and inhibin B, each with a common α subunit and a different β subunit (A: αβA; B: αβB). Activin exists in three different forms: activin A, AB and B. They are homodimeric glycoproteins composed of two β inhibin subunits: activin A: βA/βA, activin AB: βA/βB, activin B: βB/βB. Activins play an opposite role to that of inhibin, stimulating FSH release from the anterior pituitary gland.

Inhibin and activin are members of a family of growth factors, the transforming growth factor-β (TGF-β) superfamily; TGF-β is a protein found in various tissues that modulates cellular growth and differentiation and has a sequence homology with inhibin and activin. The superfamily includes Müllerian duct inhibiting substance (MIS) (a gonadal protein that causes regression of the Müllerian duct during male development), the fly decapentaplegic complex (involved in the embryonic dorsal–ventral determination) and erythroid differentiation factor (EDF) (which stimulates erythropoiesis in the Friend Strain of mice)[2,3].

Although inhibin and activin were first isolated from the gonads, an increasing number of studies have demonstrated the production of inhibin and activin in several extragonadal tissues. Inhibin α-subunit mRNA has been found in the placenta, pituitary, adrenal, spleen, kidney, brain and spinal cord[4]. The presence of the inhibin/activin βA subunit has been reported in placenta, bone marrow, spleen, brain and spinal cord. The placenta, pituitary, brain and *Xenopus* and chick embryo express the inhibin/activin βB subunit mRNA[1]. The widespread distribution supports their possible major role as growth factors. This hypothesis is furthermore supported by the evidence that activins modulate embryogenesis in mammals[5,6].

After the isolation of inhibin and activin, another FSH-suppressing hormone, termed follistatin, was isolated from follicular fluid, exerting an inhibitory effect on FSH secretion[7,8]. In contrast to inhibin, follistatin is a single-chain monomeric protein. The follistatin gene is expressed in several tissues including gonads, pituitary, bone marrow, adrenal, kidney and pancreas[9], suggesting that follistatin is implicated in several biological functions. Furthermore, the evidence that follistatin has a role as an activin-binding protein and that developing embryological tissues show an intense expression of follistatin support an involvement of follistatin in the modulation of growth factor activity[10].

This chapter focuses on the placenta and gestational tissues as sources and/or targets of inhibin, activin and follistatin. They are part of the group of placental hypophysiotropic factors, such as gonadotropin releasing hormone (GnRH), corticotropin releasing factor (CRF) and somatostatin, involved in the local control of hormonal secretion[11]. Also reviewed is the possible local action of inhibin, activin and follistatin in the gestational unit (Figure 1).

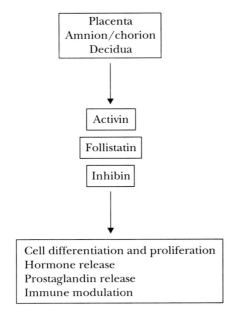

Figure 1 Intrauterine tissues of the human gestational unit produce and are targets of activin, follistatin and inhibin

Sources

Placenta

The human placenta synthesizes inhibin and activin. The trophoblast localization of mRNA or of immunoreactive inhibin α, βA, βB subunits has been achieved using techniques such as *in situ* hybridization and immunofluorescence. A different cellular distribution amongst α, βA, βB inhibin/activin subunits is recognized. The α subunit is mainly localized within the structure of the placental villi (cyto- and intermediate trophoblast, mesenchymal cells), the βB subunit is intensely stained in the outer syncytial layer and the βA subunit is distributed in both layers of placental villi[12–16]. By northern blot analysis it has been shown that α and βA inhibin subunit mRNA is expressed after the first trimester of gestation, with the highest values at term, suggesting that inhibin A and activin A are probably the major products of the human trophoblast[13]. In the rat placenta, βB-subunit mRNA is the most intensely expressed[4]. A co-localization of α and βA inhibin subunits and GnRH mRNAs

and proteins has been demonstrated in placental tissue at term[15], suggesting possible paracrine/autocrine hormonal interactions.

The human placenta also expresses follistatin mRNA, and immunoactive protein is localized in the external syncytial layer of placental villi, the same cells containing immunoreactive activin subunits, human chorionic gonadotropin (hCG) and progesterone. This cellular localization correlates with the possible action of follistatin as an activin A binding protein[17].

The mechanisms regulating inhibin secretion from human placental cells are largely similar to those described for gonadal inhibin. Placental inhibin release is increased by cAMP analogs or substances that act throughout the cAMP pathway, such as insulin, vasoactive intestinal peptide and epidermal growth factor[11,12]. Again, the addition of epidermal growth factor or prostaglandin in cultured placental cells induces inhibin secretion while TGF-β or activin decreases inhibin release[18,19]. Negative results have been shown on activin A release from cultured human placental cells: no effect is exerted by c-AMP, GnRH, dexamethasone, TGF-β or interleukin-1[20].

Decidua and fetal membranes

A growing number of studies have provided evidence that the human decidua produces and is the target organ for polypeptide hormones, suggesting an important endocrine capacity[21]. Decidual cells of zone spongiosa and zona compacta contain and synthesize inhibin and activin subunits. Both immunohistochemical and molecular data show qualitative and quantitative differences in the decidual expression of the three inhibin subunits. Inhibin α and βB mRNA levels were highest at term gestation, supporting the hypothesis that inhibin B or activin B are the preferred proteins produced by decidual cells. However, decidual cells have the ability to produce inhibin A as well as activin A and AB[22]. In particular, an intense staining of immunoactive activin A has been shown in decidual cells at term[20].

Fetal membranes (amnion and chorion) express inhibin/activin subunit mRNAs and contain immunoreactive inhibin/activin material, with some differences between the amnion and chorion[23]. Whereas amnion cells preferentially express the βB subunit, chorion cells show high levels of the α and βA subunits. The different embryological origin of these two membranes (the amnion arising from the mesoderm, and the chorion from a proliferation of the placental trophoblast) may explain the differences in intensity of hybridization to the inhibin/activin subunit probes. The local synthesis and action suggest that amnion-produced activin may act via a paracrine/autocrine mechanism[23].

In vitro effects

Inhibin and activin influence hormone secretion from cultured human placental cells. Activin increases and inhibin decreases the release of GnRH and progesterone and the release of hCG induced by GnRH[12,24,25]. A direct effect of activin on hCG release has also been shown[26]. Therefore, the modulation of hCG release by inhibin or activin is in part mediated by an effect on GnRH release. In addition, the activin-induced GnRH release is steroid hormone-related. Estradiol or estriol increases the GnRH release stimulated by activin and this effect is reversed by tamoxifen, an estrogen antagonist, or by progesterone[25]. The presence of increasing doses of progesterone significantly reduces the effect of activin on GnRH, and the progesterone antagonist RU 486 reverses this inhibitory influence[25]. A functional antagonism between inhibin and activin exists in various tissues. Indeed, the two dimers exert opposite effects on FSH release from the pituitary gland, on androgen production by the gonads, on the induction of hemoglobin synthesis in a human erythroleukemic cell line and on cell proliferation in human bone marrow[1,2]. The evidence that neither dimer influences the secretion of human placental lactogen and that moderate doses of TGF-β do not influence the release of the hormones from cultured placental cells supports the specificity of the actions of inhibin and activin in this system. Specific activin receptors are expressed by trophoblast cells and localized on syncytial cells, mediating the action of endogenous ligands[27,28]. The same receptors in cultured amnion cells explain the effect of activin A in stimulating prostaglandin E_2 (PGE$_2$) release, suggesting prostaglandin metabolism as a target for activin[23]. This effect is consistent with the view that other growth factors, such as epidermal growth factor (EGF)[29] or TGF-α[30] actively stimulate the release of PGE$_2$ from cultured human amnion cells. Considering the role of prostaglandins in human parturition and the relevance of fetal membranes as a source of prostaglandins, the increased production of prostanoids by growth factors suggests a possible role of growth factors in the mechanism of parturition.

Inhibin and activin in biological fluids

Inhibin or its precursor have been measured during pregnancy in maternal serum as well as in cord blood and in amniotic fluid. With the use of one of the inhibin radioimmunoassays, circulating inhibin levels in maternal blood have been found to increase progressively during pregnancy, showing a five-fold increase from 8 weeks and reaching maximal value at 38 weeks[31]. The Monash assay showed an initial peak in the first trimester of pregnancy (around week 10 of gestation); after 10 weeks, it fell and remained relatively low during the second trimester, with a further increase, week by week, in the third trimester[32,33]. The inhibin concentrations decreased to undetectable levels after delivery of the placenta and the disappearance curve was identical to that of estradiol and progesterone[34]. These findings suggest the placenta as the major source of inhibin production. In early pregnancy, a contribution of the corpus luteum, stimulated by luteinizing hormone (LH) or β-hCG, has been suggested as a source for maternal inhibin[33]. Immunoactive and bioactive inhibin has been found also in the umbilical cord and in amniotic fluid. While inhibin levels in umbilical cord blood are the same as those of the maternal circulation, and no

233

changes were observed whether the fetus was male or female, in the amniotic fluid the immunoreactive inhibin levels were significantly greater[33]. The source of immunoreactive inhibin in the amniotic fluid is unclear; it may be secreted by the amniotic membrane or it may be derived from the immunoreactive inhibin in fetal urine released into the amniotic cavity[31]. The evidence of high inhibin levels in pregnant women with a hydatidiform mole suggests the evaluation of plasma inhibin as a marker of trophoblastic tumor. The removal of the mole is followed by a rapid decline of inhibin levels[35].

Recent studies have shown that activin A and activin B are measurable in maternal serum, cord blood serum and amniotic fluid. The observation of different levels in the fluids suggests a different regulation between these hormones. Activin A was present in maternal serum with low levels in early pregnancy, rose 10–15-fold at the highest levels at term[36] and became undetectable within 6 h postpartum. The maternal serum activin B level was less than 100 pg/ml, and it was present in the amniotic fluid in discrete amounts. Lastly, activin B and activin A in the cord blood appear to be induced at delivery $(0.56 \pm 0.01 \text{ ng/ml})$. It is possible that activin A is contributed by the placenta, while activin B is primarily a fetal product.

In spontaneous labor, the maternal serum activin A levels increased during the early phase of labor, reaching the highest values at vaginal delivery[28]. The concentration of this hormone increased two to five-fold during vaginal delivery and at Cesarean delivery after spontaneous labor, whereas there were no changes of activin A levels in patients following elective Cesarean delivery[28].

The gestation-related changes of activin A levels in the maternal circulation correlated with the pattern of activin βA subunit mRNA levels detected in the human trophoblast[13]. Activin βA subunit mRNA levels were low in placental tissue collected during the first and second trimesters, and increased 4–8-fold in placental tissue collected at term[13]. The placenta is the likely source of circulating maternal activin A, but a fetal contribution to the rise found in the

maternal circulation at delivery cannot be excluded. In fact, there is a rapid decline of activin A levels in the postpartum period. Activin A is measurable in fetal cord blood in samples after vaginal or Cesarean delivery[36].

The significance of the activin A at term and at parturition is not clear at the moment. Activin A has been shown to regulate the release of oxytocin and adrenocorticotropic hormone (ACTH), suggesting an involvement of activin in the initiation of milk production and the neuroendocrine events of stress[2]. In addition, the local action of activin on prostaglandins or on endothelin secretion by the placenta suggests that activin may be involved in the mechanism of parturition.

Inhibin and activin in gestational diseases

The measurement of the plasma inhibin level in gestational disease is limited to the observation of high levels in hydatidiform mole, regressing after removal of the tumor[35]. High levels of activin A in maternal serum of women with preterm labor and gestational diabetes have been described[37]. In women with preterm labor, the maternal serum concentration of activin A is higher than in pregnant women at term but not in labor, indicating that parturition is associated with an increase in maternal serum activin A, regardless of gestational age. It has been seen that patients with gestational diabetes have an elevated concentration of serum activin A, which decreases after insulin therapy.

In patients with pregnancy-induced hypertension or chronic hypertension, the plasma activin A levels are lower than in pre-eclamptic patients, suggesting that it is not the hypertensive state that induces the release of activin A, but the placental or fetal changes associated with the disease[38]. The changes of activin A are more relevant in pre-eclamptic patients than in patients with different hypertensive disorders, suggesting the hypothesis that the derangement in the production of placental hormone is related to the entity of the gestational disease. This is strongly supported by the finding of an increase in activin A concentration in patients with chronic hypertension when pre-eclampsia is superimposed[38]. Moreover, the hypersecretion of several placental hormones might be explained by the proliferation of the tropho-blast that is a common finding in pre-eclamptic patients.

The factors that stimulate activin A synthesis and/or secretion in preterm labor and gestational diabetes are not known. Increased placental synthesis and/or release of activin A or a decreased clearance rate of the protein in these pathophysiological conditions are possible.

Supporting the former hypothesis, several reports indicate a hypersecretion of placental hormones in women with preterm labor, gestational diabetes or pre-eclampsia[39].

Acknowledgements

The present study has been in part supported by the Italian National Research Council (CNR), Targeted Project 'Prevention and Control Disease Factors' Subproject 'Maternal–Infant disease' contract 94.00631.PF41.

References

1. Burger, H. G., Findlay, J., Robertson, D., de Kretser, D. and Petraglia, F. (1994). Inhibin and inhibin-related proteins. In *Frontiers in Endocrinology*, Vol. 3. (Ares Serono Symposia)
2. Vale, W., Rivier, C., Hdueh, A., Campen, C., Meunier, H., Bicsak, T., Vaughan, J., Corrigan, A., Bardin, W., Sawchenko, P., Petraglia, F., Yu, J., Plotsky, P., Spiess, J. and Rivier, J. (1988). Chemical and biological characterization of the inhibition family of protein hormones. *Rec. Prog. Horm. Res.*, **44**, 1–34
3. Massague, J. (1988). The TGF-β family of growth and differentiation factors. *Cell*, **49**, 437–8
4. Meunier, H., Rivier, C., Evans, R. M. and Vale, W. (1988). Gonadal and extragonadal expression of inhibin α and β subunits in various tissues diverse functions. *Proc. Natl. Acad. Sci. USA*, **85**, 247–51
5. Thomsen, D. A., Woolf, T., Whitman, M., Sokol, S., Vaughan, J., Vale, W. and Melton, D. A. (1990). Activins are expressed in early *Xenopus* embryogenesis and can induce axial mesoderm and anterior structures. *Cell*, **63**, 485–93
6. Mitrani, E., Ziv, T., Thomsen, G., Shimoni, Y., Melton, D. A. and Bril, A. (1990). Activin can induce the formation of axial structures and is expressed in hypoblast of the chick. *Cell*, **63**, 495–501
7. Ueno, N., Ling, N., Ying, S.-Y., Esch, F., Shimasali, S. and Gullemin, R. (1987). Isolation and partial characterization of follostatin: a single-chain M_r 35.000 monomeric protein that inhibits the release of follicle-stimulating hormone. *Proc. Natl. Acad. Sci. USA*, **84**, 8282–6
8. Robertson, D. M., Klein, R., De Vos, F. L. *et al.* (1987). The isolation of polypeptides with FSH-suppressing activity from bovine follicular fluid which are structurally different to inhibin. *Biochem. Biophys. Res. Commun.*, **149**, 744–9
9. Shimasaki, S., Koga, M., Buscaglia, M. L., Simmons, D. M., Bicsak, T. A. and Ling, N. (1989). Follistatin gene expression in the ovary and extragonadal tissue. *Mol. Endocrinol.*, **3**, 651–9
10. De Paolo, L. V., Bicsak, T. A., Eikson, G. F., Shimasaki, S. and Ling, N. (1991). Follistatin and activin: a potential intrinsic regulatory system within diverse tissues. *Proc. Soc. Exp. Biol. Med.*, **117**, 500–12
11. Petraglia, F., Volpe, A., Genazzani, A. R., Rivier, J., Sawchenko, P. E. and Vale, W. (1990). Neuroendocrinology of the human placenta. *Frontiers Neuroendocrinol.*, **11**, 6–37
12. Petraglia, F., Sawchenko, P. E., Lim, A. T. W., Rivier, J. and Vale, W. (1987). Localisation, secretion and action of inhibin in human placenta. *Science*, **237**, 187–9
13. Petraglia, F., Garuti, G. C., Calzà, L., Roberts, V., Giardino, L., Genazzani, A. R. and Vale, W. (1991). Inhibin subunits in human placenta: localization and messenger ribonucleic acid levels during pregnancy. *Am. J. Obstet. Gynecol.*, **165**, 750–8
14. Merchenthaler, I., Culler, M. D., Petruz, P. and Negro-Vilar, A. (1987). Immunocytochemical localisation of inhibin in rat and human reproductive tissues. *Mol. Cell. Endocrinol.*, **54**, 239–43
15. Petraglia, F., Woodruff, T. K., Botticelli, G., Botticelli, A., Genazzani, A. R., Mayo, K. E. and Vale, W. (1991). Gonadotropin-releasing hormone, inhibin and activin in human placenta: evidence for a common cellular localization. *J. Clin. Endocrinol. Metab.*, **74**, 1184

16. de Kretser, D. M., Foulds, L. M., Hancock, M. and Robertson, D. M. (1994). Partial characterization of inhibin, activin and follistatin in term human placenta. *J. Clin. Endocrinol. Metab.*, **79**, 1–6

17. Petraglia, F., Gallinelli, A., Grande, A., Florio, P., Ferrari, S., Genazzani, A. R., Ling, N. and De Paolo, V. (1994). Local production and action of follistatin in human placenta. *J. Clin. Endocrinol. Metab.*, **79**, 502–7

18. Qu, J. and Thomas, K. (1993). Prostaglandins stimulate the secretion of inhibin from human placental cells. *J. Clin. Endocrinol. Metab.*, **77**, 556–64

19. Qu, J. and Thomas, K. (1993). Regulation of inhibin secretion in human placental cell culture by epidermal growth factor, transforming growth factors and activin. *J. Clin. Endocrinol. Metab.*, **77**, 925–31

20. Rabinovici, J., Goldsmith, P. C., Librach, C. L. and Jaffe, R. B. (1992). Localization and regulation of the activin A-dimer in human placental cells. *J. Clin. Endocrinol. Metab.*, **75**, 571

21. Jaffe, R. B. (1991). Protein hormone of the placenta, decidua and fetal membranes. In Yen, S. S. C. and Jaffe, R B. (eds.) *Reproductive Endocrinology*, pp. 758–69. (Philadelphia: W.B. Saunders)

22. Petraglia, F., Calzà, L., Garuti, G. C., Abrate, M., Giardino, L., Genazzani, A. R., Vale, W. and Meunier, H. (1990). Presence and synthesis of inhibin subunits in human decidua. *J. Clin. Endocrinol. Metab.*, **71**, 487–2

23. Petraglia, F., Anceschi, M. M., Calzà, L., Garuti, G. C., Fusaro, P., Giadino, L., Genazzani, A. R. and Vale, W. (1993). Inhibin and activin in human fetal membranes: evidence for a local effect on prostaglandin. *J. Clin. Endocrinol. Metab.*, **77**, 542–8

24. Petraglia, F., Vaughan, J. and Vale, W. (1989). Inhibin and activin modulate the release of gonadotropin-releasing hormone, human chorionic gonadotropin and progesterone from cultured human placental cells. *Roc. Natl. Acad. Sci. USA*, **86**, 5114–17

25. Petraglia, F., Vaughan, J. and Vale, W. (1990). Steroid hormones modulate the release of immunoreactive gonadotropin-releasing hormone from human placental cells. *J. Clin. Endocrinol. Metab.*, **70**, 1173–8

26. Steele, G. L., Currie, D. W., Youen, B. H. and Jia, X.-C. (1993). Acute stimulation of human chorionic gonadotropin secretion by recombinant human activin-A in first trimester human trophoblast. *Endocrinology*, **133**, 297

27. Peng, C., Huang, T. H. J., Jeung, E.-B., Donaldson, C. J., Vale, W. and Leung, P. C. K. (1993). Expression of the type II activin receptor gene in the human placenta. *Endocrinology*, **133**, 3046–9

28. Petraglia, F., Gallinelli, A., De Vita, D., Lewis, K., Mathews, L. and Vale, W. (1994). Activin at parturition: changes of maternal serum levels and evidence for binding sites in placental and fetal membranes. *Obstet. Gynecol.*, **84**, 278–82

29. Mitchell, M. D. (1987). Epidermal growth factor actions on arachidonic acid metabolism in human amnion cells. *Biochim. Biophys. Acta*, **928**, 240–2

30. Mitchell, M. D. (1987). Transforming growth factor actions on prostaglandins release from human amnion cells. *Prostaglandins Leukotrienes Essent. Fatty Acid*, **33**, 157–8

31. Qu, J., Vankrieken, L., Brulet, C. and Thomas, K. (1991). Circulating bioactive inhibin levels during human pregnancy. *J. Clin. Endocrinol. Metab.*, **72**, 862–6

32. Abe, Y., Hasegawa, Y., Miyamoto, K., Yamaguchi, M. and Igarashi, M. (1990). High concentrations of plasma immunoreactive inhibin during normal pregnancy in women. *J. Clin. Endocrinol. Metab.*, **71**, 133–7

33. Kettel, L. M., Roseff, S. J., Bangah, M. L., Bruger, H. G. and Yen, S. S. C. (1991). Circulating levels of inhibin in pregnant woman at term simultaneous disappearance with oestradiol and progesterone after delivery. *Clin. Endocrinol.*, **34**, 19–23

34. Yohkaichiya, T., Polson, D., O'Connor, A., Bishop, S., Mamers, P., McLachlan, V., Healy, D. L. and de Kretser, D. M. (1991). Concentrations of immunoactive inhibin in serum during human pregnancy: evidence for an ovarian contribution. *Reprod. Fertil. Dev.*, **3**, 671–8

35. Yohkaichiya, T., Fukaya, T., Hoshiai, H., Yajima, A. and de Kretser, D. M. (1989). Inhibin: a new circulating marker for hydatiform mole? *Br. Med. J.*, **298**, 1684–6

36. Petraglia, F., Garg, S., Florio, P., Sadik, M., Gallinelli, A., Wong, W.-L., Krummer, L., Comitini, G., Mather, J. and Woodruff, T. (1993). Activin A and activin B measured in maternal serum, cord blood serum and amniotic fluid during human pregnancy. *Endo. J.*, **1**, 323–7

37. Petraglia, F., De Vita, D., Gallinelli, A., Aguzzoli, L., Genazzani, A. R., Romero, R. and Woodruff, T. K. (1995). Abnormal concentration of maternal serum activin A in gestational diseases. *J. Clin. Endocrinol. Metab.*, **80**, 558–61

38. Petraglia, F., Aguzzoli, L., Gallinelli, A., Florio, P., Zonca, M., Benedetto, C. and Woodruff, T. (1995). Hypertension in pregnancy: changes in activin A maternal serum concentration. *Placenta*, in press

39. Tulchinsky, D. and Little, A. B. (1994). *Maternal-Fetal Endocrinology*, 2nd edn. (Philadelphia: W.B. Saunders)

Contribution of cytokines to apoptosis in the ovary and in endometrium

32

S. Tabibzadeh

Introduction

Apoptosis is a selective process for deletion of cells in various biological systems. In the ovary, apoptosis takes place in atretic follicles and during luteolysis in the corpus luteum. In endometrium, apoptosis occurs primarily in the glandular epithelium during the secretory and menstrual phases. The purpose of this review is to highlight some of the signals and molecular events that are associated with and which may participate in apoptosis in the ovary and in endometrium.

Apoptosis

The term apoptosis is derived from the Greek words *apo* meaning from and *ptosis* signifying a fall, and refers to the dropping of leaves from the trees. This term is applied to a group of characteristic structural and molecular events that distinguish this type of cell deletion from necrosis. In contrast to necrosis, which involves simultaneous deletion of a group of cells, apoptosis may occur in a single cell surrounded by a group of viable cells. There is a distinct and precise localized control over the fate of specific cells in a mixed-cell population that undergo apoptosis. A type of cell death associated with swelling, and resulting from ischemia, was called oncosis (from the Greek *onkos*, meaning swelling) by von Recklinghausen in 1910[1]. Recently, the use of this term as a specific entity has been advocated, particularly in view of its reference to swelling which allows its distinction from the shrinkage necrosis[2].

The morphological features of apoptotic cells are quite characteristic and are distinct from those occurring in the course of necrosis. The morphological changes typical of apoptosis occur in, and in some instances result from, a series of predictable molecular events which may involve transcription of new mRNA species, protein synthesis and DNA degradation. Activation of endonucleases which leads to internucleosomal fragmentation of DNA is the most common feature of apoptosis.

Apoptosis in the ovary

The Greek term *atresia* is derived from *a* meaning not and *treos* meaning perforated, and denotes the closure or obliteration of a body orifice or passage. In its strictest sense, this term is applied to the attrition of the ovarian follicles in the ovary prior to their rupture. However, atresia is more broadly defined as the attrition of the germ cells prior to the formation of follicles as well as to the degenerative changes that occur within the follicles after follicles have formed. This process which is first noted in the fetal human ovary around the 10th week of gestation, peaks between the 14th and 20th week of pregnancy and continues throughout life[3-5]. As much as 80% of germ cells have been lost by birth, and about 95% have undergone atresia by puberty[6]. The majority of the remaining number of germ cells are lost during the reproductive years with merely 400–500 follicles undergoing ovulation during this period[6]. At the time of menopause, virtually no follicles or oocytes are found in the ovary[7]. The earliest degenerative changes involve the primordial germ cells, oogonia and oocytes. Later, when follicles have formed, these changes are also seen at all stages of development of follicles both in the germ cells[8] and granulosa cells[9]. Follicular atresia is associated with degeneration of the granulosa cell layer[10,11], fragmentation of the basal lamina[12], reduced DNA synthesis[11,13], decreased estrogen production[14–17] and decreased gonadotropin binding[14,18] in ovarian follicles.

Apoptosis in the ovary was first noted by Flemming in 1885 who called this process chromatolysis[19]. This idea was reconfirmed by Gondos who, based on morphological grounds, noted that cell death is a major event during follicular atresia[8]. More recently, the identity of this type of cell death as being apoptotic in nature has been confirmed[9,20–22]. This was shown by demonstration of the fragmented DNA in the granulosa and thecal cells of atretic chicken, porcine and rat follicles[9,20,22]. This DNA fragmentation could be found in atretic but not healthy porcine[22] or rat[20] follicles. However, in bovine ovaries, apoptosis was found in the granulosa cells of atretic and some morphologically normal follicles[23]. DNA fragmentation was not found in preovulatory follicles but became apparent 1 day after ovulation in postovulatory avian follicles[21]. In some experimental models, apoptosis has been found primarily in the granulosa cells[24]. However, apoptotic DNA breakdown has been demonstrated in thecal cells from some atretic porcine follicles[22], and pyknotic nuclei have been observed in the thecal cells of sheep[25]. These findings show that apoptosis is an essential feature of follicular atresia.

During preantral follicular growth, granulosa cells replicate without displaying the ability to produce steroid hormones. However, following ovulation, granulosa cells undergo a series of changes that culminate in the formation of the corpus luteum. Following luteinization, for a short interval, luteinized granulosa/thecal cells produce progesterone until a synchronous wave of cell death leads to the regression of the corpus luteum. Luteolysis consists of a functional phase characterized by decreased progesterone production and a structural phase when the luteal cells are destroyed and removed from the corpus luteum[26]. Recently, it has been demonstrated that death of bovine luteal cells during spontaneous and prostaglandin $F_{2\alpha}$-induced luteal regression occurs by apoptosis[26].

Apoptosis in the human endometrium

The presence of basophilic granules, a quarter-to-half of the diameter of endometrial epithelial nuclei, were noted in human endometrium by Bartelmez in 1933[27]. These granules were reported to be characteristically present between the epithelium and the basement membrane. Three years after description of the process of apoptosis[28], Hopwood and Levison correctly identified these granules as the outcome of the apoptosis process[29]. It was noted that the number of apoptotic bodies became significant during the secretory, premenstrual and menstrual phases. That this process is truly apoptotic in nature was confirmed by *in situ* demonstration of fragmented DNA in the involved cells[30]. In addition, quantitation of the number of apoptotic cells confirmed that apoptosis is a menstrual cycle-dependent process. Apoptotic cells are rare in the proliferative phase of the cycle and their number progressively increases in the secretory phase and peaks in the menstrual phase. Therefore, proliferation and apoptosis of endometrial epithelium do not occur simultaneously, rather they appear in the two opposing poles of the menstrual cycle[31]. The majority of the apoptotic cells are present in the epithelial compartments and thus involves the endometrial stroma less extensively[30]. Furthermore, apoptosis occurs at a higher frequency in the basal layer and progressively diminishes towards the surface epithelium[30].

Role of systemic signals in apoptosis in the ovary and endometrium

There are two mechanisms that lead to programmed cell death. First, some biological factors transmit signals that actively induce cell death. Cytokines such as tumor necrosis factor-α (TNF-α), transforming growth factor-β

(TGF-β) and glucocorticoids are among the extracellular mediators implicated in induction of apoptosis[32–38]. Second, in other instances, the withdrawal of a trophic factor leads to cell death. Withdrawal of factors such as insulin-like growth factor-I (IGF-I)[39], epidermal growth factor (EGF)[40], b-fibroblast growth factor (FGF-b)[41], nerve growth factor (NGF)[42], interleukin (IL)-2[43,44], IL-3[44], IL-13[45], colony-stimulating factor-1 (CSF-1)[45] and steroid hormones[46–50] can lead to the apoptotic demise of cells. Within cells, two sets of proteins regulate apoptosis. One class of proteins lead to apoptosis whereas others suppress apoptosis. The intracellular proteins p53 and c-*myc* are among those implicated in apoptosis[51–54]. On the other hand, *bcl*-2 suppresses apoptosis[55–58].

Various lines of evidence suggest that many ovarian and endometrial functions are regulated by cytokines[59]. Cytokines may be appropriately defined as 'a group of factors that are released from cells and exert their functions in an intracrine, autocrine, paracrine, juxtacrine or endocrine fashion'. This functional definition may overlap with that proposed for growth factors and hormones. A characteristic feature of the cytokine family is that many of its members exhibit an overlapping set of effects in the target tissues. The available evidence links several cytokines to the apoptosis that occurs in the ovary and endometrium. This includes the TNF family of molecules, IL-6, EGF, IGF-I, TGF-α, FGF-b, leukemia inhibitory factor (LIF) and stem cell factor.

Tumor necrosis factor-α and tumor necrosis factor-α receptors

Based on sequence homology, a large family of molecules collectively called the NGF/TNF receptor family of apoptosis-inducing signaling proteins has been identified[60]. Over the past 2 years, ligands for most of the known receptors of the NGF/TNF receptor family have been identified[60]. These ligands are all type II transmembrane proteins and show homology to TNF and lymphotoxin and, therefore, belong to the TNF family of molecules.

The proteins that bind TNF-α have molecular weights of 55/60 and 75/80 kDa and are designated as TNF receptor (TNFr)-I and -II, respectively. These proteins are related, and were recently cloned[61–63]. TNF-α induces its biological effects through interaction with both of its receptors. In certain cells, the binding of TNF-α to TNFr-I or TNFr-II transmits signals that lead to apoptosis[64–66].

TNF-α is produced in the ovary[67–68]. Immunoreactive TNF-α was found in human follicular fluid (100–170 pg/ml) and in the culture medium of granulosa cells (800 pg/500 000 cells per 24 h[68]. In addition, the presence of immunoreactive TNF-α was found in the granulosa cells, granulosa–theca cells and small paraluteal cells[68]. The appearance of a greater amount of TNF-α in atretic follicles as compared to that found in the healthy antral follicles suggested that this cytokine may play a role in follicular atresia[68]. Thus far, however, no clear indication has emerged that TNF-α is implicated in atresia or apoptosis within follicles. At present, only indirect evidence exists to support the notion that TNF-α participates in apoptosis in follicular atresia. Elevated production of progesterone and decreased production of estrogen by the ovary are indicators of follicular atresia[18]. The action of TNF-α on follicles simulated the changes that are associated with follicular atresia. This cytokine increased progesterone production and slightly inhibited production of androstenedione in rat preovulatory follicles *in vitro*[69–71]. The action of the TNF-α on steroidogenesis was shown to be exerted on both healthy and atretic rat follicles[68]. Rat theca cells were found to be the target for TNF-α action[68]. Similarly, TNF-α, and to a lesser extent IL-1 and IL-2 (but not IL-6), inhibited basal and human chorionic gonadotropin (hCG)-stimulated release of progesterone and estrogen from porcine luteal cells[72].

More direct evidence links TNF-α to the apoptosis associated with luteolysis. A combination of TNF-α and interferon-γ (IFN-γ) or higher concentrations of each cytokine alone increased apoptosis in mouse luteal cells suggesting that cytokines released by macrophages and T cells within corpus luteum[73-75] may be contributing to the apoptosis of the luteal cells[76]. On the other hand, hCG acts as a luteotropin and suppresses apoptosis. *In vitro* incubation of individually dissected rabbit corpus luteum with hCG was found to inhibit apoptosis in a dose-dependent fashion[77].

T cells and macrophages constitute a major cell population in human endometrium[78-85]. Therefore, one consideration is that TNF-α, a major product of these cells, is expressed in human endometrium. Both *in situ* hybridization and immunoenzymatic labeling have shown the presence of both the mRNA and protein of TNF-α in human endometrium[86,87]. However, besides lymphoid cells, epithelial cells emerge as the major source of TNF-α in human endometrium[86,87]. Both immunohistochemical staining and Western blot analysis have failed to reveal a menstrual cycle-dependent change in the amount of TNFr-I and TNFr-II in human endometrial epithelium[88].

Northern blot analysis has demonstrated that the amount of mRNA for TNF-α is low to undetectable in the proliferative phase. The amount of TNF-α mRNA progressively increases in human endometrium during the secretory phase[89]. Consistent with this is the finding that the amount of TNF-α elaborated from human endometria is low during the proliferative phase. However, this amount progressively increases in the secretory phase and peaks during the menstrual phase[88]. The amount of TNF-α in menstrual discharge of ten individual patients was found to be significantly higher than that detected in the sera of the same patients[30]. These findings have ruled out the possibility that the TNF-α released by endometria was potentially derived from serum. In an experimental model using an endometrial epithelium cell line derived from endometrial carcinoma, TNF-α induced, in a dose- and time-dependent fashion, both the morphological features of apoptosis as well as internucleosomal DNA fragmentation[30]. Further studies have showed that TNF-α also induces apoptosis in endometrial epithelial cells derived from endometrial glands[30]. These findings suggest that TNF-α may

be implicated in the apoptosis which occurs in endometrium. Furthermore, they suggest that changes in the amount of ligand rather than receptor are responsible for the menstrual cycle-dependent changes in apoptosis in endometrial epithelium.

An important question arises as to whether the gradual rise in the amount of endometrial TNF-α during the secretory and menstrual phases is regulated by steroid hormones. The available data validate the notion that steroid hormones regulate TNF-α gene expression and/or release. In human peripheral blood mononuclear cells, estradiol down-regulated both TNF-α mRNA expression[90] and release of TNF-α[91]. The amount of spontaneously released IL-1 and TNF-α and that released after phytohemagglutinin stimulation from mononuclear cells rose 2 weeks after oophorectomy in 15 healthy premenopausal women[92]. In the absence of estrogen therapy, the highest levels of cytokines released from these cells was reached at 8 weeks postoperatively. However, 2 weeks of estrogen therapy in these women resulted in decreased levels of cytokines released from mononuclear cells[92]. 17β-Estradiol and progesterone at all concentrations ranging from 10^{-12} mol/l (2.7×10^{-4} ng/ml) to 10^{-6} mol/l (2.7×10^2 ng/ml) reduced the TNF-α released *in vitro* from the unstimulated peripheral blood mononuclear cells of postmenopausal women[91]. In contrast, 17β-estradiol did not alter the amount of TNF-α released by the mononuclear cells of men or premenopausal women[91].

The steroid regulation of TNF-α gene expression has also been examined in mouse endometrium[93,94]. In normal mice, the TNF-α mRNA was low to undetectable during proestrus, estrus and diestrus-I. However, the mRNA was detectable both in epithelial and stromal cells during diestrus-II[94]. The TNF-α protein was detectable in the epithelial cells throughout the estrous cycle, and detectable in the stromal cells only during diestrus-I[94]. Seven days after ovariectomy there was a loss of TNF-α mRNA and protein expression in endometrial cells[94]. Administration of 17β-estradiol, progesterone or 17β-estradiol plus progesterone resulted in the reappearance of the TNF-α mRNA and protein in epithelial and stromal cells of the mouse endometrium[94,95]. The TNF-α mRNA expression in the mouse endometrium after administration of 17β-estradiol was triphasic. The mRNA of TNF-α was detectable 1 and 6 h after treatment in the epithelial cells. The mRNA expression became undetectable after 24 h and reappeared 72 h later both in the epithelium and stroma[94]. In contrast, administration of progesterone alone or with 17β-estradiol resulted in an extended period of TNF-α mRNA expression[94]. The pattern of protein immunoreactivity and bioactivity in the endometrium of steroid-treated ovariectomized mice generally followed the pattern of mRNA expression[94,95]. These findings clearly show that the TNF-α mRNA and protein expression and release are subject to regulation by the steroid hormones. The inference from the available data is that production of TNF-α in human endometrium may also be regulated by the steroid hormones. However, the question remains as to how this regulation takes place in human endometrium. In humans, the rise in the amount of TNF-α production in endometrium coincides with the late secretory and menstrual phases when systemic levels of steroid hormones are falling. Therefore, it can be speculated that the TNF-α mRNA and protein expression may not only be regulated by steroid hormones but by their withdrawal as well.

As mentioned previously, 17β-estradiol withdrawal was associated with the development of apoptosis in hamster uterine epithelium[60], 17β-estradiol-sensitive human mammary cancer grown in ovariectomized nude mouse[73], granulosa cells in the rat ovary[67], and a transplantable estrogen-dependent kidney tumor. Administration of RU486 which antagonizes the action of progesterone also resulted in apoptosis in endometrium[38,76]. Consequently, the significant increase in apoptosis during the late-secretory and menstrual phases and other specific events that characterize the menstrual phase may all be attributed to the withdrawal of steroid hormones, and presumably local up-regulation of TNF-α production by endometrium. Induction of apoptosis by TNF-α in endometrial epithelial

cells *in vitro*[30] and induction of apoptosis and hemorrhage in mouse uterus by administration of a combination of TNF-α and IFN-γ[95] are consistent with this suggestion. Clearly, other studies are required to show the regulatory roles of steroid hormones on TNF-α production and release. Further studies are also needed to establish the role of TNF-α in regulation of apoptosis and in induction of manifestations of menstruation in human endometrium.

APO-1/Fas ligand and the APO-1/Fas receptor

Sequence homology has identified APO-1/Fas as a member of the NGF/TNF receptor family of molecules[96,97]. APO-1/Fas is a type I transmembrane receptor. The intracellular domain of the molecule bears homology with the so-called 'death domain' of the p55/60 of the TNF-α receptor (TNF receptor I) which is thought to be important in transmitting the apoptosis signal[34,98]. A 40-kDa ligand (FasL) for Fas protein, which has been recently identified and cloned, belongs to the tumor necrosis family of molecules[99]. Although the prime function of APO-1/Fas may be to act as a signaling surface receptor for induction of apoptosis, the protein may also be involved in proliferative events[100].

Recently, the expression of Fas protein was detected in murine oocytes and hyperstimulated eggs[101]. Induction of atresia in follicles by injection of mare's serum gonadotropin (PMSG) induced a substantial decline in the Fas mRNA and not in ribosomal RNA on day 3. Concomitant with these changes, from day 3 to 5, a two- to four-fold increase in the amount of fragmented DNA was detected. Based on the findings, it was suggested that Fas molecule may be implicated in the internucleosomal DNA fragmentation in the ovary[101].

From the various cellular constituents within endometrium, endometrial epithelial cells have emerged as the cells with prominent immunoreactivity for Fas antigen[88]. Fas antigen immunoreactivity is intense in the endometrial glands within the basal layer with immunoreactivity being progressively lost toward the surface epithelium. In the proliferative phase, cells within the stroma exhibit a weak immunoreactivity for Fas protein. However, Fas protein is expressed in stromal cells, particularly those exhibiting pre-decidualization. In the late secretory endometria, virtually all cells in the upper functional layer exhibit Fas protein. Cells within lymphoid aggregates, which primarily reside within the basal layer as well as the endothelial cells of larger vessels within basal and functional layers, also exhibit Fas protein. Whether Fas ligand participates in the induction of apoptosis in human endometrium and whether its production is regulated in a menstrual cycle-dependent fashion, similar to that of TNF-α, remains to be determined.

Other cytokines

Aside from TNF-α, it has been suggested that TGF-β1 is involved in inducing apoptosis in endometrial epithelial cells[102]. Biological activity for IL-6 has been demonstrated in the follicular fluid of patients undergoing *in vitro* fertilization[103]. The mRNA of IL-6 has been detected in the follicular aspirates and granulosa-enriched preparations derived from the same patient population[103]. Furthermore, *in situ* hybridization signals and positive immunoreactivity for IL-6 were found in the granulosa cell cultures[103]. These findings show that IL-6 produced by the granulosa cells may play a regulatory role in preovulatory follicles. One function ascribed to IL-6 is its involvement with apoptosis. Granulosa cells derived from the ovaries of PMSG-treated immature female rats and maintained *in vitro* underwent apoptosis[104]. This type of apoptosis could be suppressed by FSH[104]. On the other hand, IL-6 opposed the action of FSH and stimulated the development of apoptosis in a dose-dependent fashion[104].

Using granulosa cells derived from preovulatory follicles of PMSG-treated rats, it was demonstrated the EGF, TGF-α or FGF-b will inhibit the spontaneous onset of apoptotic DNA fragmentation. IGF-I, insulin, TGF-β or TNF-α has no effect on this event[105]. Treatment with IGF-I, FSH and hCG prevents the spontaneous onset of apoptosis in rat preovulatory follicles maintained *in vitro*[65]. Treatment with hCG increases the IGF-I mRNA levels in cultured follicles. As mentioned earlier, treatment with IGFBP-3 abolishes the suppressive effect of hCG on DNA fragmentation of the follicles suggesting that IGF-I may act as a survival factor for the ovarian follicular cells[65]. Early in vertebrate development, primordial germ cells migrate from the hindgut to the genital ridges. Following active mitotic proliferation, these cells ultimately differentiate into gametes. When maintained in culture, the primordial germ cells isolated from mouse embryos die by apoptosis[106]. Both stem cell factor and LIF markedly reduce the occurrence of apoptosis in these cells suggesting that these cytokines may be implicated in the earliest phases of atresia in the ovary[106].

Perspective

Apoptosis is indispensable to follicular atresia and luteolysis and occurs in endometrium primarily during the secretory and menstrual phases. The available evidence suggests that the actions of two main groups of signals account for the exquisite control over the process of apoptosis in the ovary and endometrium. The first group consists of signals which are systemic in nature and derived from the hypothalamic–pituitary–ovarian axis. The second group of signals consists of cytokines which locally regulate apoptosis within the ovary and endometrium. A host of cytokines are being recognized for their involvement in apoptosis in the ovary and endometrium. Since steroid hormones are among the systemic signals that regulate apoptosis, it is imperative to understand how they control the cytokine network within the ovary and endometrium. Furthermore, the function of several key molecules, such as p53, c-*myc*, *bcl*-2 that intracellularly regulate apoptosis, need to be examined in the ovary and endometrium.

Acknowledgement

This work is supported by Public Health Research Grant CA46866.

References

1. von Recklinghausen, F. (1910). *Untersuchungen über Rachitis und Osteomalacie*. (Jena Verlag Gustav Fischer)
2. Majno, G. and Joris, I. (1995). Apoptosis, oncosis, and necrosis. An overview of cell death. *Am. J. Pathol.*, **146**, 3–15
3. Hurwitz, A. and Adashi, E. Y. (1992). Ovarian follicular atresia as an apoptotic process; a paradigm for programmed cell death in endocrine tissues. *Mol. Cell. Endocrinol.*, **84**, C19–C23
4. Baker, T. G. (1963). A quantitative and cytological study of germ cells in human ovaries. *Proc. R. Soc., Lond. (Biol.)*, **158**, 417–33
5. Gondos, B., Bhiraleus, P. and Hobel, C. J. (1971). Ultrastructural observations on germ cells in human fetal ovaries. *Am. J. Obstet. Gynecol.*, **110**, 644–52
6. Himelstein-Braw, R., Byskov, A. G., Peters, H. and Faber, M. (1976). Follicular atresia in the infant human ovary. *J. Reprod. Fertil.*, **46**, 55–9
7. Hsueh, A. J. W., Billig, H. and Tsafriri, A. (1994). Ovarian follicle atresia: a hormonally controlled apoptotic process. *Endocr. Rev.*, **15**, 707–24
8. Gondos, B. (1974). Cell degeneration. Light and electron microscopic study of ovarian germ cells. *Acta Cytol.*, **18**, 504–9
9. Hughes, F. M. Jr and Gorospe, W. C. (1991). Biochemical identification of apoptosis. (programmed cell death) in granulosa cells: evidence for a potential mechanism underlying follicular atresia. *Endocrinology*, **129**, 2415–22
10. Hay, M. F., Cran, D. G. and Moor, R. M. (1976). Structural changes occurring during atresia in sheep ovarian follicles. *Cell Tissue Res.*, **169**, 515–29
11. Hirshfield, A. N. and Midgley, A. R. Jr (1978). The role of FSH in the selection of large ovarian follicles in the rat. *Biol. Reprod.*, **19**, 606–11
12. Bagavandoss, P., Midgley, A. R. Jr and Wich, M. (1983). Developmental changes in the ovarian follicular basal lamina detected by immunofluorescence and electron microscopy. *J. Histochem. Cytochem.*, **31**, 633–40
13. Greenwald, G. S. (1989). Temporal and topographic changes in DNA synthesis after induced follicular atresia. *Biol. Reprod.*, **41**, 175–81
14. Uilenbroek, J. T., Woutersen, P. J. and van der Schoot, P. (1980). Atresia of preovulatory follicles: gonadotropin binding and steroidogenic activity. *Biol. Reprod.*, **23**, 219–29
15. Terranova, P. F. (1981). Steroidogenesis in experimentally induced atretic follicles of the hamster: a shift from estradiol to progesterone synthesis. *Endocrinology*, **108**, 1885–90
16. Carson, R. S., Findlay, J. K., Clarke, I. J. and Burger, H. G. (1981). Estradiol, testosterone, and androstendione in ovine follicular fluid during growth and atresia of ovarian follicles. *Biol. Reprod.*, **24**, 105–13
17. Maxon, W. S., Haney, A. F. and Schomberg, D. W. (1985). Steroidogenesis in porcine atretic follicles: loss of aromatase activity in isolated granulosa and theca. *Biol. Reprod.*, **33**, 495–501
18. Carson, R. S., Findlay, J. K., Burger, H. G. and Trounson, A. O. (1979). Gonadotropin receptors of the ovine ovarian follicle during follicular growth and atresia. *Biol. Reprod.*, **21**, 75–87
19. Flemming, W. (1885). Über die Buildung von Richtungsfiguren in Säugethiereiern beim Untergang Graaf'scher follikel. *Arch. Anat. EntwGesch.*, 221–44
20. Palumbo, A. and Yeh, J. (1994). *In situ* localization of apoptosis in the rat ovary during follicular atresia. *Biol. Reprod.*, **51**, 888–95
21. Tilly, J. L., Kowalski, K. I., Johnson, A. L. and Hsueh, A. J. W. (1991). Involvement of apoptosis in ovarian follicular atresia and postovulatory regression. *Endocrinology*, **129**, 2799–801
22. Tilly, J. L., Kowalski, K. I., Schomberg, D. W. and Hsueh, A. J. W. (1992). Apoptosis in atretic follicles is associated with selective decreases in messenger ribonucleic acid transcripts for gonadotropin receptors and cytochrome P450 aromatase. *Endocrinology*, **131**, 1670–6
23. Jolly, P. D., Tisdal, D. J., Heath, D. A., Lun, S. and McNatty, K. P. (1994). Apoptosis in bovine granulosa cells in relation to steroid synthesis, cAMP response to FSH and LH and follicular atresia. *Biol. Reprod.*, **51**, 934–44
24. Billig, H., Furuta, I. and Hseuh, A. J. W. (1994). Gonadotropin releasing hormone (GnRH) directly induces apoptotic cell death in the rat ovary. Biochemical and *in situ* detection of DNA fragmentation in granulosa cells. *Endocrinology*, **134**, 245–52
25. O'Shea, J. D., Hay, M. F. and Cran, D. G. (1978). Ultrastructural changes in the theca interna during follicular atresia. *J. Reprod. Fertil.*, **44**, 183–7
26. Jeungel, J. L., Gaverick, H. A., Johnson, A. L., Youngquist, R. S. and Smith, M. F. (1993). Apoptosis during luteal regression in cattle. *Endocrinology*, **132**, 249–54
27. Bartelmez, G. W. (1933). The histological studies of the menstruating mucous membrane of

the human uterus. *Carnegie Institute Contrib. Embryol.*, **24**, 141–86

28. Kerr, J. F. R., Wyllie, A. H. and Currie, A. R. (1972). Apoptosis: a basic biological phenomenon with wide-ranging implications in tissue kinetics. *Br. J. Cancer*, **26**, 239–57

29. Hopwood, D. and Levison, D. A. (1975). Atrophy and apoptosis in the cyclical human endometrium. *J. Pathol.*, **119**, 159–66

30. Tabibzadeh, S., Kong, Q. F., Satyaswaroop, P. G., Zupi, E., Marconi, D., Romanini, C. and Kaput, S. (1994). Distinct regional- and menstrual cycle-dependent distribution of apoptosis in human endometrium. Potential regulatory role of T cells and TNF-α. *Endocrine*, **2**, 87–95

31. Tabibzadeh, S. (1995). Signals and molecular pathways involved in apoptosis with special emphasis on human endometrium. *Hum. Reprod.*, in press

32. Wyllie, A. H. and Morris, R. G. (1982). Hormone-induced cell death. Purification and properties of thymocytes undergoing apoptosis after glucocorticoid treatment. *Am. J. Pathol.*, **109**, 78–87

33. Tartaglia, L. A., Rothe, M., Hu, Y.-F. and Goeddel, D. V. (1993). Tumor necrosis factor's cytotoxic activity is signaled by the p55 TNF receptor. *Cell*, 213–16

34. Tartaglia, L. A., Ayers, T. M., Wong, G. H. W. and Goeddel, D. V. (1993). A novel domain within the 55kd TNF receptor signals cell death. *Cell*, **74**, 845–53

35. Lin, J.-K. and Chou, C.-K. (1992). *In vitro* apoptosis in the human hepatoma cell line induced by transforming growth factor-β1. *Cancer Res.*, **52**, 385–8

36. Oberhammer, F. A., Pavelka, M., Sharma, S., Tiefenbacher, R., Purchio, A. F., Bursch, W. and Schulte-Hermann, R. (1992). Induction of apoptosis in cultured hepatocytes and in regressing liver by transforming growth factor-β1. *Proc. Natl. Acad. Sci. USA*, **89**, 5408–12

37. Yanaghihara, K. and Tsumuraya, M. (1992). Transforming growth factor-β1 induces apoptotic cell death in cultured human gastric carcinoma cells. *Cancer Res.*, **52**, 4042–5

38. Rotello, R. J., Lieberman, R. C., Lepoff, R. B. and Gerschenson, L. E. (1992). Characterization of uterine epithelium apoptotic cell death kinetics and regulation by progesterone and RU486. *Am. J. Pathol.*, **140**, 449–56

39. Barres, B. A., Hart, I. K., Coles, H. S., Burne, J. F., Voyvodic, J. T., Richardson, W. D. and Raff, M. C. (1992). Cell death and control of cell survival in the oligodendrocyte lineage. *Cell*, **70**, 31–46

40. Hassell, J. R. and Pratt, R. M. (1977). Elevated levels of cAMP alters the effect of epidermal growth factor *in vitro* on programmed cell death in the secondary palatal epithelium. *Exp. Cell Res.*, **106**, 55–62

41. Araki, S., Shimada, Y., Kaji, K. and Hayashi, H. (1990). Apoptosis of vascular endothelial cells by fibroblast growth factor deprivation. *Biochem. Biophys. Res. Commun.*, **168**, 1194–200

42. Raff, M. C., Barres, B. A., Burne, J. F., Coles, H. S., Ishizaki, Y. and Jacobson, M. D. (1993). Programmed cell death and the control of cell survival: lessons from the nervous system. *Science*, **262**, 695–700

43. Duke, R. C. and Cohen, J. J. (1986). IL-2 addiction; withdrawal of growth factor activates a suicide program in dependent cells. *Lymphokine Res.*, **5**, 289–99

44. Otani, H., Erdos, M. and Leonard, W. J. (1993). Tyrosine kinase(s) regulate apoptosis and bcl-2 expression in a growth factor-dependent cell line. *J. Biol. Chem.*, **268**, 22733–6

45. Williams, G. T., Smith, C. A., Spooner, E., Dexter, T. M. and Taylor, D. R. (1990). Haemopoietic colony stimulating factors promote cell survival by suppressing apoptosis. *Nature (London)*, **343**, 76–9

46. Wyllie, A. H., Kerr, J. F. R. and Currie, A. R. (1973). Cell death in the normal neonatal rat adrenal cortex. *J. Pathol.*, **111**, 255–61

47. Berges, R. R., Furuya, Y., Remington, L., English, H. F., Jacks, T. and Isaacs, J. T. (1993). Cell proliferation, DNA repair, and p53 function are not required for programmed death of prostatic glandular cells induced by androgen ablation. *Proc. Natl. Acad. Sci. USA*, **90**, 8910–14

48. Martin, L. and Finn, C. A. (1968). Hormonal regulation of cell division in epithelial and connective tissues of the mouse uterus. *J. Endocrinol.*, **41**, 363–71

49. Martin, L., Finn, C. A. and Trinder, G. (1973). Hypertrophy and hyperplasia in the mouse uterus after oestrogen treatment: an autoradiographic study. *J. Endocrinol.*, **56**, 133–44

50. Sandow, B. A., West, N. B., Norman, R. L. and Brenner, R. M. (1979). Hormonal control of apoptosis in hamster uterine luminal epithelium. *Am. J. Anat.*, **156**, 15–36

51. Change, F., Syrjanen, S., Tervahauta, A. and Syrjanen, K. (1993). Tumourigenesis associated with the p53 tumour suppressor gene. *Br. J. Cancer*, **68**, 653–61

52. Askew, D. S., Ashmun, R. A., Simmons, B. C. and Cleveland, J. L. (1991). Constitutive c-myc expression in an IL-3-dependent myeloid cell line suppresses cell cycle arrest and accelerates apoptosis. *Oncogene*, **6**, 1915–22

53. Evan, G. I., Wyllie, A. H., Gilbert, C. S., Littlewood, T. D., Land, H., Brooks, M., Waters, C. M., Penn, L. Z. and Hancock, D. C. (1992). Induction of apoptosis in fibroblasts by c-myc protein. *Cell*, **69**, 119–28

54. Shi, Y., Glynn, J. M., Guilbert, J., Cotter, T. G., Bissonnett, R. P. and Green, D. R. (1992). Role of c-myc in activation-induced apoptotic cell death in T cell hybridomas. *Science*, **257**, 212–14

55. Hockenbery, D., Nunez, G., Milliman, C., Schreiber, R. D. and Korsmeyer, S. J. (1990). bcl-2 is an inner mitochondrial membrane protein that blocks programmed cell death. *Nature (London)*, **348**, 334–6

56. Wang, F., Riley, J. C. M. and Behrman, H. R. (1993). Immunosuppressive levels of glucocorticoid block extrauterine luteolysis in the rat. *Biol. Reprod.*, **49**, 66–73

57. Bissonnette, R. P., Echeverri, F., Mahboudi, A. and Green, D. R. (1992). Apoptotic cell death induced by c-myc is inhibited by bcl-2. *Nature (London)*, **359**, 552–4

58. Fanidi, A., Harrington, E. A. and Evan, G. I. (1992). Cooperative interaction between c-myc and bcl-2 proto-oncogenes. *Nature (London)*, **359**, 554–6

59. Tabibzadeh, S. (1994). Cytokines and hypothalamic–pituitary–ovarian–endometrial axis. *Hum. Reprod.*, **9**, 947–67

60. Beutler, B. and Van Huffel, C. (1994). Unraveling function in the TNF ligand and receptor families. *Science*, **264**, 667–8

61. Kohno, T., Brewer, M. T., Baker, S. L., Schwartz, P. E., King, M. W., Hale, K. K., Squires, C. H., Thompson, R. C. and Vannice, J. L. (1990). A second tumor necrosis factor receptor gene product can shed a naturally occurring tumor necrosis factor inhibitor. *Proc. Natl. Acad. Sci. USA*, **87**, 8331–5

62. Schall, J. S., Lewis, M., Koller, K. J., Lee, A., Rice, G. C., Wong, G. W., Gatanga, T., Granger, G. A., Lentz, R., Raab, H., Kohr, W. J. and Goeddel, D. V. (1990). Molecular cloning and expression of a receptor for human tumor necrosis factor. *Cell*, **61**, 361–70

63. Smith, C. A., Davis, T., Anderson, D., Solam, L., Beckman, M. P., Jerzy, R., Dower, S. K., Cosman, D. and Goodwin, R. G. (1990). A receptor of tumor necrosis factor defines an unusual family of cellular and viral proteins. *Science*, **248**, 1019–23

64. Mangan, D. F. and Wahl, S. M. (1991). Differential regulation of human monocyte programmed cell death (apoptosis) by chemotactic factors and pro-inflammatory cytokines. *J. Immunol.*, **147**, 3408–12

65. Higuchi, M. and Aggarwal, B. B. (1993). p80 form of the human tumor necrosis factor receptor is involved in DNA fragmentation. *Fed. Eur. Biochem. Soc.*, **331**, 252–5

66. Grell, M., Zimmerman, G., Husler, D., Pfizenmaier, K. and Scheurich, P. (1994). TNF receptors TR60 and TR80 can mediate apoptosis via induction of distinct signal pathways. *J. Immunol.*, **153**, 1963–72

67. Roby, K. F. and Terranova, P. F. (1989). Localization of tumor necrosis factor (TNF) in rat and bovine using immunocytochemistry and cell blot: evidence for granulosal production. In Hirshfield, A. N., (ed.) *Growth Factors and the Ovary*, pp. 273–8. (New York: Plenum Press)

68. Roby, K. F. and Terranova, P. F. (1990). Effects of tumor necrosis factor-alpha *in vitro* on steroidogenesis of healthy and atretic follicles of the rat: theca as a target. *Endocrinology*, **126**, 2717–18

69. Roby, K. F. and Terranova, P. F. (1988). Tumor necrosis factor-α alters follicular steroidogenesis *in vitro*. *Endocrinology*, **123**, 2952–4

70. Adashi, E. Y., Resnick, C. E., Jeffrey, B. S., Packman, N., Hurwitz, A. and Payne, D. W. (1990). Cytokine-mediated regulation of ovarian function: tumor necrosis factor-α inhibits gonadotropin-supported progesterone accumulation by differentiating and luteinized murine granulosa cells. *Am. J. Obstet. Gynecol.*, **162**, 889–99

71. Fukuoka, M., Yasuda, K., Fujiwara, H., Kanazaki, H. and Mori, T. (1992). Interactions between interferon-γ, tumor necrosis factor-α, and interleukin-1 in modulating progesterone and oestradiol production by human luteinized granulosa cells in culture. *Hum. Reprod.*, **7**, 1361–4

72. Pitzel, L., Jarry, H. and Wuttke, W. (1993). Effects and interactions of prostaglandin F2α, oxytocin, and cytokines on steroidogenesis of porcine luteal cells. *Endocrinology*, **132**, 751–6

73. Adams, E. C. and Hertig, A. T. (1969). Studies on the human corpus luteum. I. Observation on the ultrastructure of development and regression of the luteal cells during the menstrual cycle. *J. Cell. Biol.*, **41**, 696–715

74. Bulmer, D. (1964). The histochemistry of ovarian macrophages in the rat. *J. Anat.*, **98**, 313–19

75. Brannstrom, M., Pascoe, V., Norman, R. J. and McClure, N. (1994). Localization of leukocyte subsets in the follicle wall and in the corpus luteum throughout the menstrual cycle. *Fertil. Steril.*, **61**, 488–95

76. Jo, T., Tomiyama, T., Ohashi, K., Saji, F., Tanizawa, O., Ozaki, M., Yamamoto, R., Yamamoto, T., Nishizawa, Y. and Terada, N. (1995). Apop-

tosis of cultured mouse luteal cells induced by tumor necrosis factor-α and interferon-γ. *Anat. Rec.*, **241**, 70–6

77. Dharmarajan, A. M., Goodman, S. B., Tilly, K. I. and Tilly, J. L. (1994). Apoptosis during functional corpus luteum regression: evidence of a role for chorionic gonadotropin in promoting luteal cell survival. *Endocr. J.*, **2**, 295–303

78. Kamat, B. and Isaacson, D. M. (1987). The immunocytochemical distribution of leukocytic subpopulations in human endometrium. *Am. J. Pathol.*, **127**, 66–73

79. Marshal, R. J. and Jones, D. B. (1988). An immunohistochemical study of lymphoid tissue in human endometrium. *Int. J. Gynecol. Pathol.*, **7**, 225–35

80. Morris, H., Edwards, J., Tiltman, A. and Malcolm, E. (1985). Endometrial lymphoid tissue. An immunohistological study. *J. Clin. Pathol.*, **38**, 644–52

81. Sen, D. K. and Fox, H. (1967). The lymphoid tissue of the endometrium. *Gynaecologia*, **163**, 371–8

82. Tabibzadeh, S. S. (1990). Proliferative activity of lymphoid cells in human endometrium throughout the menstrual cycle. *J. Clin. Endocrinol. Metab.*, **70**, 437–43

83. Tabibzadeh, S. S. (1990). Evidence of T cell activation and potential cytokine action in human endometrium. *J. Clin. Endocrinol. Metab.*, **71**, 645–9

84. Tabibzadeh, S. and Satyaswaroop, P. G. (1989). Sex steroid receptors in lymphoid cells of human endometrium. *Am. J. Clin. Pathol.*, **91**, 656–63

85. Tabibzadeh, S. S. and Poubouridis, D. (1990). Expression of leukocyte adhesion molecules in human endometrium. *Am. J. Clin. Pathol.*, **93**, 183–9

86. Tabibzadeh, S. (1991). Ubiquitous expression of TNF-α/cachectin in human endometrium. *Am. J. Reprod. Immunol.*, **26**, 1–5

87. Hunt, J. S., Chen, H.-L., Hu, X.-L. and Tabibzadeh, S. (1992). Tumor necrosis factor-α mRNA and protein in human endometrium. *Hum. Reprod.*, **47**, 141–7

88. Tabibzadeh, S., Babaknia, A., Liu, R., Zupi, E., Marconi, D. and Romanini, C. (1995). Site and menstrual cycle-dependent expression of proteins of the TNF receptor family, and bcl-2 oncoprotein and phase specific production of TNF-α in human endometrium. *Hum. Reprod.*, **10**, 277–86

89. Philippaeaux, M.-M. and Piguet, P. F. (1993). Expression of tumor necrosis factor-α and its mRNA in the endometrial mucosa during the menstrual cycle. *Am. J. Pathol.*, **143**, 480–6

90. Loy, R. A., Loukides, J. A. and Polan, M. L. (1992). Ovarian steroids modulate human monocyte tumor necrosis factor alpha messenger ribonucleic acid levels in cultured human peripheral monocytes. *Fertil. Steril.*, **58**, 733–9

91. Ralston, S. H., Russell, R. G. and Gowen, M. (1990). Estrogen inhibits release of tumor necrosis factor from peripheral blood mononuclear cells in postmenopausal women. *J. Bone Min. Res.*, **5**, 983–8

92. Pacifici, R., Brown, C., Puscheck, E., Friedrich, E., Slatopolsky, E., Maggio, D., McCracken, R. and Avioli, L. V. (1991). Effect of surgical menopause and estrogen replacement on cytokine release from human blood mononuclear cells. *Proc. Natl. Acad. Sci. USA*, **88**, 5134–8

93. De, M., Sanford, T. R. and Wood, G. W. (1992). Interleukin-1, interleukin-6, and tumor necrosis factor alpha are produced in the mouse uterus during the estrous cycle and are induced by estrogen and progesterone. *Dev. Biol.*, **151**, 297–305

94. Roby, K. F. and Hunt, J. S. (1994). Mouse endometrial tumor necrosis factor-α messenger ribonucleic acid and protein: localization and regulation by estradiol and progesterone. *Endocrinology*, **135**, 2780–9

95. Shalaby, M. R., Laegried, W. W., Ammann, A. J. and Liggitt, H. D. (1989). Tumor necrosis factor-α associated uterine endothelial injury *in vivo*. Influence of dietary fat. *Lab. Invest.*, **61**, 564–70

96. Oehm, A., Behrmann, I., Falk, W., Pawlita, M., Maier, G., Klas, C., Li-Weber, M., Richards, S., Dhein, J., Trauth, B. C., Postingl, H. and Krammer, P. H. (1992). Purification and molecular cloning of the APO-1 antigen, a new member of the TNF/NGF receptor superfamily: Sequence identity with the Fas antigen. *J. Biol. Chem.*, **267**, 10709–15

97. Itoh, N., Yonehara, A., Ishi, A., Yonehara, M., Mizushima, S.-I., Sameshima, M., Hase, A., Seto, Y. and Nagata, S. (1991). The polypeptide encoded by the cDNA for human cell surface antigen Fas can mediate apoptosis. *Cell*, **66**, 233–43

98. Itoh, N. and Nagata, S. (1993). A novel protein domain required for apoptosis. *J. Biol. Chem.*, **25**, 10932–7

99. Suda, T., Takashashi, T., Golstein, P. and Nagata, S. (1993). Molecular cloning and expression of the Fas ligand, a novel member of the tumor necrosis factor family. *Cell*, **75**, 1169–78

100. Alderson, M. R., Armitage, R. J., Marashovsky, E., Tough, T. W., Roux, E., Schooley, K., Ramsdell, F. and Lynch, D. H. (1993). Fas transduces

activation signals in normal human T-lymphocytes. *J. Exp. Med.*, **178**, 2231–5

101. Guo, M. W., Mori, E., Xu, J. P. and Mori, T. (1994). Identification of Fas antigen associated with apoptotic cell death in murine ovary. *Biochem. Biophys. Res. Commun.*, **203**, 1438–46

102. Rottelo, R. J., Lieberman, R. C., Purchio, A. F. and Gerschenson, L. E. (1991). Coordinated regulation of apoptosis and cell proliferation by transforming growth factor-β1 in cultured uterine epithelial cells. *Proc. Natl. Acad. Sci. USA*, **88**, 3412–15

103. Machelon, V., Emilie, D., Lefevre, A., Nome, F., Durand-Gasselin, I. and Testart, J. (1994). Interleukin-6 biosynthesis in human preovulatory follicles: some of its potential roles at ovulation. *J. Clin. Endocrinol. Metab.*, **79**, 633–42

104. Hughes, F. M. Jr, Fong, Y.-Y. and Gorospe, W. C. (1995). Interleukin-6 stimulates apoptosis in FSH-stimulated rat granulosa cells *in vitro*. Development and utilization of an *in vitro* model. *Endocrinology*, in press

105. Tilly, J. L., Kowalski, K. I., Johnson, A. L. and Hsueh, A. J. W. (1992). Epidermal growth factor and basic fibroblast growth factor suppress the spontaneous onset of apoptosis in cultured rat granulosa cells and follicles by a tyrosine kinase-dependent mechanism. *Mol. Endocrinol.*, **6**, 1942–50

106. Pesce, M., Farrace, M. G., Piacentini, M., Dolci, S. and De Felici, M. (1993). Stem cell factor and leukemia inhibitory factor promote primordial germ cell survival by suppressing programmed cell death (apoptosis). *Development*, **118**, 1089–94

Cytokines and spermatogenesis 33

C. Piquet-Pellorce, E. Gomez, C. Cudicini, J. P. Stephan, N. Dejucq and B. Jégou

Introduction

Spermatogenesis is under the control of both pituitary hormones, luteinizing hormone (LH) and follicle stimulating hormone (FSH), and of a complex communication system between the various somatic cell types and the different generations of germ cells[1,2]. Several types of testicular interactions have been demonstrated: direct cell–cell interactions involving adhesion molecules, specialized junctions or phagocytosis of cellular materials, and indirect interactions via soluble factors. Among the latter, several factors, collectively named cytokines and known to be able to regulate both cellular proliferation and differentiation and to modulate cell function, have been identified within the testis. This review will focus on such factors and summarize the present knowledge concerning cytokines and cytokine receptors which have been found in the testis, as well as their putative roles.

Cytokines are glycoproteins which were originally discovered in the immune system[3]. They have now been localized and seem to be involved in virtually every organ. Alternative terms used for molecules belonging to this family such as interleukins, growth factors, neurotrophic factors, became inappropriate because they reflected only part of their actions. These factors can affect cell proliferation positively or negatively, they can direct cellular differentiation and modulate cell function. Each cytokine interacts with many different cell types and exhibits pleiotropic functions depending on the target cell. Conversely, a single cell often responds to multiple cytokines; the cellular response to different cytokines can be different, as expected, but can also be similar. Indeed, functional redundancy of cytokines is an intriguing feature

which started to be understood with the study of their receptors. High affinity cytokine receptors are generally formed by the association of two or more subunits, one binding the ligand with low affinity, the other transducing the signal. These transducing subunits have been shown to be shared between receptor complexes to various factors[4–6]. Furthermore, most cytokine receptor subunits share structural domains which are very similar in their extracellular portion[7, 8], this is another reason to bring together all their ligands into a unique family.

Testicular cytokines

Over the past few years, a number of cytokines have been identified in the testis, as well as in isolated testicular cell types or secretions[2,9]. Testicular cytokine levels have been monitored using various bio- and immuno-assays, combined with immunocytolocalization, when possible. Occasionally, binding experiments with radiolabelled ligands have been performed to identify and to localize receptors. Cytokine and receptor gene expression have also been investigated by Northern blot analysis and, in some cases, by *in situ* hybridization. Current data on cytokines and their putative roles in the testis are summarized in Table 1. This comprehensive list exhibits, beside each cytokine identified, its sites of production and putative action on the three major testicular cell types: Leydig cells, Sertoli cells and germ cells. In parallel, specific receptor expression on each cell type is indicated. Our laboratory has been more specifically involved in research on interleukin 1 (IL-1), interleukin 6 (IL-6) and interferons.

Table 1 Cytokines, major paracrine regulators of testicular functions

Cytokines	Producing cell types	Potential targets and roles						References
		Leydig cells		Sertoli cells		Germ cells		
		Receptor	Effects	Receptor	Effects	Receptor	Effects	
IL-1	L, S, G	+	↓ steroidogenesis ↑ proliferation	+	↑ IL-6 production	?	↑ DNA synthesis	10–19
IL-6	L, S	?		?	modulate transferrin production	?	↓ DNA synthesis	20–23
TNFα	G		modulate function		modulate function	+	↑ PGC survival	24–26
c-kit ligand	S	+	?				↑ SG proliferation	27–32
Interferons	S, G, P	+	↓ steroidogenesis		↓ function			33–35
TGFα/EGF	L, S, G, P	+	↑ steroidogenesis ↓ other functions	+	↑ proliferation ↑ function	+	mitogen	36–39
TGFβ	L, S, P	+	↓ function	+	↓ function			40–42
IGF-1	L, S, P	+	↑ function	+	↑ function ↑ proliferation	+	↑ SG proliferation	43–46
FGF	L, S, G, P	+	↓ function	+	↑ proliferation ↑ function	?	↑ gonocyte survival	47–50
NGF	G	+	↓ function	+	?			51, 52
PDGF	L, S	+	↓ steroidogenesis	+	?			53–55
Activin	L, S	+		+	pseudo-tubular aggregation	+	↑ SG proliferation	56–58
Inhibin	L, S	+	↑ steroidogenesis	+		+	↓ SG proliferation	59–62

TNFα, tumor necrosis factor α; TGFα/EGF, transforming growth factor α/epidermal growth factor; TGFβ, transforming growth factor β; IGF-I, insulin-like growth factor-I; FGF, fibroblast growth factor; NGF, nerve growth factor; PDGF, platelet-derived growth factor; G, germ cells; L, Leydig cells; S, Sertoli cells; P, peritubular cells; PGC, primordial germ cells; SG, spermatogonia; ↑, stimulation; ↓, inhibition; +, presence; ?, to be determined

Interleukin 1

High levels of IL-1 were observed in both rat and human testis[63, 64]. We have demonstrated that Sertoli cells constitute an important source of IL-1α[11]. Recently, it has been established that rat germ cells also produce IL-1α[16] (and unpublished results from our laboratory). Conversely, according to Lin and colleagues[14], IL-1 produced by Leydig cells is essentially of β type. IL-1 production by Sertoli cells increases with sexual maturation since IL-1 concentration is higher in media conditioned by Sertoli cells from 45-day-old rats than from 35-day-old rats. Immature Sertoli cells from 20-day-old rats do not constitutively produce IL-1 (or only very low levels)[11,64]. As macrophages, the main IL-1 producer within the immune system, Sertoli cells can be stimulated to secrete IL-1 by lipopolysaccharides and by phagocytosis of latex beads. According to Gérard and colleagues[65], a physiological stimulus might be the phagocytosis of residual bodies. The pattern of IL-1 production in the seminiferous tubules argues for a role of this cytokine in the regulation of DNA replication in germ cells. In fact, IL-1 secretion in the rat is undetectable at stage VII of the seminiferous epithelium cycle, but increases to reach a maximum during stages VIII and IX–X[12]. Moreover, in vitro, IL-1α stimulates DNA synthesis in spermatogonia at stage I of the cycle and meiotic DNA synthesis at stage VII and VIII–IX[13]. Altogether, these results suggest that IL-1 could be a mediator involved in the synchronization of the seminiferous tubule cycle; i.e. as spermatozoa are released, residual body phagocytosis would trigger Sertoli cells to produce IL-1, which in turn would stimulate DNA synthesis in preleptotene spermatocytes. More recent investigations using an in vitro two-compartment culture system, indicate that IL-1 is equally and constitutively produced via the apical and basal poles of the Sertoli cell, but when stimulated, these cells specifically direct IL-1 secretion at the pole which has been activated[66]. Identification of IL-1 receptor type I and/or II mRNAs in Sertoli, peritubular and Leydig cells[67] argues for multicellular targets of IL-1 in the testis. Furthermore, IL-1 has been shown to affect Leydig cell proliferation and function in vitro[15,17], and to induce acute inflammation-like changes in the testicular microcirculation[68].

Interleukin 6

IL-1 is a well known inducer of IL-6 production in many cell types such as macrophages, endothelial cells, fibroblasts and keratinocytes[69]. This prompted us to investigate IL-6 production within the rat testis. We found that Sertoli cells, but not germ cells or peritubular cells, secrete IL-6[20]. The production of this cytokine increases with age and is stimulated by phagocytosis, lipopolysaccharides and IL-1. Precise kinetic studies and the use of a specific anti-IL-1α antibody enabled us to demonstrate that phagocytosis-induced IL-6 release by Sertoli cells is in fact mediated by IL-1 production[70]. Moreover, IL-1 induced IL-6 secretion by Sertoli cells is mediated by lipoxygenase activation[70]. Interestingly, the pattern of IL-6 bi-directional secretion by Sertoli cells is completely different from that of IL-1. Constitutive IL-6 production occurs essentially at the apical pole, but can only be stimulated from the basal pole of the cell[66]. IL-6 production varies according to the different stages (I–XIV, c.f.2) of the seminiferous epithelium. High levels of IL-6 have been detected at stages XIII, XIV and I–V, while stages VII–VIII featured low levels of expression. Investigations of IL-6 effects on DNA synthesis in seminiferous tubules have shown a clear inhibition of the onset of meiotic DNA replication[21]. Therefore, in contrast to IL-1, IL-6 appears to be a negative regulator of germ cell DNA replication. These two cytokines, closely regulated during the cycle, are presumably important regulators of spermatogenesis.

Interferons

Another aspect of cytokine involvement in testis, of special interest with regards to the problem of sexually transmissible diseases, is antiviral defence. Our group has recently identified interferons in purified testicular cells[34]. Interferon α protein and corresponding mRNA are produced spontaneously by pachytene spermatocytes and early spermatids *in vitro*. Surprisingly, addition of the Sendai virus increases their production only in early spermatids. Moreover, the presence of the virus in purified testicular cell cultures also induces interferon α expression in peritubular and Sertoli cells. Activated Sertoli cells were shown to be the most potent producers of interferon α. However, only early spermatids were found to produce interferon γ protein and mRNA, whether the different purified testicular cells were cultured in the presence of the virus or not. In addition to their putative role in the defence against viral attacks, it is likely that testicular interferons may also be involved in the paracrine regulation of the spermatogenic process. For instance, *in vitro* studies have already demonstrated that interferons inhibit steroid production by both Leydig and Sertoli cells[33, 35]. Furthermore, their well known antiproliferative effect on numerous cell types[71] is of primary interest with regard to the regulation of spermatogonial proliferation.

Conclusion

A list of cytokines which have been detected within the testis is provided in this paper. However, it is worth noting that some cytokines, still not identified in the testis, have nevertheless already been reported to affect testicular cell function *in vitro*. For instance, IL-2 appears to be able to inhibit testosterone production by Leydig cells[33]. This correlates well with the suppression of plasma testosterone in IL-2-treated patients and the germ cell depletion observed in IL-2-transgenic mice[72]. Another example is the ability of leukemia inhibitory factor to promote survival and growth of primordial germ cells[73], gonocytes as well as Sertoli cells (de Miguel and colleagues, submitted). It is therefore most probable that further investigations will soon reveal the existence of other cytokines in the testis and their involvement in the paracrine regulation of spermatogenesis. Alternatively, they could indicate new endocrine regulatory pathways of testicular function via cytokines secreted elsewhere in the body. Indeed, most organs beside the immune system are able to produce such cytokines, which could act on somatic testicular cells and, therefore, indirectly affect germ cells.

Acknowledgements

We are grateful to Anne-Marie Touzalin for her excellent technical assistance. This project was funded by INSERM, MRES, DRED, Région Bretagne.

References

1. Jegou, B. and Sharpe, R. M. (1993). Paracrine mechanism in testicular control. In de Kretser, D. M. (ed.) *Molecular Biology of the Male Reproductive System*, pp. 271–310. (New York: Academic Press)
2. Jegou, B. (1993). The Sertoli-germ cell communication network in mammals. *Int. Rev. Cytol.*, **147**, 25–96
3. Arai, J., Lee, F., Miyajima, A., Miyatake, S., Arai, N. and Yokoto, T. (1990). Cytokines: coordinators of immune and inflammatory responses. *Ann. Rev. Biochem.*, **59**, 783–836
4. Miyajima, A., Hara, T. and Kitamura, T. (1992). Common subunits of cytokine receptors and the functional redundancy of cytokines. *TIBS*, **17**, 378–82
5. Stahl, N. and Yancopoulos, G. D. (1993). The alphas, betas, and kinases of cytokine receptor complexes. *Cell*, **74**, 587–90
6. Cosman, D. (1993). The hematopoietin receptor superfamily. *Cytokine*, **5**, 95–106
7. Bazan, J. F. (1990). Structural design and molecular evolution of a cytokine receptor superfamily. *Proc. Natl. Acad. Sci. USA*, **87**, 6934–8

8. Bazan, J. F. (1990). Haemopoietic receptors and helical cytokines. *Immunol. Today*, **11**, 350–4

9. Niederberger, C. S., Shubhada, S., Kim, S. J. and Lamb, D. J. (1993). Paracrine factors and the regulation of spermatogenesis. *World J. Urol.*, **11**, 120–8

10. Khan, S. A., Söder, O., Syed, V., Gustafsson, K., Lindh, M. and Ritzén, E. M. (1987). The rat testis produces large amounts of an interleukin-1-like factor. *Int. J. Androl.*, **10**, 494–503

11. Gérard, N., Syed, V., Bardin, C. W., Genetet, N. and Jegou, B. (1991). Sertoli cells are the site of interleukin-1α synthesis in rat testis. *Mol. Cell Endocrinol.*, **82**, R13–R16

12. Söder, O., Syed, V., Callard, G. V., Toppari, J., Pöllänen, P., Parvinen, M., Fröysa, B. and Ritzén, E. M. (1991). Production and secretion of an interleukin-1-like factor is stage-dependant and correlates with spermatogonial DNA synthesis in the rat seminiferous epithelium. *Int. J. Androl.*, **14**, 223–31

13. Parvinen, M., Söder, O., Mali, P., Fröysa, B. and Ritzén, E. M. (1991). In vitro stimulation of stage-specific deoxyribonucleic acid synthesis in rat seminiferous tubule segments by Interleukin-1α. *Endocrinology*, **129**, 1614–20

14. Lin, T., Wang, D. and Nagpal, M. L. (1993). Human chorionic gonadotropin induces interleukin-1 gene expression in rat Leydig cells *in vivo*. *Mol. Cell. Endocrinol.*, **95**, 139–45

15. Khan, S. A., Khan, S. J. and Dorrington, J. H. (1992). Interleukin-1 stimulates deoxyribonucleic acid synthesis in immature rat Leydig cell *in vitro*. *Endocrinology*, **131**, 1853–7

16. Haugen, T. B., Landmark, B. F., Josefsen, G. M., Hansson, V. and Högset, A. (1994). The mature form of interleukin-1α is constitutively expressed in immature male germ cells from rat. *Mol. Cell. Endocrinol.*, **105**, R19–23

17. Calkins, J. H., Sigel, M. M., Nankin, H. R. and Lin, T. (1988). Interleukin-1 inhibits Leydig cell steroidogenesis in primary culture. *Endocrinology*, **123**, 1605–10

18. Takao, T., Mitchell, W. M., Tracey, D. E. and De Souza, E. B. (1990). Identification of Interleukin-1 receptors in mouse testis. *Endocrinology*, **127**, 251–64

19. Cunningham, E. T. Jr, Wada, E., Carter, D. B., Tracey, D. E., Battey, J. F. and De Souza, E. B. (1992). Distribution of type I interleukin-1 receptor messenger RNA in testis: an *in situ* histochemical study in the mouse. *Neuroendocrinology*, **56**, 94–9

20. Syed, V., Gérard, N., Kaipia, A., Bardin, C. W., Parvinen, M. and Jégou, B. (1993). Identification, ontogeny, and regulation of an interleukin-6-like (IL-6) factor in the rat testis. *Endocrinology*, **132**, 293–9

21. Hakovirta, H., Syed, V., Jégou, B. and Parvinen, M. (1995). Function of Interleukin-6 as an inhibitor of meiotic DNA synthesis in rat seminiferous epithelium. *Mol. Cell. Endocrinol.*, **108**, 193–8

22. Boockfor, F. R. and Schwartz, L. K. (1991). Effects of interleukin-6, interleukin-2 and tumor necrosis factor α on transferrin release from Sertoli cells in culture. *Endocrinology*, **129**, 256–62

23. Boockfor, F. R., Wang, D., Lin, T., Nagpal, M. L. and Spangelo, B. L. (1994). Interleukin-6 secretion from rat Leydig cells in culture. *Endocrinology*, **134**, 2150–5

24. De, S. K., Chen, H. L., Pace, J. L., Hunt, J. S., Terranova, P. F. and Enders, G. C. (1993). Expression of Tumor Necrosis Factor-α in mouse spermatogenic cells. *Endocrinology*, **131**, 3091–9

25. Xiong, Y. and Hales, D. B. (1993). The role of tumor necrosis factor-α in the regulation of mouse Leydig cell steroidogenesis. *Endocrinology*, **132**, 2438–44

26. Mauduit, C., Jaspar, J. M., Poncelet, E., Charlet, C., Revol, A., Franchimont, P. and Benahmed, M. (1993). Tumor necrosis factor-α antagonizes follicle-stimulating hormone action in cultured Sertoli cells. *Endocrinology*, **133**, 69–76

27. Tajima, Y., Onoue, H., Kitamura, Y. and Nishimune, Y. (1991). Biologically active kit ligand growth factor is produced by mouse Sertoli cells and is defective in Sl[d] mutant mice. *Development*, **133**, 1031–5

28. Sorrentino, V., Giorgi, M., Geremia, R., Besmer, P. and Rossi, P. (1991). Expression of the c-kit proto-oncogene in the murine male germ cells. *Oncogene*, **6**, 149–51

29. Godin, I., Doed, R., Cooke, J. S., Zsebo, K., Dexter, M. and Wylie, C. C. (1991). Effects of the *steel* gene product on mouse primordial germ cells in culture. *Nature*, **352**, 807–9

30. Rossi, P., Mavrail, G., Albanesi, C., Charlesworth, A., Geremie, R. and Sorrentino, V. (1992). A novel *c-kit* transcript potentially encoding a truncated receptor originates within a Kit gene intron in mouse spermatids. *Dev. Biol.*, **152**, 203–7

31. Yoshinga, K., Nishikawa, S., Ogawa, M. and Hayashi, S. I. (1991). Role of *c-kit* in mouse spermatogenesis: identification of spermatogonia as a specific site of *c-kit* expression and function. *Development*, **113**, 689–99

32. Manova, K., Nocka, K., Besmer, P. and Bachvarova, R. F. (1990). Gonadal expression of *c-kit* encoded at the W locus of the mouse. *Development*, **100**, 1057–69

33. Meikle, A. W., Cardoso-de-Sousa, J. C., Dacosta, N., Bishop, D. K. and Samlowski, W. E. (1992). Direct and indirect effects of murine inter-

leukin-2, gamma interferon and tumor necrosis factor on testosterone synthesis in mouse Leydig cells. *J. Androl.*, **13**, 437–43

34. Dejucq, N., Dugast, I., Ruffault, A., Van der Meide, P. H. and Jégou, B. (1995). Interferon α and γ expression in the rat testis. *Endocrinology*, in press

35. Branca, A. A., Franke, M. A., Sluss, P. M. and Reichert, L. E. Jr (1987). Interferon inhibits FSH-stimulated estradiol production in rat Sertoli cell cultures. *Med. Sci. Res.*, **15**, 739

36. Skinner, M. K., Takacs, K. and Coffey, R. J. (1989). Transforming growth factor-alpha gene expression and action in the seminiferous tubule: peritubular cell-Sertoli cell interactions. *Endocrinology*, **124**, 845–54

37. Avallet, O., Vigier, M., Chatelain, P. G. and Saez, J. M. (1991). Regulation by growth factors of Leydig cell differentiated function. *J. Steroid. Biochem. Mol. Biol.*, **40**, 453–64

38. Radhakrishnan, B., Oke, B. O., Papadopoulos, V., Diaugustine, R. P. and Suarez-Quian, C. A. (1992). Characterization of epidermal growth factor in mouse testis. *Endocrinology*, **131**, 3091–9

39. Tsutsumi, O., Kirachi, H. and Oka, A. (1986). A physiological role of epidermal growth factor in male reproductive function. *Science*, **233**, 975–7

40. Lin, T., Blaisdell, J. and Haskell, J. F. (1987). Transforming growth factor-β inhibits Leydig cell steroidogenesis in primary culture. *Biochem. Biophys. Res. Commun.*, **146**, 387–94

41. Mullaney, B. P. and Skinner, M. K. (1993). Transforming growth factor-β (β1, β2 and β3) gene expression and action during pubertal development of the seminiferous tubule: potential role at the onset of spermatogenesis. *Mol. Endocrinol.*, **7**, 67–76

42. Morera, A. M., Esposito, G., Ghiglieri, C., Chauvin, M. A., Hartman, D. J. and Benahmen, M. (1992). Transforming growth factor-beta-1 inhibits gonadotropin action in cultured porcine Sertoli cells. *Endocrinology*, **130**, 831–6

43. Vanelli, B. G., Natali, A., Barni, T., Serio, M., Orlando, C. and Balboni, G. (1988). Insulin-like growth factor-I (IGF-I) and IGF-I receptor in human testis: an immunohistochemical study. *Fertil. Steril.*, **49**, 666–9

44. Lin, T., Haskell, J. F., Vinson, N. and Terracio, L. (1986). Characterization of insulin and insulin-like growth factor I receptors of purified Leydig cells and their role in steroidogenesis in primary culture: a comparative study. *Endocrinology*, **119**, 1641–7

45. Borland, K., Mita, M., Oppeneimer, C., Blinderman, L. A., Massague, J., Hall, P. F. and Czech, M. P. (1984). The actions of insulin-like growth

factors I and II on cultured Sertoli cells. *Endocrinology*, **114**, 240–6

46. Söder, O., Baqng, P., Wabab, A. and Parvinen, M. (1992). Insulin-like growth factors selectively stimulate spermatogonial, but not meiotic, deoxyribonucleic acid synthesis during rat spermatogenesis. *Endocrinology*, **131**, 2344–50

47. Mullaney, B. P. and Skinner, M. K. (1992). Basic fibroblast growth factor (bFGF) gene expression and protein production during pubertal development of the seminiferous tubule; follicle-stimulating hormone-induced Sertoli cell bFGF expression. *Endocrinology*, **131**, 2928–34

48. Han, I. S., Sylvester, S. R., Kim, K. U., Schelling, M. E., Venkateswaran, S., Blanckaert, N. D., McGuinness, M. P. and Griswold, M. D. (1993). Basic fibroblast growth factor is a testicular cell product which may regulate Sertoli cell function. *Mol. Endocrinol.*, **7**, 889–97

49. Sordoillet, C., Chauvin, M. A., Revol, A., Morera, A. M. and Benhamed, M. (1988). Fibroblast growth factor is a regulator of testosterone secretion in cultured immature Leydig cells. *Mol. Cell. Endocrinol.*, **58**, 283–6

50. Resnick, J. L., Bixler, L. S., Cheng, L. and Donovan, P. J. (1992). Long-term proliferation of mouse primordial germ cells in culture. *Nature*, **359**, 550–1

51. Ayer-LeLièvre, C., Olson, L., Ebendal, T., Hallbrook, F. and Persson, H. (1988). Nerve growth factor mRNA and protein in the testis and epididymis of mouse and rat. *Proc. Natl. Acad. Sci. USA*, **85**, 2628–32

52. Person, H., Ayer-Lelievre, C., Söder, O., Villar, M. J., Metsis, M., Olson, L., Ritzén, M. and Hokfelt, T. (1990). Expression of β-nerve growth factor receptor mRNA in Sertoli cells downregulated by testosterone. *Science*, **247**, 704–7

53. Murono, E. P. and Washburn, A. L. (1990). Platelet derived growth factor inhibits 5α-reductase and D5-3β-hydroxysteroid dehydrogenase activities in cultured immature Leydig cells. *Biochem. Biophys. Res. Commun.*, **169**, 1229–34

54. Gnessi, L., Emidi, A., Farini, D., Scarpa, S., Modesti, A., Ciampani, T., Silvestroni, L. and Spera, G. (1992). Rat Leydig cells bind platelet-derived growth factor through specific receptors and produce platelet-derived growth factor-like molecules. *Endocrinology*, **130**, 2219–24

55. Loveland, K. L., Zlatic, K., Steinoakley, A., Risbridger, G. and de Kretser, D. M. (1995). Platelet-derived growth factor ligand and receptor subunit mRNA in the Sertoli and Leydig cells of the rat testis. *Mol. Cell. Endocrinol.*, **108**, 155–9

56. Grootenhuis, A. J., Steebergen, J., Timmerman, M. A., Dorsman, A. N. R. D., Shaaper, W. M. M.,

Meloen, R. M. and de Jong, F. M. (1989). Activin. *J. Endocrinol.*, **122**, 293–301

57. Woodruff, T. K., Borre, J., Atti, K. M., Cox, E. T., Rice, G. C. and Mather, J. P. (1992). Stage-specific binding of inhibin and activin to sub-populations of rat germ cells. *Endocrinology*, **130**, 871–81

58. de Winter, J. P., Themmen, A. P. N., Hooger-Brugge, J. W., Klaij, I. A., Grootegoed, J. A. and de Jong, F. H. (1992). Activin receptor mRNA present in pachytene spermatocytes and early spermatids (not late spermatids). *Mol. Cell. Endocrinol.*, **83**, R1–R8

59. Le Gac, F. and de Kretser, D. M. (1982). Inhibin production by Sertoli cell cultures. *Mol. Cell. Endocrinol.*, **28**, 487–98

60. van Dissel-Emiliani, F. M. F., Grootenhuis, A. J., de Jong, F. H. and de Rooij, D. G. (1989). Inhibin reduces spermatogonial numbers in testis of adult mice and chinese hamsters. *Endocrinology*, **125**, 1899–1903

61. Lin, T., Calkins, J. K., Morris, P. L., Vale, W. and Bardin, C. W. (1989). Regulation of Leydig cell function in primary culture by inhibin and activin. *Endocrinology*, **125**, 2134–40

62. Risbridger, G. P., Clements, D., Robertson, D. M., Drummond, A. E., Muir, J., Berger, H. G. and de Kretser, D. M. (1989). Immuno- and bioactive inhibin an inhibin alpha-subunit expression in rat Leydig cell cultures. *Mol. Cell. Endocrinol.*, **66**, 119–22

63. Khan, S. A., Schmidt, K., Hallin, P., Di Pauli, R., De Geyter, C. H. and Nieschlag, E. (1988). Human testis cytosol and ovarian follicular fluid contain high amounts of interleukin-1-like factor(s). *Mol. Cell. Endocrinol.*, **58**, 221–30

64. Syed, V., Söder, O., Arver, S., Lindh, M. and Ritzén, E. M. (1988). Ontogeny and cellular origin of an IL-1-like factor in the reproductive tract of male rats. *Int. J. Androl.*, **11**, 437–47

65. Gérard, N., Syed, V. and Jégou, B. (1992). Lipopolysaccharide, latex beads and residual bo-dies are potent activators of Sertoli cell inter-leukin-1α production. *Biochem. Biophys. Res. Commun.*, **185**, 154–61

66. Cudicini, C., Touzalin, A. M., Ballet, F. and Jégou, B. (1994). Sertoli cell vectorial production of IL-1α and IL-6. Miniposter no. 63. Presented at *8th European Workshop on Molecular and Cellular Endocrinology of the Testis*, March, De Panne, Belgium

67. Gomez, E., Lejeune, H., Staerman, F., Lobel, B., Saez, J. and Jégou, B. (1994). Expression of IL receptor mRNAs in rat and human testicular cells. Miniposter no. 53. Presented at *8th European Workshop on Molecular and Cellular Endocrinology of the Testis*, March, De Panne, Belgium

68. Bergh, A. and Söder, O. (1990). Interleukin-1β, but not interleukin-1α, induces acute inflamma-tion-like changes in the testicular microcircula-tion of adult rats. *J. Reprod. Immunol.*, **17**, 155–65

69. Hirano, T., Akira, S., Taga, T. and Kishimoto, T. (1990). Biological and clinical aspects of inter-leukin 6. *Immunol. Today*, **11**, 443–9

70. Syed, V., Stephan, J. P., Gérard, N., Le grand, A., Parvinen, M., Bardin, C. W. and Jégou, B. (1995). Residual bodies activates Sertoli cell IL-1α release which triggers IL-6 production by an autocrine mechanism through the lipoxygenase pathway. *Endocrinology*, **136**, 3070–8

71. Clemens, M. J. and MacNurlan, M. A. (1985). Regulation of cell proliferation and differentia-tion by Interferons. *Biochem. J.*, **226**, 345–60

72. Otha, M., Mitomi, T., Kimura, M., Habu, S. and Katsuki, M. (1990). Anomalies in transgenic mice carrying the human interleukin-2 gene. *Tokai, J. Exp. Clin. Med.*, **15**, 307–15

73. Cheng, L., Gearing, S. P., White, L. S., Compton, D. L., Schooley, K. and Donovan, P. J. (1994). Role of Leukemia Inhibitory Factor and its re-ceptor in mouse primordial germ cell growth. *Development*, **120**, 3145–53

The human sex determination pathway: news and views

34

M. Desclozeaux, S. Soullier, P. Jay, B. Boizet, F. Poulat and Ph. Berta

Introduction

In humans, as in all mammals, sex determination is under the control of a genetic switch mechanism. The chromosomal location of such a switch became evident in the early 1960s by the cytogenetic analysis of patients with abnormal sex chromosome constitution. We all know that a normal female has two X chromosomes and a normal male one X and one Y chromosome. However, in the absence of a Y chromosome, patients with only an X chromosome (Turner's syndrome) will develop as females, and patients carrying multiple X chromosomes in the presence of a Y chromosome will develop as males (Klinefelter's syndrome). So, it was postulated that, in the presence of a dominant switch located on the Y chromosome, human embryos will develop as male, while in its absence they will develop as female.

Sex determination in mammals: first rules

Alfred Jost's[1] pioneering experiments on rabbit embryos demonstrated that the hormonal product of the fetal testis is able to induce male development. Early castration of a male embryo will result in the development of female ducts as well as female external genitalia. Conversely, from the same castration of a female, no phenotype modification will result, implying that the ovaries are not necessary for female differentiation. Masculinization of the testis depends on the production of two distinct hormones by the supporting cells: testosterone produced by the Leydig cells and anti-Müllerian hormone produced by the Sertoli cells. The sex of the third cell type of the testis, the germ cell, is independent of the chromosomal constitution.

To conclude, sexual differentiation is the result of a two-step process sex determination which corresponds to the choice between testis or ovary during embryonic life and sex differentiation which is under the control of the hormones produced by the gonads.

Furthermore, as previously mentioned, the basis of sex determination in humans is chromosomal:

(1) The presence of a Y chromosome: male phenotype,

(2) The absence of a Y chromosome: female phenotype.

In recent decades, this observation has opened a new field of research with the long quest for a putative dominant factor located on the Y chromosome and called TDF (testis determining factor) in humans and TDY (testis determining Y gene) in mice.

Primary localization of TDF on the Y chromosome

From the cytogenetic analysis of sterile patients with deletion of the Y chromosome, it was clear that TDF must be located on the Y short arm (Figure 1). Later, a more precise location came from the study of sex-reversed patients, i.e. 46,XX males. About 1 in 20 000 new-born males have a 46,XX karyotype and yet most of them are the result of an abnormal X–Y cross-over during paternal meiosis, leading to the exchange of sex-specific sequences between the

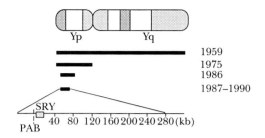

Figure 1 The historical search for the testis determining factor (TDF) during recent decades and the evolution of its localization

two chromosomes[2]. The molecular analysis of the DNA fragments transferred by such a mechanism has permitted the construction of a deletion map of the Y short arm and the location of TDF in this arm, in the sex-specific part adjacent to the pseudo-autosomal boundary[3]. In 1989, the description of four new XX individuals, three XX males and one XX true hemaphrodite, carrying less than 60 kb of Y-specific DNA inherited from their paternal X, defined the minimal portion of the Y chromosome necessary to confer a male phenotype[4].

Cloning of the sex determining region Y chromosome (SRY) gene

The four XX individuals were then shown to carry only 35 kb of Y-derived DNA immediately adjacent to the pseudoautosomal boundary. Out of this 35 kb, only one clone, PY 53.3, was shown to be unique on the Y chromosome and to be evolutionarily conserved to the Y of diverse mammals[5]. The longer open reading frame, termed SRY (sex determining region, Y), encodes a 204 amino acid protein. This SRY gene consists of a small intronless sequence coding for a protein containing a centrally located 'high mobility group' (HMG) domain or HMG box[6]. The HMG box shows sequence conservation with a heterogenous group of nuclear proteins with diverse functions including transcriptional activation. Although HMG box sequences of different SRY cloned in a growing number of mammals appear to be relatively conserved,

there is little similarity between them outside the HMG motif. The superfamily of genes coding for proteins with such a domain is already large[7] and now includes a sub-family of genes with more than 50% identity with the HMG box, a sub-family today termed SOX (SRY-box containing genes)[8]. If, for most of these SOX genes, their function remains unknown, some of them could be involved in different cell determination processes, and one of them, as mentioned later in this review could even contribute to the sex determination pathway.

Evidence equating SRY with testis determining factor

The location of SRY within this minimum sex-determination portion of the Y chromosome known to confer maleness in humans and conservation on the Y chromosome of other entherian and methaterian mammals[5,9] are both consistent with SRY being the TDF. Other evidence came from the mutational analysis of SRY in XY females. Such individuals with a Y chromosome but without testes must have a defect in the sex determination pathway. Thus approximately 15–20% of XY females with pure gonadal dysgenesis have mutations in SRY, the majority being *de novo*[10]. All mutations in the SRY open reading frame have been found in the HMG box motif and probably affect DNA binding ability. So, it is obvious that, for the majority of XY females, sex reversal is the result of mutations in other genes of the sex determination cascade, or could be the result of a delay in the timing of SRY action (default in SRY control or in its putative partners).

If the *de novo* mutations found in some XY sex-reversed females provide proof that SRY is required for sex determination, these results do not give an indication on the number of Y located genes necessary for testis induction. This answer has come from the demonstration that some transgenic XX, Sry⁺ mice have developed a normal male phenotype although the animal was sterile[11]. Curiously, no XX mice transgenic for the human SRY were sex-reversed, suggesting that SRY function is not tightly conserved, which might not be as predicted for such a crucial function.

SRY protein: first biochemical properties

DNA binding

The sequence of the SRY protein suggests that SRY may bind DNA via its HMG box; this has been confirmed[12-14]. Some of the mutations found in SRY, within the HMG domain, were shown to abolish DNA binding. If SRY has sequence-specific DNA binding activity, the linear sequence is not specific enough to permit the identification of potential target genes under the control of SRY. It is worth noting that the DNA binding of SRY also induced DNA bending of approximately 85°[15]. This bending could facilitate protein–protein interactions to allow the assembly of a multiprotein complex, thereby inducing the positive or negative control of downstream genes.

Nuclear localization

The subcellular localization of SRY protein has recently been specified[16]. The nuclear localization signal shared by most of the other members of the HMG box superfamily has been delineated in the molecule using a mutational approach.

Conclusion

The human SRY, when compared to mice Szy, has lost its activation domain[17]. Thus, it appears to be a non-conventional transcription factor since classical bi-functional structure of transcription factors is not observed.

Only hypotheses can be made on the mode of action of the SRY protein:

(1) All the SRY function is restricted to the HMG box, which, when bound on its targets will induce either the local fusion of DNA to allow either the binding of other transcription factors (SRY with a positive regulatory function), to block a transcription

process (SRY with a negative regulatory function), or SRY could use these two ways as a mode of control of downstream genes.

(2) When bound to DNA, SRY could interact with partner protein(s) which could replace the regulator domain lost during evolution.

(3) The binding induced by SRY could facilitate the assembly of a multiprotein complex, which will regulate gene expression.

These three possibilities will need to be evaluated, and will contribute to the identification of the upstream and downstream genes, identification is necessary to reconstruct the whole process of sex determination in humans.

Other TDFs

Upstream

As previously mentioned, SRY must be expressed at the appropriate critical time and in the correct location during embryogenesis. Genes controlling SRY expression and located anywhere in the genome (except on the Y chromosome) still need to be identified.

Downstream

Mutations in such downstream genes could cause XY sex reversal even with a functional SRY protein. If none of the downstream genes have been shown to be controlled directly by SRY, the candidate genes recently discovered are the result of cytogenetic or molecular analysis of sex-reversed patients. The position of these genes in the sex determination cascade still requires elucidation. These genes could be:

(1) Candidate genes, not cloned to date, at chromosome 9p[18], or 10q[19];

(2) WT-1, the Wilms tumor suppressor gene at 11p13. This tumor is found in Denys–Drash syndrome along with XY gonadal dysgenesis. Denys–Drash patients have point mutations in WT1[20];

(3) SOX9 at chromosome 17q25, a recently described gene involved in campomelic dwarfism as well as in sex reversal[21];

(4) SF-1 which encodes an orphan receptor controlling directly the anti-Müllerian hormone gene[22].

(5) A candidate gene located in the DSS ('Dosage Sensitive Sex Reversal') locus at Xp[23]. If DSS is not needed for testis development, two active copies result in ovarian development in XY individuals. One possibility is that DSS is required for ovarian development but must be repressed in order to allow the testes to develop.

Conclusions

Understanding the mechanisms by which gonadal determination and differentiation occur has fundamental importance in biology but also practical implications in clinical medicine. If SRY is clearly equivalent to TDF, it only provides a start point from which to reconstruct the whole process of sex determination and explains only a small proportion of sex-reversed individuals.

Thus, although the isolation of the SRY gene has closed an era of investigation for TDF, new questions now come to the fore, about the mode of SRY action, the possible existence of SRY partners, the nature of the preceding and the subsequent steps in the sex determination cascade.

References

1. Jost, A. (1953). Problems of fetal endocrinology: the gonadal and hypophysial hormones. *Rec. Prog. Horm. Res.*, **8**, 379–418
2. Weissenbach, J., Levilliers, J., Petit, C., Rouyer, F. and Simmler, M. (1987). Normal and abnormal interchanges between the human X and Y chromosomes. *Development*, **101** (Suppl.), 67–74
3. Vergnaud, G., Page, D. C., Simmler, M. C., Brown, L., Rouyer, F., Noel, B., Botstein, D., de la Chapelle, A. and Weissenbach, J. (1986). A deletion map of the human Y chromosome based on DNA hybridization. *Am. J. Hum. Genet.*, **38**, 109–24
4. Palmer, M. S., Sinclair, A. H., Berta, P., Ellis, N. A., Goodfellow, P. N., Abbas, N. E. and Fellous, M. (1989). Genetic evidence that ZFY is not the testis-determining factor. *Nature (London)*, **342**, 937–9
5. Sinclair, A. H., Berta, P., Palmer, M. S., Hawkins, J. R., Griffiths, B. L., Smith, M. J., Foster, J. W., Frischauf, A. M., Lovell-Badge, R. and Goodfellow, P. N. (1990). A gene from the human sex-determining region encoding a protein with homology to a conserved DNA-binding motif. *Nature (London)*, **346**, 240–4
6. Jantzen, H. M., Admon, A., Bell, S. P. and Tjian, R. (1990). Nucleolar transcription factor hUBF contains a DNA-binding motif with homology to HMG proteins. *Nature (London)*, **344**, 830–6
7. Laudet, V., Stehelin, D. and Clevers, H. (1993). Ancestry and diversity of the HMG box superfamily. *Nucleic Acids Res.*, **21**, 2493–501
8. Berta, P., Goze, C. and Poulat, F. (1993). Mais que sont les gènes SOX? *Médecine/Sciences*, **11**, 1247–8
9. Foster, J. W., Brennam, F. E., Hampikian, G. K., Goodfellow, P. N., Sinclair, A. H., Lovell, B. R., Selwood, L., Renfree, M. B., Cooper, D. W. and Graves, J. A. (1992). Evolution of sex determination and the Y chromosome: SRY-related sequences in marsupials. *Nature (London)*, **359**, 531–3
10. Berta, P., Hawkins, J. R., Sinclair, A. H., Taylor, A., Griffiths, B. L., Goodfellow, P. N. and Fellous, M. (1990). Genetic evidence equating SRY and the testis determining factor. *Nature (London)*, **348**, 448–50
11. Koopman, P., Gubbay, J., Vivian, N., Goodfellow, P. N. and Lovell-Badge, R. (1991). Male development of chromosomally female mice transgenic for Sry. *Nature (London)*, **351**, 117–21
12. Harley, V. R., Jackson, D. I., Hextall, P. J., Hawkins, J. R., Berkovitz, G. D., Sockanathan, S., Lovell-Badge, R. and Goodfellow, P. N. (1992). DNA binding activity of recombinant SRY from normal males and XY females. *Science*, **255**, 453–6
13. Nasrin, N., Buggs, C., Kong, X. F., Carnazza, J., Goebl, M. and Alexander-Bridges, M. (1991).

DNA-binding properties of the product of the testis-determining gene and a related protein. *Nature (London)*, **354**, 317–20

14. Poulat, F., Guichard, G., Goze, C., Heitz, F., Calas, B. and Berta, P. (1992). Synthesis of a large peptide mimicking the DNA binding properties of the sex determining protein, SRY. *FEBS Lett.*, **309**, 968–71

15. Giese, K., Cox, J. and Grosscheld, R. (1992). The HMG domain of lymphoid enhancer factor 1 binds DNA and facilitates assembly of functional nucleoprotein structures. *Cell*, **69**, 185–95

16. Poulat, F., Girard, F., Chevron, M. P., Goze, C., Rebillard, X., Calas, B., Lamb, N. and Berta, P. (1995). Nuclear localization of the testis determining gene product SRY. *J. Cell. Biol.*, **128**, 737–48

17. Dubin, R. A. and Ostrer, H. (1994). Sry is a transcriptional activator. *Mol. Endocrinol.*, **8**, 1182–92

18. Bennett, C. P., Docherty, Z., Robb, S. A., Ramani, P., Hawkins, J. R. and Grant, D. (1993). Deletion 9p and sex reversal. *J. Med. Genet.*, **30**, 518–20

19. Wilkie, A. O. M., Campbell, F. M., Daubeney, P., Grant, D. B., Daniels, R. J., Mullarkey, M., Affara, N. A., Fitchett, M. and Huson, S. M. (1993). Complete and partial XY sex reversal associates with terminal deletion of 10q – report of 2 cases and literature-review. *Am. J. Med. Genet.*, **46**, 597–600

20. Pelletier, J., Bruening, W., Kashtan, C. E., Mauer, S. M., Manivel, J. C., Striegel, J. E., Houghton, D. C., Junien, C., Habib, R., Fouser, L., Finer, R. N., Silverman, B. L., Haber, D. A. and Houseman, D. (1991). Germline mutations in the Wilm's tumor suppressor gene are associated with abnormal urogenital development in Denys-Drash syndrome. *Cell*, **67**, 437–47

21. Foster, J. W., Dominguez-Steglich, M. A., Guioli, S., Kwok, C., Weller, P. A., Stevanovic, M., Weissenbach, J., Mansour, S., Young, I. D., Goodfellow, P. N., Brook, J. D. and Schafer, A. J. (1994). Campomelic dysplasia and autosomal sex reversal caused by mutations in an SRY-related gene. *Nature*, **372**, 525–30

22. Shen, W. H., Moore, C. C. D., Ikeda, Y., Parker, K. L. and Ingraham, H. A. (1994). Nuclear receptor steroidogenic factor 1 regulates the Müllerian inhibiting substance gene: a link to the sex determination cascade. *Cell*, **77**, 651–61

23. Zanaria, E., Muscatelli, F., Bardoni, B., Strom, T. M., Guioli, S., Worley, K. A., Lalli, E., Moser, C., Walker, A. P., McCabe, E. R., Fraccaro, M., Zuffardi, O. and Camerino, G. (1994). An unusual member of the nuclear hormone receptor superfamily responsible for X-linked adrenal hypoplasia congenita. *Nature (London)*, **372**, 635–41

Molecular genetics of the androgen receptor

35

C. Sultan, S. Lumbroso, N. Poujol, C. Belon and J.-M. Lobaccaro

Introduction

The incongruity of a female phenotype in the presence of testes made the androgen insensitivity syndrome (AIS) a disorder of great fascination for physicians. Wilkins[1] was the first to recognize how the clinical features of one of his patients were the result of end organ resistance to androgen while Morris[2] gave a detailed summary of the features of the testicular feminization syndrome. Migeon, 20 years ago, provided evidence that AIS resulted from defective androgen receptor function in androgen target cells[3]. Since the cloning of the androgen receptor gene and its sequencing, there has been an explosion of data regarding the molecular genetics of AIS.

The two androgens, testosterone and 5α-dihydrotestosterone, are indispensable for normal male sexual differentiation[4]. Androgen action at the target cell level is accomplished via the androgen receptor which belongs to the steroid, thyroid hormone and retinoic acid receptor family[5]. The human androgen receptor is expressed in cultured genital skin fibroblasts, and demonstration of impaired ligand binding in fibroblasts is the most reliable means of diagnosing AIS[6]. Since the androgen receptor gene has been cloned, the tools of molecular biology have made it possible to identify mutations with the androgen receptor gene from patients with different phenotypes of androgen insensitivity. Such techniques include restriction fragment-length polymorphism analysis and enzymatic amplification of the various exons of the androgen receptor gene to detect large-scale changes in the gene structure[7]. Screening procedures such as denaturing gradient gel electrophoresis

(DGGE) or single strand conformation polymorphism (SSCP) assay, along with sequencing of the gene, allow identification of subtle changes responsible for mis-sense or nonsense mutations[8,9]. Measurements of androgen receptor mRNA have been useful in identifying mutations that cause AIS by altering the expression levels or the size of the mRNA[10]. Transfection of constructs expressing the mutant androgen receptor in mammalian cells is the main approach for demonstrating the causative role of the mutation in the development of androgen insensitivity[7].

Structure of the human androgen receptor and mechanism of androgen action

The androgen receptor belongs to the subfamily of steroid hormone receptors within a larger family of nuclear proteins that are likely to have evolved from a common ancestral gene[5]. The androgen receptor contains an N-terminal region, which is variable in length and has a role in transcriptional activation, a central cysteine-rich DNA-binding domain and a C-terminal ligand-binding domain (Figure 1). The primary structure of the human androgen receptor has been determined from molecular cloning and characterization of the cDNA encoding the human androgen receptor[11-13]. This sequence reveals an open reading frame of 2730 nucleotides encoding a protein of 910 amino acids residues with a calculated molecular mass of 99 kDa. The human androgen receptor gene has been localized to the Xq11-12 position[14].

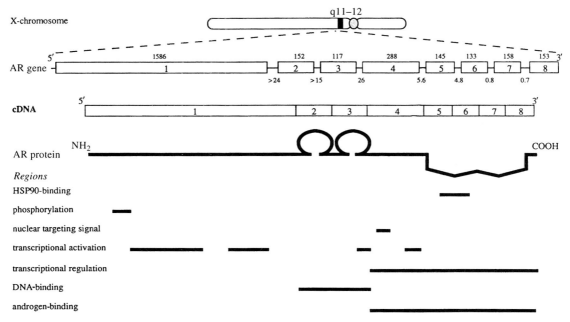

Figure 1 Structural organization of the eight exons of the androgen receptor (AR) gene and schematic figure of the androgen receptor showing the three domains common to all members of the nuclear receptor family

The gene is estimated to be approximately 90 kb and is composed of eight exons[15]. The N-terminal domain is encoded by the large exon 1 and contains segments encoding glutamine and glycine homopolymeric stretches[12]. The first and second zinc-finger structures of the central DNA-binding domain are encoded by exons 2 and 3, respectively. The androgen-biding domain is encoded by sequences in exons 4 to 8. Furthermore, silent mutations have been described demonstrating a heterogeneity within the androgen receptor gene[16] (and personal data).

The transactivating N-terminal domain

Although this N-terminal domain is termed a transactivator, its function has not been delineated in great detail. However, it is clear that the N-terminal domain contains sequence information to optimize the transactivation capability of the receptor and to specify gene recognition in transcriptional regulation. The transactivating domains among the different members of the nuclear receptor superfamily have the least conserved amino acid sequences and, consequently, they represent the most immunogenic parts of the proteins[17]. The biological function of the poly-Gln region or the other poly-Gly and -Pro motifs of the transactivation domain is not known. Similar repeats, however, have been identified in other steroid receptors and in a number of transcription-regulating proteins, particularly in the homeotic gene product[18].

The DNA-binding domain

Steroid receptors recognize specific DNA sequences with a functional domain that encompasses 66–68 amino acid residues. This cysteine-rich region appears to fold into two so-called zinc-finger structures, with one zinc atom being tetrahedrally co-ordinated with four cysteines in each case[5]. Recent data from the crystallization of the glucocorticoid receptor have indicated that the first zinc-finger (N-terminal) specifies DNA recognition of the receptor[19], while the second zinc-finger is mainly responsible for

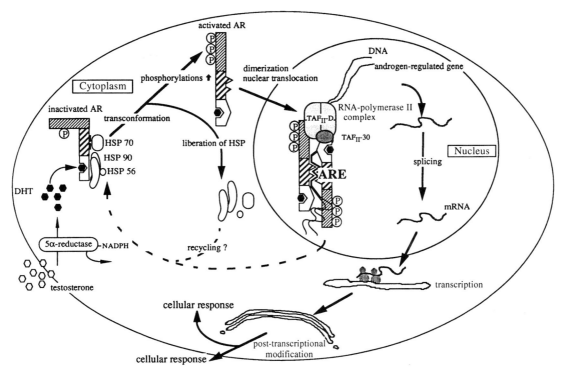

Figure 2 Theoretical view of androgen action in target cells. TAF_{II}-D is a complex of transcriptional activating factor, TAF_{II}-30, a part of TAF_{II}-D. In the absence of androgens, the androgen receptor (AR) is inactivated by the association with the different heat-shock proteins (HSP). In the presence of androgens (testosterone, open hexagon, or 5α-dihydrotestosterone (DHT), black hexagon), there is a transconformation of the receptor, transfer of the androgen–androgen receptor complex to the nucleus, fixation to the androgen-responsive elements (ARE) and, lastly, the expression of the target gene

dimerization of two receptor molecules during their association with DNA[20]. The DNA-binding domain interacts with *cis*-acting elements of the regulated genes (androgen-responsive elements) which are 15-nucleotide-long palindromic sequences located in the flanking region of the gene[21].

The C-terminal and androgen-binding domain

The C-terminal regions of the nuclear receptors are involved in ligand-binding and in the interaction with heat-shock proteins such as HSP90[22-24]. Although the two physiologically active androgens, testosterone and 5α-dihydrotestosterone, interact directly with the androgen receptor and mediate hormonal responses[25], conversion of testosterone to the more potent

agonist 5α-dihydrotestosterone in certain tissues is required for the androgen action to occur[4]. This requirement is particularly clear during male sexual development, when formation of 5α-dihydrotestosterone is mandatory for virilization of external genitalia and development of the prostate gland. Virilization of the Wolffian duct structures is, however, thought to be mediated by testosterone[4].

The actions of androgens on target cells occur via the classical steroid receptor pathway (Figure 2). The process of androgen receptor transformation into a tight nuclear-binding form has been studied extensively. Most investigations[22-24] have focused on *in vitro* transformation of androgen receptor and have shown that the untransformed (i.e. non-DNA-binding) receptor is associated with several heat-shock proteins. The transformation of the receptor to the tight nuclear-binding form is a multistep process that involves the dissociation of the heat-shock proteins from the receptor[23]. The complex androgen-activated androgen receptor is thus able to migrate into the nucleus and interact with the androgen-responsive elements[26]. The mechanism by which the receptor causes gene activation involves N-terminal sequences of the protein, but the molecular details of this activation process remain to be elucidated. Protein–protein interactions are likely to occur with other transcription factors[26]. Both promoter and host cell specificity appear to influence the requirement for the N-terminal domain in transcriptional activation, suggesting that this region interacts with cell-specific transcription factors[26].

Genetic abnormalities of the human androgen receptor gene in AIS

Androgen insensitivity syndromes are X-linked disorders resulting from androgen action defects in target cells[27]. Patients have been classified both by clinical phenotype and on the basis of androgen receptor abnormalities as assessed by a variety of *in vivo* and *in vitro* tests. Phenotype patients range from males who are phenotypically female (complete androgen insensitivity syndrome, CAIS) to men who are slightly under-virilized (partial androgen insensitivity syndrome, PAIS) or infertile[28]. Individuals with CAIS usually come to medical attention because of an inguinal hernia or primary amenorrhea after puberty. The phenotype is female except that axillary and pubic hair are diminished or absent. The external genitalia are normal, and the vagina is short and blind or absent. Female internal genital structures are usually absent. PAIS covers a large spectrum of ambiguous genitalia: partial fusion of the labioscrotal folds, perineoscrotal hypospadias or severe hypospadias, and usually some clitoromegaly at birth. At puberty, pubic hair growth is sparse, and gynecomastia develops. Underdeveloped Wolffian duct derivatives are usually present. Cryptorchidism is common, and the testes are usually

small and the production of sperm is decreased or absent[4]. This clinical spectrum is paralleled by an equally wide range of receptor abnormalities that can be grouped into four broad categories on the basis of the level and character of androgen binding in cultured genital skin fibroblasts: (1) receptor-binding negative, (2) receptor-binding reduced, (3) qualitative-binding abnormality, and (4) receptor-binding positive[29]. Genetic alterations detected within the androgen receptor gene allow a classification of androgen insensitivity based on the defects of the androgen receptor gene[30]: mutations that cause large-scale alterations of the structure of the androgen receptor gene or mRNA (e.g. macro- and microdeletions, micro-insertions, stop codon) and mutations that alter the primary structure of the androgen receptor (e.g. missense mutations).

Mutations that cause large-scale alterations of the androgen receptor gene or mRNA

Genomic Southern blot analysis or polymerase chain reaction (PCR) to examine the androgen receptor gene structure in affected members of families with AIS has demonstrated that this mechanism does not appear to account for a large percentage of patients – only seven deletions have been reported to date among 200 patients screened for AIS[31,32]. In our experience, we have found a partial deletion in one family with CAIS[33] among 100 unrelated patients with AIS[34] (and unpublished data).

A second mechanism is an anomaly in the intron regions. Ris-Stalpers and colleagues[35] first reported an aberrant splicing site within exon 4 which led to a shorter androgen receptor of 41 amino acids. This seems to be due to a cryptic splice donor activation. Similarly, Evans and co-workers[36] found a mutation in the exon 3/intron 3 junction causing CAIS.

Lastly, the third mechanism found to cause large-scale alterations of the gene is a single nucleotide change introducing premature termination codons into the coding sequence of the androgen receptor gene. The resulting androgen receptor is truncated at the C-terminus

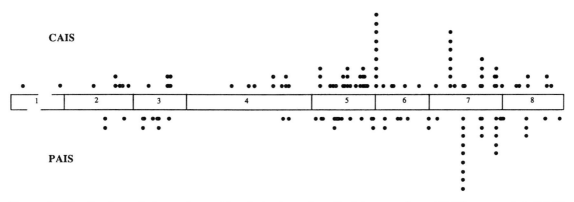

Figure 3 Distribution of the amino acid substitutions described in complete (CAIS) or partial (PAIS) androgen insensitivity syndrome

and, therefore, is inactive in hormone binding and in assays of transcriptional activation. To date, 11 nonsense mutations have been described in CAIS. This mechanism has been recently described in the *Tfm* mouse[37,38]. Zoppi and co-workers[39] also recently described an interesting stop codon occurring in the NH$_2$-terminal domain. *In vitro* mutagenesis showed that the synthesis of the mutant androgen receptor is initiated downstream of the stop codon at reduced levels and that each molecule is thus functionally impaired. The same mechanism was described in the *Tfm* rat by Gaspar and co-workers[40].

Mutations that alter the primary structure of the androgen receptor

The main mechanism that causes AIS is a single nucleotide change that introduces an amino acid substitution into the coding sequence of the androgen receptor gene. To date, around 180 mutations have been reported within the androgen receptor gene[32] (Figure 3). Among these, our group have described 16 missense mutations. In the DNA-binding domain, seven amino acid substitutions have been described in patients with PAIS or CAIS: Gly568Trp[41], Cys579Tyr[31], Val581Phe[42], Arg585Lys, Ala596Thr, Arg60Lys[43] and Leu616Pro[31]. In the androgen-binding domain, nine substitutions have been described: Leu707Arg, Met734Thr[31],

a *de novo* Gly–Val substitution at position 743[9], a Phe–Val substitution at position 754 which created a new *Mae* III restriction site[44], Asp676Glu, a silent substitution Gly595Gly and Arg855Cys[31] in patients with CAIS. In two patients with PAIS, we found Arg840His[45] and a silent substitution Ser888Ser[31].

Prenatal and carrier diagnosis of AIS

The screening of carriers and prenatal diagnosis of AIS in high-risk families is impossible unless the mutation has been identified. Once the mutation has been described and correlated to the disease, sequencing of the suspected exon of the 46,XX probands or the 46,XY fetus ascertains whether they are carrying the affected chromosome. In one family with PAIS, we performed an exclusion diagnosis of PAIS (submitted data) by sequencing of the trophoblastic DNA. In some cases, point mutation creates or abolishes a restriction site – in these conditions prenatal and carrier diagnoses are easier and more rapid[42,44,46]. However, when the mutation has not been identified, it is necessary to look for one of the two androgen receptor gene polymorphisms. Brown and colleagues[14] described a moderate-frequency Hind III polymorphism which proved useful in identifying the affected X chromosomes in one family with PAIS[47]. Moreover, this polymorphism allowed us to perform prenatal diagnosis of PAIS[41]. Lubahn and co-workers[12] described a polymorphic tandem CAG repeat in the first exon. Its frequency has been estimated to be 55–85%[48,49]. Our group was the first to prenatally predict the exclusion of androgen insensitivity syndrome in two families[49]: in the first family, three members were affected by PAIS, and in the second, the propositus had CAIS. In both cases, the expectation of normal male sexual development was confirmed by the detection of normal external fetal genitalia by ultrasonography at week 20.

Androgen receptor gene mutation and prostate cancer

In prostate cancer, several somatic point mutations have been described in patients with advanced cancers[50–53]. Newmark and co-workers[50] described a Val–Met substitution at position 730 in the androgen-binding domain. This amino acid is also involved in the binding of the inactivated androgen receptor with the heat-shock protein. Newmark and co-workers hypothesize that this mutation might be involved in the development or progression of prostate cancer. Likewise, a Thr877–Ala substitution located in the androgen-binding domain was described in the cancer cell line LNCaP[54]. This mutation is responsible for the pharmaco-resistance observed in these cells. Gaddipati and colleagues[52] found this 'LNCaP mutation' in 25% of advance stage cancers. Very little is known about the molecular changes in prostatic carcinomas, which progress from a pharmaco-dependent to a pharmaco-independent stage[55]. Under these conditions, it would be interesting to screen somatic point mutations of the androgen receptor gene in the tumors of patients with prostate cancer before and after the development of pharmaco-independence, in order to study the potential role of the androgen receptor mutation in the progression of the cancer.

Androgen receptor gene mutation and male breast cancer

Wooster and co-workers[56] recently reported an Arg–Gln substitution at position 607 in the and-rogen receptor gene in two brothers with breast cancer and PAIS. In one out of thirteen patients with breast cancer, we found an androgen receptor gene mutation in exon 3 encoding for a part of the DNA-binding domain[57]. Sequencing showed a G–A point mutation at nucleotide 2185 responsible for an Arg–Lys substitution at position 608. This patient was referred to the Department of Endocrinology for PAIS. There are two main hypotheses to explain the development of breast cancer linked to mutations of the androgen receptor. One possibility is that the mutated androgen receptor acquires the ability to bind to estrogen response elements and thus to activate estrogen-regulated genes. This region of the binding domain, however, has never been involved in the specificity of the binding to the response elements[58]. Nevertheless, a tri-dimensional structure modification cannot be ruled out. In vitro band shift studies may give more information on the potential binding of the mutated androgen receptor at position 608 to estrogen response elements. The second hypothesis is the loss of a protective effect of androgens. This explanation seems to be reinforced by other studies[59–61]. Moreover, Couture and co-workers[62] recently demonstrated an androgen receptor-mediated stimulation of 17β-hydroxysteroid dehydrogenase activity by androgens in ZR-75-1 human breast cancer cells. They observed that treatment with an androgen can increase oxidation of the active estradiol into the weak estrogen estrone, thus decreasing the observed tendency in breast tumors to accumulate estradiol from estrone due to a higher reductive 17β-hydroxysteroid dehydrogenase activity[63].

Androgen receptor gene mutation and Kennedy's disease

La Spada and colleagues[64] showed that Kennedy's disease, an adult-onset neurodegenerative disorder, is due to the expansion of the normal poly-Gln tract (tandem CAG repeat) from 14–32 to more than 40. Furthermore, this X-linked spinal and bulbar muscular atrophy is associated inconsistently with mild androgen insensitivity. This extension of the CAG repeat is the most puzzling of all human androgen receptor mutations defined to date[65,66]. In some patients, androgen receptor abnormalities have been described by immunohistochemical analysis[67]. It would be interesting to study the role of the length of the CAG repeat on the transactivation capacity of the androgen receptor by direct mutagenesis and, thus, to analyze the specific role of androgens in motor neuron growth, development and regeneration[68].

Conclusion

Significant progress has been made in delineating the mutations that cause AIS. It appears that the androgen receptor is the nuclear receptor that presents the greatest number of 'natural' mutants. The mechanisms causing AIS are heterogeneous, and in most cases the mutation in each family is distinctive. The mutations seem not to be distributed by chance but occur in specific areas of the androgen receptor gene. However, important questions remain unanswered. Since it appears that different mutations can cause the same phenotype, a major challenge will be to elucidate how the different phenotypes are correlated with the genetic mutation detected.

From the studies to date, a number of findings on the molecular genetics of the androgen receptor have been established:

(1) Molecular analysis of the androgen receptor gene has revealed that there are a wide variety of molecular defects underlying the clinical and biochemical heterogeneity of AIS.

(2) All androgen receptor defects appear to disturb the androgen receptor ability to regulate transcription of its target genes.

(3) Androgen receptor gene sequence and studies of androgen receptor function *in vitro* do not explain every aspect of AIS.

(4) The same mutation can be associated with different phenotypes from different families, and even within the same families.

(5) Other genetic determinants may influence androgen action within its target cells.

(6) Markedly different molecular defects (major deletion, premature termination, single amino acid substitution in the androgen receptor protein) can produce the same phenotype.

(7) The effects of a change upon tertiary structure of the protein is likely to be involved in some aspects of AIS.

(8) Detection of potential carriers and prenatal diagnosis may be performed simply and rapidly when the mutation is identified in the family.

(9) Molecular studies might possibly facilitate prediction of androgen responsiveness in some cases of PAIS.

(10) Mutations provide new insights into the molecular mechanism of action of the androgen receptor in humans.

References

1. Wilkins, L. (1950). *The Diagnosis and Treatment of Endocrine Disorders in Childhood and Adolescence.* (Springfield, IL: Charles C. Thomas)
2. Morris, J. M. (1953). The syndrome of testicular feminization in male pseudohermaphrodites. *Am. J. Obstet. Gynecol.*, **65**, 1192–1211
3. Keenan, B. S., Meyer, W. J., Hadjian, A. J., Jones, H. W. and Migeon, C. J. (1974). Syndrome of androgen insensitivity in man: absence of 5α-dihydrotestosterone binding protein in skin fibroblasts. *J. Clin. Endocrinol. Metab.*, **38**, 1143–6

4. Griffin, J. E. (1992). Androgen resistance – the clinical and molecular spectrum. *N. Engl. J. Med.*, **326**, 611–18

5. Evans, R. M. (1988). The steroid and thyroid hormone receptor superfamily. *Science*, **240**, 889–95

6. Sultan, C. (1986). Androgen receptors and partial androgen insensitivity in male pseudohermaphrodism. *Ann. Génét. (Paris)*, **29**, 5–10

7. French, F. S., Lubahn, D. B., Brown, T. R., Simental, J. A., Quigley, C. A., Yarbrough, W. G., Tan, J., Sar, M., Joseph, D. R., Evans, B. A., Hughes, I. A., Migeon, C. J. and Wilson, E. M. (1990). Molecular basis of androgen insensitivity. *Recent Prog. Horm. Res.*, **46**, 1–38

8. Brown, T. R., Lubahn, D. B., Wilson, E. M., French, F. S., Migeon, C. J. and Corden, J. L. (1990). Functional characterisation of naturally occurring mutant androgen receptors from subjects with complete androgen insensitivity. *Mol. Endocrinol.*, **4**, 1759–72

9. Lobaccaro, J. M., Lumbroso, S., Berta, P., Chaussain, J. L. and Sultan, C. (1993). Complete androgen insensitivity syndrome associated with a *de novo* mutation of the androgen receptor gene detected by single strand conformational polymorphism. *J. Steroid Biochem. Mol. Biol.*, **44**, 211–16

10. Marcelli, M., Tilley, W. D., Zoppi, S., Griffin, J. E., Wilson, J. D. and McPhaul, M. J. (1991). Androgen resistance associated with a mutation of the androgen receptor at amino-acid 772 (Arg-Cys) results from a combination of decreased messenger ribonucleic acid levels and impairment of receptor function. *J. Clin. Endocrinol. Metab.*, **73**, 318–25

11. Chang, C., Kokontis, J. and Liao, S. (1988). Structural analysis of complementary DNA and amino acid sequences of human and rat androgen receptors. *Proc. Natl. Acad. Sci. USA*, **85**, 7211–15

12. Lubahn, D. B., Joseph, D. R., Sar, M., Tan, J., Higgs, H., Larson, R. E., French, F. S. and Wilson, E. M. (1988). The human androgen receptor: complementary deoxyribonucleic acid cloning, sequence analysis and gene expression in prostate. *Mol. Endocrinol.*, **2**, 1265–75

13. Trapman, J., Klaassen, P. and Kuiper, G. J. (1988). Cloning, structure and expression of a cDNA encoding the human androgen receptor. *Biochem. Biophys. Res. Commun.*, **153**, 241–8

14. Brown, C. J., Goss, S. J., Lubahn, D. B., Joseph, D. R., Wilson, E. M., French, F. S. and Willard, H. F. (1989). Androgen receptor locus on the human X chromosome: regional localization to Xq11-12 and description of a DNA polymorphism. *Am. J. Hum. Genet.*, **44**, 264–9

15. Kuiper, G. G. J. M., Faber, T. W., van Rooij, H. C. J., van der Korput, J. A. G. M., Ris-Stalpers, C., Klaassen, P., Trapman, J. and Brinkmann, A. O. (1989). Structural organization of the human androgen receptor gene. *J. Mol. Endocrinol.*, **2**, R1–R4

16. McPhaul, M. J., Marcelli, M., Zoppi, S., Griffin, J. E. and Wilson, J. D. (1993). Genetic basis of endocrine disease 4. The spectrum of mutations in the androgen receptor gene that causes androgen resistance. *J. Clin. Endocrinol. Metab.*, **76**, 17–23

17. Wilson, C. M., Griffin, J. E., Wilson, J. D., Marcelli, M., Zoppi, S. and McPhaul, M. J. (1992). Immunoreactive androgen receptor expression in subjects with androgen resistance. *J. Clin. Endocrinol. Metab.*, **75**, 1474–8

18. Scott, M. P. and Carroll, S. B. (1987). The segmentation and homeotic gene network in early Drosophila development. *Cell*, **51**, 689–98

19. Luisi, B. F., Xu, W. X., Otwinowski, Z., Freedman, L. P., Yamamoto, K. R. and Sigler, P. B. (1991). Crystallographic analysis of the interaction of the glucocorticoid receptor with DNA. *Nature (London)*, **352**, 497–505

20. Freedman, L. P. (1992). Anatomy of the steroid receptor zinc finger region. *Endocr. Rev.*, **13**, 129–45

21. Ham, J., Thomson, A., Needham, M., Webb, P. and Parker, M. (1988). Characterization of response elements for androgens, glucocorticoids and progestins in mouse mammary tumor virus. *Nucleic Acids Res.*, **16**, 5263–76

22. Nemoto, T., Ohara-Nemoto, Y. and Ota, M. (1992). Association of the 90-kDa heat shock protein does not affect the ligand-binding ability of androgen receptor. *J. Steroid Biochem. Mol. Biol.*, **42**, 803–12

23. Veldscholte, J., Berrevoets, C. A., Zegers, N. D., Vanderkwast, T. H., Grootegoed, J. A. and Mulder, E. (1992). Hormone-induced dissociation of the androgen receptor-heat-shock protein complex – use of a new monoclonal antibody to distinguish transformed from nontransformed receptors. *Biochemistry*, **31**, 7420–7430

24. Marivoet, S., Vandijck, P., Verhoeven, G. and Heyns, W. (1992). Interaction of the 90-kDa heat shock protein with native and *in vitro* translated androgen receptor and receptor fragments. *Mol. Cell. Endocrinol.*, **88**, 165–74

25. Sultan, C., Migeon, B. R., Rothwell, S. W., Maes, M., Zerhouni, N. and Migeon, C. J. (1980). Androgen receptors and metabolism in cultured human fetal fibroblasts. *Pediatr. Res.*, **13**, 67–9

26. Simental, J. A., Sar, M., Lance, M. V., French, F. S. and Wilson, E. M. (1991). Transcriptional

activation and nuclear targeting signals of the human androgen receptor. *J. Biol. Chem.*, **266**, 510–18

27. Meyer, W. J., Migeon, B. R. and Migeon, C. J. (1975). Locus on human chromosome for dihydrotestosterone receptor and androgen insensitivity. *Proc. Natl. Acad. Sci. USA*, **72**, 1469–72

28. Sultan, C., Lobaccaro, J. M., Lumbroso, S., Boudon, C., Poujol, N., Belon, C. and Dumas, R. (1995). Molecular aspects of sex differentiation – applications in pathological conditions. In Bergadà, C. and Moguilevsky, J. A. (eds.) *Puberty: Basic and Clinical Aspects*. (Firenze: Academic Press)

29. Marcelli, M., Tilley, W. D., Zoppi, S., Griffin, J. E., Wilson, J. D. and McPhaul, M. J. (1992). Molecular basis of androgen resistance. *J. Endocrinol. Invest.*, **15**, 149–59

30. McPhaul, M. J., Marcelli, M., Tilley, W. D., Griffin, J. E. and Wilson, J. D. (1991). Androgen resistance caused by mutations in the androgen receptor gene. *FASEB J.*, **5**, 2910–15

31. Sultan, C., Lumbroso, S., Poujol, N., Belon, C., Boudon, C. and Lobaccaro, J. M. (1993). Mutations of the androgen receptor gene in androgen insensitivity syndrome. *J. Steroid. Biochem. Mol. Biol.*, **46**, 519–30

32. Patterson, M. N., Hughes, I. A., Gottlieb, B. and Pinsky, L. (1994). The androgen receptor gene mutations database. *Nucleic Acids Res.*, **22**, 3560–2

33. Lobaccaro, J.-M., Lumbroso, J. M., Poujol, N., Georget, V., Brinkmann, A. O., Malpuech, G. and Sultan, C. (1995). Complete androgen insensitivity syndrome due to a new frameshift deletion in exon 4 of the androgen receptor gene: functional analysis of the mutant receptor. *Mol. Cell. Endocrinol.*, **111**, 21–8

34. Lobaccaro, J. M., Belon, C., Chaussain, J. L., Job, J. C., Toublanc, J. E., Battin, J., Rochiccioli, P., Bernasconi, S., Bost, M., Bozzola, M., Bouccekine, N., Burési, C., Chaabouni, H., Hachicha, M., Larget-Piet, L., Leconte, P., Limal, J. M., Magnin, G., Malpuech, G., Moraine, C., Nivelon, J. L., Ranke, M., Schonberg, D., Vander-Schueren, M., Moustarih, R., Terraza, A. and Sultan, C. (1992). Molecular analysis of the androgen receptor gene in 52 patients with complete or partial androgen insensitivity syndrome: a collaborative study. *Horm. Res.*, **37**, 54–9

35. Ris-Stalpers, C., Kuiper, G. G. J. M., Faber, P. W., Schweikert, H. U., van Rooij, H. C. J., Zegers, N. D., Hodgins, M. B., Degenhart, H. J., Trapman, J. and Brinkmann, A. O. (1990). Aberrant splicing of androgen receptor mRNA results in non-functional receptor protein in a patient with androgen insensitivity. *Proc. Natl. Acad. Sci. USA*, **87**, 7866–70

36. Evans, B. A. J., Ismail, R. A., France, T. and Hugues, I. A. (1991). Analysis of the androgen receptor gene structure in a patient with complete androgen insensitivity syndrome. *J. Endocrinol.*, **129**, 65

37. He, W. E., Kumar, M. V. and Tindall, D. J. (1991). A frameshift mutation in the androgen receptor gene causes complete androgen insensitivity in the testicular-feminized mouse. *Nucleic Acids Res.*, **19**, 2373–8

38. Charest, N. J., Zhou, Z., Lubahn, D. B., Olsen, K. L., Wilson, E. M. and French, F. S. (1991). A frameshift mutation destabilizes androgen receptor messenger RNA in the Tfm mouse. *Mol. Endocrinol.*, **5**, 573–81

39. Zoppi, S., Wilson, C. M., Harbison, M. D., Griffin, J. E., Wilson, J. D. and McPhaul, M. J. (1992). Complete testicular feminization caused by an amnio-terminal truncation of the androgen receptor with downstream initiation. *J. Clin. Invest.*, **91**, 1105–21

40. Gaspar, M. L., Meo, T., Bourgarel, P., Guenet, J. L. and Tosi, M. (1991). A single base deletion in the Tfm androgen receptor gene creates a short-lived messenger RNA that directs internal translation initiation. *Proc. Natl. Acad. Sci. USA*, **88**, 8606–10

41. Lobaccaro, J.-M., Belon, C., Lumbroso, S., Olewniczack, G., Carré-Pigeon, F., Job, J.-C., Chaussain, J.-L., Toublanc, J.-E. and Sultan, C. (1994). Molecular prenatal diagnosis of partial androgen insensitivity syndrome based on the Hind III polymorphism of the androgen receptor gene. *Clin. Endocrinol.*, **40**, 297–302

42. Lumbroso, S., Lobaccaro, J.-M., Belon, C., Martin-Coignard, D., Chaussain, J.-L. and Sultan, C. (1993). A new mutation within the DNA-binding domain of the androgen receptor gene in a family with complete androgen insensitivity syndrome and positive receptor-binding activity. *Fertil. Steril.*, **60**, 814–19

43. Lobaccaro, J. M., Lumbroso, S., Belon, C., Galtier-Dereure, F., Bringer, J., Lesimple, T., Namer, M., Cutuli, B. F., Pujol, H. and Sultan, C. (1993). Androgen receptor gene mutation in male breast cancer. *Hum. Mol. Genet.*, **2**, 1799–802

44. Lobaccaro, J.-M., Lumbroso, S., Ktari, R., Dumas, R. and Sultan, C. (1993). An exonic point mutation creates a *Mae* III site in the androgen receptor gene of a family with complete androgen insensitivity syndrome. *Hum. Mol. Genet.*, **2**, 1041–3

45. Lumbroso, S., Lobaccaro, J. M., Belon, C., Boulot, P., Amram, S. and Sultan, C. (1994). Molecular prenatal exclusion of Reifenstein syndrome. *Eur. J. Endocrinol.*, **130**, 327–32

46. Sai, T., Seino, S., Chang, C., Trifiro, M., Pinsky, L., Mhartre, A., Kaufman, M., Lambert, B., Trapman, J., Brinkmann, A. O., Rosenfield, R. L. and Liao, S. (1990). An exonic point mutation of the androgen receptor gene in a family with complete androgen insensitivity. *Am. J. Hum. Genet.*, **46**, 1095–100

47. Lobaccaro, J. M., Belon, C., Ruiz-Pacheco, R., Heinrichs, C., van Regemorter, N., Terraza, A. and Sultan, C. (1991). Genetic association of Hind III polymorphism with the androgen receptor gene in partial androgen insensitivity syndrome. *Ann. Génét. (Paris)*, **34**, 9–13

48. Sleddens, H. F. B. M., Oostra, B. A., Brinkmann, A. O. and Trapman, J. (1992). Trinucleotide repeat polymorphism in the androgen receptor gene (AR). *Nucleic Acids Res.*, **20**, 1427

49. Lobaccaro, J. M., Lumbroso, S., Carré-Pigeon, F., Chaussain, J.-L., Toublanc, J.-E., Job, J.-C., Olewniczack, G., Boulot, P. and Sultan, C. (1992). Prenatal prediction of androgen insensitivity syndrome using exon 1 polymorphism of the androgen receptor gene. *J. Steroid. Biochem. Mol. Biol.*, **43**, 659–63

50. Newmark, J. R., Hardy, D. O., Tonb, D C., Carter, B. S., Epstein, J. I., Isaacs, W B., Brown, T. R. and Barrack, E. R. (1992). Androgen receptor gene mutations in human prostate cancer. *Proc. Natl. Acad. Sci. USA*, **89** 6319–23

51. Suzuki, H., Sato, N., Watabe, Y., Masai, M., Seino, S. and Shimazaki, J. (1993). Androgen receptor gene mutations in human prostate cancer. *J. Steroid Biochem. Molec. Biol.*, **46**, 759–65

52. Gaddipati, J. P., Mcleod, D. G., Heidenberg, H. B., Sesterhenn, I. A., Finger, M. J., Moul, J. W. and Srivastava, S. (1994). Frequent detection of codon 877 mutation in the androgen receptor gene in advanced prostate cancers. *Cancer Res.*, **54**, 2861–4

53. Schoenberg, M. P., Hakimi, J. M., Wang, S. P., Bova, G. S., Epstein, J. I., Fischbeck, K. H., Isaacs, W. B., Walsh, P. C. and Barrack, E. R. (1994). Microsatellite mutation (Cag(24-> 18)) in the androgen receptor gene in human prostate cancer. *Biochem. Biophys. Res. Commun.*, **198**, 74–80

54. Vedscholte, J., Ris-Stalpers, C., Kuiper, G. G. J. M., Jenster, G., Berrevoets, C., Claassen, E., van Rooij, H. C. J., Brinkmann, A. O. and Mulder, E. (1990). A mutation in the ligand binding domain of the androgen receptor of human LNCaP cells affects steroid binding characteristics and response to anti-androgens. *Biochem. Biophys. Res. Commun.*, **173**, 534–40

55. Culig, Z., Klocker, H., Eberle, J., Kaspar, F., Hobisch, A., Cronauer, M. V. and Bartsch, G. (1993). DNA sequence of the androgen receptor in prostatic tumor cell lines and tissue specimens assessed by means of the polymerase chain reaction. *Prostate*, **22**, 11–22

56. Wooster, R., Mangion, J., Eeles, R., Smith, S., Dowsett, M., Averill, D., Barrett-Lee, P., Easton, D. F., Ponder, B. A. J. and Stratton, M. R. (1992). A germline mutation in the androgen receptor gene in two brothers with breast cancer and Reifenstein syndrome. *Nature Genet.*, **2**, 132–4

57. Lobaccaro, J. M., Lumbroso, S., Belon, C., Galtier-Dereure, F., Bringer, J., Lesimple, T., Heron, J.-F., Pujol, H. and Sultan, C. (1993). A second instance of male breast cancer linked to a germline mutation of the androgen receptor gene. *Nature Genet.*, **5**, 109–10

58. Mader, S., Kumar, V., de Vermeuil, H. and Chambon, P. (1989). Three amino acids of the estrogen receptor are essential with ability to distinguish an estrogen from a glucocorticoid-response element. *Nature (London)*, **338**, 271–4

59. Thomas, D. B., Jimenez, L. M., McTiernan, A., Rosenblatt, K., Stalsberg, H., Stemhagen, A, Thompson, W. D., McCrea Curnen, M. G., Satariano, W., Austin, D. F., Greenberg, R. S., Key, C., Lolonel, L. N. and West, D. W. (1992). Breast cancer in men: risk factors with hormonal implications. *Am. J. Epidemiol.*, **135**, 734–48

60. Mabuchi, K., Bross, D. S. and Lessler, I. I. (1985). Risk factors for male breast cancer. *J. Natl. Cancer Inst.*, **74**, 371–5

61. Crichlow, R. W. and Spencer, W. G. (1990). Male breast cancer. *Surg. Clin. North Am.*, **70**, 1165–77

62. Couture, P., Thériault, C., Simard, J. and Labrie, F. (1993). Androgen receptor-mediated stimulation of 17β-hydroxysteroid dehydrogenase activity by dihydrotestosterone and medroxyprogesterone acetate in ZR-75-1 human breast cancer cells. *Endocrinology*, **132**, 179–85

63. McNeil, M., Reed, M. J., Beranek, P. A., Bonney, R. C., Ghilchick, M. W., Robinson, D. J. and James, V. H. T. (1986). A comparison of the *in vivo* uptake and metabolism of 3H-oestrone and 3H-oestradiol by normal breast and breast tumor tissues in post-menopausal women. *Int. J. Cancer*, **38**, 193–6

64. La Spada, A. R., Wilson, E. M., Lubahn, D. B., Harding, A. E. and Fischbeck, K. (1991). Androgen receptor gene mutations in X-linked spinal and bulbar muscular atrophy. *Nature (London)*, **352**, 77–9

65. Biancalana, V., Serville, F., Pommier, J., Julien, J., Hanauer, A. and Mandel, J. L. (1992). Moderate instability of the trinucleotide repeat in spino bulbar muscular atrophy. *Hum. Mol. Genet.*, **1**, 255–8

66. Yamamoto, Y., Kawai, H., Nakahara, K., Osame, M., Nakatsuji, Y., Kishimoto, T. and Sakoda, S. (1992). A novel primer extension method to detect the number of CAG repeats in the androgen receptor gene in families with X-linked spinal and bulbar muscular atrophy. *Biochem. Biophys. Res. Commun.*, **182**, 507–13

67. Matsuura, T., Demura, T., Aimoto, Y., Mizuno, T., Moriwaka, F. and Tashiro, K. (1992). Androgen receptor abnormality in X-linked spinal and bulbar muscular atrophy. *Neurology*, **42**, 1724–6

68. Goldstein, L. A. and Sengelaub, D. R. (1992). Timing and duration of dihydrotestosterone treatment affect the development to motoneuron number and morphology in sexually dimorphic rat spinal nucleus. *J. Comp. Neurol.*, **326**, 147–57

Molecular biology of the human androgen receptor

36

L. Pinsky, P. Kazemi-Esfarjani, L. K. Beitel and M. A. Trifiro

Basic molecular biology

The human androgen receptor is encoded by a gene (hAR) > 90 kb[1] at Xq11–12[2]. The complementary DNA (cDNA) ($\approx$ 10.6 kb) contains an open reading frame ($\approx$ 2.7 kb) flanked by a 1.1 kb 5'-untranslated region (5'-UTR) and by a very long, 6.8 kb, 3'-UTR[3]. There are two major sites of transcription initiation 13 base pairs (bp) apart[3] and two functionally equivalent polyadenylation signals[3]. The promoter area is 'TATA' and 'CAAT'-free but GC-rich, and contains both a Sp 1-binding site and a 44-bp sequence that includes four repeats of the pentanucleotide GGGGA[4]. Sp 1 binding at -46/-37 controls the use of the upstream transcription initiation site[5]. The purine-rich segment (-75/-119) can bind specific nuclear proteins[6]. A region further upstream (-380/-530) underlies AR transactivation by cAMP, and contains a putative cAMP response element[6].

The human androgen receptor is a ligand-activated, phosphorylated[7], DNA-binding, transcriptional factor (a 'nuclear receptor'). In effect, it is a 'one-stop' signal transduction system: a C-terminal module, the androgen-binding domain (ABD), receives the 'signal'; a central module, the DNA-binding domain (DBD), binds it to a sequence of regulatory nucleotides (an androgen response element, ARE), usually upstream from the promoter of a nearby target gene; a N-terminal module modulates the amplitude and specificity of its transcriptional regulatory effect on a given gene.

The hAR is composed of eight exons[1]. Exon 1 encodes the 5'-UTR and the ($\approx$ 550 amino acids) N-terminal region of the AR that contains a polymorphic (CAG)$_n$CAA (polyglutamine) tract (n = 11–33) starting at residue 58, and a polymorphic (GGN)$_n$ (polyglycine) tract (n = 12–29) near its C-terminal. Exons 2 and 3 encode the 67 amino acid DBD. Exons 4–7 and a bit of exon 8 encode the 252 amino acid ABD. The C-terminal flank of the DBD encodes a bipartite nuclear localization signal that is rich in arginine and lysine[8].

The androgen receptor's ABD has a set of subsidiary functions: heat shock protein (HSP) binding[9]; nuclear localization[8], dimerization[10]; transregulation[11]. Likewise, by homology with the glucocorticoid receptor[11], it is very likely that the androgen receptor's DBD contributes to dimerization, and to transregulation itself.

A simplified, operational view of its life cycle begins with the cytoplasmic form of the androgen receptor that binds a number of chaperone proteins, the most prominent being HSP-90 and HSP-59[9]. Probably, they stabilize the androgen receptor and/or keep it in an androgen-binding configuration. Once the androgen receptor has bound an androgen, the chaperones dissociate, and the androgen–receptor complex traverses the nuclear membrane. In the nucleus it dimerizes with another androgen–receptor complex either before, or in conjunction with, their binding to an ARE (a pair of imperfectly palindromic hexanucleotide repeats, separated by three spacer nucleotides). The union of paired androgen–receptor complexes with an ARE mediates a serial process that usually culminates in transcriptional activation of an androgen target gene. This depends on interactions between upstream DNA-bound regulatory factors and the downstream transcription initiation com-

275

plex, but its details are essentially unknown. For instance, androgen–receptor complexes may facilitate protein–protein interactions by acting as direct bridges. Or they may bend DNA so that upstream factors can contact components of the transcription initiation complex directly. Transcriptional repression of a target gene by androgen–receptor complexes is not well understood. For instance, how androgen down-regulates androgen receptor mRNA in LNCaP cells is unknown[12]. Competition, 'squelching' and 'quenching' mechanisms have been proposed[13]. In some of them, protein–protein, not protein–DNA, interaction is crucial[13].

Molecular biology as revealed by mutation of the gene

Little is known about the conformation of the ABD, and nothing about the stereochemistry of its androgen-binding 'pocket'. Missense mutations throughout the breadth of the ABD impair androgen binding. Hence, widely dispersed amino acid components of the ABD must contribute to the structural integrity of the 'pocket'. Importantly, some ABD missense mutants diminish equilibrium androgen-binding affinity *and* increase the rate of androgen–receptor complex dissociation[14]. Others do one[15] or the other[14]. The reason(s) for this difference are not clear. Some ABD mutants with low affinity for androgen increase androgen receptor degradation alone[15] or with diversion to a non-androgen-binding state[16]. Indeed, some missense mutations alter androgen binding in an androgen-selective way[14]. Hence, different missense mutations must alter the pocket in subtly different ways. No ABD missense mutant is known to affect solely an ABD subsidiary function. Thus, the structural substrates for the ABD subsidiary functions are intimately intertwined with those for androgen binding itself.

Missense ABD mutants yield three degrees of androgen insensitivity according to the external genitalia: *complete or incomplete,* when the external genitalia are female or near-female; *partial,* when the external genitalia are appreciably ambiguous; *mild,* when the external genitalia are

male or near-male. Within families, external genitalia usually vary little. In rare families, external genitalia may vary from complete to mild androgen insensitivity. Among families with the same mutation, external genitalia phenotype may vary by one degree. Thus, para-receptor factors influence external genitalia phenotype significantly. Yet, among families, alternative missense mutations at single codons may yield reproducibly different degrees of androgen insensitivity[17]. Impaired spermatogenesis is not an obligate feature of mild androgen insensitivity[18], nor is gynecomastia[19]. Yet either may be the only sign of constitutional mild androgen insensitivity. Therefore, the overall transcriptional regulatory competence of a particular mutant androgen receptor depends on the transcriptional cofactor environments of a given set of target genes.

The normal unliganded ABD has a conformation that renders it a transcriptional repressor. Among the supporting evidence are three facts. First, an androgen receptor with a sufficiently long C-terminal ABD deletion (for example, Δ715–919) is constitutively transactive when cotransfected into an androgen receptor-free host cell together with an androgen-responsive reporter gene[8]. (Parenthetically, because of androgen receptor protein or mRNA[20] instability, 46,XY humans with germline nonsense mutations that should produce comparable C-terminally truncated androgen receptors have complete androgen insensitivity.) Second, androgen, but not anti-androgen, protects a 30-kDa fragment, corresponding to the ABD, when *in vitro* synthesized androgen receptor is exposed to partial proteolysis[21]. Third, the missense mutation, Thr877Ala, permits the androgen receptor in LNCaP cells to form complexes with the pure anti-androgen, hydroxyflutamide, that are fully transactive[22]; normal androgen receptor-hydroxyflutamide complexes cannot even bind ARE normally[10].

Some germline missense mutations in the DBD of the human androgen receptor cause complete androgen insensitivity[23]; others cause partial androgen insensitivity[24]. Interestingly, none is known to cause mild androgen insensitivity. These genotype–phenotype correlations will help to elucidate the physiological significance of the physico-chemical interaction(s) between a particular DBD mutant and a set of AREs.

No missense mutations in the N-terminal modulatory domain of the human androgen receptor have been proven to be pathogenic. Eight of ten point mutations we have detected in this region are of the nonsense variety, or are deletions, insertions that frameshift to premature translation termination.

Artificial mutant androgen receptors in which the polyglutamine (polyGln) tract of the N-terminal modulatory domain is deleted cleanly[25], or nearly so[26], are transcriptionally hyperactive in various cotransfection systems. In view of previous reports that androgen receptors with N-terminal[27] or interstitial[28] deletions removing the polyGln tract are transcriptionally inferior, the foregoing observation is provocative in three respects. First, it indicates that a polyGln tract collaborates with the flanking sequence when it contributes to the overall activity of the modulatory domain. Second, it suggests that a normal-size polyGln tract can repress the transactivity of a polyGln-free androgen receptor. Third, it provides one explanation, transactivational inferiority, for the mild androgen insensitivity that accompanies spinobulbar muscular atrophy (Kennedy syndrome) when the polyGln tract is expanded to $n \geq 40$[25].

Finally, contrary to conventional dogma, it has become clear that the three major structural modules of the androgen receptor are not functionally autonomous. Alterations in the N-terminal modulatory domain affect androgen binding[15], dimerization[10] and nuclear translocation[8]. Likewise, alterations in the DNA-binding domain may affect androgen binding[23]. Thus, the trimodular approach to analysing androgen receptor structure–function relations is useful but simplistic: a full understanding requires recognition of the intimate functional interaction among its three modules.

References

1. Kuiper, G. G. J. M., Faber, P. W., van Rooij, H. C. J., van der Korput, J. A. G. M., Ris-Stalpers, C., Klaassen, P., Trapman, J. and Brinkmann, A. O. (1989). Structural organization of the human androgen receptor gene. *J. Mol. Endocrinol.*, **2**, R1–4
2. Brown, C. J., Goss, S. J., Lubahn, D. B., Joseph, D. R., Wilson, E. M., French, F. S. and Willard, H. F. (1989). Androgen receptor locus on the human X chromosome: regional localization to Xq11-12 and description of a DNA polymorphism. *Am. J. Hum. Genet.*, **44**, 264–9
3. Faber, P. W., van Rooij, H. C. J., van der Korput, H. A. G. M., Baarends, W. M., Brinkmann, A. O., Grootegoed, J. A. and Trapman, J. (1991). Characterization of the human androgen receptor transcription unit. *J. Biol. Chem.*, **266**, 10743–9
4. Tilley, W. D., Marcelli, M. and McPhaul, M. J. (1990). Expression of the human androgen receptor gene utilizes a common promoter in diverse human tissues and cell lines. *J. Biol. Chem.*, **265**, 13776–81
5. Faber, P. W., van Rooij, H. C. J., Schipper, H. J., Brinkmann, A. O. and Trapman, J. (1993). Two different, overlapping pathways of transcription initiation are active on the TATA-less human androgen receptor promoter. *J. Biol. Chem.*, **268**, 9296–301
6. Mizokami, A., Yeh, S.-Y. and Chang, C. (1994). Identification of 3', 5'-cyclic adenosine monophosphate response element and other *cis*-acting elements in the human androgen receptor gene promoter. *Mol. Endocrinol.*, **8**, 77–88
7. Kuiper, G. G. J. M., de Ruiter, P. E., Trapman, J., Boersma, W. J. A., Grootegoed, J. A. and Brinkmann, A. O. (1993). Localization and hormonal stimulation of phosphorylation sites in the LNCaP-cell androgen receptor. *Biochem. J.*, **291**, 95–101
8. Zhou, Z.-X., Sar, M., Simental, J. A., Lane, M. V. and Wilson, E. M. (1994). A ligand-dependent bipartite nuclear targeting signal in the human androgen receptor. *J. Biol. Chem.*, **269**, 13115–23

9. Smith, D. F. and Toft, D. O. (1993). Steroid receptors and their associated proteins. *Mol. Endocrinol.*, **7**, 4–11

10. Wong, C.-I., Zhou, Z.-X., Sar, M. and Wilson, E. M. (1993). Steroid requirement for androgen receptor dimerization and DNA binding. *J. Biol. Chem.*, **268**, 19004–12

11. Tsai, M.-J, and O'Malley, B. W. (1994). Molecular mechanisms of action of steroid/thyroid receptor superfamily members. *Annu. Rev. Biochem.*, **63**, 451–86

12. Krongard, A., Wilson, C. M., Wilson, J. D., Allman, D. R. and McPhaul, M. J. (1991). Androgen increases androgen receptor protein while decreasing receptor mRNA in LNCaP cells. *Mol. Cell. Endocrinol.*, **76**, 79–88

13. Levine, M. and Manley, J. L. (1989). Transcriptional repression of eukaryotic promoters. *Cell*, **59**, 405–8

14. Kazemi-Esfarjani, P., Beitel, L. K., Trifiro, M., Kaufman, M., Rennie, P., Sheppard, P., Matusik, R. and Pinsky, L. (1993). Substitution of valine-865 by methionine or leucine in the human androgen receptor causes complete or partial androgen insensitivity, respectively with distinct androgen receptor phenotypes. *Mol. Endocrinol.*, **7**, 37–46

15. Zhou, Z.-X., Lane, M. V., Kemppainen, J. A., French, F. S. and Wilson, E. M. (1995). Specificity of ligand-dependent androgen receptor stabilization: receptor domain interactions influence ligand dissociation and receptor stability. *Mol. Endocrinol.*, **9**, 208–18

16. Beitel, L. K., Kazemi-Esfarjani, P., Kaufman, M., Lumbroso, R., DiGeorge, A. M., Killinger, D. W., Trifiro, M. A. and Pinsky, L. (1994). Substitution of arginine-839 by cysteine or histidine in the androgen receptor causes different receptor phenotypes in cultured cells and coordinate degrees of clinical androgen resistance. *J. Clin. Invest.*, **94**, 546–54

17. Patterson, M. N., Hughes, I. A., Gottlieb, B. and Pinsky, P. (1994). The androgen receptor gene mutations database. *Nucleic Acids Res.*, **22**, 3560–2

18. Tsukada, T., Inoue, M., Tachibana, S., Nakai, Y. and Takebe, H. (1994). An androgen receptor mutation causing androgen resistance in undervirilized male syndrome. *J. Clin. Endocrinol. Metab.*, B **79**, 1202–7

19. Pinsky, L., Kaufman, M. and Killinger, D. W. (1989). Impaired spermatogenesis is not an obligate expression of receptor-defective androgen resistance. *Am. J. Med. Genet.*, **32**, 100–4

20. Urlaub, G., Mitchell, P. J., Ciudad, C. J. and Chasin, L. A. (1989). Nonsense mutations in the dihydrofolate reductase gene affect RNA processing. *Mol. Cell. Biol.*, **9**, 2868–80

21. Kallio, P. J., Janne, O. A. and Plavimo, J. J. (1994). Agonists, but not antagonists, alter the conformation of the hormone-binding domain of androgen receptor. *Endocrinology*, **134**, 998–1001

22. Veldscholte, J., Berrevoets, C. A., Brinkmann, A. O., Grootegoed, J. A. and Mulder, E. (1992). Anti-androgens and the mutated androgen receptor of LNCaP cells: differential effects on binding affinity, heat-shock protein interaction, and transcription activation. *Biochemistry*, **31**, 2393–9

23. Beitel, L. K., Prior, L., Vasiliou, D. M., Gottlieb, B., Kaufman, M., Lumbroso, R., Alvarado, C., McGillivray, B., Trifiro, M. and Pinsky, L. (1994). Complete androgen insensitivity due to mutations in the probable α-helical segments of the DNA-binding domain in the human androgen receptor. *Hum. Mol. Genet.*, **3**, 21–7

24. Klocker, H., Kaspar, F., Eberle, J., Uberreiter, S., Radmayr, C. and Bartsch, G. (1992). Point mutation in the DNA binding domain of the androgen receptor in two families with Reifenstein syndrome. *Am. J. Hum. Genet.*, **50**, 1318–27

25. Kazemi-Esfarjani, P., Trifiro, M. A. and Pinsky, L. (1995). Evidence for a repressive function of the long polyglutamine tract in the human androgen receptor: possible pathogenetic relevance for the $(CAG)_n$ expanded neuronopathies. *Hum. Mol. Genet.*, **4**, 523–7

26. Chamberlain, N. L., Driver, E. D. and Miesfeld, R. L. (1994). The length and location of CAG trinucleotide repeats in the androgen receptor N-terminal domain affect transactivation function. *Nucleic Acids Res.*, **22**, 3181–6

27. Simental, J. A., Sar, M., Lane, M. V., French, F. S. and Wilson, E. M. (1991). Transcriptional activation and nuclear targeting signals of the human androgen receptor. *J. Biol. Chem.*, **266**, 510–18

28. Jenster, G., van der Korput, H. A. G. M., van Vroonhoven, C., van der Kwast, T. H., Trapman, J. and Brinkmann, A. O. (1991). Domains of the human androgen receptor involved in steroid binding, transcriptional activation, and subcellular localization. *Mol. Endocrinol.*, **5**, 1396–404

The clinical and molecular spectrum of disorders of the androgen receptor

37

J. E. Griffin, J. D. Wilson and M. J. McPhaul

The androgen resistance syndromes are single-gene disorders of phenotypic sexual development in 46,XY individuals who have bilateral testes, normal regression of the Müllerian ducts and normal testosterone secretion. The known molecular defects responsible for androgen resistance involve either the steroid 5α-reductase 2 enzyme or the androgen receptor[1].

Steroid 5α-reductase 2 deficiency is an autosomal recessive disorder characterized by a distinct phenotype in which Wolffian structures are male in character but the urogenital sinus and external genitalia are female. At the time of expected puberty, some virilization of the external genitalia occurs, and axillary and pubic hair develop. The breasts remain male in character. The testes are well developed, but spermatogenesis is usually diminished. Testosterone production, estrogen production and serum testosterone levels are in the normal male range. Dihydrotestosterone levels are low. Approximately 50 families with the disorder have been reported, and the specific mutation in the enzyme has been characterized in the majority[2]. This disorder is to be distinguished from the receptor disorders, the subject of this review.

Disorders of androgen receptor function cause a spectrum of phenotypic abnormalities in genetic males, ranging from phenotypic women with complete testicular feminization to minimally affected men. Although the various syndromes differ in their clinical manifestations, they have similar X-linked inheritance and hormonal profiles.

Subjects with complete testicular feminization have a female phenotype, except that axillary and pubic hair are diminished or absent. The external genitalia are those of a normal woman, and the vagina is short and blind-ending. Except for the testes, internal genital structures are usually absent. The testes may be located in the abdomen, along the course of the inguinal canal or in the labia majora. Spermatogenesis is incomplete or absent, and Leydig cells are normal. Affected individuals undergo a normal pubertal growth spurt and feminization.

Incomplete testicular feminization resembles the complete disorder except that there is partial fusion of the labioscrotal folds and usually some clitoromegaly at birth. At puberty, pubic hair develops, the clitoris enlarges, and female breasts develop. Wolffian duct derivatives are usually present.

Reifenstein's syndrome encompasses several forms of incomplete male pseudohermaphroditism. The predominant phenotype is male, and the usual manifestation is perineoscrotal hypospadias in a child or severe gynecomastia and hypospadias in an adult. However, the spectrum in a single family may range from infertile men with gynecomastia to individuals with such severe defects in virilization that a pseudovagina is present and gender assignment is female. Axillary and pubic hair are normal, but chest and facial hair are minimal. Cryptorchidism is common, the testes are small, and sperm production is decreased or absent. Some individuals have defects in Wolffian duct derivatives such as absence or hypoplasia of the vas deferens.

The infertile male syndrome is a disorder of phenotypically normal men in whom isolated infertility is the only consistent manifestation of androgen resistance. Although some men in families with Reifenstein's syndrome have only azoospermia, this syndrome appears to also occur in men without a family history of the disorder. Evaluation of men with normal external genitalia, apparently normal Wolffian structures, and infertility due to azoospermia or severe oligospermia, has revealed that an androgen receptor abnormality is present in a fraction of them[1].

The undervirilized fertile male syndrome is manifested by gynecomastia, a small penis, decreased beard and body hair, a normal male urethra, and normal sperm density but usually decreased ejaculate volume. The family history is often positive, and some affected men are fertile[1].

The most recently recognized manifestation of an androgen receptor disorder is the late development of gynecomastia with or without oligospermia, testicular atrophy and impotence in men with X-linked spinobulbar muscular atrophy (also called Kennedy's disease) (see reference 3 for review). These men have a hormonal pattern similar to that in disorders of the androgen receptor (see below).

The endocrine profile has been best characterized in complete testicular feminization but is similar in all disorders of the androgen receptor. Serum testosterone concentrations and rates of testosterone production by the testes are normal or higher than normal. The elevated testosterone production is caused by increased luteinizing hormone secretion, which results from defective feedback regulation due to androgen resistance at the hypothalamic–pituitary level. The increased secretion of luteinizing hormone also leads to increased testicular estrogen secretion. Variable androgen resistance coupled with enhanced estrogen production is presumably responsible for the varying degrees of defective virilization and enhanced feminization in different subjects.

Androgen receptor binding in fibroblasts grown from biopsies of individuals from 130 families with androgen resistance has been studied in our laboratory[1]. In 33 families, binding was absent or nearly absent, most commonly in association with complete testicular feminization. In 56 families, the receptor binding was qualitatively abnormal, usually manifested as thermolability or rapid dissociation, and as-

sociated with variable phenotypes. A decreased amount of apparently normal receptor was present in subjects in 18 families, usually in those with a predominant male phenotype. In 23 families with variable phenotypes, androgen receptor binding was normal in spite of endocrine and phenotypic evidence of androgen resistance.

The cloning of the complementary DNA (cDNA) for the human androgen receptor made it possible to characterize mutations in the gene[1]. Specific mutations have been identified in many patients. Southern blotting was used to identify large deletions, and exon amplification by polymerase chain reaction followed by sequencing has been used to detect point mutations. Assessment of functional capacity using a steroid response element with a reporter gene has also proved useful in characterizing mutant receptors.

Most of the subjects in whom genetic mutations have been identified have complete testicular feminization. The diverse mechanisms responsible include partial or complete gene deletions, mutations that result in aberrant splicing of androgen receptor messenger RNA (mRNA), and nucleotide replacements that cause either the introduction of premature termination codons or amino acid substitutions[1].

Single amino acid substitutions are most common in two regions of the receptor protein: the DNA-binding domain and the hormone-binding domain. Mutations in the DNA-binding domain are responsible for the 'no abnormality identified' category identified in the fibroblast studies. Mutations in this region impair binding of the hormone–receptor complex to DNA and result in a receptor incapable of modulating the activity of a reporter gene. Amino acid substitutions in the hormone-binding domain of the receptor cause a variety of ligand binding abnormalities ranging from absent androgen binding to qualitatively abnormal androgen binding. Fewer genetic mutations have been reported in patients with incomplete testicular feminization and Reifenstein's syndrome. All defects to date have been traced to single amino acid substitutions within the receptor protein with resultant impairment in receptor function. However, these mutant receptors are less severely impaired in activating a reporter gene than those of patients with complete testicular feminization. Point mutations resulting in single amino acid substitutions in the hormone-binding domain have also been reported for individuals with the infertile male syndrome[4] and the undervirilized fertile male syndrome[5].

The most unexpected alteration in the androgen receptor has been in patients with spinobulbar muscular atrophy. In this disorder, the usual 20 glutamine repeat homopolymeric region is expanded to 40 or more glutamines[3]. Initial studies of receptor binding revealed no change or a decreased amount of qualitatively normal androgen binding, but it is now clear that this change is associated with a modest decrease in transactivation[3,6]. How this decrease in androgen receptor function and the associated mild clinical androgen resistance relate to the progressive degeneration of anterior motor neurons is unclear[3].

Excluding spinobulbar muscular atrophy, the distribution of types of mutations are approximately: deletions (including small-scale)

11%; splicing abnormalities 3%; premature termination codons 10%; and amino acid substitutions 76%. About 85% of the amino acid substitutions are in the hormone-binding domain, and the remainder are in the DNA-binding domain[1].

Although it is established that mutations in the androgen receptor gene cause the different phenotypes characteristic of the androgen resistance, by interfering with receptor function to different degrees, patients may have identical mutations but distinctive phenotypes[1]. The level or timing of androgen receptor expression, the rate of testosterone synthesis or metabolism, and a variety of other factors could all be invoked as possible explanations. In support of the possible role of hormone metabolism in affecting receptor function, androgen levels influence the stability of the hormone–receptor complex and receptor function[7]. Studies of mutant androgen receptors with amino acid substitutions in the hormone-binding domain reveal that transactivation is enhanced by increased hormone concentrations, increased frequency of hormone addition, and the presence of nonmetabolizable androgen analogs[7].

References

1. Griffin, J. E., McPhaul, M. J., Russell, D. W. and Wilson, J. D. (1995). The androgen resistance syndromes: steroid 5α-reductase 2 deficiency, testicular feminization, and related disorders. In Scriver, C. R., Beaudet, A. L., Sly, W. S. and Valle, D. (eds.) *Metabolic and Molecular Bases of Inherited Disease*, 7th edn., pp. 2967–98. (New York: McGraw-Hill)
2. Wilson, J. D., Griffin, J. E. and Russell, D. W. (1993). Steroid 5α-reductase 2 deficiency. *Endocr. Rev.*, **14**, 577–93
3. Trifiro, M. A., Kazemi-Esfarjani, P. and Pinsky, L. (1994). X-linked muscular atrophy and the androgen receptor. *Trends Endocrinol. Metab.*, **5**, 416–21
4. Yong, E. L., Ng, S. C., Roy, A. C., Yun, G. and Ratnam, S. S. (1994). Pregnancy after hormonal correction of severe spermatogenic defect due to

mutation in androgen receptor gene. *Lancet*, **344**, 826–7
5. Tsukada, T., Inque, M., Tachibana, S., Nakai, Y. and Takebe, H. (1994). An androgen receptor mutation causing androgen resistance in undervirilized male syndrome. *J. Clin. Endocrinol. Metab.*, **79**, 1202–7
6. Chamberlain, N. L., Driver, E. D. and Miesfeld, R. L. (1994). The length and location of CAG trinucleotide repeats in the androgen receptor N-terminal domain affect transactivation function. *Nucleic Acids Res.*, **22**, 3181–6
7. Marcelli, M., Zoppi, S., Wilson, C. M., Griffin, J. E. and McPhaul, M. J. (1994). Amino acid substitutions in the hormone-binding domain of the human androgen receptor alter the stability of the hormone receptor complex. *J. Clin. Invest.*, **94**, 1642–50

Anti-Müllerian hormone in normal and malignant granulosa cells

R. Rey, C. Lhommé, J.-M. Bidart and N. Josso

38

Introduction

Anti-Müllerian hormone (AMH), also known as Müllerian inhibiting substance (MIS) or factor (MIF), a 140-kDa homodimeric glycoprotein that belongs to the transforming growth factor β (TGF-β) family, is encoded by a 2.75 kb gene located on the short arm of chromosome 19[1]. In the male, AMH is responsible for the regression of Müllerian ducts, which give rise in the female to the uterus, the Fallopian tubes and the upper part of the vagina. AMH is secreted from the earliest stages of testicular differentiation up to puberty, representing a specific marker of immature Sertoli cells. The timing of AMH secretion during fetal development is very important as Müllerian ducts become insensitive to AMH after the 8th fetal week[1].

Ovarian production of AMH

Granulosa cells of the ovary and testicular Sertoli cells share many structural and functional characteristics[2]. Production of AMH in the ovary can be visualized in the cytoplasm of granulosa cells of developing follicles by immunocytochemistry (Figure 1). In the mouse, AMH transcripts are first observed six days after birth by *in situ* hybridization[3]. The pattern of AMH production by the ovary is related to the degree of follicular maturation rather than to the age of the animal. As the follicle grows, the immunoreactivity of the granulosa cells close to the basal membrane progressively fades, while that of those lining the antrum and the cumulus oophorus increases[4,5]. Just before ovulation, AMH becomes undetectable in cumulus cells[3,5].

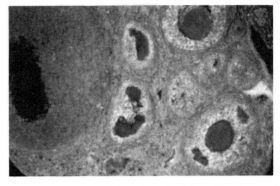

Figure 1 Immunohistochemical localization of AMH in an ovarian follicle of an adult female mouse

AMH production by granulosa cells is low compared to that of immature Sertoli cells; however, ovarian and testicular AMH have similar anti-Müllerian activity when tested at similar concentrations in a bioassay[1].

Using an enzyme-linked immunoassay (ELISA), we measured AMH levels in the serum of 59 normal women. Serum AMH was undetectable or very low (less than 5 ng/ml) prior to menopause and then became undetectable[6].

Biological effects of AMH in the ovary

It is easy to understand why the fetal ovary does not produce AMH. In bovine freemartins, i.e. heterosexual twins united by placental anastomoses, high AMH levels are present in both fetuses, inducing Müllerian duct and ovarian regression in the female fetus[1]. Transgenic female mice expressing high amounts of AMH

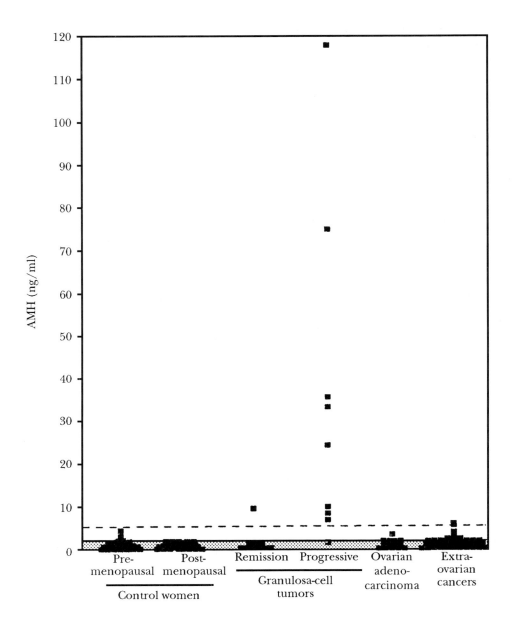

Figure 2 Serum AMH levels in normal women and in patients with ovarian and extra-ovarian cancers. The shaded area indicates the limit of sensitivity of our assay (2 ng/ml), which is not exceeded in postmenopausal or ovariectomized women. The dotted line (5 ng/ml) indicates the highest level observed in normal premenopause[6]

in gonadal and non-gonadal tissues lack a uterus and have ovaries which progressively lose germ cells and either disappear or develop cordlike structures resembling testicular seminiferous tubules[7,8]. AMH represses aromatase activity in the fetal and immature ovary[9,10] . In the post-natal ovary, AMH also decreases the expression of luteinizing hormone receptors in the granulosa cells[10], and opposes epidermal growth factor-induced progesterone biosynthesis[11]. The negative effect of AMH on these markers of granulosa-cell differentiation suggests that it may be implicated in the control of ovarian follicle maturation, a hypothesis supported by the fact that the AMH receptor is expressed in granulosa cells[12].

AMH production by granulosa-cell tumors

Granulosa-cell tumors belong to a relatively rare category of ovarian tumors, the sex-cord stromal tumors; yet, they account for 6–10% of all ovarian cancers and may recur, even many years after surgical treatment. When the tumor recurs, the prognosis is poor unless the diagnosis is made when its size is still small. Thus, the availability of a serum marker is of great importance. Increased levels of serum AMH have been reported in three patients with a granulosa-cell tumor by Gustafson and co-workers[13]. In order to investigate further the sensitivity and specificity of serum AMH as tumor marker, we studied serum AMH levels during up to 44 months of follow-up in patients with a diagnosis of granulosa-cell tumor, as well as in women with other types of ovarian and extra-ovarian cancers. Serum AMH was between 6.8 and 117.9 ng/ml in eight of nine patients with a progressive granulosa-cell tumor and undetectable in the remaining case (Figure 2). Serum AMH fell to undetectable values after successful treatment (Figure 3a), but remained high when the tumor was resistant to chemotherapy (Figure 3b). In three cases, serum AMH rose again up to two years before a clinical recurrence of the tumor could be detected (Figure 3c). Serum AMH was within control levels, i.e. less than 5 ng/ml before and undetectable after menopause, in 93% of patients with other ovarian or extra-ovarian cancers (Figure 2). In the remaining 7%, serum AMH was very close to normal values (< 5.9 ng/ml). When compared with inhibin, a well-accepted marker for granulosa-cell tumors[14], serum AMH and inhibin levels were significantly correlated during

progressive disease. However, during clinical remission, while serum AMH was undetectable in

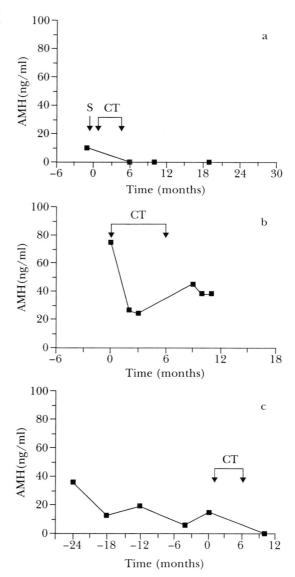

Figure 3 Serum AMH levels during follow-up in patients with a diagnosis of granulosa-cell tumor. (a) Patient successfully treated by surgery (S) and chemotherapy (CT); (b) patient in whom a resistance to chemotherapy (CT) was observed; (c) patient with a recurrence of a granulosa-cell tumor that became clinically detectable two years after the elevation of serum AMH[6]. Time 0 indicates the date of clinical diagnosis

the follow-up of ten of 11 patients, serum inhibin levels fluctuated between normal and elevated levels more frequently. Therefore, AMH seem slightly more specific as a marker of granulosa-cell tumors. The reason for this could be that while AMH is synthesized exclusively by the ovarian follicle, inhibin is also produced by the pituitary, adrenal and bone marrow[15].

In summary, serum AMH appears to be a sensitive, specific and reliable marker of granulosa-cell tumors, proving useful in the evaluation of the efficacy of treatment and for the early detection of recurrences.

Acknowledgements

This work has been supported in part by CRC no. 95.4, Institut Gustave Roussy, Villejuif, France, and by the Association de Recherche sur le Cancer (ARC), France

References

1. Josso, N., Cate, R. L., Picard, J. Y., Vigier, B., di Clemente, N., Wilson, C., Imbeaud, S., Pepinsky, R. B., Guerrier, D., Boussin, L., Legeai, L. and Carré-Eusèbe, D. (1993). Anti-Müllerian hormone, the Jost factor. In Bardin, C. W. (ed.) *Recent Progress in Hormone Research*, pp. 1–59. (San Diego: Academic Press)

2. Vigier, B., Picard, J. Y., Tran, D., Legeai, L. and Josso, N. (1984). Production of anti-Müllerian hormone: another homology between Sertoli and granulosa cells. *Endocrinology*, **114**, 1315–20

3. Münsterberg, A. and Lovell-Badge, R. (1991). Expression of the mouse anti-Müllerian hormone gene suggests a role in both male and female sex differentiation. *Development*, **118**, 613–24

4. Bézard, J., Vigier, B., Tran, D., Mauléon, P. and Josso, N. (1987). Immunocytochemical study of anti-Müllerian hormone in sheep ovarian follicles during fetal and postnatal development. *J. Reprod. Fertil.*, **80**, 509–16

5. Ueno, S., Takahashi, M., Manganaro, T. F., Ragin, R. C. and Donahoe, P. K. (1989). Cellular localization of Mullerian inhibiting substance in the developing rat ovary. *Endocrinology*, **124**, 1000–6

6. Rey, R., Lhommé, C., Marcillac, I., Lahlou, N., Duvilland, P., Josso, N. and Bidart, J. (1995). Anti-Müllerian hormone as a serum marker of granulosa-cell tumors of the ovary: comparative study with serum α-inhibin and estradiol. *Am. J. Obstet. Gynecol.*, in press

7. Behringer, R. R., Cate, R. L., Froelick, G. J., Palmiter, R. D. and Brinster, R. L. (1990). Abnormal sexual development in transgenic mice chronically expressing Müllerian inhibiting substance. *Nature*, **345**, 167–70

8. Lyet, L., Louis, F., Forest, M. G., Josso, N., Behringer, R. R. and Vigier, B. (1995). Ontogeny of reproductive abnormalities induced by deregulation of anti-Müllerian hormone expression in transgenic mice. *Biol. Reprod.*, **52**, 444–54

9. Vigier, B., Forest, M. G., Eychenne, B., Bézard, J., Garrigou, O., Robel, P. and Josso, N. (1989). Anti-Müllerian hormone produces endocrine sex-reversal of fetal ovaries. *Proc. Natl. Acad. Sci. USA*, **56**, 3684–8

10. di Clemente, N., Goxe, B., Rémy, J. J., Cate, R. L., Josso, N., Vigier, B. and Salesse, R. (1994). Effect of AMH upon aromatase activity and LH receptors of granulosa cells of rat and porcine immature ovaries. *Endocrine*, **2**, 553–8

11. Kim, J. H., Seibel, M. M., MacLaughlin, D. T., Donahoe, P. K., Ransil, B. J., Hametz, P. A. and Richards, C. J. (1992). The inhibitory effects of Mullerian-inhibiting substance on epidermal growth factor induced proliferation and progesterone production of human granulosa-luteal cells. *J. Clin. Endocrinol. Metab.*, **75**, 911–17

12. di Clemente, N., Wilson, C. A., Faure, E., Boussin, L., Carmillo, P., Tizard, R., Picard, J. Y., Vigier, B., Josso, N. and Cate, R. L. (1994). Cloning, expression and alternative splicing of the receptor for anti-Müllerian hormone. *Mol. Endocrinol.*, **8**, 1006–20

13. Gustafson, M. L., Lee, M. M., Scully, R. E., Moncure, A. C., Hirakawa, T., Goodman, A., Muntz, H. G., Donahoe, P. K., MacLaughlin, D. T. and Fuller, A. F. (1992). Müllerian inhibiting substance as a marker for ovarian sex-cord tumor. *N. Engl. J. Med.*, **326**, 466–71

14. Burger, H. G. (1994). Inhibin as a tumour marker. *Clin. Endocrinol.*, **41**, 151–3

15. Vale, W., Bilezikjian, L. M. and Rivier, C. (1994). Reproductive and other roles of inhibins and activins. In Knobil, E. and Neill, J. D. (eds.) *The Physiology of Reproduction*, pp. 1861–78. (New York: Raven Press)

4

Androlology

Management of male problems   39

S. Gordts, M. Vercruyssen, P. Roziers, J. Donnez, S. Bassil and R. Campo

Introduction

After the introduction of intracytoplasmic sperm injection as a treatment for extreme male subfertility problems and the excellent results reported by Palermo and colleagues[1], several centers worldwide have successfully applied this technique in their program of assisted reproduction. Owing to the high success rates obtained after intracytoplasmic sperm injection[1–8], which are sometimes better than the results obtained by some centers after normal *in vitro* fertilization (IVF) for non-male problems, it has been suggested that all techniques of assisted reproduction should be replaced by intracytoplasmic sperm injection, and some authors question the value of andrological examinations and therapy.

This attitude is dangerous, however. Even though the results obtained after intracytoplasmic sperm injection are excellent, and it is very inviting to widen the scale of indications, the technique remains intrusive and bypasses the normal fertilization selection processes.

A complete semen analysis is fundamental, although these preliminary parameters have not always answered our expectations in the past, resulting in some lack of confidence in the 'standard' semen analysis. The introduction of strict criteria for evaluation of sperm morphology[9] expressed the need to have more reliable data to predict the fertilization outcome in assisted reproduction.

Andrology laboratories now offer more functional and biochemical tests, such as assessment of the spontaneous acrosome reaction, the capacity of sperm–zona binding with the hemizona assay, evaluation of different sperm preparation methods and analysis of the presence of antisperm antibodies. Research is

continuing to develop more specific tests with a higher predictive value of fertilization outcome. In this regard, the testing of the presence of mannose binding sites on sperm is very promising, and correlates well with the potential of sperm to bind to the ZP3 sperm receptor molecule on the zona pellucida[10]. Now, more than ever, there is an urgent need for close collaboration between andrology laboratories and clinics of assisted reproduction.

Semen preparation techniques

Sperm preparation can be achieved by several methods. Currently, the most frequently employed are the swim-up procedure and the use of a Percoll gradient. The swim-up technique selects spermatozoa on the basis of their motility, with the Percoll gradient, the selection is based upon density. The use of Percoll has been found to be advantageous by Hall and co-workers[8], although they reported no benefit in the use of Percoll when the morphology was < 5%. These findings are in contrast with the data of Sapienza and associates[11], who found no difference between swim-up and Percoll-treated semen samples when the initial sperm quality was poor. The selection of morphologically normal sperm was even better after swim-up ($p = 0.05$). It is also interesting in this study that, in cases of initial poor semen quality, the fertilization rates in sibling oocytes were significantly higher after insemination with Percoll-treated sperm than after swim-up (51.3% vs. 37.8%), confirming that morphology alone is unlikely to offer a 100% prognosis. These higher fertilization rates after Percoll separation may be explained by the findings of Aitken[12], who postulated that the use of Percoll protects against the excessive formation of free oxygen radicals.

As there is some evidence that the timing of the acrosome reaction is important for the ability of penetrating the zona pellucida[13], evaluation of this acrosome reaction process is important; a premature spontaneous acrosome reaction will have a negative effect on the fertilization process. In our laboratory we performed an evaluation of the percentage of spontaneous acrosome reactions during different techniques of sperm preparation: layering technique, layering technique and follicular fluid, swim-up technique and a 40–90 Percoll gradient. The percentage of acrosome-reacted sperm was respectively 17.2, 14.6, 32.7 and 21%. A positive correlation was found between the percentage of non-acrosome reacted spermatozoa and the fertilization rate[14].

Selection of the method of assisted reproduction

In cases of mild or moderate male subfertility, the use of intrauterine insemination can be considered as a valuable treatment before a couple is referred to an *in vitro* fertilization program. In cases of 'unexplained' infertility, intrauterine insemination can detect male factor problems. In the study of Depypere and colleagues[15], the pregnancy rate per cycle after intrauterine insemination following the use of a Percoll gradient was 18.4% vs. 8.1% after treatment of sperm with the swim-up technique. This study also demonstrated that pregnancies were usually obtained after three or four cycles with intrauterine insemination, and that couples who failed to conceive within this period received little or no benefit from continuing the treatment.

To increase pregnancy rates per cycle, we demonstrated that a mild ovulation induction with human menopausal gonadotropin (hMG) was favorable, whereas the use of clomiphene citrate alone and with human chorionic gonadotropin (hCG) had no advantage over a spontaneous cycle (24% vs. 13%)[16]. Peterson

and associates[17] concluded that a course of four cycles of intrauterine insemination with hMG was beneficial and should be the first-line therapy before IVF treatment was attempted.

In cases of moderate male subfertility it is not always easy to decide whether a more costly and time-consuming microfertilization technique or a 'heavy' insemination protocol should be preferred. Several reports now demonstrate good fertilization rates after the use of a heavy insemination concentration technique in which spermatozoa are added at a concentration of 1×10^6/ml per oocytes, reporting fertilization rates of 50–60%[18–22] in cases of moderate to severe male subfertility. A higher concentration of added sperm is recommended to compensate for the loss in fertilizing potential of the sperm. This has clearly been demonstrated in our data of subzonal sperm insertion (Figure 1). When morphology is < 14%, up to 15 sperm can be inserted subzonally without a great impact on the polyspermic fertilization rate, whereas in cases of normal morphology, the percentage of abnormally fertilized oocytes immediately increases to 22% with the insertion of 3–5 spermatozoa[23].

In our own series of 44 couples in which sibling oocytes were used for intracytoplasmic sperm injection or heavy insemination concentration, the fertilization rates were 57% and 32%, respectively, and fertilization was obtained in 85% and 41% of the cycles, respectively. These data are in accordance with the findings of Baker and colleagues[24]. In our study, pregnancy rates were not impaired by the use of high sperm concentrations (Table 1).

In view of the excellent results now obtained after intracytoplasmic sperm injection, the place of subzonal insemination, with its comparatively low and inconsistent fertilization rate and the risk of a high polyspermic fertilization rate, can be questioned. With the use of the laser, it should in the future become possible to simplify the methods of micromanipulation. An ultraviolet laser combined with an optical trapping infrared laser system requires no special training and no micromanipulators and is less time-consuming. In an experimental study, we

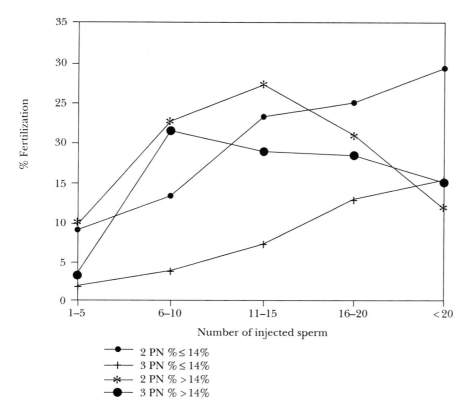

Figure 1 Number of subzonally inserted sperm correlated with the morphology and influence upon monospermic and polyspermic fertilization rate. PN, pronuclei

Table 1 Intracytoplasmic sperm injection (ICSI) and microdrop insemination (MD) in a first attempt for 44 couples with sperm morphology of < 14%

	ICSI	MD	MD + ICSI
Number of oocytes	326	303	
Number of fertilized oocytes	187 (57%)*	97 (32%)*	
Number of embryo transfers	27	7	
Number of mixed embryo transfers	–	–	13
Number of replaced embryos	75	16	41
Number of pregnancies/embryo transfers	9 (33%)	3 (43%)	5 (41%)
Implantation rate (%)	16	21	20.5

*$p < 0.001$

evaluated the usefulness of such a system (PALM laser, Wolfsrathausen, Germany) in mouse gametes[25,26]. At this time, intracytoplasmic sperm injection is the treatment of choice in cases of severe male subfertility, and must be used in cases of persistent failure of IVF, extreme oligo-, astheno- and teratozoospermia, probably with a cut-off level of 5% of normal forms.

Our results after intracytoplasmic sperm injection are listed in Table 2. Analyzing the quality of embryos[27] obtained after intra-

Table 2 Results from 103 intracytoplasmic sperm injection (ICSI) cycles

Number of patients	96
Number of cycles	103
Number of aspirated oocytes	1110
Number of injected oocytes	797
Number of degenerated oocytes	58 (7.3%)
Number of fertilized oocytes	547 (74%)
Number of fertilized oocytes 3PN	10 (1.8%)
Number of embryo transfers	95
mixed	6
only ICSI	89
Number of pregnancies per transfer	24 (27%)
Number of pregnancies per cycle	24 (23%)
Number of transferred embryos	175
Implantation rate per embryo	17%
Number of successful pregnancies	18 (19% of embryo transfers)
single	13
twin	5
Number of abortions	4 (17%)
Biochemical pregnancies	2 (8%)

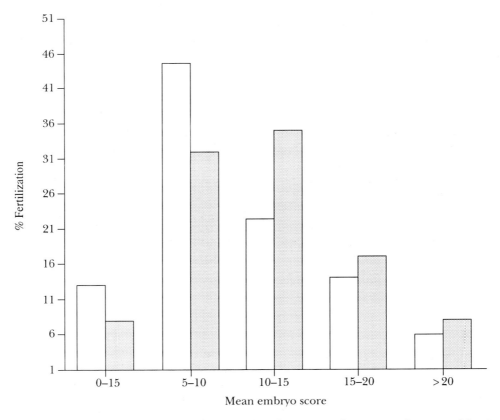

Figure 2 Quality of transferred embryos expressed as the mean embryo score after normal *in vitro* fertilization (hollow bars): 312 cycles and 630 embryos; and after intracytoplasmic sperm injection (shaded bars): 103 cycles and 280 embryos

cytoplasmic sperm injection, we found no difference in quality compared with the embryos obtained after IVF for non-male subfertility (Figure 2).

Discussion

The excellent results obtained after intracytoplasmic sperm injection[1,2] have now been reproduced by several other groups[4-8]. Because of its efficacy and reproducibility in terms of fertilization and pregnancy rates in cases of male subfertility, this technique is superior to any other form of micromanipulation. It guarantees fertilization and embryo transfer in nearly 90% of the started cycles, comparable with the data of our normal IVF population. In our study, none of the sperm parameters correlated with the success of intracytoplasmic sperm injection. Only in cases of total immotility of the sperm was the choice of viable sperm completely random. Using this technique we are now able to treat severe cases of male subfertility, impossible a decade ago. Injection of epididymal and testicular sperm has proven to result in good fertilization rates and pregnancy rates[3,28].

Although from the reported data in the literature[3] and from our own experience, there is no increased congenital malformation rate of the offspring, it is still unclear whether there might be a higher abnormality rate later in life which is not manifest at birth, or perhaps in the next generation. At this stage, it would be unwise to feel completely confident with the safety of the procedure. The data presented by Pang and co-workers[29], indicating an incidence of chromosomal aberrations of 19.6% in sperm from oligo–astheno–teratozoospermic patients compared with only 1.45% in sperm from fertile donors, needs our attention and questions the safety of the intracytoplasmic injection technique.

Using this technique, we must also be aware of the potentiality of injecting foreign DNA into the oocyte. Contamination may occur at several levels: microtools, polyvinylpyrrolidone solution, improperly prepared sperm and the possible danger of virus contamination.

Direct intracytoplasmic sperm injection is a palliative treatment for male subfertility, leaving the etiological factor unsolved. In most men the underlying cause of a defect in spermatogenesis is not known. Mutations and chromosomal aberrations may be the cause of fertilization failure. It is not impossible that such defects are passed through to the next generation, when direct sperm injection is used. In cases of moderate male subfertility, we therefore recommend use of a heavy insemination concentration technique at a first attempt or division of sibling oocytes for heavy insemination concentration and intracytoplasmic sperm injection. We agree with Tucker and associates[21] that we have to use the simplest and least expensive procedure to provide infertile couples with the highest long-term chance of conceiving healthy children. The challenge for the future will be to develop highly accurate andrological tests to predict the fertilizing potential of human spermatozoa, thus enabling us to treat couples by intracytoplasmic sperm injection only when it is strictly necessary.

References

1. Palermo, G., Joris, H., Devroey, P. and Van Steirteghem, A. C. (1992). Pregnancies after intracytoplasmic injection of single spermatozoa into an oocyte. *Lancet*, **340**, 17–18
2. Van Steirteghem, A. C., Liu, J., Joris, H., Nagy, Z., Janssenswillen, C., Tournaye, H., Derde, M.-P., Van Assche, E. and Devroey, P. (1993). Higher success rate by intracytoplasmic sperm injection than by subzonal insemination. Report of a second series of 300 consecutive treatment cycles. *Hum. Reprod.*, **8**, 1055–60
3. Van Steirteghem, A. C., Nagy, P., Liu, J., Joris, H., Smitz, J., Camus, M. and Devroey, P. (1994).

Intracytoplasmic sperm injection–ICSI. *Reprod. Med. Rev.*, **3**, 199–207

4. Payne, D., Flaherty, S. P., Jeffrey, R., Warnes, G. M. and Matthews, C. D. (1994). Successful treatment of severe male factor infertility in 100 consecutive cycles using intracytoplasmic sperm injection. *Hum. Reprod.*, **9**, 2051–7

5. Hamberger, L., Sjögren, A., Lundin, K., Söderlund, B. and Nilsson, L. (1993). Microfertilization techniques – Scandinavian experience. In Gordts, S. (ed.) *Current Status of Micromanipulation*, pp. 85–9. (Leuven: Drukkerij Nauwlaerts)

6. Tucker, M. J., Wright, G., Morton, P. C., Mayer, M. P., Ingargiola, P. E. and Jones, A. E. (1995). Practical evolution and application of direct intracytoplasmic sperm injection for male factor and idiopathic fertilization failure infertilities. *Fertil. Steril.*, **63**, 820–7

7. Gordts, S., Vercruyssen, M., Roziers, P., Bosmans, E., Campo, R. and Bassil, S. (1995). Intracytoplasmic sperm injection: embryo quality and the effect of training. Presented at the *IXTH World Congress on In Vitro Fertilization and Alternate Assisted Reproduction*, Vienna, April 3–7. *JARGE*, **12**, 848

8. Hall, J. A., Fishel, S. B., Timson, J. A., Dowell, K. and Klentzeris, L. D. (1995). Human sperm morphology evaluation pre- and post-Percoll gradient centrifugation. *Hum. Reprod.*, **10**, 342–6

9. Kruger, T. F., Acosta, A. A., Simmons, K. F., Swanson, R. J., Matta, J. F., Veeck, L. L., Morshedi, M. and Brugo, S. (1987). New method of evaluating sperm morphology with predicted value for human *in vitro* fertilization. *Urology*, **30**, 248–51

10. Benoff, S., Cooper, G. W., Hurley, I. R. and Hershlag, A. (1995). Calcium-ion channel blockers and sperm fertilization. *Rev. Ass. Reprod.*, **5**, 2–13

11. Sapienza, F., Verheyen, G., Tournaye, H., Janssens, R., Pletincx, I., Derde, M. and Van Steirteghem, A. (1993). An auto-controlled study in *in-vitro* fertilization reveals the benefit of Percoll centrifugation to swim-up in the preparation of poor-quality semen. *Hum. Reprod.*, **8**, 1856–62

12. Aitken, R. (1994). A free radical theory of male infertility. *Reprod. Fertil. Dev.*, **6**, 19–24

13. Tesarik, J. (1989). Appropriate timing of the acrosome reaction is a major requirement for the fertilizing spermatozoon. *Hum. Reprod.*, **4**, 957–61

14. Bassil, S., Stallaert, S., Verougstraete, J. C., Pensis, M., Donnez, J. and Gordts, S. (1995). Acrosome status according to the sperm preparation technique in *in vitro* fertilization. Presented at the *IXth World Congress on In Vitro Fertilization and Alternate Assisted Reproduction*, Vienna, April 3–7. *JARGE*, 12, 46S

15. Depypere, H., Millingos, S. and Comhaire, F. (1995). Intrauterine insemination in male subfertility: a comparative study of sperm preparation using a commercial Percoll kit and conventional sperm wash. *Eur. J. Obstet. Gynecol.*, in press

16. Depypere, H. T., Gordts, S., Campo, R. and Comhaire, F. (1994). Methods to increase the success rate of artificial insemination with donor semen. *Hum. Reprod.*, **9**, 661–3

17. Peterson, C. M., Hatasaka, H. H., Jones, K. P., Poulson, A. M., Carell, D. T. and Urry, R. L. (1994). Ovulation induction with gonadotropins and intrauterine insemination compared with *in vitro* fertilization and no therapy: a prospective, nonrandomized, cohort study and meta-analysis. *Fertil. Steril.*, **62**, 535–44

18. Fiorentino, A., Magli, M., Fortini, D., Feliciani, E., Ferrarretti, A., Dale, B. and Gianaroli, L. (1994). Sperm : oocyte ratios in an *in vitro* fertilization (IVF) program. *J. Assist. Reprod. Genet.*, **11**, 97–103

19. Hall, J., Fishel, S., Green, S., Fleming, S., Hunter, A., Stoddart, N., Dowell, K. and Thornton, S. (1995). Intracytoplasmic sperm injection versus high insemination concentration *in vitro* fertilization in cases of very severe teratozoospermia. *Hum. Reprod.*, **10**, 493–6

20. Ombelet, W., Fourie, F., Ie, R., Vandeput, H., Bosmans, E., Cox, A., Janssen, M. and Kruger, T. (1994). Teratozoospermia and *in vitro* fertilization; a randomized prospective study. *Hum. Reprod.*, **9**, 1479–84

21. Tucker, M., Wiker, G. and Massey, J. (1993). Rational approach to assisted fertilization. *Hum. Reprod.*, **8**, 1778

22. Hershlag, A., Cooper, G. W. and Benoff, S. (1995). Pregnancy following discontinuation of a calcium channel blocker in the male partner. *Hum. Reprod.*, **10**, 599–606

23. Gordts, S., Garcia, G., Vercruyssen, M., Roziers, P., Campo, R. and Swinnen, K. (1993). Subzonal insemination: a prospective randomized study in patients with abnormal sperm morphology. *Fertil. Steril.*, **60**, 307–13

24. Baker, H. W. G., Liu, D. Y., Bourne, H. and Lopata, A. (1993). Diagnosis of sperm defects in selecting patients for assisted fertilization. *Hum. Reprod.*, **8**, 1778–85

25. Gordts, S., Enginsu, E., Bassil, S., Pensis, M., Calmpo, R., Schütze, K. and Donnez, J. (1995). Combined use of an ultraviolet and infrared laser beam in the micromanipulation of mouse gametes. Presented at the *IXth World Congress on In Vitro Fertilization and Alternate Assisted Reproduction*, Vienna, April 3–7. *JARGE*, **12**, 108S

26. Enginsu, E., Schütze, K., Bellanca, S., Pensis, M., Campo, R., Bassil, S., Donnez, J. and Gordts, S.

(1995). Micromanipulation of mouse gametes with laser micro beam and optical tweezers. *Hum. Reprod.*, **10**, in press

27. Steer, C., Mills, C., Tan, S., Campbell, S. and Edwards, R. (1992). The cumulative embryo score: a predictive embryo scoring technique to select the optimal number of embryos to transfer in an *in-vitro* fertilization and embryo transfer programme. *Hum. Reprod.*, **7**, 117–19

28. Schoysman, R., Vanderzwalmen, P., Nijs, M., Segal, L., Segal-Bertin, G. and Geerts, L. (1993). Pregnancy after fertilisation with human testicular spermatozoa. *Lancet*, **342**, 1237

29. Pang, M. G., Zackowski, J. L., Hoegermann, S. F., Moon, S. Y., Cuticchia, A. J., Acosta, A. A. and Kearns, W. G. (1995). Presented at the *IXth World Congress on In Vitro Fertilization and Alternate Assisted Reproduction*, Vienna, April 3–7. *JARGE*, **12**, 53S

Assessment of sperm concentration 40

F. Comhaire, B. Depoorter, L. Vermeulen and F. Schoonjans

Necessity for sperm counting

New methods for treating infertile couples in whom the male factor is the major cause, can achieve pregnancies even in the absence of spermatozoa in the ejaculate (azoospermia). Hence, the question can be raised why sperm counting is still necessary.

In order to answer this question, we need to review the different purposes of semen analysis. First, we try to establish whether the semen sample originates from a man who is potentially fertile, subfertile, or infertile when trying to attain pregnancy through vaginal intercourse. Second, in case sperm quality is deficient, we wish to use the result of semen analysis to decide towards which mode of treatment the couple should be directed. Third, semen analysis may give information on the cause of the infertility helping us to select optimal treatment.

In addition, semen analysis may predict the probability of success of a particular treatment modality. It is also an increasingly important tool for research into the mechanisms of male reproduction, and the exact pathogenetic defects which cause its failure. Finally, sperm analysis is highly sensitive in revealing unfavorable environmental influences, as has been demonstrated from retrospective studies indicating dramatic deterioration of male reproductive capacity.

The next challenge is to select the method of semen analysis which will give the most accurate information to answer the questions raised above. Clearly, there is no such single test method and except for the occurrence of a normal pregnancy with the delivery of a healthy child, it is impossible to assess all the functions and the genetic content of spermatozoa.

Nevertheless, modern techniques of semen analysis including cytological, biochemical, microbiological and *in vitro* functional methods have made it possible to perform a battery of complementary tests assessing most aspects of spermatozoon 'efficiency'.

But what is the role of sperm counting in this context? In fact, its role is limited. It is important to know whether or not spermatozoa are present, and whether their number is 'few' or 'many', but sperm concentration has a rather poor power to discriminate between potentially fertile, subfertile or infertile semen. It is sperm motility that is the more important characteristic when *in vivo* conception (either through intercourse or through intrauterine insemination) is concerned, and sperm morphology when *in vitro* fertilization is performed.

Sperm concentration is useful for diagnostic purposes. Indeed, the total sperm output per ejaculate gives reliable information on the amount and functional state of the seminiferous epithelium. If sperm transport is not hindered, there is a close correlation between sperm output and testicular volume. The absence of such correlation, e.g. the finding of a low sperm output in a man with normal testicular volume, suggests sperm transport to be impaired either inside or outside the testes. The therapeutic approach in the latter cases will differ from that in cases where low sperm concentration is associated with decreased testicular volume.

Sperm concentration is also a useful marker of the general condition of the seminiferous epithelium, particularly in epidemiological studies, and for the evaluation of methods of male contraception.

Pitfalls in sperm counting

Semen is a viscous mixture of secretory products of different glands in which the spermatozoa are suspended. The concentration of spermatozoa not only depends on the number of cells produced, but also on the amount of fluid in which these are suspended. Because the latter varies considerably between men, and also in the same man at different ejaculations, sperm concentration presents important changes independent of the production capacity of the testes. Therefore, it is the total output of spermatozoa per ejaculate that must be taken into account when the functional state of the testes needs to be evaluated. However, it is the concentration per ml of ejaculate which is more important when the fertilizing potential of semen must be assessed, since the latter determines the number of spermatozoa in direct contact with cervical mucus.

Due to its viscous and often inhomogeneous composition, semen may contain remarkably different sperm numbers per aliquot tested. This inhomogeneity may cause discrepant results in sperm counting when smaller aliquots of semen are tested. The basic rules of statistics leave no doubt that testing an aliquot of only 5 or 10 µl out of an ejaculate with a volume of for example 3 ml can give no more than an approximate estimation of the composition of the entire sample.

In addition, there are certain pitfalls depending on the rheological characteristics of semen, and which result in important variability of the aspirated and transferred volume during pipetting. The use of automatic pipettes with negative pressure is accurate when the aspirated liquid is perfectly fluid, but will result in the transfer of a lower volume when seminal plasma is manipulated, and of an even lower average volume in case of whole semen. Also, the variability of the transferred amount is higher, and the error is not systematic, but differs between samples. Therefore, only positive displacement pipettes may be used when semen is handled.

Other problems arise from purely technical causes, such as the imprecision of certain counting chambers, variability in the depth of such chambers depending on the viscosity of the semen sample and the pressure exerted on the cover glass. Errors during visual counting are difficult to detect, and mathematical errors in the calculation of sperm concentration based on the number of cells and number of squares counted, the dilution factor, and the depth of the chamber, are more common than suspected.

Recommended techniques for sperm counting

Two techniques have proved efficient for conventional counting of sperm concentration, namely the hemocytometer method and the use of disposable fixed-depth counting chambers. The first is the more precise method, because a larger aliquot of semen is used, but errors may result during dilution, and from incorrect visual counting or calculation. The method using the disposable chambers with fixed depth has the advantage not to require sperm dilution, reducing mathematical errors. However, the aliquot of semen tested is smaller, so that errors due to the small volume's failure to represent the concentration of the entire sample will be greater.

Counting of sperm concentration using the hemocytometer method

Semen must be diluted whenever the hemocytometer method is applied. The dilution medium consists of 50 g $NaHCO_3$, 10 ml of a 35% (v/v) formalin solution, and distilled water to a final volume of 1000 ml. Optionally, 5 ml of saturated aqueous gentian violet can be added, but this is not required when phase contrast microscopy is used.

If preliminary examination of the sample suggests sperm concentration to be high (> 100 million/ml) or low (< 20 million/ml), then the dilution must be adjusted (Figure 1). For samples with concentration estimated between 20 and 100 million/ml, a 1 : 20 dilution

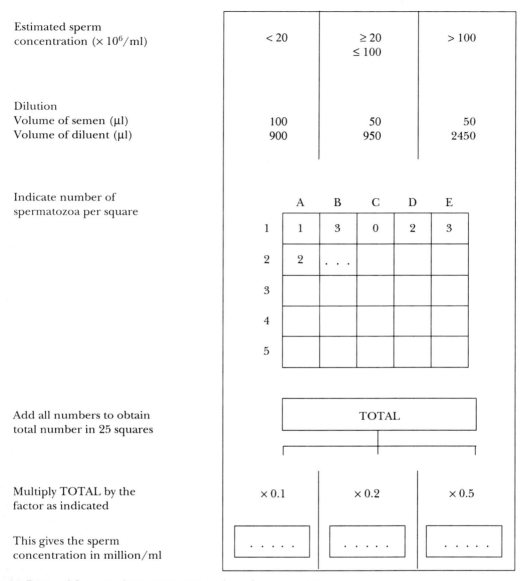

Figure 1 Protocol for counting spermatozoa using a hemocytometer

is used, which is obtained by adding 50 µl of well-mixed semen to 950 µl of diluent. Samples with higher concentration are diluted 1 : 50 by adding 50 µl of semen to 2450 µl of diluent, and samples with allegedly low sperm concentration of < 20 million/ml are diluted 1 : 10 by mixing 100 µl of semen to 900 µl of diluent. Specimens must be diluted in small glass tubes, and thoroughly mixed by hand and by vortex. A fixed volume is transferred onto a Neubauer or Burker counting chamber, and covered with a cover slip. The hemocytometer is allowed to rest for a few minutes, preferably in a moist chamber to minimize drying. During this time the immobilized spermatozoa form a sediment. Counting is performed under a bright light or phase

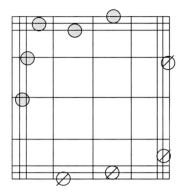

Figure 2 Neubauer hemocytometer grid, one of the 25 larger squares divided into 16 smaller squares; spermatozoa lying on the dividing line between two adjacent squares are only counted on the upper and left sides (shaded circles)

contrast microscope at magnification 100–400 ×, and only spermatozoa, which are morphologically mature germinal cells with tails, are counted.

The procedure for counting is as follows: the central square of the improved Neubauer hemocytometer contains 25 large squares with each containing 16 smaller squares. It is recommended that the number of spermatozoa present in the 25 large squares are counted. If a spermatozoon lies on the line dividing two adjacent squares, it should be counted only if it is on the upper or left side of the square being assessed (Figure 2). In order to calculate the concentration of spermatozoa in the original sample in millions per ml, the number of spermatozoa counted in 25 large squares must be multiplied by 0.1 if a dilution 1 : 10 has been used, or by 0.2 if diluted 1 : 20, or by 0.5 in case the sample was diluted 1 : 50.

It is recommended to perform a duplicate count using a second aliquot of semen and the same dilution. Ideally, the result of both counts should not be more than 5% apart. In reality, the difference is often larger due to inhomogeneity of the semen sample and pipetting or dilution errors. However, differences exceeding 10% indicate inadequate counting, and the procedure must be repeated.

Sperm concentration assessment using disposable fixed-depth counting chambers

An alternative procedure to determine sperm concentration uses special sperm counting chambers. Reusable chambers such as those by Makler or Howell can be used without dilution of the semen sample, but they may lack precision resulting from differences in the depth of the chamber due to overfilling or hyperviscosity of the sample. Counting errors up to 70% may occur, and the chambers are relatively expensive and require thorough and time-consuming cleaning.

We have assessed the accuracy of several fixed-depth disposable counting chambers (Disposlide Tecnolos, Alkmaar, The Netherlands; Microcell, Conception Technologies, La Jolla, USA) and recommend the following technique for their adequate use. The chamber is filled by applying 5 µl of undiluted semen against the edge of the cover slip. The semen enters the chamber by capillary force. A special calibration grid must be introduced in the ocular, since the disposable slides themselves do not contain such a grid. Once the calibration factor has been calculated, it can be applied for all subsequent counting procedures, if these are performed under the same optical conditions, i.e. with the same oculars and objective. Cells must be counted in the central part of the chamber, avoiding the inlet and outlet area.

Comparison between the hemocytometer and disposable counting chambers

In a comparative study we have recorded a correlation coefficient of $r = 0.95$ between sperm concentration measured by the hemocytometer and the disposable fixed-depth counting chamber. The coefficient of variation assessed by repeated counting of ten aliquots of each of ten different semen samples was 5.9% with the hemocytometer method, and 7.6% with the disposable counting chamber. Also, counting of standard suspensions of micro beads (Hamilton-Thorn, Danvers, USA) gave similar results in the two methods.

The time needed for sperm counting with the disposable chamber was only one third of that needed when the hemocytometer was used. In addition, the disposable chamber permits the simultaneous assessment of sperm motility, since spermatozoa do not need to be immobilized. The gain of time favorably balances against the negligible loss of precision when disposable chambers are used.

Conclusion

Although there is important variability between sperm concentration in different ejaculates of the same person, and although the clinical meaning of small variations in sperm concentration is doubtful, each laboratory must assess this concentration as accurately as possible. However, the latter should be performed keeping in mind that the time spent to collect this information must not be excessive, since it is probably more important to invest more time in measuring other sperm characteristics, such as motility, morphology, biochemistry, functional quality, etc. Therefore, sperm counting using disposable fixed-depth chambers is probably the method of first choice for the routine laboratory.

Biochemical aspects of semen analysis 41

W. H.-B. Schill, F.-M. Köhn, R. Henkel and G. Haidl

Introduction

The use of biochemical markers in the diagnostic investigation of male infertility provides specific information about anatomical and functional disturbances at the level of the accessory sex glands and the epididymis, the occurrence of acute and chronic male genital tract inflammation, and the fertilizing capacity of human spermatozoa. Thus, biochemical markers in andrology are important complementary tools for the proper diagnosis of fertility disorders. In contrast to bioassays, the use of marker substances has the advantage that these are objective methods which are subject to common conditions of laboratory methods including quality control.

The following biochemical markers can be used in clinical andrology to determine and identify:

(1) Sperm fertilizing capability (aniline blue, acrosin, reactive oxygen species (ROS));

(2) Male genital tract inflammation (elastase, C'3 complement component, coeruloplasmin, IgA, IgG);

(3) Accessory sex gland and epididymal dysfunction and obstruction (fructose, α-glucosidase, acid phosphatase, prostatic specific antigen (PSA)).

Some of these markers are part of the routine program of an andrological laboratory, others are sophisticated methods which will only be performed in selected patients.

Sperm fertilizing capacity

Apart from the light microscopy determination of acrosomal malformations, the assessment of a disturbed acrosomal function is considered to be an important diagnostic parameter to estimate the fertilizing capacity of a sperm population[1]. The following biochemical methods are available:

(1) Determination of acrosin activity;

(2) Aniline blue staining;

(3) Determination of reactive oxygen species.

Acrosin activity

Determination of acrosin, which is one of the best characterized sperm-specific enzymes, is a suitable approach to evaluate the fertilizing capacity of human spermatozoa. Acrosin is a serine proteinase which is located within the acrosome; it is considered to be the major penetration enzyme required for zona penetration, through limited proteolysis of zona proteins. Another important function is its ability to bind to the zona pellucida. Acrosin is apparently also involved in capacitation and acrosome reaction. In addition, it may act as a sperm-stimulating agent during intrauterine sperm migration when it is released from the acrosome of dead spermatozoa, since it is able to liberate kinins from kininogen. Kinins have been demonstrated to enhance sperm metabolism and sperm motility *in vitro*[2].

Several methods have been described to assess the acrosin activity in human spermatozoa[3]. A very simple method is the determination of the proteolytic potential of spermatozoa on gelatin plates[4]. Acrosin is released by hyperosmolaric rupture of the acrosome and leads to halo formation during incubation in a humid

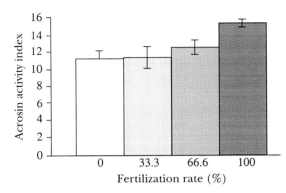

Figure 1 Correlation between mean acrosin activity index (± SEM) and fertilization rate in 110 patients attending the IVF program at the University of Giessen, Germany. The acrosin activity index is calculated from halo diameter and halo formation rate by multiplication of both these values and subsequent division by 100. The four groups differ significantly by Mann–Whitney test ($p = 0.0003$)

chamber at 37°C. Halo formation is predominantly brought about by living spermatozoa, which is supported by correlation with the eosin test ($r = 0.619$). The more dead spermatozoa that are identified, the lower the halo formation rate. No acrosin is available in cases of globozoospermia. The method of gelatinolysis is advantageous in that the equipment is simple and acrosin activity can be determined in individual spermatozoa. It shows good correlation with the biochemical assay[5].

Figure 1 shows a comparison of fertilization rates and acrosin activity index calculated from halo diameter and halo formation rate in an *in vitro* fertilization (IVF) program (110 patients). Normal acrosin activity indices are observed in men with high fertilization rates, whereas the halo diameters and halo formation rates are smaller in most cases of poor fertilization ($< 50\%$)[4]. Thus, the method may give information about the fertilizing potential of a sperm population. Patients showing a normal acrosin activity index but low fertilization probably have defects other than impaired acrosin activity (e.g. impaired acrosome reaction, impaired spermoolemma interaction or disturbance of chromatin decondensation). This is also a reason why statistical calculations show a low sensitivity

(26%), whereas high specificity (98%) and a high predictive value (positive predictive value 90%, negative predictive value 74%) exist for human IVF outcome[4].

A more sophisticated method is the spectrophotometric determination of acrosin after acid extraction from the sperm acrosome, performed in the presence of synthetic acrosin inhibitors to avoid autoactivation from proacrosin. Proacrosin is the zymogen form predominating in epididymal and freshly ejaculated spermatozoa. This method allows the determination of active, non-zymogen acrosin, proacrosin, and total acrosin, activity[3]. In most sperm populations, acrosin activity shows normal values and a wide overlap of the range of acrosin levels. In contrast, significantly lower acrosin activity is observed in patients with severe teratozoospermia and polyzoospermia, the latter with an average of -60%[3]. By immunological methods, it was shown that the acrosomal membrane integrity is severely disturbed in most spermatozoa from polyzoospermic men. Thus, polyzoospermic patients correspond to men with severe oligozoospermia who show reduced fertility compared to normozoospermic controls. This supports the concept that acrosin determination may be a useful parameter to predict the fertilizing potential of spermatozoa[2].

In conclusion, assessment of acrosin should be considered in selected cases of teratozoospermia, particularly to confirm the diagnosis of globozoospermia. Acrosin activity should also be determined in polyzoospermic patients to recognize severe acrosomal dysfunctions. In addition, the demonstration of sufficient amounts of acrosin in men from couples with idiopathic sterility, in cases of unknown male sterility factor and before *in vitro* fertilization may exclude severe disturbances of the sperm acrosome.

Aniline blue staining for determination of chromatin condensation

During spermatogenesis, lysine-rich histones are normally replaced by protamines. This process is prerequisite for the later occurring decondensation to form a male pronucleus during oocyte fertilization. In case of disturbed chromatin condensation, histones persist and can be identified by staining with acid aniline blue[6]. Since nuclear proteins play a significant role in chromatin condensation, this method is an attempt to discriminate between fertile men and those suspected of being infertile[7,8], using nuclear maturity as a parameter. Disturbed chromatin condensation is often observed in combination with an increased number of acrosomal defects[9]. In cases of > 50% aniline blue-positive spermatozoa, a protamine gene defect has been discussed. According to studies by Dadoune and co-workers[10] and Hofmann and colleagues[9], a normal ejaculate should contain at least 75% unstained spermatozoa which indicates normal chromatin condensation. This corresponds to a normal nuclear maturation of ejaculated spermatozoa.

Preliminary results in 33 men participating in an IVF program showed a close correlation ($r = 0.825$) between normal chromatin condensation and fertilization rate[11]. This indicates that normal chromatin condensation is mandatory to induce fertilization. Thus, aniline blue staining is highly predictive and may be used as an easily performable laboratory test which should precede all methods of assisted reproduction. However, its value is apparently restricted to conventional IVF procedures, since a recent study assessing chromatin condensation in spermatozoa used for intracytoplasmic sperm injection (ICSI) failed to predict the outcome of fertilization[12]. In this context, it should be mentioned that Henkel and co-workers[13] showed that glass wool filtration has a selective capacity to enrich the number of normal chromatin condensed spermatozoa, suggesting its beneficial effect for the various procedures of assisted reproduction.

Reactive oxygen species Since the first report by McLeod[14] on the influence of reactive oxygen species (ROS) on human spermatozoa, it is now believed that oxidative stress is associated with male infertility[15,16]. Spermatozoa have a much higher content of polyunsaturated fatty acids in their membranes than somatic cells. Therefore, they are particularly susceptible to oxidation by ROS, which cause lipid peroxidation. In extreme cases this might result in a dramatic loss of normal sperm function, e.g. markedly reduced motility[17] and penetration in the zona-free hamster ovum penetration test[16,18] or impaired membrane integrity[19], thus indicating decreased fertilizing capability of spermatozoa. In addition, oxidative damage to spermatozoa is closely correlated with inflammatory processes in the genital tract and occurrence of leukocytes, particularly granulocytes, that generate at least 100 times more ROS than spermatozoa themselves[20]. In addition, a high positive correlation between reactive oxygen species and elastase ($r = 0.6132$, $p = 0.0001$), a specific parameter of inflammation, has been found.

Several authors revealed that 30–40% of ejaculates from infertile men generate excessive levels of ROS[21,22]. Particularly oligozoospermic patients tend to have high ROS production by spermatozoa[23]. From a clinical point of view it is, therefore, important to determine semen samples that produce excessive amounts of ROS and to separate leukocytes and damaged spermatozoa from those sperm cells which still do not show signs of lipid peroxidation. Because of the sensitivity of spermatozoa to oxidative damage, sperm separation should be performed very carefully, preferably by means of density gradient centrifugation with Percoll or glass wool filtration. Both methods have been shown to maintain normal sperm function with regard to motility and penetration into zona-free hamster oocytes[16,17,24].

Male genital tract inflammation

From a clinical point of view, differential diagnosis of chronic male genital tract inflammations and non-inflammatory complaints such as vegetative urogenital syndrome or anogenital symptom complex is mandatory. Chronic inflammatory processes need antibiotic-antiphlogistic therapy, whereas complaints of the autonomic nervous system should be treated quite differently, either with tranquilizers or by different psychosomatic techniques. To prove an inflammatory semen pattern, $> 1 \times 10^6$ peroxidase-positive round cells (neutral granulocytes) per ml, known as leukocytospermia, indicate the existence of a reproductive tract infection. However, the absence of leukocytes does not exclude the possibility of an accessory sex gland infection. Therefore, biochemical markers have been suggested as sensitive indicators of an inflammatory reaction[25].

An enzyme immunoassay for determination of elastase in seminal plasma as a specific inflammatory parameter of polymorphonuclear granulocytes (PMN) enables the diagnosis of an asymptomatic male genital tract inflammation[26]. In addition, sequential determinations allow the control of the course of the disease during and after therapy.

Apart from elastase measurements, a permeable blood-seminal plasma barrier, indicating an adnexal disturbance, can provide valuable information about an accessory sex gland infection. Particularly helpful is the quantitative determination of the complement component C'3 and coeruloplasmin. Normally, C'3 complement component is only detectable in traces or not at all, in seminal plasma. During an inflammatory reaction, transudation from the blood is increased, and both C'3 complement component and coeruloplasmin are found in significantly elevated amounts in semen samples[25].

Determination of granulocyte elastase

Granulocyte elastase is determined in cell-free seminal plasma according to the method by Neumann and Jochum[27], using an enzyme-linked immunoabsorbent assay provided by E. Merck, Darmstadt, Germany. Due to the relatively rapid reaction of extracellularly liberated elastase with its major inhibitor, α_1-proteinase inhibitor (α_1 PI), the enzyme can only be detected in body fluids in an inactive, complexed form (E-α_1 PI). PMN elastase levels above 1000 ng/ml are diagnostic of leucocytospermia[28]. Thus, clinically asymptomatic inflammations can be measured by PMN elastase in semen[29]. Recent investigations with an exact

quantification of granulocyte elastase in 305 andrological patients confirmed its high specificity and sensitivity to distinguish inflammatory from non-inflammatory male adnexal affections[30].

Quantitative determination of C'3 complement component and coeruloplasmin

C'3 complement component and coeruloplasmin can be quantified in human seminal plasma by radial immunodiffusion (Partigen®, Behringwerke, Marburg, Germany). An increase in coeruloplasmin in seminal plasma is only seen during a significant inflammatory semen reaction, whereas C'3 complement determinations seem to be much more sensitive[25]. An increase in seminal plasma IgA and IgG has also been found to give relative information about a genital tract inflammation, but is not as sensitive and specific as determination of granulocyte elastase in seminal plasma.

Determination of accessory sex gland secretory function

The secretory capacity of the seminal vesicles, the prostate and the epididymis can be determined by means of various biochemical markers, e.g. fructose, prostatic specific antigen (PSA) and neutral α-glucosidase[31]. A low secretory function or its absence due to an occlusion is reflected in a low total output of the specific markers; therefore, they may be used for the assessment of both accessory sex gland secretory function and location of an obstruction.

Fructose

Fructose in semen is determined, according to the WHO laboratory manual, by means of a colorimetric reaction with indole[31]. An enzymatic assay using spectrophotometry may also be performed. In case of azoospermia caused by congenital absence of the vasa deferentia, low fructose levels indicate an associated dysgenesis of the seminal vesicles. Fructose levels are also low in cases of postinflammatory atrophy of the seminal vesicle epithelium or relative androgen deficiency. Oral androgen medication (e.g. 120 mg testosterone undecanoate or 75 mg mesterolone) allows differentiation between an androgen-sensitive and an androgen-resistant form of seminal vesicle insufficiency. In cases of ejaculatory duct obstruction or agenesis of the vasa deferentia and seminal vesicles, semen samples are characterized by low volume, low pH and absence of fructose; this indicates that the ejaculate consists exclusively of prostatic fluid.

α-glucosidase

Determination of L-carnitine as a common epididymal marker has been abandoned. Assessment of neutral α-glucosidase, which originates from the corpus and cauda epididymidis, has been found to give more reliable and reproducible results, is simpler, cheaper and less time-consuming[31]. Distal ductal obstruction shows significantly decreased α-glucosidase values.

Unfortunately, functional disturbances at the level of the epididymis cannot be characterized by the α-glucosidase assay. In case of an occlusion at the level of the rete testis, α-glucosidase activity in seminal plasma is found within the normal range. Recently, increased amounts of macrophages in semen have been shown to be associated with chronic epididymitis. Future research will hopefully provide more specific and sensitive markers of epididymal function.

Prostatic gland secretion

To give a reliable measure of the prostatic gland secretion, several marker substances can be used, including zinc, citric acid and prostatic acid phosphatase[31]. For clinical purposes, however, determination of prostatic gland secretions is of no great diagnostic value to determine the location of an obstruction. On the other hand, assessment of the specific prostatic marker PSA, a kallikrein-like protease, may give information about inflammatory reactions and tumor cells in the prostate[32,33]. PSA can be

determined in semen and serum by means of a commercial radioimmunoassay. This determination is used as a screening test to exclude prostatic cancer or chronic inflammatory processes within the prostatic tissue. However, despite a considerable decrease of the prostatic secretory function by infectious agents, the total amount of markers in semen may be still within the normal range.

In conclusion, biochemical markers of seminal plasma allow assessment of the functional state of the accessory sex glands and will help to determine the location of obstructive azoospermia. Thus, absence of fructose in combination with a low pH and a low ejaculate volume allows recognition of men with obstructions in the periphery, because pure prostatic fluid with an acid pH around 6.4 and a low semen volume with or without traces of fructose are observed in these cases. Future investigations will also clarify whether other biochemical markers (e.g. the testis-specific marker transferrin, acridine orange as marker of the stability of sperm DNA, the cholesterol/phospholipid ratio as marker of human sperm capacitation) have any diagnostic relevance for clinical andrology.

Summary

Determination of markers of sperm function, accessory sex gland secretion and asymptomatic male genital tract inflammation is of considerable diagnostic value in the evaluation of male infertility. The introduction of biochemical tests into the analysis of male factor has the advantage that standardized assays with a coefficient of variation characteristic of clinical chemistry are performed, in contrast to biological test systems with a larger variability. Biochemical parameters may be used in clinical practice to evaluate the sperm fertilizing capacity (acrosin, aniline blue, ROS), to characterize male accessory sex gland secretions (fructose, α-glucosidase, PSA), and to identify men with asymptomatic genital tract inflammation (elastase, C'3 complement component, coeruloplasmin, IgA, IgG, ROS).

References

1. Schill, W.-B., Henkel, R., Sanchez, R., Khanaga, O., Turley, H., Haidl, G. and Gips, H. (1994). Sperm function tests: do they have any predictive value? *Hum. Reprod.*, **9** (Suppl. 4), 94–5

2. Schill, W.-B. (1991). Some disturbances of acrosomal development and function in human spermatozoa. *Hum. Reprod.*, **6**, 969–78

3. Schill, W.-B. (1990). Determination of active, non-zymogen acrosin, proacrosin and total acrosin in different andrological patients. *Arch. Dermatol. Res.*, **282**, 335–42

4. Henkel, R., Muller, C., Miska, W., Schill, W.-B., Kleinstein, J. and Gips, H. (1995). Determination of the acrosin activity of human spermatozoa by means of a gelatinolytic technique: a simple, predictive method useful for IVF. *J. Androl.*, **16**, 272–7

5. Schill, W.-B. (1981). Acrosin and seminal plasma proteinase inhibitors in the diagnostic workup of male infertility. In Insler, V. and Bettendorf, G. (eds.) *Advances in Diagnosis and Treatment of Infertility*, pp. 321–37. (North Holland, New York: Elsevier)

6. Terquem, A. and Dadoune, J. P. (1983). Aniline blue staining of human spermatozoa chromatin: evaluation of nuclear maturation. In André, J. (ed.) *The Sperm Cell*, pp. 249–52. (The Hague: Martinus Nijhoff)

7. Auger, J., Mesbah, M., Huber, C. and Dadoune, J. P. (1990). Aniline blue staining as a marker of sperm chromatin defects associated with different semen characteristics discriminates between proven fertile and suspected infertile men. *Int. J. Androl.*, **13**, 452–62

8. Hofmann, N. and Hilscher, B. (1991). Use of aniline blue to assess chromatin condensation in morphologically normal spermatozoa in normal and infertile men. *Hum. Reprod.*, **6**, 979–82

9. Hofmann, N., Hilscher, B. and Bierling, C. (1990). Quantitative Untersuchungen der Korrelation von Störungen der Chromatinkondensierung mit der Spermatozoenmorphologie (Quantitative studies on the correlation between disturbed chromatin condensation and sperm morphology). *Fertilitat*, **6**, 208–13

10. Dadoune, J. P., Mayaux, M. J. and Guilhard-Moscato, M. L. (1988). Correlation between defects of chromatin condensation of human spermatozoa stained by aniline blue and semen characteristics. *Andrologia*, **20**, 211–17

11. Haidl, G. and Schill, W.-B. (1994). Assessment of sperm chromatin condensation: an important test for prediction of IVF outcome. *Arch. Androl.*, **32**, 263–6

12. Van Ranst, H., Bocken, G., Desmet, B., Joris, H., Vankeleccm, A. S., Liu, J., Nagy, Z. P. and Van Steirteghem, A. C. (1994). Chromatin condensation assessment in spermatozoa used for intracytoplasmic sperm injection. *Hum. Reprod.*, **9** (Suppl. 4), 24

13. Henkel, R., Franken, D. R., Lombard, C. J. and Schill, W.-B. (1994). Selective capacity of glass wool filtration for the separation of human spermatozoa with condensed chromatin: a possible therapeutic modality for male factor cases? *J. Assist. Reprod. Genet.*, **11**, 395–400

14. McLeod, J. (1943). The role of oxygen in the metabolism and motility of human spermatozoa. *Am. J. Physiol.*, **138**, 512–8

15. Aitken, R. J. and Clarkson, J. S. (1987). Cellular basis of defective sperm function and its association with the genesis of reactive oxygen species by human spermatozoa. *J. Reprod. Fertil.*, **81**, 459–69

16. Aitken, R. J., Clarkson, J. S. and Fishel, S. (1989). Generation of reactive oxygen species, lipid peroxidation, and human sperm function. *Biol. Reprod.*, **40**, 183–97

17. Mortimer, D. (1991). Sperm preparation techniques and iatrogenic failure of *in-vitro* fertilization. *Hum. Reprod.*, **6**, 173–6

18. Aitken, R. J. and West, K. M. (1990). Analysis of the relationship between reactive oxygen species production and leukocyte infiltration in fractions of human semen separated on Percoll gradients. *Int. J. Androl.*, **13**, 433–51

19. Gavella, M., Lipovac, V. and Marotti, T. (1991). Effect of pentoxifylline on superoxide anion production by human sperm. *Int. J. Androl.*, **14**, 320–7

20. Ford, W. C. L. (1990). The role of oxygen free radicals in the pathology of human spermatozoa: implications of IVF. In Matson, P. L. and Lieberman, B. A. (eds.) *Clinical IVF Forum: Current Views in Assisted Reproduction*, pp. 123–39. (Manchester, UK: University Press)

21. Iwasaki, A. and Gagnon, C. (1992). Formation of reactive oxygen species in spermatozoa of infertile patients. *Fertil. Steril.*, **31**, 531–7

22. Agarwal, A., Ikemoto, J. and Loughlin, K. R. (1994). Relationship of sperm parameters with levels of reactive oxygen species in semen specimens. *J. Urol.*, **152**, 107–10

23. Aitken, R. J., Clarkson, J. S., Hargreave, T. B., Irvine, D. S. and Wu, F. C. W. (1989). Analysis of

the relationship between defective sperm function and the generation of reactive oxygen species in cases of oligozoospermia. *J. Androl.*, **10**, 214–20

24. Rana, N., Jeyendran, R. S., Holmgren, W. J., Rotman, C. and Zaneveld, L. J. D. (1989). Glass wool-filtered spermatozoa and their oocyte penetrating capacity. *J. In Vitro Fertil. Embryo Transfer*, **6**, 280–4

25. Schiessler, H., Jochum, M., Friesen, A., Schill, W.-B. and Hofstetter, A. (1984). Granulozyten-Elastase im Ejakulat als Entzündungsparameter bei Adnex-Affektionen. In Schirren, C. and Semm, K. (eds.) *Fortschritte der Fertilitätsforschung*, edn. 12, pp. 157–63. (Berlin: Grosse Verlag)

26. Jochum, M., Pabst, W. and Schill, W.-B. (1986). Granulocyte elastase as a sensitive diagnostic parameter of silent male genital tract inflammation. *Andrologia*, **18**, 413–19

27. Neumann, S. and Jochum, M. (1984). Elastase-α_1-proteinase inhibitor complex. In Bergmeyer, H. U., Bergmeyer, J. and Grassl, M. (eds.) *Methods of Enzymatic Analysis*, 3rd ed., pp. 184–95. (Weinheim: Verlag Chemie)

28. Wolff, H. and Anderson, D. J. (1988). Evaluation of granulocyte elastase as a seminal plasma marker for leukocytospermia. *Fertil. Steril.*, **50**, 129–32

29. Wolff, H., Bezold, G., Zebhauser, M. and Meurer, M. (1991). Impact of clinically silent inflammation on male genital tract organs as reflected by biochemical markers in semen. *J. Androl.*, **12**, 331–4

30. Reinhardt, A., Haidl, G. and Schill, W.-B. (1995). Granulozytenelastase – Bedeutung für die andrologische Diagnostik (Granulocyte elastase – significance for andrological diagnosis). *Fertilitat*, in press

31. World Health Organization (1992). *Laboratory Manual for the Examination of Human Semen and Sperm-cervical Mucus Interaction*, 3rd edn. (Cambridge: University Press)

32. Kirby, R. S., Kirby, M. G., Feneley, M. R., McNicholas, T., McLean, A. and Well, J. A. (1994). Screening for carcinoma of the prostate: a GP based study. *Br. J. Urol.*, **74**, 64–71

33. Lehmann, K., Simmler, F., Schmucki, O. and Hauri, D. (1994). PSA in prostatic fluid. *Urologe A*, **33**, 232–4

Fertilization capacity

42

A. Veiga

Introduction

Male factor infertility is considered to be the cause of a couple's infertility in 40% of cases. Sperm samples were originally evaluated with very simple and subjective semen analyses. As andrology has developed, the examination and evaluation of the infertile male has incorporated more objective and useful tests. These include tests to assess sperm quality as well as tests to predict sperm fertilizing ability.

Assessment of sperm quality

It is very important to establish standards of normality for routine sperm sample analysis and the World Health Organization (WHO)[1] has clearly defined these. At least two samples have to be analyzed to classify the patient as normozoospermic, oligozoospermic, asthenozoospermic, teratozoospermic, oligoasthenoteratozoospermic, azoospermic or aspermic[2].

Traditional manual/visual semen analysis methods evaluate the quantitative and qualitative aspects of sperm production. They include sperm concentration, motility, vitality and morphology assessments.

Sperm concentration determination

The hemocytometer method is still the most accurate for determining sperm concentration, with a coefficient of variation of approximately 10%. Recently, specially designed counting chambers such as the Makler chamber (Sefi Medical Instr., Haifa, Israel) or the disposable ones such as Cell-VU chambers (Fertility Tech. Inc., Natick, MA, USA) or MicroCell chambers (Conception Technologies, La Jolla, CA, USA) are available, but although they may simplify the routine work in the laboratory, important evaluation errors can be made with their use.

Sperm motility assessment

A preparation of sperm is made and at least 200 spermatozoa are counted. The percentage of each grade of motility is established. The WHO classifies motility grading as follows:

(1) Grade a: rapid progressive motility;

(2) Grade b: slow progressive motility;

(3) Grade c: non-progressive motility;

(4) Grade d: immotility.

Sperm viability

Live and dead sperm are distinguished using sperm vitality staining techniques with eosin or other commercially available stains.

Sperm morphology

Papanicolaou staining, as well as a variety of commercially available stains, may be used to evaluate sperm morphology. Spermatozoa are scored for head, midpiece and tail abnormalities.

Recently, very strict criteria (Tygerberg criteria) have been used by some teams to assess sperm morphology[3]

CASA

Computer assisted sperm analysis (CASA) instruments have been developed in recent years to allow a more objective and automated method for semen analysis. These systems are supposed to provide more accurate measurements of sperm concentration and motility. They offer clear advantages and unfortunately some disadvantages. Each laboratory must find the most appropriate tool for sperm analysis, depending on its own necessities and criteria.

Correlation of sperm count, motility, vitality and morphology with sperm fertilizing ability

An association between sperm count and motility parameters and fertility has been established by many authors and the use of CASA has confirmed this relationship objectively[4].

Sperm morphology, assessed either with WHO or strict criteria, has been correlated with *in vitro* fertilization rates[5].

Specific fertilizing ability tests

A number of tests to evaluate sperm fertilizing ability have recently been developed. They are based on the concept of sperm function and physiology. Some of those most used are: the sperm penetration assay (SPA or hamster test), hemizona assay (HZA), hypo-osmotic swelling test (HOS test), Immunobead assay, human sperm survival test, sperm–cervical mucus interaction, biochemical sperm evaluation, transmission electron microscopy (TEM) observation and chromosomal studies on semen or testicular biopsy. Patient chromosomal status is also helpful.

Sperm penetration assay

First described by Yanagimachi and colleagues in 1976[6], the hamster oocyte penetration assay measures the ability of acrosome reacted human spermatozoa to fuse with the membrane of the hamster oocyte and initiate nuclear decondensation. It is very important to follow the methodology adequately (capacitation of the sperm population, WHO recommendations) and be aware of the fact that this bioassay does not measure aspects such as the capacity to

penetrate the cervical barrier or to bind to the zona pellucida. Occasionally, false-positive results, as well as false-negative results, occur. Despite hundreds of reports using this assay, there is still considerable controversy regarding its variability and predictive value[7]. When the test is performed in the presence of calcium ionophore A23187, the results obtained correlate best with fertility. A sperm sample is considered SPA-positive when the penetration rate is > 14%.

Hemizona assay

This test involves microdissection of the zona pellucida into equal halves and testing of the binding on each matching half with the same number of test and control spermatozoa[8]. The test is only available through *in vitro* fertilization (IVF) programs and has been shown to be a good predictive tool for fertilization[9].

A new test based on the number of spermatozoa penetrating the zona pellucida has been designed to identify patients whose spermatozoa fail to achieve this. This parameter correlates significantly with the *in vitro* fertilization rate[10].

Hypo-osmotic swelling test

The HOS test assesses the functional integrity of the sperm cell membrane[11]. When the membranes are intact and exposed to a hypo-osmotic solution, they swell and assume different forms. It has been shown that the correlation between fertilization and the HOS test is very high, with low false-positive results (12%) and low false-negative results (7.7%)[12]. The HOS test is considered positive when > 50% swelling is observed.

Immunobead test

This test is useful to detect anti-sperm antibodies on spermatozoa. Immunobeads are polyacrylamide spheres with covalently bound rabbit and anti-human immunoglobulins (IgG, IgA and IgM)[13]. The husband's sperm as well as the wife's biological fluids should be tested. The test is considered positive when > 20% of motile spermatozoa show Immunobead binding. Anti-sperm antibodies may affect fertility, but no conclusive data support this hypothesis completely.

Human sperm survival test

This test has been used in most IVF programs to evaluate the number of spermatozoa recovered after the use of different sperm preparation techniques (swim-up, Percoll gradients, etc.) and to assess the percentage of motile spermatozoa present after a 24-h incubation. It helps in detecting men with normal sperm samples and sperm with poor survival rates after incubation. Recovery and survival tests correlate with fertilization and even with pregnancy rates after IVF[14].

Sperm–cervical mucus interaction

Cervical mucus is receptive to sperm migration for a limited time during the menstrual cycle. *In vitro* sperm–cervical mucus interaction measures the capacity of motile sperm to penetrate through cervical mucus by means of sperm motility and also in the presence of anti-spermatozoal antibodies. This test and also cross-hostility tests are used for further evaluation of abnormal post-coital tests[15,16].

Biochemical sperm studies

Prostatic secretions such as acid phosphatase, citrate and zinc, seminal vesicle secretion (fructose) and epididymal secretions such as carnitine and α-1-4 glucosidase allow determination of the origin of certain endocrine and metabolic disorders as well as inflammatory diseases (whether or not they are related to infection) and occlusions of the genital tract[17].

Electron microscopy

Transmission electron microscopy is the only way to assess the structural condition of the sperm organelles responsible for motility, penetrating ability and fertilizing competence. This specific and complex sperm evaluation[18] is useful in different situations:

(1) When there is a discrepancy between a normal or almost normal sperm sample and a normal female factor associated with a prolonged history of infertility or with a SPA with zero or very low penetration rate;

(2) When the morphological evaluation of sperm suggests congenital defects;

(3) When micromanipulation techniques have failed (some authors propose evaluating sperm through TEM before using micromanipulation techniques); and

(4) When the asthenozoospermia is unknown and a flagellar defect is suspected.

The complexity of the technique limits its use to specialized laboratories where TEM as well as trained personnel are available[19].

Chromosomal analysis

Chromosomal abnormalities are more frequent in infertile men than in the general population. Spermatogenic failure can be caused by sex chromosome abnormalities as well as by structural autosomal rearrangements.

Cytogenetic investigation of the patient and of meiosis in sperm[20] or in testicular biopsy[21] may explain the unknown origin of certain cases of male infertility.

Acrosome reaction

The acrosome reaction is an exocytosis process in the spermatozoon that is necessary for successful penetration of the oocyte. No fertilization can take place if spermatozoa have not undergone the acrosome reaction.

A number of investigations have recently been performed to determine the predictive value of the acrosome reaction inducibility in spermatozoa, its diagnostic significance and

313

clinical application[22]. The most widely used technique for assessment of the acrosome reaction is the triple stain[23]. A number of biochemical and biological stimulators of the acrosome reaction have been described. Different studies evaluating the acrosome reaction potential of spermatozoa (spontaneous or induced) show controversial results[24,25], even though low percentages of acrosome reacted spermatozoa may be indicative of subfertility. Studies correlating the acrosome reaction and *in vivo* fertilization are needed, to provide more conclusive results.

In conclusion, sperm fertilizing ability cannot be tested by a unique procedure. Each laboratory has to perform as many tests as its methodology and trained personnel permit, to try to establish the expectancy of fertilization of a given sperm sample. Micromanipulation techniques, especially intracytoplasmic sperm injection, today represent a very useful tool for treating male infertility, but we must not forget the importance of patient evaluation to determine the origin and causes of the infertility in each case.

References

1. World Health Organization (1992). *WHO Laboratory Manual for the Examination of Human Semen and Sperm–Cervical Mucus Interaction*, 3rd edn. (Cambridge: Cambridge University Press)
2. Elliasson, R. (1971). Standards for investigation of human semen. *Andrologie*, **3**, 49–64
3. Kruger, T. F., Ackerman, S. B., Simmons, K. F., Swanson, R. J., Brugo, S. and Acosta, A. A. (1987). A quick reliable staining technique for sperm morphology. *Arch. Androl.*, **18**, 275
4. Auger, J., Serres, C., Wolf, J. P. and Jouannet, P. (1994). Mouvement des spermatozoides et fécondation. *Contracept. Fertil. Sex.*, **22**, 314–18
5. Kruger, T. F., Acosta, A., Simmons, K., Swanson, R. J., Matta, J. F. and Oehninger, S. (1988). Predictive value of abnormal sperm morphology in *in vitro* fertilization. *Fertil. Steril.*, **49**, 112–17
6. Yanagimachi, R., Yanagimachi, H. and Rogers, B. J. (1976). The use of zona free animal ova as a test system for the assessment of the fertilizing capacity of human spermatozoa. *Biol. Reprod.*, **15**, 471–6
7. Aitken, J. (1994). On the future of the hamster oocyte penetration assay. *Fertil. Steril.*, **62**, 17–19
8. Burkman, L. J., Coddington, C. C., Franken, D. R., Kruger, T. F., Rosenwaks, Z. and Hodgen, G. D. (1988). The hemizona assay (HZA): development of a diagnostic test for the binding of human spermatozoa to the human hemizona pellucida to predict fertilization potential. *Fertil. Steril.*, **49**, 688–97
9. Oehninger, S., Coddington, C. C., Scott, R., Franken, D. R., Burkman, L. J., Acosta, A. A. *et al.* (1989). Hemizona assay: assessment of sperm disfunction and prediction of *in vitro* fertilization outcome. *Fertil. Steril.*, **51**, 665–70
10. Liu, D. Y. and Baker, H. W. (1994). A new test for the assessment of sperm–zona pellucida penetration: relationship with results of other sperm tests and fertilization *in vitro*. *Hum. Reprod.*, **9**, 489–96
11. Jeyendran, R. S., Van der Ven, H. H., Perez-Pelaez, M., Crabo, B. G. and Zanenveld, L. J. D. (1984). Development of an assay to assess the functional integrity of the human sperm membrane and its relationship to the other semen characteristics. *J. Reprod. Fertil.*, **70**, 219–28
12. Van der Ven, H. H., Jeyendran, R. S., Al-Hasani, S. *et al.* (1986). Correlation between swelling hypoosmotic medium (hypoosmotic swelling test) and *in vitro* fertilization. *J. Androl.*, **7**, 190
13. Clarke, G. N., Elliot, P. J. and Smaila, C. (1985). Detection of sperm antibodies in semen using the Immunobead test: a survey of 813 consecutive patients. *Am. J. Reprod. Immunol. Microbiol.*, **7**, 118–23
14. Stovall, D. W., Guzick, D. S., Berga, S. L., Krasnow, J. S. and Zeleznik, A. J. (1994). Sperm recovery and survival: two tests that predict *in vitro* fertilization outcome. *Fertil. Steril.*, **62**, 1244–9
15. Alexander N. J. (1981). Evaluation of male infertility with an *in vitro* cervical mucus penetration test. *Fertil. Steril.*, **36**, 201–8
16. Overstreet, J. W. (1986). Evaluation of sperm–cervical mucus interaction. *Fertil. Steril.*, **45**, 324–6
17. Cohen-Bacrie, P. (1993). Exploration biochimique du sperme humain. *Contracept. Fertil., Sex.*, **21**, 891–2

18. Stefanini, M., De Martino, C. and Zamboni, L. (1967). Fixation of ejaculated sperm for electron microscopy. *Nature (London)*, **216**, 173–4

19. Zamboni, L. (1992). Sperm, structure and its relevance to infertility. *Arch. Pathol. Lab. Med.*, **116**, 325–44

20. Vidal, F., Templado, C., Navarro, J., Brusadin, S., Marina, S. and Egozcue, J. (1982). Meiotic and synaptonemal complex studies in 45 subfertile males. *Hum. Genet.*, **60**, 301–4

21. Evans, E. P., Breckon, G. and Ford, C. E. (1964). An air drying method for meiotic preparations from mammalian testes. *Cytogenetics.*, **3**, 403–6

22. De Jonge, C. J. (1994). The diagnostic significance of the induced acrosome reaction. *Reprod. Med. Rev.*, **3**, 159–78

23. Talbot, P. and Chacon, R. (1981). A triple stain technique for evaluating normal aerosome reactions of human sperm. *J. Exp. Zool.*, **215**, 201–8

24. Fenichel, P. (1994). Fonction acrosomique et fertilite masculine. *Contracept. Fertil. Sex.*, **22**, 675–81

25. Yovich, J., Edirisinghe, W. R. and Yovich, J. (1994). Use of the acrosome reaction to ionophore challenge test in managing patients in an assisted reproduction program: a prospective double blind, randomized controlled study. *Fertil. Steril.*, **61**, 902–10

Cryopreservation of semen

43

G. Ragni and W. Vegetti

Introduction

More than 200 years have passed since the first attempts to freeze human semen[1], 45 years since the discovery of the cryoprotective properties of glycerol[2]. The first infants born of donated frozen spermatozoa are more than 40 years old by now[3].

In spite of this long history of cryopreservation of semen, there are still technical and biological problems. Refinements of the technology have constantly increased the yield and have almost completely overcome the risks and the complications of using frozen sperm, but there is still a difference of 25–30% between the qualities of the sperm before and after freezing. This might be due either to damage of the sperm by cryoprotective agents or to the freezing and thawing processes.

The purpose of this paper is to review the current state of the art of cryopreservation of human semen with the emphasis on where the trend is leading.

Cryoprotective media

Fewer than 15% of the cell population normally survives the freezing and thawing of human semen unless a cryoprotective agent has been added. There are several damaging factors when the spermatozoon is frozen, even though it has a low water content. These include: thermal shock; formation of ice crystals; dehydration, due to loss of fluid from the cell secondary to formation of ice; increased salt concentration after the water has frozen; and osmotic shock.

For effective cryopreservation, the concentration of cryoprotectant must be sufficient to control the rise in salt concentration and to increase the unfrozen volume during cooling.

The discovery by Polge and colleagues[2] in 1949 of the cryoprotective properties of glycerol led to the current successful cryopreservation of human sperm. Glycerol is now used almost universally at a volume of 5–10%[4].

However, glycerol is also quite toxic. Toxic effects with concentrations of less than 2% have been reported[5], and there is a decrease in the number of motile sperm as the concentration of glycerol is increased[6]. The toxic effects of glycerol are probably due to modifications of the structure of the plasma membrane, and at high concentrations it may also inhibit energy metabolism[7].

In recent years more complex cryoprotectives have been used in attempts to improve the recovery of functional spermatozoa after freezing[8,9]. These extenders contain the following, in various combinations:

(1) Egg yolk (non-permeable molecules), to preserve the integrity of the cell membranes, especially the lipoproteins;

(2) Citrate, after it became recognized that seminal fluid is a bicarbonate–citrate buffer;

(3) Sugar such as saccharose, to keep the osmotic pressure of the extracellular fluids constant at different temperatures;

(4) Test-tris or Hepes buffered solution; and

(5) Penicillin, streptomycin, to prevent cryopreservation of bacteria.

In one comparative study of eight possible media[10], containing only glycerol or the various extenders in glycerol (citrate, egg yolk, Test-tris, fructose, glucose, Hepes), the best post-thaw motility was achieved with Test-tris + citrate + egg yolk + fructose in 6% glycerol. In another comparative study of 12 possible media[11], the best was judged to be that used by the French National Sperm bank: egg yolk + citrate + dextrose–glycine medium in 7.5% glycerol.

This illustrates the amount of energy that has been applied to looking for ever less toxic cryopreservatives, but today we still do not have a medium that prevents the damage resulting from the freezing procedure.

Freezing and thawing procedures

The other major problem in cryopreservation of semen is the procedure used for freezing and thawing. It has already been mentioned that one of the major mechanisms of sperm damage is formation of ice crystals. The critical period for this is between 0° and −10°C. Essentially, two procedures with some variations have been proposed: rapid freezing and slow, controlled freezing.

The rapid method, first proposed in 1963 by Sherman[12], is very cheap and practical and uses the neck of the nitrogen container itself. The straws are left in contact with nitrogen vapors for 8–30 min and then directly immersed in the liquid nitrogen at −196°C. Exposure of straws to nitrogen vapor in a vertical position can result in cooling rates that vary considerably from one part of the straw to another[13]. Therefore, it is important to place the straws in a horizontal position, parallel to the surface of the liquid nitrogen, at no less than 10 cm above the surface[14].

For the slow method, expensive programmable biological freezers in which the semen is gradually cooled at computer-controlled rates, with loss of 1–10°C per min, must be used to arrive at a determined temperature, usually about −80°C, before the semen is placed in the liquid nitrogen. Some investigators have said that the computer-controlled freezing methods preserve sperm quality better than vapor freezing[13,15,16], but others have found no

beneficial effects, at least for human spermatozoa[14,17,18].

Since there is still controversy about the usefulness of the programmed freezing, in view of the differences in cost, the practicality and the time required, we might think that this technique should be reserved for particularly low-quality spermatozoa, for example, abnormal semen from patients with testicular tumors or with Hodgkin's disease[16].

Thawing procedures are simple: the straws are taken out of the liquid nitrogen and left at room temperature (22°C) for a few minutes or immersed in a 37°C chamber for 30 s to 10 min (more rapid 37°C thawing).

Systematic studies of the effects of thawing on sperm survival have not been reported recently, but only minor differences in the effects of the two procedures have been found[14].

Effects of the preparation procedure on semen frozen for assisted reproductive technology

Cryopreserved semen has been used successfully for supracervical insemination or *in vitro* fertilization (IVF), but when the spermatozoa are prepared for these procedures, it is necessary to remove the toxic cryoprotectant medium by dropwise dilution with medium followed by centrifugation in order to perform a swim-up procedure. As an alternative, the thawed spermatozoa can be stratified on a Percoll gradient.

There have been only a few reports of the effects of the dilution and the washing plus centrifugation of thawed spermatozoa. Graczykowski and Siegel[19] found considerably lower motility of thawed spermatozoa after swim-up (7% as compared with 33% motile sperm for fresh spermatozoa after swim-up). Verheyen and associates[14] found a 50% decrease in motility of thawed spermatozoa after dilution and washing.

Therefore, removal of the cryoprotective medium causes osmotic shock that markedly decreases the final quality of the semen, in addition to the deleterious effects on the freezing and thawing.

Damage to spermatozoa

Whatever procedure of freezing is used, there is damage to the cells, producing either structural or functional changes. Damage to human spermatozoa can be recognized immediately after thawing as a loss in motility. Ultrastructural changes in the spermatozoa can be seen by electron microscopy, in both the peripheral membrane and the acrosome[20–22].

Huret[23] studied the nuclear chromatin and observed that nuclear stability of the frozen spermatozoa was equivalent to that of fresh sperm, while Royere and colleagues[24] found, instead, overcondensed sperm chromatin after freezing and thawing, which might delay paternal nuclear decondensation during fertilization.

A reassuring study[25] of the effects of freezing on the frequency or the type of chromosomal anomalies in the spermatozoon indicated that cryopreservation has no effect on the overall incidence, the type or the distribution of chromosomal abnormalities in human sperm. The freezing–thawing processes also appear to have no discernible effects on the sex ratio.

Conclusions

In conclusion, on the basis of the data in the literature, we can say that currently used freezing techniques are adequate for normal semen. In addition, unlike the situation for embryos, and even more so for oocytes, the large numbers of cells can provide success even with low cryosurvival rates.

The situation for abnormal semen is different. At present there is still a 25–35% difference between the potentials for fertility of fresh and frozen semen, a difference that has not been decreased in the last 20 years.

The basic and applied investigations that are now increasing, especially in the field of freezing of embryos and oocytes, may, we hope, provide information useful for the better cryopreservation of human semen.

References

1. Spallanzani, L. (1776). In *Opuscoli di Fisica Animale e Vegetabile, Opuscolo II.* Osservazioni e sperienze intorno ai vermicelli spermatici dell'uomo e degli animali. (Modena)
2. Polge, C., Smith, A. U. and Parkes, A. S. (1949). Revival of spermatozoa after vitrification and dehydration at low temperature. *Nature (London)*, **164**, 666
3. Bunge, R. G. and Sherman, J. K. (1953). Fertilizing capacity of frozen human spermatozoa. *Nature (London)*, **172**, 767
4. Pilikian, S., Czyba, J. C. and Guerin, J. F. (1982). Effect of varous concentrations of glycerol on post-thaw motility and velocity of human spermatozoa. *Cryobiology*, **19**, 147–53
5. Tulandi, T. and McInnes, R. A. (1984). Vaginal lubrificant: effect of glycerol and egg white on human sperm motility and progression *in vitro*. *Fertil. Steril.*, **41**, 151–3
6. Critser, J. K., Huse-Benda, A. R., Aaker, D. V., Arneson, B. W. and Ball, G. D. (1988). Cryopreservation of human spermatozoa. III. The effect of cryoprotectant on motility. *Fertil. Steril.*, **50**, 314–20
7. McLaughlin, E. A., Ford, W. C. L. and Hull, M. G. R. (1992). The contribution of the toxicity of a glycerol-egg yolk-citrate cryopreservative to the decline in human sperm motility during cryopreservation. *J. Reprod. Fertil.*, **95**, 749–54
8. Mahadevan, M. and Trounson, A. O. (1983). Effect of cryoprotective media and dilution methods on the preservation of human spermatozoa. *Andrologia*, **15**, 355–66
9. Prins, G. S. and Weidel, L. (1986). A comparative study of buffer systems as cryoprotectants for human spermatozoa. *Fertil. Steril.*, **46**, 147–9
10. Weidel, L. and Prins, G. S. (1987). Cryosurvival of human spermatozoa frozen in eight different buffer systems. *J. Androl.*, **8**, 41–7
11. Brotherton, J. (1990). Cryopreservation of human semen. *Arch. Androl.*, **25**, 181–95
12. Sherman, J. K. (1963). Improved methods of preservation of human spermatozoa by freezing and freeze-drying. *Fertil. Steril.*, **14**, 49–54
13. McLaughlin, E. A., Ford, W. C. L. and Hull, M. G. R. (1990). A comparison of the freezing of human semen in the uncirculated vapour above

liquid nitrogen and in a commercial semi-programmable freezer. *Hum. Reprod.*, **5**, 724–8

14. Verheyen, G., Pletincx, I. and Van Steirteghem, A. (1993). Effect of freezing method, thawing temperature and post-thaw dilution/washing on motility (CASA) and morphology characteristics of high-quality human sperm. *Hum. Reprod.*, **8**, 1678–84

15. Serafini, P. and Marrs, R. P. (1986). Computerized staged-freezing technique improves sperm survival and preserves penetration of zona-free hamster ova. *Fertil. Steril.*, **45**, 854–8

16. Ragni, G., Caccamo, A. M., Dalla Serra, A. and Guercilena, S. (1990). Computerized slow-staged freezing of semen from men with testicular tumors or Hodgkin's disease preserves sperm better than standard vapor freezing. *Fertil. Steril.*, **53**, 1072–5

17. Thachill, J. V. and Jewett, M. A. S. (1981). Preservation technique for human semen. *Fertil. Steril.*, **35**, 546–8

18. Wolf, D. P. and Patton, P. E. (1989). Sperm cryopreservation: state of the art. *J. In Vitro Fertil. Embryo Transfer*, **6**, 325–7

19. Graczykowski, J. W. and Siegel, M. S. (1991). Motile sperm recovery from fresh and frozen-thawed ejaculates using a swim-up procedures. *Fertil. Steril.*, **55**, 841–3

20. Mahadaven, M. and Trounson, A. O. (1984). Relationship of fine structure of sperm head to fertility of frozen human semen. *Fertil. Steril.*, **41**, 287–93

21. Bharthelemy, C., Royere, D., Hamamah, C., Lebos, C., Tharanne, M. J. and Lansac, J. (1990). Ultrastructural changes in membranes and acrosome of human sperm during cryopreservation. *Arch. Androl.*, **25**, 29–40

22. Oettle, E. E., Clarke, U. A., McLoughlin, J., Levin, M. R., Wiswedel, K. and Kruger, T. F. (1992). Ultrastructural parameters of fertile cryopreserved human semen. *Arch. Androl.*, **29**, 151–6

23. Huret, J. L. (1984). Effect of cryopreservation on the nuclear decondensation ability of human spermatozoa. *Arch. Androl.*, **12**, 33–8

24. Royere, D., Hamamah, S., Nicolle, J. C., Barthelemy, C. and Lansac, J. (1988). Freezing and thawing alter chromatin stability of ejaculated human spermatozoa. *Gamete Res.*, **21**, 51–7

25. Chernos, J. E. and Martin, R. H. (1989). A cytogenetic investigation of effects of cryopreservation on human sperm. *Am. J. Hum. Genet.*, **45**, 766–77

Paternal age and development

44

M. Auroux

Introduction

As with aging of the ovaries, aging of the testes not only influences the individual, but through the gametes, also affects offspring. The first signs of testicular aging appear quite early[1]. In fact, from around the age of 30, vascularization starts to deteriorate, as witnessed by a decrease in the number of capillaries; the basement membrane of the seminiferous tubules, which constitute one of the major elements in the blood–testis barrier, begin to thicken, and the number of Sertoli cells decreases. Diminishing endocrine function appears some ten years later and in point of fact shows significant inter-individual variations.

These modifications are accompanied by a slow decrease in the number of spermatozoa, with changes in their quality concerning both

their shape and motility[2] (Figure 1). For any given maternal age, a progressive decrease in male fertility can be observed. Gamete quality is also low for very young males, as seen in mice[3] and bulls[4]. Gamete quality is therefore at a maximum around 30 years of age (Figure 1). One important point, of particular significance when considering the effects of age in men on the quality of their offspring, is the fact that sperm quality is genetically determined[5]. This suggests that the messages which determine this quality improve between puberty and 30 years of age, thereafter decreasing.

Paternal age and conceptus development

Paternal aging may be responsible, in spermatozoa, for chromosomal abnormalities of structure and number, sometimes leading to abnormalities in children. This aging may also be the source of dominant or recessive mutations leading to the appearance in descendants of certain specific syndromes or functional changes, which are sometimes very subtle, concerning for example certain cerebral mechanisms.

Chromosomal abnormalities

In a normal male population of 30 years of age, approximately 5% of spermatozoa show non-disjunction of meotic origin leading to aneuploidia[6-8]. Some authors report 5–10% of trisomy 21 is therefore of male origin[9,10], but, in this case, the role of paternal age is somewhat controversial, being considered as observable for some[11-13] and inexistent for others[10,14,15]. According to Hassold[16], 50% of cases of

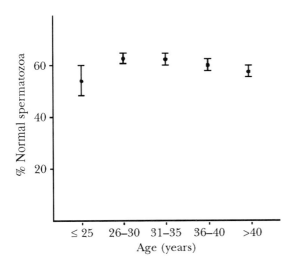

Figure 1 Variations in the percentage of normal morphological spermatozoa as a function of subject's age[2]

Klinefelter's syndrome are also due to male aging, while on the other hand, other aneuploidies such as trisomies 13 and 18, 47,XXX and 47,XYY or 45,X monosomia are not linked to paternal age.

In relation to chromosomal structural anomalies, a correlation has been shown between their incidence and increases in age[6]. Over 44 years of age, for example, 13% of gametes carry structural abnormalities. However, these abnormalities do not seem to affect the offspring[6]. Finally, according to Hook and colleagues[17], paternal aging is accompanied in the fetus by an increase in the rate of balanced reciprocal translocations.

Dominant and recessive syndromes

It has been known for some time that paternal aging is associated with certain dominant autosomal mutations, giving rise to macroscopic malformations such as achondroplasia[18], Apert's disease, Marfan's syndrome, fibrodysplasia ossificans, aniridia, bilateral retinoblastoma, Crouzon's, Lesch–Nyhan's, Treacher–Collin's and Wardenburg's syndromes, ooculo–dento–digital syndrome, renal polycystic kidney disease, polyposis coli, progeria and tuberous sclerosis[19-21]. Despite the low frequency of these syndromes, according to Friedman[19] their total frequency reaches 0.3–0.5% of births at a paternal age of 40 or over, which places the risk at the level of trisomy 21 for women between 35 and 40 years of age. While Hook and Regal contest these estimations, which they consider as only reflecting the upper limits of the phenomena[15], Lian and colleagues[22], studying almost 7500 newborn children with abnormalities, showed that the risk of congenital abnormalities was 2%

with 20-year-old fathers, 2.4% at 40 and 2.6% at 50 years of age. This increase of 0.6% is similar to Friedman's results. Dominant autosomal mutations may also be the cause of more subtle abnormalities than malformations, such as Recklinghausen's neurofibromatosis, which is the most frequent syndrome (1 out of 3000 births) which seems to be associated with paternal age (Table 1)[23].

For some authors, it seems that X-linked recessive mutations may equally be the result of paternal aging, such as hemophilia A or Duchenne's myopathy. In these cases, the first mutation would occur in the maternal grandfather and be transmitted by his daughters, appearing in 50% of his grandsons[24].

The origin of mutations

The mutations mentioned above may be due to exogenous factors (radiation, chemical products, etc.) or to endogenous factors. The latter are generally not taken into account despite the fact that they relate to the characteristics of spermatogenesis. The probability of the appearance of gene related abnormalities is in fact much higher in males than females. This is explained by the fact that, as we know, the phases of cell multiplication are at the origin of gene mutations and in particular cause recopying of the mistakes of genetic messages[24]. In the female, the oogonia multiply during the fetal phase and it is from this stock that, with no further multiplication, oocytes are periodically supplied after puberty. In males, on the contrary, the spermatogonia, which multiply during the fetal phase and then stop, multiply without interruption from puberty up to an advanced age (over 80 years of age), even if production

Table 1 Paternal age and Recklinghausen's neurofibromatosis[23]

	General population*	*Recklinghausen's neurofibromatosis*		
		Carey (1979)	*Riccardi (1984)*	*Kaplan (1987)*
Average paternal age (all children)	29.1 ± 0.3 years	32	32.8	34.9
Average maternal age (all children)	26.9 ± 0.3 years	27.5	27.4	27.8

*Institut National de la Statistique et des Etudes Economiques (France)

gradually decreases. During the period of full sexual activity the rythm is about 23 multiplications per year. The spermatozoa of a 28-year-old man will therefore have a history of approximately 380 cell divisions since puberty, and those of a 38-year-old, approximately 540[24]. In the light of these facts, the increase in the risk of mutation is obvious.

Modifications in cerebral function

As well as the specific abnormalities which we have just discussed, paternal age seems to be involved in subtle and continuous changes in the quality of the conceptus. In fact, we have shown that for a fixed maternal age, paternal aging gives rise to a progressive decrease in the learning capacity in the offspring of animals

(Figure 2)[25], and in man, to decreased success in psychometric tests, which were administered to young 18-year-old recruits before joining the army in France[26].

An initial study carried out by our team included more than 1700 recruits. The effects of paternal aging appear from 30 years of age. Conversely, we observed that very young paternal age (post-puberty) led to similar effects, with the first generation offspring showing improved performance with increasing paternal age, up to 30 years of age. The overall curve of success rate in the tests takes the form of a parabola with the peak corresponding to 30 years of paternal age (Figure 3). When paternal age is kept constant, there is no relationship between the scores obtained and the age of the mother, indicating that maternal age does not influence the variables examined.

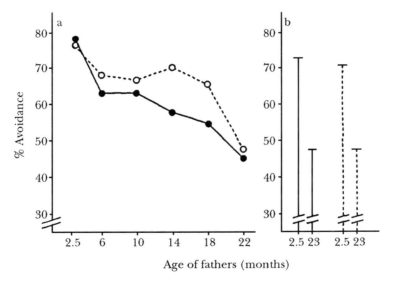

Figure 2 (a) The same group of rats successively crossed at 2.5, 6, 10, 14, 18 and 22 months with 2.5-month females, yielded offspring which as adults (2.5 months) were less and less capable of avoiding noxious stimulation following neutral sensory stimulation (sound and light). The males were more affected than the females from the start, with the latter significantly affected by the phenomenon only when paternal age reached 22 months (this may be considered as corresponding to 65–70 years in man). For the moment there is no clear genetic explanation for this sex-based effect. It is noteworthy that the greater male fragility implied by this result also exists in man, in so far as mentally retarded populations contain significantly more males than females[36], which may be attributed to the fragility of the X chromosome. (b) 2.5- and 23-month rats simultaneously crossed with 2.5-month females yielded offspring with a learning capacity which was significantly decreased when the father was older (experiment carried out to confirm the previous finding[25]). Male offspring, solid line; female offspring, dashed line

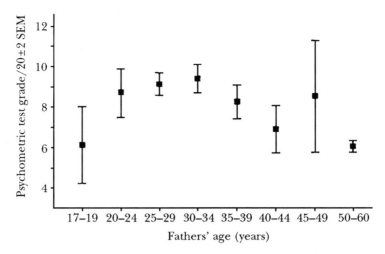

Figure 3 Paternal age and the quality of progeny. Paternal age at birth affected the probability of success on psychometric tests for 18-year-old young men ($p < 0.04$). The curve is parabolic. There are no differences between the means of the observed and the theoretical values of the calculated parabola[26]

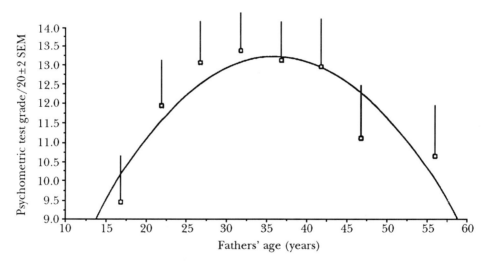

Figure 4 Paternal age and offspring quality. Preliminary results of the survey in progress. The first 5000 cases analyzed yield a curve similar to that in Figure 3 (unpublished)

The first survey was carried out in Nancy, in 1985, and to explain the curve, we may suppose that a cohort effect introduced a bias. The study was therefore repeated in another region with a greater number of subjects and with a much larger population base, namely the greater Paris area. This study was spread out over 1989 and 1990 and involved 12 000 recruits.

Analysis of the first 5000 subjects yielded the same type of curve as in the initial study (Figure 4) (unpublished). These data obviously go beyond the context of pathological abnormalities, including general factors which may influence the quality of the conceptus. In the light of this, it is necessary to identify the role of cultural factors and to verify the neutral effect of maternal age. These constitute part of the aims of the second part of our study which will include the 12 000 cases. If, however, we apply the genetic hypothesis to the data already available, the shape of the curve indicates that the sperm genome may be characterized by subtle improvements from puberty, with a maximum quality being reached around 30 years of age, followed by deterioration. As has been observed, the qualitative characteristics of spermatozoa reach a maximum around 30 years of age[2]. Given that we know that the morphology of sperm is genetically determined[5], such a pattern of development would suggest an improvement in factors related to information transmission in the ascending part of the curve and a deterioration concerning these factors in the descending part of the curve. The question may then be asked as to whether analogous phenomena may affect information other than that which determines gamete phenotype, that is to say, which determine an individual's phenotype.

A deterioration in the information factors in the descending part of the curve may be easily explained by the aging phenomena which, in so far as they affect somatic cells, no doubt also affect the spermatogonia, given the presence in them of DNA repair systems[27]. Other recent studies[28] have indicated that mitochondrial DNA is more fragile than nuclear DNA concerning mutations, and, in particular, in relation to those caused by free radicals, which cumulate with age. The fact that these modifications lead to a decrease in the possibility of oxidative phosphorylation in the mitochondria suggest another possible effect of aging in the male, even if the sperm mitochondria only represent 0.1% of the zygote mitochondria.

Concerning the type and subtle nature of the disorders observed, we must compare them to results already obtained by provoking experimental mutations in the male rat using mutagenic antimitotics such as cyclophosphamide: the offspring derived from these rats showed changes in learning ability, emphasized in the males, by a degradation in some biochemical substrates of memory[29].

It is more difficult to explain the improvement in information factors in the ascending part of the curve. However, the role currently attributed to the cytoplasm in the final organization of gamete DNA[30–33], allows us to suppose a kind of breaking-in period of variable duration which would precede genome maturity. Within this context we have recently carried out a study in the mouse which showed that on the one hand spontaneous movements and exploratory movements were significantly less for animals with post-puberal fathers (6 weeks) (Figure 5,

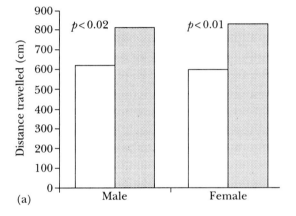

(a)

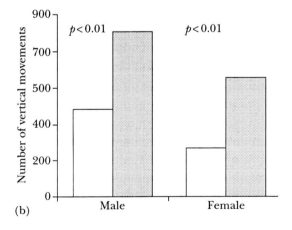

(b)

Figure 5 (a) Average spontaneous movements (distance travelled) and (b) exploratory behaviors (number of vertical movements) for 12-week male and female adult mice in an open-field test over a 5-min period, as a function of paternal age at conception (6 weeks, unshaded and 16 weeks shaded) and fixed maternal age (12 weeks) (unpublished)

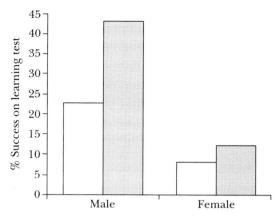

Figure 6 Percentage of adult mice (12 weeks) according to sex, succeeding on a learning test (conditioned avoidance reaction) as a function of paternal age at conception (6 weeks, unshaded or 16 weeks, shaded) with a fixed maternal age (12 weeks). The differences are significant for the male mice ($p < 0.01$) but not the female mice (unpublished)

unpublished), and on the other hand, that the learning capacity of mice from 6-week-old fathers was less than those with 16-week-old fathers (Figure 6, unpublished).

Concerning the absence of effects of maternal age, if confirmed, this may be explained by the different and complementary roles played by female and male genomes in the development of the conceptus[34,35]. If the information supplied by the father and mother is not the same, we can conclude that changes in one or other genome will not have the same effects, and that paternal information plays a dominant part in the characteristics which we have examined.

Conclusion

It would seem that paternal age influences both the appearance of specific syndromes and the determination of the most detailed potential of the conceptus. If the latter effects are confirmed, one aspect of the problem which becomes very important is the fact that paternal aging would influence not only the appearance of particular medical conditions, but would act along a qualitative continuum which would concern the general population. Whether the factors involved are psychosocial, genetic, or both, it is important to identify them because as well as behavioral effects, they may also influence other parameters such as the defense mechanisms of the organism, morbidity, aging in the individual, etc. Their clarification would be as important as that of environmental toxins, in an attempt to obtain, within a non-pathological context and for a given genetic patrimony, maximum quality conceptuses.

Acknowledgement

We thank Miss N. Hatilip for her kind and effective secretarial assistance.

References

1. Auroux, M. (1991). Evolution de la fertilité masculine en fonction de l'âge et risques pour la progéniture. *Contracept. Fertil. Sex.*, **19**, 945–9
2. Schwartz, D., Mayaux, M. J., Spira, A., Moscato, M. L., Jouannet, P., Czyglik, F. and David, G. (1981). Study of a group of 484 fertile men, Part II: relation between age (20–59) and semen characteristics. *Int. J. of Androl.*, **4**, 450–6
3. Albert, M. and Roussel, C. (1984). Strain differences in the concentration, mobility and morphology of epididymal sperm in relation to puberty in mice. *Int. J. Androl.*, **7**, 334–47
4. Lunstra, D. D. and Echternkamp, S. E. (1982). Puberty in beef bulls: acrosome morphology and semen quality in bulls of different breeds. *J. Anim. Sci.*, **55**, 638–48
5. Burgoyne, P. S. (1975). Sperm phenotype and its relationship to somatic and germ line genotype: a study using mouse aggregation chimeras. *Dev. Biol.*, **44**, 63–76
6. Martin, R. H. and Rademaker, A. W. (1987). The effect of age on the frequency of sperm chromosomal abnormalities in normal men. *Am. J. Hum. Genet.*, **41**, 484–92

7. Martin, R. H., Balkan, W., Burns, K., Rademaker, A. W., Lin, C. C. and Rudd, N. L. (1983). The chromosome constitution of 1000 human spermatozoa. *Hum. Genet.*, **63**, 305–9

8. Brandriff, B., Gordon, L., Ashworth, L., Watchmaker, G., Moore II, D., Wyrobek, A. J. and Carrano, A. V. (1985). Chromosomes of human sperm: variability among normal individuals. *Hum. Genet.*, **70**, 18–24

9. Sherman, S. L., Takaesu, N., Freeman, S., Philipps, C., Blackston, R. D., Keats, B. J., Jacobs, P. A., Cockwell, A. E., Kurnite, D., Uchida, I. and Hassold, T. J. (1990). Trisomy 21: association between reduced recombination and non-disjunction. *Am. J. Hum. Genet.*, **47**, A 97

10. Stylianos, E. and Antonarakis, M. D. (1991). The Down syndrome collaborative group. Parental origin of the extra chromosome in trisomy 21 as indicated by analysis of DNA polymorphisms. *N. Engl. J. Med.*, **324**, 872–6

11. Stene, J., Fischer, G., Stene, E., Mikkelsen, M. and Petersen, E. (1977). Paternal age effect in Down's syndrome. *Ann. Hum. Genet.*, **40**, 299–306

12. Matsunaga, E., Tonomura, E., Oishi, A. and Kikuchi, Y. (1978). Reexamination of paternal age effect in Down's syndrome. *Hum. Genet.*, **40**, 259–68

13. Thepot, F., Wack, T., Selva, J., Czyglik, F. and Mayaux, M. J. (1993). Age paternal et issues de grossesses. Expérience des CECOS. *Contracept. Fertil. Sex.*, **21**, 388–90

14. Roth, M. P., Stoll, C., Taillemite, J. L., Girard, S. and Boue, A. (1983). Paternal age and Down's syndrome diagnosed prenatally: no association in French data. *Prenat. Diagn.*, **3**, 327–35

15. Hook, E. B. and Regal, R. R. (1984). A search for a paternal-age effect upon cases of 47, + 21 in which the extra chromosome is of paternal origin. *Am. J. Hum. Genet.*, **36**, 413–21

16. Hassold, T. J. (1991). The origin of non-dysjunction in humans. Presented at the *Meeting of the International Human Genetics Society*, Washington, October

17. Hook, E. B., Schreinemachers, D. M., Wiley, A. M. and Cross, P. K. (1984). Inherited structural cytogenetic abnormalities detected incidentally in fetuses diagnosed prenatally: frequency, paternal age associations, sex-ratio trends, and comparison with rates of mutants. *Am. J. Hum. Genet.*, **36**, 422–43

18. Penrose, L. S. (1955). Paternal age and mutation. *Lancet*, **ii**, 312–13

19. Friedman, J. M. (1981). Genetic disease in the offspring of older fathers. *Obstet. Gynecol.*, **57**, 745–9

20. Cohen, F. L. (1986). Paternal contribution to birth defects. *Nurs. Clin. North. Am.*, **21**, 49–64

21. Bordson, B. L. and Leonardo, V. S. (1991). The appropriate upper age limit for semen donors: a review of the genetic effects of paternal age. *Fertil. Steril.*, **56**, 397–401

22. Lian, Z. H., Zack, M. M. and Erickson, J. D. (1986). Paternal age and the occurrence of birth defects. *Am. J. Hum. Genet.*, **39**, 648–60

23. Kaplan, J. and Toutain, A. (1987). La maladie de Recklinghausen. In Briard, M. L., Kaplan, J., Le Merrer, M. and Frezal, J. (eds.) *3e Seminaire de Genetique Clinique: affections dominantes à expression variable et Conseil Génétique*, pp. 42–52, (Paris: Necker)

24. Vogel, F. and Rathenberg, R. (1975). Spontaneous mutation in man. *Adv. Hum. Genet.*, **5**, 223–318

25. Auroux, M. (1983). Decrease of learning capacity in offspring with increasing paternal age in the rat. *Teratology.*, **27**, 141–8

26. Auroux, M., Mayaux, M. J., Guihard-Moscato, M. L., Fromantin, M., Barthe, J. and Schwartz, D. (1989). Paternal age and mental functions of progeny in man. *Hum. Reprod.*, **4**, 794–7

27. Lee, I. P. (1983). Adaptive biochemical repair responses toward germ cell DNA damage. *Am. J. Int. Med.*, **4**, 135–47

28. Wallace, D. C. (1992). Mitochondrial genetics: a paradigm for aging and degenerative diseases? *Sciences*, **256**, 628–32

29. Auroux, M., Dulioust, E., Selva, J. and Rince, P. (1990). Cyclophosphamide in the F_0 male rate: physical and behavioral changes in three successive adult generations. *Mutat. Res.*, **229**, 189–200

30. Campbell, J. H. and Zimmermann, E. G. (1982). Automodulation of genes: a proposed mechanism for persisting effects of drugs and hormones in mammals. *Neurobehav. Toxicol. Teratol.*, **4**, 435–9

31. Campbell, J. H. (1987). Automodulation of genes: explanation for lasting effects seen in functional neuroteratology? In *15th International Summer School of Brain Research: Neurochemistry of Functional Neuroteratology*, Amsterdam, August

32. Reik, W., Walter, J., Gurtmann, I., Feil, R., Surani, A., Sasaki, H., Klose, J. and Allen, N. (1993). Imprinting in development and disease. In *9th Annual Meeting of European Society of Human Reproduction and Embryology*, Thessaloniki, June

33. Krumlauf, R., Marshall, H., Monchev, S., Sham, M. H. and Studer, M. (1993). Transgenic approaches to the role of Hox homeobox genes in craniofacial development. In *21st Annual Conference of the European Teratology Society*. Lyon, September

34. Barton, S. C., Surani, M. A. H. and Norris, M. L. (1984). Role of paternal and maternal genome in mouse development. *Nature*, **311**, 374–6

35. Sepienza, C., Peterson, A. C., Rossant, J. and Balling, R. (1987). Degree of methylation of transgenes is dependent on gamete of origin. *Nature*, **328**, 251–4

36. Anthenaise, M. and Salbreux, R. (1979). Prévalence de la déficience mentale profonde chez l'enfant. *Neuropsy. Enfance Adolesc.*, **27**, 45–8

Acquired immunodeficiency syndrome and donor insemination

45

K. S. Moghissi

Therapeutic donor artificial insemination (TDI) was first performed in 1884 by William Pancoast in Philadelphia, Pennsylvania. The indication for this procedure was therapy resistant azoospermia. In the United States, it is estimated that 75 000 TDI are performed each year resulting in over 15 000 live births. In some countries, such as, France and Denmark, government controlled national services for TDI have been established with excellent results. A major complication of TDI is the transmission of sexually transmitted diseases (STD) from the donor semen to the recipient. There is ample documentation that the ejaculate can carry bacteria and viruses and that these organisms are capable of infecting a recipient through insemination, just as they do as a consequence of coital activity. STDs that are likely to infect women undergoing TDI include those due to *Neisseria gonorrhoea, Treponema pallidum, Chlamydia trachomatis, Mycoplasma hominis, Ureaplasma urealyticum*, streptococcal species and *Trichomonas vaginalis*. Several viral infections are also known to be transmitted to the female recipient through TDI. They include cytomegalovirus, hepatitis B virus and human immunodeficiency virus (HIV). Clearly the most lethal of these infections is HIV. HIV has been cultured from the semen of patients with AIDS. Vertical transmission of HIV from infected mother to the fetus has also been documented. Therefore, both the recipients of donor semen containing HIV and their offspring are at risk for AIDS.

The first report of transmission of HIV through TDI appeared in 1985 from Australia. Four women who had been inseminated between 1982 and 1984 were found to be seroposi-

tive. All four cases were inseminated with cryopreserved semen. A woman from New York who was inseminated with semen from five HIV infected donors between 1984 and 1985 was the first reported case from the United States. Subsequently, seven cases of TDI associated HIV transmission occurring in five infertility clinics were reported to the Los Angeles Country Department of Health Services in California. Three cases occurred in clinics located in Los Angeles County, one in Arizona and two in Vancouver, British Columbia. These seven women represented 3.52% of the 199 patients who were artificially inseminated with semen from five identified HIV infected semen donors. Risk factors for HIV acquisition through TDI have not been identified. Also, the relationship between the frequency of TDI procedures and the risk of HIV infection remains unclear and is probably related to intrinsic properties of the donor, the host, or viral infectivity and virulence. To prevent transmission of HIV through TDI, guidelines have been developed by professional societies and government agencies in several countries. In the United States, the American Fertility Society (now, the American Society for Reproductive Medicine) developed its first set of guidelines for semen donor insemination in 1980. These guidelines were subsequently revised three times. The last revision, in 1991, recommended that donors belonging to high-risk groups for STD including HIV be excluded by careful historical screening and the criteria for selection of donors include, among others, a physical examination and evaluation for STDs, as well as, HIV.

Available data indicate that pregnancy rates using frozen semen are lower than with fresh semen. Sexually transmitted diseases is a risk with both fresh and frozen semen. Since it is possible for the HIV to be transmitted by fresh semen before the donor has become seropositive, a process which may take up to 3 months or longer to occur after initial infection. The potential for transmission of AIDS by fresh semen cannot be eliminated entirely. Therefore, the American Society for Reproductive Medicine (ASRM) recommends that only frozen semen be used for TDI, and that all frozen specimens should be quarantined for 180 days and the donor retested and found to be seronegative for HIV before the specimen is released and used. This position is consistent with that of the Food and Drug Administration (FDA) and Center for Disease Control (CDC) guidelines.

As polymerase chain reaction technology becomes more readily available and cost effective for direct evaluation of semen for the presence of HIV, it will be possible to alter these guidelines.

Are semen quality and male fertility at risk?

B. Jégou

46

Introduction

Over the last decades, there has been growing concern among the public about the threat to human and animal health represented by chemical and radioactive materials introduced into the environment. A new wave of concern has recently arisen that not only the health of individuals may be at risk but, also, their fertility.

Are male reproductive disorders increasing?

Semen quality in men

Since 1974, there has been a stream of data claiming that there exists a secular trend in the decline of sperm counts[1-16]. At the same time, however, this assumption has been repeatedly challenged[17-24]. The most recent data published have not avoided the development of controversy. It may be surprising that, after 20 years of research, so important a matter has not been settled. This reflects the very real difficulty there is in measuring objectively possible changes in male fertilizing capacity and in male reproductive disorders.

In 1992, Carlsen and colleagues[10] published a meta-analysis of a total of 61 papers containing data on semen characteristics in healthy fertile men, covering the period 1938–90. The study included 14 947 men and concluded that the seminal plasma volume declined from 3.4 ml in 1940 to 2.75 ml in 1990, and that, during the same period, the average sperm density dropped from $113 \times 10^6/\mathrm{ml}$ to $66 \times 10^6/\mathrm{ml}$. In this meta-analysis, Carlsen and co-workers[10] paid particular attention to avoiding certain methodological bias. For example, they restricted their analysis to data obtained using hemocytometers, thereby excluding reports using computer assisted or flow cytometer methods which are known to vary greatly from one laboratory to another. They also omitted studies based on data from infertile couples. Despite these precautions, their report has generated strong criticism[21-23]. The main criticism is that selection bias may have occurred, since the 61 studies may not be representative of the corresponding populations; the methods of semen analysis varied from one laboratory to another; data distribution is unequal, as data are scarce in the period 1950–70; and also, linear regression was used for statistical analysis. Carlsen and colleagues[10] have responded to these criticisms[13].

One of the major merits of the study by Carlsen and colleagues[10] is that it has generated a renewed and vivid interest in the hypothesis that semen quality has declined world-wide since the 1940s. It has prompted several groups to evaluate their data on semen quality obtained during recent years. At present, the strongest argument which favors this allegation is based on a report by Auger and colleagues[14] which claims that, during the past 20 years, the mean concentration of sperm has decreased by 2.1% per year in the Paris area ($89 \times 10^6/\mathrm{ml}$ in 1973 vs. $60 \times 10^6/\mathrm{ml}$ in 1992) whereas, during the same period, the percentages of motile and normal spematozoa decreased by 0.6% and 0.5% per year, respectively. The particular strengths of this study are that all the data included (corresponding to 1351 men) originated from the same geographical area; the same equipment was used over the study period; few changes had occurred in the laboratory staff; the method of study did not change and was verified over the 20-year period; the authors integrated important parameters such as donor age and the duration of sexual abstinence; and the authors were able to use the year of birth of the donors, instead of the year of donation of the semen, as in previous studies.

Recently, other papers claiming a degradation in sperm characteristics during the past two decades in Scotland, Belgium and England have also been published by laboratories which used the same semen analysis techniques throughout the period[11,15,16]. Conversely, during the same period, no changes were found in Finland[20], in Toulouse, France (Bujan and colleagues, submitted) and in Wisconsin, USA, in a 10-year prospective study, suggesting that geographical differences may exist in the phenomenon[19].

It can always be said that all studies claiming a decline in semen are retrospective and that prospective studies in the general population would be much better. Prospective studies would certainly be invaluable in this domain and should be encouraged, but it is very naive to believe, as Sherins does[24], that all the bias encountered in the retrospective studies would be avoided. In fact, it is most likely that attempts to develop such prospective trials would encounter great reticence in the general population if the study required semen collection. Therefore, any prospective study in this domain would favor participation bias; this was recently experienced by Spira and collaborators (personal communication). Furthermore, prospective studies ought to last several decades and it does not seem reasonable to wait for their completion before initiating research into the origin of the possible decline in semen quality.

Genitourinary abnormalities in humans

The secular changes reported here do not seem to be restricted to semen characteristics as, according to converging sources, the incidence of testicular cancer, hypospadia, cryptorchidism or

even prostate and breast cancer in men may have been increasing during the past 50 years, in many different countries[25,26].

Male reproduction disorders in animals

Most interesting is the fact that, at the same time as alarming observations are made in humans, the development of reproductive disorders resulting from exposure to xenobiotics have been observed in wildlife[27,28]. Thus, an increased rate in the incidence of cryptorchidism and a drop in semen quality have been observed in the North American wild panther[29], very serious reproductive disorders have been seen in Florida alligators and various changes in male reproduction have also been recorded in other mammals and in fish, birds, reptiles and even gasteropod species[26].

An interesting approach to study the secular trends in male reproductive function would be to perform retrospective or prospective studies among domesticated animals, e.g. bull, ram, stallion, dog. To our knowledge, no such experiments have been undertaken yet. Although the development of such studies would provide important information, genetic selection in breeding animals over the last decades may have more or less counterbalanced the possible secular changes in semen characteristics.

Is the quality of male reproductive function linked to quality of the environment?

It has been suggested that an etiological link exists between the apparent decline in semen quality and reproductive disorders in humans[10,25,30]. At present, arguments are too scarce to conclude unequivocally on this matter. However, it is a stimulating working hypothesis as there are arguments to support it: both semen and genitourinary abnormalities have been found to occur in panthers[29], in mice and probably in humans exposed *in utero* to estrogens[26]; the Finnish population, which displays the highest sperm counts in Europe[20], is the one which presents the lowest rate of testicular cancer[31], hypospadia[32] and male breast cancer[33]; conversely, the Danish population, whose sperm counts are about half that of the Finnish, presents the highest incidence in male reproductive disorders[25,26].

A particular susceptibility of individuals to chemicals may render them more vulnerable to alterations in their environment. However, it is unlikely that genetic factors are directly responsible for the degradation in male reproductive health, as the incidence in abnormalities has arisen rapidly and over the same period, in different parts of the world. It is more likely that the great vulnerability of the testis to chemical agents or physical (radiation, heat) factors explains that changes in the environment may be at the origin of the negative trends observed.

Among the man-made substances which may interfere with reproductive parameters, great attention has been focused on the so-called endocrine disrupters that are in daily use in industry, agriculture or in the home. Their estrogenic or anti-androgenic actions may well interfere with normal fetal gonadal development and with postnatal testicular function[26,27,30]. Among the thousands of chemicals in use, just a handful have been tested in this respect and identified as estrogen-like substances (e.g. organochlorine pesticides, dioxins, alkylphenol polyethoxylates and polychlorinated biphenyl (PCBs)). Very few others have been reported to behave like androgens[34].

In addition to these chemicals, many others probably not behaving like hormones can also interfere with the development and function of the male reproductive system. In addition, elevated temperatures (e.g. ceramists in industry), the trend in the increased exposure to radiation (medical, occupational) and changes in life style (e.g. stress) may have also contributed separately, additionally or synergistically to the degradation of male reproductive health.

Does a decline in semen quality mean declined fertility?

In the wild, chemical pollution and its consequence on the reproductive function

have already endangered some animal populations[26,27,28,29].

In humans, it is well known that, except in extreme situations, a change in sperm concentration, even if important, does not automatically result in a change in fertility. The best illustration of this is the very high variability (up to 75%) that can be observed among semen samples from a healthy fertile man[35]. It is, therefore, very unlikely that an average decline of 20–50% in sperm counts would automatically result in a drop in fertility in the general population. What could happen is that, as a consequence of the decline in semen characteristics which apparently occurs within all ranges of sperm concentrations, the population of subfertile men would increase[10]. Therefore, increasing numbers of couples may have trouble conceiving and may require medical assistance, with its attendant psychological, economical and social costs.

The principle of precaution

As the reality of the secular decline in male reproductive health is very difficult to establish unequivocally, it is most likely that the controversy on the subject will persist. The scientist confronted with this problem has several options open to him: either he remains a passive witness or he contributes to the 'sterile' controversy, or he actively makes his own the 'principle of precaution': there is now enough disturbing evidence in vertebrates and more specifically in mammals, including humans, to believe that alarm is justified and to initiate and/or participate research in this domain.

Acknowledgements

The author thanks P. Jouannet, A. Spira, L. Bujan, R. Mieusset, J. F. Bourgoin, R. E. Chapin, E. Ben-Hassel and the 'Group of Copenhagen'[26] for helpful discussions.

References

1. Nelson, C. M. K. and Bunge, R. G. (1974). Semen analysis: evidence for changing parameters of male fertility potential. *Fertil. Steril.*, **25**, 503–7

2. Rehan, *et al.* (1975). The semen of fertile men. Statistical analysis of 1300 men. *Fertil. Steril.*, **26**, 492–502

3. James, W. H. (1980). Secular trend in reported sperm counts. *Andrologia.*, **12**, 381–8

4. Leto, S. and Frensilli, F. J. (1981). Changing parameters of donor semen. *Fertil. Steril.*, **36**, 766–70

5. Bostofte, E., Serup, J. and Rebbe, H. (1983). Has the fertility of Danish men declined through the years in terms and semen quality? A comparison of semen qualities between 1952 and 1972. *Int. J. Fertil.*, **28**, 91–5

6. Osser, S., Liedholm, P. and Ranstam, J. (1984). Depressed semen quality: a study over two decades. *Arch. Androl.*, **12**, 113–16

7. Menkveld, R. *et al.* (1986). Possible changes in male fertility over a 15-year period. *Arch. Androl.*, **17**, 143–4

8. Murature, D. A. *et al.* (1987). Phthalate esters and semen quality parameters. *Biomed. Environ. Mass Spectrom.*, **14**, 473–7

9. Bendvold, E. (1989). Semen quality in Norwegian men over a 20-year period. *Int. J. Fertil.*, **34**, 401–4

10. Carlsen, E., Giwercman, A., Keiding, N. and Skakkebaek, N. E. (1992). Evidence for decreasing quality of semen during the past 50 years. *Br. Med. J.*, **305**, 609–13

11. Van Waeleghem, K., De Clercq, N., Vermeulen, L., Schoojans, F. and Comhaire, F. (1994). Deterioration of sperm quality in young Belgian men during recent decades. *Hum. Reprod.*, **9** (Suppl. 4), 73 (abstr.)

12. Skakkebaek, N. E. and Keiding, N. (1994). Changes in semen and the testis. *Br. Med. J.*, **309**, 1316–17

13. Keiding, N. *et al.* (1994). Falling sperm quality (letter). *Br. Med. J.*, **309**, 131

14. Auger, J., Kunstmann, J. M., Czyglik, F. and Jouannet, P. (1995). Decline in semen quality among fertile men in Paris during the past 20 years. *N. Engl. J. Med.*, **322**, 281–5

15. Irvine, D. S. (1994). Failing sperm quality (letter) *Br. Med. J.*, **309**, 476

16. Ginsburg, J., Okolo, S., Prelevic, G. and Hardiman, P. (1994). Residence in London area and sperm density. *Lancet*, **343**, 230

17. Macleod, J. and Wang, Y. (1979). Male fertility potential in terms of semen quality: a review of the past, a study of the present. *Fertil. Steril.*, **31**, 103–16

18. David, G. *et al.* (1979). Sperm counts in fertile and infertile men. *Fertil. Steril.*, **31**, 453–5

19. Wittmaack, F. M. and Shapiro, S. S. (1992). Longitudinal study of semen quality in Wisconsin men over one decade. *Wis. Med. J.*, **91**, 477–9

20. Suominen, J. and Vierula, M. (1993). Semen quality of Finnish men. *Br. Med. J.*, **306**, 1579

21. Bromwich, P., Cohen, J., Stewart, I. and Walker, A. (1994). Decline in sperm counts: an artefact of changed reference range of 'normal'? *Br. Med. J.*, **309**, 19–22

22. Farrow, S. (1994). Falling sperm quality: fact or fiction? *Br. Med. J.*, **309**, 1–2

23. Olsen, W. O., Bodner, K. M., Ramlow, J. M., Ross, C. E. and Lipshultz, L. I. (1995). Have sperm counts been reduced 50 percent in 50 years? A statistical model revisited. *Fertil. Steril.*, **63**, 887–93

24. Sherins, R. J. (1995). Are semen quality and male fertility changing? *N. Engl. J. Med.*, **332**, 327–8

25. Giwercman, A., Carlsen, E., Keiding, N. and Skakkebaek, N. E. (1993). Evidence for increasing incidence of abnormalities of the human testis: a review. *Environ. Health Perspect.*, **101** (Suppl. 2), 65–71

26. Toppari, J., Larsen, J. C., Christiansen, P., Giwercman, A., Grandjean, P., Guillette, L. J., Jégou, B., Jensen, T. K., Jouannet, P., Keiding, N., Leffers, H., McLachlan, J. A., Meyer, O., Müller, J., Rajpert-De Meyts, E., Scheike, T., Sharpe, R., Sumpter, J. and Skakkebaek, N. E. (1995). In *Male Reproductive Health and Environmental Chemicals*, Miljoprojekt nr 290. (Denmark: Ministry of Environmental and Energy)

27. Colborn, T. and Clement, C. (1992). *Chemically-induced Alterations in Sexual and Functional Development: The Wildlife/Human Connection.* (Princeton: Princeton Scientific Publishing)

28. Colborn, T., vom Saal, F. S. and Soto, A. M. (1993). Developmental effects of endocrine-disrupting chemicals in wildlife and human. *Environ. Health Perspect.*, **101**, 378–84

29. Facemire, C. F., Gross, T. S. and Guillette, L. J. J. (1995). Reproductive impairment in the Florida panther: nature or nurture? *Environ. Health Perspect.*, **103** (Suppl. 4), in press

30. Sharpe, R. M. and Skakkebaek, N. E. (1993). Are oestrogens involved in falling sperm counts and

disorders of the male reproductive tract? *Lancet*, **341**, 1392–5

31. Adami, H., Bergström, R., Möhner, M., Zatonski, W., Storm, H., Ekbom, A., Tretli, S., Teppo, L., Ziegler, H., Rahu, M., Gurevicius, R. and Stengrevics, A. (1994). Testicular cancer in nine Northern European countries. *Int. J. Cancer*, **59**, 33–8

32. World Health Organization (1991). Impact of the environment on reproductive health. **38**, 425–6

33. Ewertz, M., Holmberg, L., Karjalainen, S., Tretli, S. and Adami, H. O. (1989). Incidence of male breast cancer in Scandinavia, 1943–1982. *Int. J. Cancer*, **43**, 27–31

34. Kelce, W. R., Stone, C. R., Laws, S. C., Gray, L. E., Kemppainen, J. A. and Wilson, E. M. (1995). Persistent DDT metabolite p,p′-DDE is a potent androgen receptor antagonist. *Nature (London)*, **375**, 581–5

35. Scherins, R. J. (1974). Clinical aspects of treatment of male infertility with gonadotropins: testicular response of some men given hCG with and without pergonal. In Mancini, R. E. and Martini, L. (eds.) *Male Fertility and Sterility, Proceedings of the Serono Symposia*, Vol. 5, pp. 545–65. (London: Academic Press)

5

Reproductive surgery

Risks and benefits of endoscopic surgery in reproductive medicine

47

I. A. Brosens

Introduction

Soon after the introduction of laparoscopy in gynecological practice in the 1950s, Raoul Palmer developed the endoscopic technique of tubal sterilization, giving women the choice of controlling their fertility permanently and by a more acceptable method than by laparotomy. For decades operative laparoscopy in gynecology was used for this indication and also for the treatment of lesser degrees of pelvic endometriosis and adhesions. The introduction of videoendoscopy together with surgical lasers in the 1980s caused a sudden increase in the number of procedures performed by laparoscopy. Today, if endoscopic surgery is no more than a method of access to perform established techniques, the progress has been revolutionary for the industry and to some extent beneficial for the patient, but problematic for the gynecologist. The critical question that must be answered is whether or not the use of endoscopic surgery is progress and means better medical care for the patient with an improved benefit/risk ratio. The claimed benefits have been simplified by stating that the minimally invasive access is less traumatic and leads to a lower morbidity and shorter recovery period. Frequently, the surgical procedure is claimed to be the same procedure as that performed in the open abdomen. Minimally invasive surgery is, however, a misnomer and should be called minimal access surgery as it is in no way a guarantee for atraumatic surgery. In many cases the procedure is sufficiently different to be considered as a new experimental technique. Therefore, a rigorous evaluation is needed to ascertain and establish the grade of safety and efficacy in comparison to the established procedure before such a technique can be accepted as a standard procedure.

The present paper intends to discuss, first, the risks and, second, the benefits which have been formulated since the introduction of videoendoscopic surgery.

What are the risks?

Therapeutic inappropriateness

It has been suggested that endoscopic surgery promotes unnecessary and incomplete surgery. Gynecological surgery has been notoriously bedevilled with procedures of doubtful or unproven benefit to the patient. Some of these procedures have now been revived. Patients are likely to accept laparoscopy more readily than laparotomy, and gynecologists may be tempted to reason that the potential benefit may outweigh the risk and discomfort of the procedure for the patient. Using the same vein of reasoning, procedures of questionable or doubtful benefit are readily performed at the time of diagnostic laparoscopy. It is evident that any surgical procedure performed at the time of endoscopy carries a surgical risk and that the appropriateness of each procedure must be based on scientific evidence independent of the method of access.

Incomplete surgery may be a specific problem of endoscopic surgery because of the loss of depth perception, the absence of palpation and the limited degree of manipulation. In general, incomplete as well as excessive surgery is a consequence of inadequate diagnosis and surgical inexperience. Laparoscopy is a powerful diagnostic tool and the illumination, the magnification, the angle of access to the pelvis and the use of angled scopes all add to the improved visibility and identification of pathology. Full pelvic exploration can require adhesiolysis and mobilization to detect and localize pathology. Explorative surgery as a combination of diagnosis and surgery is an important aspect of reproductive surgery and can more readily be performed by endoscopic techniques than by laparotomy.

On the other hand, some new surgical techniques such as endometrial ablation and laparoscopic myomectomy are likely to be associated with incomplete surgery as a consequence of inadequate diagnosis. The risk exists that endometrial ablation is a symptomatic treatment and that underlying myometrial pathology such as adenomyosis or myomas are not removed. The failure to recognize the type of myometrial pathology could even delay the diagnosis and definitive treatment of uterine malignancies such as leiomyosarcoma[1].

High levels of complications

There is much concern about the increased rate of complications in endoscopic surgery. According to large survey studies the risk of serious complications of diagnostic laparoscopy decreased in the 1980s due to increased experience. With the dramatic increase of operative procedures in recent years and the problem of inadequate training of surgeons or gynecologists, the current risk of injury or complications of operative laparoscopy may exceed that of laparotomy for some new procedures. Serious specific complications have been observed in hysteroscopic and laparoscopic procedures. Unfortunately, the current risk is not known as there is no register or other systematic way to acquire such information. Publications by experienced laparoscopists tend to underestimate the complication rates, while surgeons who have experienced an unusually high rate of complications are not likely to publish their results. Complications are more likely to be increased by the introduction of new surgical procedures, e.g. in the retropubic, rectovaginal or lateral

pelvic spaces or when laparoscopic surgery is performed in older patients who have underlying or associated medical problems. Initiatives which are taken to set up registers to monitor the rate of complications in the average situation are at present the most realistic approach to obtain data.

Results are no better

No firm data have been brought forward to support the view that the results of endoscopic surgery are better than after laparotomy. A prospective randomized study of the surgical treatment of ectopic pregnancy showed less increase in adhesion formation after laparoscopy than after laparotomy, but there was no significant difference in pregnancy rate[2]. This may be explained by the relatively small number of patients in such studies, but more likely by the fact that the fertility outcome after ectopic pregnancy is determined by the underlying condition of the tubal mucosa rather than by the surgical technique or the damage due to trophoblast invasion.

The problems of availability and training

The claim made 10 years ago by DeCherney[3] that laparotomy is on the way out has unfortunately been interpreted by some enthusiasts to mean that every physician in every hospital should and can perform any pelvic procedures by endoscopy in a safe and effective fashion. There is undoubtedly an increasing number of gynecologists performing an increasing number of endoscopic procedures in a safe and effective way but there are important limiting factors in this evolution.

The first is the cost of hardware and the expense of equipment, maintenance and supply which can be too high for hospitals in many countries around the world. Expensive equipment such as lasers or sophisticated, non-reusable instruments have been promoted by the industry but are not affordable and frequently not worth the money. Fortunately, improvement of electrosurgical and mechanical instrumentation has significantly reduced the costs of endoscopic equipment to a level comparable to that of conventional surgery.

The most important limiting factor is the training and accreditation. Specialists were not exposed to operative laparoscopy during their training and the organization of training in endoscopic surgery in the curriculum of the resident and the criteria for accreditation and the postaccreditation monitoring have not been established. Recently, specific guidelines have been given for surgeons in the state of New York following a plethora of patient injuries after laparoscopic cholecystectomy. These guidelines recommend three phases:

(1) A practical course with extensive individual training;

(2) Participation as an assistant surgeon in a number of cases performed by an expert to acquire knowledge of the risks of the procedure as well as familiarization with the instrumentation;

(3) Performance of the procedure as the responsible surgeon under the direct supervision of an expert laparoscopist in a number of cases depending on the progression in skill of the surgeon. In case of a practising specialist, the last stage can be performed most efficiently by assisting the trainee in his or her hospital.

The majority of the problems of accreditation concern the availability of qualified staff, the duration of training which may vary considerably between individuals, the objective evaluation of the trainee and the medico-legal responsibility of the perceptor or supervisor.

What are the benefits?

New access, old technique

Endoscopic treatment of ectopic pregnancy is a typical example of new access, old technique. The access by laparoscopy is new but the surgical procedure of linear salpingotomy is an old technique. It is well accepted that the technique of salpingotomy can be applied with the same results, not better or worse, by laparoscopy as by the open abdomen method.

Minimal access surgery can be described as progress when equal results and no higher complication rate are obtained when compared to standard open abdomen procedures. This has been shown to be the case for procedures such as tubal sterilization, tubal pregnancy, benign ovarian cyst within certain criteria, adhesiolysis and endometriosis. Today endoscopic surgery can be considered as the gold standard procedure in these cases.

Endoscopic access and surgical exploration

The endoscopic approach provides new tools for the exploration of the pelvis at the time of surgery. First, the illumination, magnification and versatility of the scopes give an improved visibility. Second, endoscopic techniques allow the access and examination of structures such as the Fallopian tube mucosa, ovarian cysts, endometriomas, pseudocysts and subperitoneal spaces. The endoscopic technology not only allows confirmation of the diagnosis, but, in addition, localization of the more exact pathology. The anatomopathology or macroscopic description of the pathological specimen performed by the pathologist in the laboratory and the selection of the site for biopsies can be advantageously performed *in situ* by the endoscopic surgeon. The combination of laparoscopy and organ-endoscopy has been particularly useful in the surgical management of ovarian endometriomas and tubal diseases.

The hemorrhagic ovarian cyst in the young woman remains a major diagnostic and surgical challenge. Excessive as well as incomplete surgery can aggravate the problem and compromise the fertility outcome. Excessive surgery such as excision of a hemorrhagic functional cyst in a young woman increases the risk of ovarian adhesive disease, while inadequate surgery increases the risk of recurrence or fails to detect nuclear atypia or neoplastic changes. The surgical exploration of the hemorrhagic ovarian cyst by combining laparoscopy and ovarioscopy allows accurate identification of the surgical pathology and a decision about the surgical procedure with minimal ovarian damage: hemorrhagic functional and neoplastic cysts are differentiated, endometrial implants are localized in endometriomas and guided biopsies provide more representative tissue than random biopsies or resected specimen. The endoscopic anatomopathology improves the selection of the appropriate surgical procedure. In tubal infertility, the combination of laparoscopy and salpingoscopy is a powerful technique for the assessment of tubal pathology and the selection between reconstructive surgery and *in vitro* fertilization (IVF). Third, surgical exploration is frequently needed in pelvic conditions associated with adhesions such as endometriosis or tubal disease to confirm the diagnosis, to localize the pathology and to identify the stage of the disease. The combination of endoscopic inspection and surgical exploration allow avoidance of not only the trauma of laparotomy but more importantly unnecessary organ trauma.

Endoscopic access and microsurgical techniques

The major surgical benefit that has been claimed for endoscopic surgery is that the procedure is less traumatic and associated with less postoperative adhesion formation. Minimal access can, however, not be equated with minimal tissue trauma. Excessive trauma can be inflicted in the same way as in open abdomen surgery. Unfortunately, much of the instrumentation is not designed for reconstructive but for ablative surgery. Even manipulation of the ovaries has been shown to inflict surface epithelium damage. There is good evidence that endoscopic surgery can be followed by a lower risk of *de novo* adhesion formation than open abdomen surgery but on the condition that the principles of atraumatic surgery are respected.

The question of whether endoscopic surgery is progress since microsurgery was introduced in gynecology was recently discussed in an editorial of the Fertility and Sterility journal. One of its most senior promotors Victor Gomel[4] concluded that microsurgery in gynecology is more a way of surgery than the use of magnification. It is a way of tissue handling, identification of surgical pathology and surgical restraint not to damage healthy tissue.

Conclusion

Despite the limitations and criticisms, the development of endoscopic surgery has been a major progress in reproductive surgery. The progress, however, does not depend on the feasibility of certain procedures by a few skilled surgeons but on the efficiency and safety of the procedure for all patients. The 'new access' with 'old techniques' is used in many procedures. The results are no better and no worse than after laparotomy but the patients benefit from less trauma, less pain, shorter hospitalization stay and faster recovery. However, it is also evident that the new access changes the application of the old techniques sufficiently to create specific problems which must be correctly assessed. In spite of the specific problems the complication rates are not unacceptably high. Incomplete and excessive surgery is in the first place a result of incomplete diagnosis. The *endoscopic access and surgical exploration* constitute major progress in defining pathology more accurately before undertaking surgery. The endoscopic exploration of the ovaries and Fallopian tubes permits detection and localization of pathology before surgery is performed. Determination of the stage of severe diseases such as in pelvic inflammatory disease or endometriosis is frequently not possible until extensive adhesiolysis is performed. The attribute of minimally invasive surgery is abused unless *the new access is combined with microsurgical techniques.* Microsurgery in gynecology is not only the use of magnification but a way of performing surgery. It is the combination of the accurate identification of the pathology and the surgical restraint not to damage healthy tissue.

References

1. Leibsohn, S., d'Ablaing, G., Mishell, D. R. and Schlaerth, J. B. (1990). Leiomyosarcoma in a series of hysterectomies performed for presumed uterine leiomyomas. *Am. J. Obstet. Gynecol.*, **162**, 968–76

2. Lundorff, P., Thorburn, J., Hahlin, M., Lindblom, B. and Kallfelt, B. (1991). Adhesion formation after laparoscopic surgery in tubal pregnancy: a randomized trial versus laparotomy. *Fertil. Steril.*, **55**, 911–15

3. DeCherney, A. H. (1985). 'The leader of the band is tired'. *Fertil. Steril.*, **44**, 299–302

4. Gomel, V. (1995). From microsurgery to laparoscopic surgery: a progress. *Fertil. Steril.*, **63**, 464–8

Endoscopic surgery of peritoneal, ovarian and rectovaginal septum endometriosis

48

J. Donnez, M. Nisolle, M. Smets and S. Bassil

Introduction

It is generally believed that endometriosis is caused by the implantation of retrograde menstrual endometrial cells, or by metaplasia. In the pelvis, three different forms of endometriosis[1] must be considered:

(1) Peritoneal;

(2) Ovarian; and

(3) Rectovaginal septum.

The early manifestations of the peritoneal form of the disease are believed to be subtle or non-colored lesions such as white lesions (white opacification, yellow–brown patches or hemosiderin patches). The presence of a lower mitotic activity in white lesions[2] suggests that this type of lesion is a latent form of the disease. The presence of a scanty stroma and poor stroma vascularization are two other arguments. Red lesions (red vesicles, polypoid lesions, red flame-like lesions, hypervascularized areas or even petechial peritoneum)[1–4] are more active forms of the disease. Recent experimental studies in the baboon[5] have suggested that these lesions undergo active remodelling, some disappearing, while other new lesions are formed. In women, our hypothesis is that red lesions are more aggressive and progress to the so-called typical or black lesions which must be considered as an enclosed implant surrounded by fibrosis. Red lesions have recently been proved to be a very active form of the disease[2].

Ovarian chocolate-colored fluid cysts are, according to the hypothesis of Hughesdon[6], the consequence of the invagination of superficial implants into the ovary. Endometriosis can also develop in the ovaries and this type of cystic ovarian endometriosis must be considered as another severe form of endometriosis, often related to infertility.

A third form of the disease is 'deep-infiltrating endometriosis of the rectovaginal septum'. Sampson[7] defined cul-de-sac obliteration as 'extensive adhesions in the cul-de-sac, obliterating its low portion and uniting the cervix or the lower portion of the uterus to the rectum; with adenoma of the endometrial type invading the cervical and the uterine tissue and probably also (but to a lesser degree) the anterior wall of the rectum.' Cul-de-sac obliteration secondary to endometriosis implies the presence of deep fibrotic retrocervical endometriosis beneath the peritoneum. Treatment options for pain or infertility secondary to cul-de-sac obliteration include ovarian suppression therapy with danazol or gonadotropin releasing hormone agonists, or surgery[5, 8–10]. For existing infertility or the preservation of fertility, reconstructive surgery can be considered either via laparotomy, microsurgery or laparoscopy, depending on the skill and experience of the surgeon.

At laparotomy, deep fibrotic retrocervical endometriosis is commonly managed by bowel resection, assuming that the major portion of the lesion infiltrates the anterior rectum. In such cases, the deep fibrotic lesion is mobilized, starting with the posterior uterus and progressing downward to the rectum where it appears

345

to be attached. But recently, some gynecologists[8,11-13] have developed the endoscopic technique.

Peritoneal endometriosis

The endoscopic use of the laser is not new in medicine, and several types of operative procedures have been carried out with the CO_2 laser laparoscope for the treatment of reproductive pathology. The most frequent indication is endometriosis, which can be vaporized by means of CO_2 laser laparoscopy with highly satisfactory postoperative pregnancy rates. Laser surgeons have removed endometriosis with great precision from the reproductive structure. There are at least three advantages of laser laparoscopy over conventional operative laparoscopy: precise destruction of diseased tissue, minimal bleeding and minimal damage to the adjacent normal tissue. Tissue reaction and postoperative adhesion formation have been shown to be no greater than with conventional methods. But vaporization of the endometriotic peritoneal lesion or of the endometriotic cyst wall provokes residual carbon charring. Expensive high-power operating lasers are required for the vaporization of tissue without residual carbon charring. The SwiftLase® (Sharplan, Model 757) allows a char-free ablation, even when using a 30-W operating laser.

Peritoneal endometriotic implants

In general, a power setting of 40–50 W is used. The debulking of endometriotic implants is best performed using a continuous firing mode. If a lesion is overlying a vital structure such as the ureter, urinary bladder, colon, or larger blood vessels, a retroperitoneal injection of fluid (aquadissection and aquaprotection) provides safer vaporization of the lesions. This duration allows a 100–200 µm depth of vaporization, thus substantially limiting the depth of penetration. Vaporizing an endometriotic implant provokes the bubbling of old blood, followed by a curdy white material representing vaporization of the stromal layer. After the endometriotic lesion has

been vaporized, retroperitoneal fat is encountered, and the appearance of bubbling confirms the complete vaporization of the lesion. Absorption of the CO_2 laser by water (contained in fatty tissue) for a few seconds after the complete destruction of the implants prevents deeper penetration of the laser beam.

Ovarian endometriosis

Ovarian endometriosis < 3 cm

Ovarian endometriosis is treated during first-look laparoscopy if a penetration of no more than 3 cm into the ovary is observed and if the cyst diameter is no larger than 3 cm. Small (< 1 cm in diameter) endometriotic implants of the ovary were vaporized until follicles containing fluid were encountered or no further pigmented tissue was seen. Large (< 3 cm in diameter) endometriomas were destroyed as follows. A 3–4 mm portion of the top of the cyst was excised, the chocolate-colored material was aspirated, and the cyst was washed out with irrigation fluid. After washing, the interior wall of the cyst was examined carefully to confirm the absence of any intracystic lesion suspected to be malignant (ovarian cystoscopy). With a power setting of 40 W and continuous mode application, the interior wall of the cyst was then vaporized to destroy the mucosal lining of the cyst. The vaporization continued until no further pigment could be seen. After copious irrigation, the ovaries were left open.

Ovarian endometriosis > 3 cm

In our series of 2912 patients with endometriosis, ovarian endometriosis larger than 3 cm in diameter were found in 481 patients. During diagnostic laparoscopy, the endometrial cyst was washed out with irrigation fluid (saline solution), and a biopsy was taken. Then, gonadotropin releasing hormone (GnRH) agonist (Zoladex®, ICI, UK) therapy was given for 12 weeks to decrease the cyst size. A decrease of 50% in cyst diameter was observed after drainage followed by a 12-week course of GnRH

Table 1 Scores (revised American Fertility Society classification) and ovarian cyst diameter after drainage and GnRH agonist therapy

	Scores	
	First look	Second look
Total	43.4 ± 2.1	33.2 ± 2.1
Implants	27.1 ± 2.1	16.9 ± 1.7
Adhesions	16.3 ± 2.7	16.3 ± 2.7
Cyst diameter (mm)	47.3 ± 6.2	21.7 ± 3.8

agonist (Table 1). Drainage alone (if not associated with GnRH agonist) was ineffective; indeed, 12 weeks after drainage, the ovarian cyst diameter was found to be unchanged when compared to the diameter observed before drainage[14]. Thereafter, a second-look laparoscopy was carried out. If the diameter of the residual endometrial cyst was < 3 cm after GnRH agonist therapy (233 patients), the interior wall of the cyst was vaporized as previously described. If the diameter of the residual cyst was > 3 cm after GnRH agonist therapy, another technique was proposed. In this series, the range of the ovarian cyst sizes was 3–8 cm. A portion of the ovarian cyst was first removed by making a circular cut over the protruded ovarian cyst portion, using the CO_2 laser. Partial cystectomy was then carried out. Ovarian cystoscopy was performed for evaluation of the interior cyst wall, and a biopsy was taken. The residual endometrial cyst wall was then vaporized with the CO_2 laser, equipped with the SwiftLase. At the end of the procedure, copious irrigation of the pelvic cavity was carried out to prevent deposits of carbon and glue[15]. Thereafter, 100–200 ml of 32% Dextran 70 was instilled into the peritoneal cavity in all patients of both groups. Recently, the closure of the ovarian edges has been performed using special new titanium clips (Endohernia®, Autosuture). The clips permit an excellent approximation of ovarian edges. Very often, two clips are sufficient to close the ovary.

Results

The operating time varied from 45 to 80 min. Vaporization of the mucosal lining was facili-

tated by the preoperative therapy (GnRH agonist administered subcutaneously). Indeed, the interior wall of the endometrial cyst seen during ovarian cystoscopy was found to be less hemorrhagic and more atrophic than before therapy. These data were confirmed by ovarian biopsy. An endometriotic lesion was considered 'active' when typical glandular epithelium was either proliferative, or completely unresponsive to hormonal therapy with typical stroma[16]. Such a lesion was found significantly more often (84% of cases, $p < 0.001$) before GnRH agonist therapy than after such therapy (44% of cases) (Table 2).

Pregnancy rates

The cumulative pregnancy rates were analyzed in a consecutive series of 407 patients with ovarian endometriosis (American Fertility Society (AFS) moderate, $n = 305$; AFS severe, $n = 102$). A pregnancy rate of more than 55% was achieved in moderate endometriosis and 44% in severe endometriosis. The majority (95%) of pregnancies occurred during the first 10 months after surgery.

Ovarian cystectomy

Ovarian cystectomy, a frequently performed procedure, can be accomplished laparoscopically in most cases[17]. The procedure begins with adhesiolysis. Once the cyst is mobilized, the cortex is grasped with a forceps introduced through a second trocar. The cortex is incised using laser or scissors. The cyst wall is then exposed. The incision is enlarged with scissors, and

Table 2 Ovarian endometrial cyst biopsy: incidence of 'active' endometriosis, mitotic index and epithelial height in active endometriosis ovarian foci

	First look	Second look
Active endometriosis (%)	88	44*
Mitotic index (%)	0.2	0.06*
Epithelial height (μm)	16.0 ± 4.9	17.2 ± 4.8

*Significantly different ($p < 0.001$) from other values

aquadissection can be used to separate the cyst wall from the ovarian stroma. Recent histological studies have suggested that some cortex surrounding the endometrioma and containing follicles is removed together with the endometrioma capsule, because of the absence of a real plane of cleavage. If the cyst is opened and spillage occurs, peritoneal irrigation must be performed in order to remove the chocolate-colored fluid. Ovarioscopy and careful evaluation of the internal cyst[18] wall allow the surgeon to exclude the presence of malignant lesions. The ovary usually does not require suturing.

The reduction of both cyst size and internal wall thickness observed in our study after the GnRH agonist therapy make the laparoscopic management of large endometrial cysts possible. The cumulative pregnancy rate achieved after combined (GnRH agonist and endoscopy) therapy was similar to that obtained after microsurgery and allows us to propose this form of therapy in the management of large endometriomas. The size of the cyst also has little bearing on the operability in reconstructive surgery. The most important criteria on operability is the extent of adhesions and some authors have suggested that a stage V needs to be considered in the AFS classification. Moreover, the recurrence rate of ovarian endometriomas was low (8%) although Fayez and Vogel[19] reported a 22% incidence of deep ovarian endometriosis at second-look laparoscopy after laparoscopic stripping of ovarian endometriomas in cases of very large cysts and/or friable cysts walls. Using the same laparoscopic procedure, Canis and colleagues[20] reported a 7% incidence of deep ovarian endometriosis at second-look laparoscopy in cases of endometriomas of > 3 cm. They suggest an additional vaporization or fulguration when the ovarian stripping is not satisfactory.

We recommend the vaporization technique for the internal wall of the endometrioma because the active implants are located on the surface of the cyst. Another argument in favor of this technique is the frequent absence of a thickened capsule around the endometrial cyst which makes capsule removal difficult and re-sponsible for the simultaneous removal of numerous ovocytes.

Rectovaginal septum endometriosis

A series of 231 cases of rectovaginal septum endometriosis is presented here (Table 3). The main symptom was severe pelvic pain in 180 women. The other 51 suffered pelvic pain and infertility. In cases of infertility, all patients underwent an evaluation of ovulation, cervical mucus–sperm interaction (postcoital test) and male factor (defined as < 15 million sperm per ml using a Makler counting chamber). Preoperative radiography of the colon was carried out in order to evaluate the involvement of the rectal surface. Profile radiography of an air contrast barium enema offers the best evaluation of the infiltration of the rectal anterior wall.

The surgical techniques have evolved gradually but all of them involve the separation of the anterior rectum from the posterior vagina and the excision or ablation of the endometriosis in that area. Aquadissection, scissor dissection and electrosurgery with an unmodulated (cutting) current are used by some authors[8], while others[11] prefer the use of the CO_2 laser.

Table 3 Technical aspects and complications in a series of 231 cases of rectovaginal septum endometriosis

Technical aspects	
Duration (min)	64 (45–120)
Hospitalization (days)	2.8 (2–5)
Laparoscopic bowel resection	none
Complications	
Rectal perforation	3 (1.3%)
Delayed hemorrhage (< 24 h postoperative)	2 (1.0%)
Urinary retention	3 (1.3%)
Ureteral injury	none
Late complication	none
Long-term results (n = 151, follow-up > 1 year)	
Recurrence of severe pelvic pain (n = 151)	2 (1.5%)
Fertility (n = 48)	25 (52%)

Whenever extensive endometriotic involvement of the cul-de-sac was suspected preoperatively, either because of the clinical presentation or from another physician's operative record, a mechanical bowel preparation was administered only on the afternoon before surgery to induce brisk, self-limiting diarrhea that rapidly cleanses the bowel without disrupting the electrolytic balance. In cases of endometriotic lesions of the rectal anterior wall, a bowel preparation was proposed as for conventional bowel resection. Cul-de-sac obliteration was partial when rectal tenting was visible, but a protrusion of the sponge in the posterior vaginal fornix was identified between the rectum and the inverted U of the uterosacral ligaments. But sometimes, a deep-infiltrating lesion of the rectovaginal septum is only barely visible by laparoscopy.

Surgical technique

Deep fibrotic nodular endometriosis involving the cul-de-sac required an excision of the nodular fibrotic tissue from the posterior vagina, rectum, posterior cervix and uterosacral ligaments[21]. A sponge on a ring forceps was inserted into the posterior vaginal fornix and a dilatator (Hegar 25) was placed in the rectum. In addition, a cannula was inserted into the endometrial cavity markedly to antevert the uterus. The peritoneum covering the cul-de-sac of Douglas was opened between the 'adenomyotic' lesion and the rectum. This approach is possible even when anterior rectal muscularis infiltration is present. Careful dissection was then carried out using the aquadissector and the CO_2 laser for sharp dissection until the rectum was completely freed and identifiable below the lesion. Excision of the fibrotic tissue on the side of the rectum was attempted only after the rectal dissection was complete. A partial rectal resection was never performed in our series. In cases of deep-infiltrating lesions, the vaginal wall is more or less penetrated by the adenomyosis and excision of a part of the vagina is essential. Dissection was performed accordingly, not only with the removal of all visible endometriotic lesions, but also the vaginal mucosa with at least a 0.5 cm disease-free margin. Lesions extending totally through the vagina were treated with *en bloc* laparoscopic resection from the cul-de-sac to the posterior vaginal wall; the pneumoperitoneum was maintained and the posterior vaginal wall was closed vaginally.

In our series of 231 cases, laparoscopic rectal perforation occurred in three cases. Perforation was diagnosed at the time of the laparoscopy. In one case, the rectum was repaired by laparotomy and in the two other cases by colpotomy.

In cases of full-thickness rectal lesions provoking menstrual rectorrhagia, translaparoscopic rectal resection can also be performed according to the technique of Nezhat and colleagues[11]. In our series of 231 cases, laparoscopic dissection was successfully performed in all cases, even when the radiography of the colon showed bowel involvement. During the same period, three cases of rectal endometriosis and three cases of sigmoid colon endometriosis were diagnosed. These six patients had no nodules of the septum, but had bowel wall endometriosis which provoked menstrual rectorrhagia. In these six cases, laparotomy and bowel resection were performed.

Histology

Deep vaginal endometriosis associated with pelvic endometriosis can take the form of nodular or polypoid masses involving the posterior vaginal fornix. The differential diagnosis of vaginal endometriosis, particularly of the superficial type, includes vaginal adenosis of the tuboendometrial variety, but the latter lacks endometrial stroma and the characteristic inflammatory response of endometriosis[22].

Histologically, scanty endometrial type stroma and glandular epithelium are disseminated in muscular tissue. These very similar histological descriptions lead to the suggestion that the so-called endometriotic nodule of the rectovaginal septum is in fact just like an adenomyoma or an adenomyotic nodule. Sometimes, the 'invasion' of the muscle by a very active glandular epithelium proved that the stroma is not necessary for the invasion in this particular type of pathology called adenomyosis.

Comments

In the pelvis, three different forms of endometriosis must be considered:

(1) Peritoneal;

(2) Ovarian; and

(3) Rectovaginal septum.

By evaluation of the mitotic activity and the stromal vascularization, we have recently proved[2] that peritoneal red lesions were the most aggressive form of the disease and progress to the so-called typical or black lesion which must be considered as an enclosed implant surrounded by fibrosis. The white lesions are the latent or quiescent form of the disease[3]. The red lesions can invade the retroperitoneal space by

infiltration. The three-dimensional evaluation[1] demonstrated the pluri-ramified aspect of the glandular structures.

For us, there are two different types of 'deep-infiltrating endometriosis':

(1) *True deep-infiltrating endometriosis* caused by the invasion of a very active peritoneal lesion deep in the retroperitoneal space. In cases of lateral peritoneal invasion, uterosacral ligaments can be involved as well as the anterior wall of the rectosigmoid bowel junction resulting in retraction and adhesions and secondary obliteration of the cul-de-sac.

(2) *Pseudo deep-infiltrating endometriosis or adenomyosis* of the rectovaginal septum. This lesion originates from the rectovaginal septum tissue and consists essentially of smooth muscle with active glandular epithelium and scanty stroma.

References

1. Donnez, J., Nisolle, M. and Casanas-Roux, F. (1992). Three-dimensional architectures of peritoneal endometriosis. *Fertil. Steril.*, **57**, 980–3
2. Nisolle, M., Casanas-Roux, F., Anaf, V., Mine, J. M. and Donnez, J. (1993). Morphometric study of the stromal vascularization in peritoneal endometriosis. *Fertil. Steril.*, **59**, 681–4
3. Donnez, J. and Nisolle, M. (1988). Appearances of peritoneal endometriosis. In *Proceedings of the IIIrd International Laser Surgery Symposium*, Brussels
4. Nisolle, M., Paindaveine, B., Bourdon, A., Berliere, M., Casanas-Roux, F. and Donnez, J. (1990). Histologic study of peritoneal endometriosis in infertile women. *Fertil. Steril.*, **53**, 984–8
5. Koninckx, P. D. (1993). Deeply infiltrating endometriosis. In Brosens, I. and Donnez, J. (eds.) *Endometriosis: Research and Management*, pp. 437–46. (Carnforth, UK: Parthenon Publishing)
6. Hughesdon, P. E. (1957). The structure of endometrial cysts of the ovary. *J. Obstet. Gynaecol. Br. Emp.*, **64**, 481–7
7. Sampson, J. A. (1922). Intestinal adenomas of endometrial type. *Arch. Surg.*, **5**, 217
8. Reich, H., McGlynn, F. and Salvat, J. (1991). Laparoscopic treatment of cul-de-sac obliteration secondary to retrocervical deep fibrotic endometriosis. *Reprod. Med.*, **36**, 516
9. Shaw, R. W., Fraser, H. M. and Boyle, H. (1983). Intranasal treatment with luteinizing hormone-releasing agonist in women with endometriosis. *Br. Med. J.*, **287**, 1167–9
10. Donnez, J., Nisolle, M. and Casanas-Roux, F. (1990). Endometriosis-associated infertility: evaluation of preoperative use of danazol, gestrinone and buserelin. *Int. J. Fertil.*, **42**, 128
11. Nezhat, C., Nezhat, F. and Pennington, E. (1992). Laparoscopic treatment of lower colorectal and infiltrative rectovaginal septum endometriosis by the technique of video laparoscopy. *Br. J. Obstet. Gynaecol.*, **99**, 664–7
12. Canis, M., Wattiez, A., Pouly, J. L., Bassil, S., Bouquet de Joliniere, J., Chapron, C., Manhes, H., Mage, G. and Bruhat, M. A. (1993). Laparoscopic treatment of endometriosis. In Brosens, I. and Donnez, J. (eds.) *Endometriosis: Research*

and Management, pp. 407–17. (Carnforth, UK: Parthenon Publishing)

13. Donnez, J., Nisolle, M., Casanas-Roux, F. and Clerckx, F. (1993). Endometriosis: rationale for surgery. In Brosens, I. and Donnez, J. (eds.) *Endometriosis: Research and Management*, pp. 385–95. (Carnforth, UK: Parthenon Publishing)

14. Donnez, J., Nisolle, M., Gillerot, S., Anaf, V., Clerck, F. and Casanas-Roux, F. (1994). Ovarian endometrial cyst: the role of gonadotropin-releasing hormonal agonist and/or drainage. *Fertil. Steril.*, **62**, 63–6

15. Donnez, J. and Nisolle, M. (1991). Laparoscopic management of large ovarian endometrial cyst: use of fibrin sealant. *J. Gynecol. Surg.*, **7**, 163–7

16. Nisolle, M., Casanas-Roux, F. and Donnez, J. (1988). Histologic study of ovarian endometriosis after hormonal therapy. *Fertil. Steril.*, **49**, 423–6

17. Canis, M., Mage, G., Manhes, H., Pouly, J. L., Wattiez, A. and Bruhat, M. A. (1989). Laparoscopic treatment of endometriosis. *Acta Obstet. Gynecol. Scand.*, **150**, 15

18. Brosens, I. and Gordon, A. (1989). Endometriosis: ovarian endometriosis. In Brosens, I. and Gordon, A. (eds.) *Tubal Infertility*, pp. 313–17. (London: Gower, Med. Publishing)

19. Fayez, J. A. and Vogel, M. S. (1991). Comparison of different treatment methods of endometriosis by laparoscopy. *Obstet. Gynecol.*, **78**, 660–5

20. Canis, M., Mage, G., Wattiez, A., Chapra, C., Pouly, J. L. and Bassil, S. (1992). Second look laparoscopy after laparoscopic cystectomy of large endometriomas. *Fertil. Steril.*, **58**, 617–19

21. Donnez, J., Nisolle, M., Casanas-Roux, F., Anaf, V. and Smets, M. (1994). Laparoscopic treatment of rectovaginal septum endometriosis. In Donnez, J. and Nisolle, M. (eds.) *An Atlas of Laser Operative Laparoscopy and Hysteroscopy*, pp. 75–85. (Carnforth, UK: Parthenon Publishing)

22. Zaloudek, C. and Norris, H. J. (1987). Mesenchymal tumors of the uterus. In Kurman, R. (ed.) *Blaustein's Pathology of the Female Genital Tract*, pp. 373. (Berlin: Springer-Verlag)

Laparoscopic procedures for treatment of infertility related to polycystic ovarian syndrome

49

J. Cohen

Introduction

Wedge resection of ovaries was proposed by Stein in 1935[1] and for a long time it was the only treatment of polycystic ovaries (PCO). When treatment by antiestrogens was initiated (clomifene citrate in 1960) and when the beneficial results of these treatments were known, the surgical technique which had the inconvenience of peri-ovarian adhesion formation disappeared. Recently, numerous publications[2-6] have indicated the interest in laparoscopic techniques (biopsy, cauterization, multi-electrocoagulation, laser, etc.) in cases of non-response to the medical treatments. The first attempts were in France using Raoul Palmer's ovarian biopsy forceps[7,8].

Biopsy

The first publication concerning pregnancies obtained after laparoscopic ovarian biopsies with the Palmer forceps dates back to 1972. At this time Cohen, Audebert, De Brux and Giorgi[9] mentioned 21 pregnancies after 51 successive ovarian biopsies. They came to the conclusion that this procedure had a therapeutic effect on some ovarian infertilities.

In 1989, Cohen[3] reported 778 ovarian biopsies performed between 1971 and 1987 with a pregnancy rate (PR) of 31.8%, distributed as 36.6% in less than 3 months, 32.2% between 3 and 8 months and 31% over this delay.

As early as 1972, numerous French authors confirmed spontaneous pregnancies after laparoscopic ovarian biopsy. Among those publications are Sykes (63% PR for 70 cases), Mintz (44% PR for 157 cases), Tescher (23% PR for 85 cases), Chassagnard (23% PR for 92 cases), Devaut (33% PR for 32 cases), Scarpa (55% PR for 29 cases) and Fouquet (50% PR for 100 biopsies). Diquelou[10] practised 68 ovarian biopsies. He obtained 13 pregnancies in a period of 3 months (19%) and 24 pregnancies in 12 months (35%). The rate of success was 34% in PCO and 40% in unexplained infertilities. As early as 1972, Cohen and colleagues[7] indicated that there was no relationship between pathological examination of the biopsied ovary and the occurrence of a pregnancy.

In the 778 cases of Cohen[3] the authors observed three complications due to the ovarian biopsy. There were two cases of ovarian hemorrhage linked to the trauma of ovarian blood vessels which had been impossible to coagulate. One case was treated by immediate laparotomy and the second one by delayed laparotomy for hematocele. There was one bowel perforation due to an electric spark, leading to a perforation at the 9th day postlaparoscopy. It was treated by a simple suture. In all the other cases where ovarian bleeding occurred during the biopsy, hemostasis could be obtained either by cauterization or by pressure on the two sides of the biopsy with the forceps.

The authors could observe the appearance of the biopsied ovary a few years later (on the occasion of Cesarean sections, ectopic pregnancy or iterative laparoscopy). The appearance usually observed is that of a simple depression on the surface of the ovary. In no case have adhesions on the biopsied zona been observed.

Electrocautery

In 1984 Gjoannaess[11] proposed the use of laparoscopic multi-electrocauterization in the treatment of polycystic ovarian syndrome (PCOS). The ovulation rate was 92% and the pregnancy rate 69%. In a publication of 1989[4], with a follow-up of 10 years, the same author reports the outcome of pregnancy of 89 women pregnant after electrocauterization. The abortion rate was 15%, which is less than after clomifene or wedge resection. In a recent publication, Gjoannaess[12] reports the results from 252 women with PCOS treated with ovarian electrocauterization during the years 1979–91: ovulation was obtained in 92% of the total series, and pregnancy in 84%. The response was influenced by body weight, with an ovulation rate of 96–97% for the slim and moderately obese women, decreasing to 70% in the very obese ones.

Greenblatt and Casper[5] proposed cauterization with small scissors. Eight to ten punctures are made on each ovary with a current of 4 A, until there is penetration of the cortex. Six cases of PCO have been studied, compared to six controls with regular cycles. Three to four days after laparoscopy a decrease of androsterone, testosterone, estradiol and luteinizing hormone (LH) was observed only in the PCO group. An increase of follicle stimulating hormone (FSH) is also observed. These modifications are independent of anesthesia or laparoscopy as they do not appear in the control group. Four of six PCO women became pregnant during the same month.

Sumioki and associates[13] propose a multiple punch resection-cautery with monopolar forceps carried out on six to ten surface follicles. The authors estimate that this technique reduces ovarian volume by a tenth. Seven cases were observed. Four days after laparoscopy a decrease of LH, a diminution of LH pulse amplitude and a decrease of androgens were observed. FSH and prolactin were not modified.

The modifications observed persisted at the 6th week postlaparoscopy. Four of the six women became pregnant between 12 and 44 weeks after the operation.

Pellicer and Remohi[6] have treated 76 patients with PCOS. Of these, 58 had electrocautery and six laser vaporization. All patients failed to respond to clomifene or human menopausal gonadotropin (hMG) treatment. Thirty-three patients had anovulatory cycles. The pregnancy rate after laparoscopic treatment was 52.6% and the ovulation rate 67.1%.

Armar and Lachelin[14] made a study of 50 PCO women treated over a period of 3 years and 3 months. Diathermy was applied to each ovary for 4 s at a time in four separate places. Forty-three women (86%) ovulated in an average time of 23 days (± 6.2) and 33 women became pregnant (50 pregnancies with eight spontaneous abortions). The abortion rate of 14% is very low; of the 22 women who had no pelvic abnormality other than PCO, 19 (86%) had one or more successful pregnancies.

Campo and Felli[15] treated 23 PCO women who failed to become pregnant with many kinds of ovulation induction. The technique was either multiple laparoscopic biopsies or a longitudinal incision on the surface of the ovary. Of these patients, 56% ovulated and 13 pregnancies occurred (with 8% abortion).

Kovacs and Buckler[16] treated ten PCO patients with ovarian electrocautery on ten different points on each ovary. Seven women ovulated. The author observed a significant and persistent fall in serum testosterone levels and a transient fall with subsequent rise in inhibin.

Abdel Gadir and Mowafi[17] consider the laparoscopic electrocautery of ovaries as 'the' treatment of PCO. They divided 88 patients who failed to respond to clomifene into three groups: group A, electrocautery; group B, hMG; and group C, pure FSH. After treatment the ovulation rates (as shown by estradiol and ultrasound) were A, 71.4%; B, 70.6%; and C, 66.7%. The pregnancy rates were 9.5%, 12.6% and 8.8%, respectively. The spontaneous abortion rates were 21.4%, 53.3% and 40%, respectively. The birth rates were 37.9%, 23.3% and 20.7%, respectively. The authors concluded that ovarian electrocautery is the best choice in PCOS.

Balen and Jacobs[18] carried out a prospective study comparing unilateral or bilateral laparoscopic diathermy. Unilateral ovarian diathermy resulted in ovulation from both ovaries.

Laparoscopic laser

Laparoscopic laser drilling has been introduced and used in the treatment of PCO within the last 15 years. In the mind of the promoters, laser provides controllable power density, desirable depth of penetration and predictable thermo-damage of surrounding tissues. It may also diminish the risk of adhesions.

A few series have been published in which all types of laser have been used: carbon dioxide (CO_2), argon and YAG. With YAG laser Huber and colleagues[19] performed three to five drills on each ovary (5–10 mm long and 4 mm deep). He obtained five spontaneous ovulations in the eight patients treated. For the other three, clomifene induced ovulation, contrary to the results obtained before laparoscopy.

Daniell and Brown[20,21] treated 85 PCO women with different models of laser. They were bad responders to clomifene. During laparoscopy, ovarian vaporization was performed by argon, CO_2 or potassium titanyl phosphate (KTP). A two-puncture technique was used to drain all the visible small subcapsular follicles of each ovary and to drill randomly placed craters in the ovarian stroma. Ovulation occurred spontaneously in 71% of patients. Postoperatively, 56% conceived within 6 months of laparoscopy.

Ostzrenski[22] used translaparoscopic CO_2 laser ovarian wedge resection. The free ovarian surface was vaporized to a width of 1 cm. There was a 92% pregnancy rate and an 8% postsurgical adhesion rate, among the 12 cases that were incorporated into the study.

Donesky and Adashi[23] provided an up-to-date review in 1995. Twenty-nine relevant studies were identified in the English language. Pregnancies after laparoscopic ovulation induction procedures have been reported in an average of 55% of treated subjects (range 20–65%).

Results and complications

The results are presented in Table 1. They are similar irrespective of the technique: means of 50% spontaneous ovulation and 50% pregnancy were obtained. The main risk of the technique could be postoperative adhesions, but Gjoannaess[11] has found no adhesions during Cesarean sections of pregnant patients. In a study by Dabirashrafi and colleagues[24], 17 women were electrocauterized and eight second-look laparoscopies were performed, with no adhesions. In a second group of 21 patients

Table 1   Results of treatments for polycystic ovarian syndrome in terms of spontaneous ovulation and pregnancy

Authors	Year	Technique	Spontaneous ovulation (%)	Pregnancies (%)
Cohen et al.[9]	1972	biopsy	–	41
Gjoannaess[12]	1984	cauterization	92.0	84
Greenblatt and Casper[5]	1987	cauterization	71.0	56.0
Cohen et al.[7]	1988	cauterization	–	31.8
Huber et al.[19]	1988	laser	41.7	–
Daniell[20]	1989	laser	83.8	66.7
Sumioki et al.[13]	1988	biopsy	93.8	50.0
Abdel Gadir and Mowafi[17]	1990	cauterization	26.5	43.8
Pellicer and Remohi[6]	1992	cauterization laser	67.1	52.6
Ostrzenski[22]	1992	laser	92	92
Armar and Lachelin[14]	1993	cauterization	86	66
Campo et al.[15]	1993	resection	56	56

who have all had a second-look laparoscopy, four minimal adhesions and one moderate (according to the American Fertility Society classification) were observed.

Gurgan and associates[25] reported a review of 12 publications concerning adhesion formation as a complication of laparoscopic treatment of PCOS. Adhesion formation rates, as assessed by second-look laparoscopy, ranged from 0–100%. The mean adhesion score of the group treated with CO_2 laser was significantly higher than that of the electrocautery group.

Mode of action of laparoscopic procedures

The first postoperative endocrine alterations were described by Greenblatt and Casper[5] and Sumioki and co-workers[13]. They observed a significant decrease of LH and androgen levels during the days immediately after surgery. The decrease is persistent after 6 weeks and is sufficient to explain how the endocrinological disorders of PCO are corrected and how pregnancies occur. The two groups of authors agree that the trauma of the ovary is enough to induce a decrease in the production of local androgens, followed by a fall in estradiol, and a decrease of the positive feedback on LH.

Greenblatt and Casper[5] ascribe an important role to inhibin. Sakata and associates[26] studied nine anovulatory patients having PCO submitted to a laparoscopic cauterization of ovaries. The levels of bioactive LH, immunoreactive LH, FSH, androstenedione and testosterone were studied before and after cauterization and in five controls. Eight women ovulated spontaneously and three became pregnant. The authors noticed a decrease of androgens as well as immunoreactive LH and they were the first to point out a decrease of bioactive LH.

Pellicer and Remohi[6], studying 13 anovulatory patients after cauterization, confirmed the decrease in levels of LH, testosterone and androstenedione ($p < 0.05$). Meanwhile, the levels of insulin and insulin-like growth factor-1 remained unchanged.

Campo and colleagues[15] confirmed the rapid decrease in the levels of androstenedione and plasmatic testosterone in all cases after cauterization of the ovaries. However, the variations of these levels were not linked to the clinical successes. For these authors there was no variation in the levels of LH. In contrast, the mean values of FSH and its pulsatility increased significantly in the patients who became pregnant.

It seems that all the authors agree that ovarian traumas lead to a significant and immediate decrease of androgens, and a secondary increase of FSH which could be related to a decrease of intraovarian inhibin. However, the most difficult aspect of the problem is how to explain that a physical trauma induces endocrine modifications. As all the authors did not perform the same technique (multiperforation, single or multibiopsy, laser), one might conclude that it is not the volume of the injured tissues which plays a part. The only factor in common is the ovarian burn.

Mio and associates[27] have shown, in 18 patients with PCO, that only with transvaginal ultrasound-guided follicular aspiration could they obtain an 87–100% ovulation rate per patient and 50% pregnancy rate. A significant decrease of basal LH was observed. This method, simpler and less invasive, may be revolutionary, if further experiments confirm its efficacy.

One may consider again the two hypotheses already formulated in 1983[2]:

(1) Either the burning of the ovary provokes a secondary revascularization inducing an increase in the concentration of gonadotropins by surface unity; or

(2) Electrocoagulation stimulates the ovarian nerves which transmit the excitation to the superior centers.

Cohen[28] put forward the hypothesis that drainage of androgens and inhibin from surface follicles could inhibit the excessive collagenization of overlying ovarian cortex and facilitate a softening of the ovaria tunica. Neighboring follicles that are not undergoing atresia may then

356

mature and gain access to the ovarian surface, facilitating normal ovulation. It remains a mystery as to how laparoscopic techniques bring about the resolution of an endocrinological dysfunction. What is sure, though, is that laparoscopic techniques suppress less ovarian tissue that the wedge resection, but act in the same way.

Conclusions

There are considerable data assessing the impact of the laparoscopic treatment of polycystic ovarian syndrome on the resumption of ovulation and the rate of pregnancy in infertile patients (> 50%). A significant difficulty encountered in the evaluation of the studies is their lack of uniformity. There was a great variation in the diagnosis criteria used to define polycystic ovarian syndrome. None of the studies included a treatment-independent control group. Some of the patients became pregnant with a medical treatment after laparoscopy (the same treatment being inefficient beforehand).

However, laparoscopic techniques have the advantages over surgical wedge resection of cost savings and fewer postoperative adhesions. They have the advantages over gonadotropin therapy of serial repetitive ovulatory events resulting from a single treatment, no increased risk of ovarian hyperstimulation or multiple pregnancies and a lower incidence of spontaneous abortion.

The possible adverse effects (postoperative adhesions, bowel lesions) indicate that the technique must be performed by a well-trained gynecologist. This procedure must not be considered as the first-line treatment. Clomifene citrate remains the first line of therapy for the anovulatory patient with polycystic ovarian syndrome. For the resistant patients, the laparoscopic techniques have many advantages over gonadotropin therapy, and must be offered. When a gynecologist diagnoses polycystic ovarian syndrome (ultrasound imaging or hormonal results), and performs a laparoscopy for infertility, cauterization of the ovaries may be performed at the same time in order to avoid a secondary surgical laparoscopy. This treatment option deserves further study by means of randomized controlled trials.

References

1. Stein, I. F. and Leventhal, M. L. (1935). Amenorrhea associated with bilateral polycystic ovaries. *Am. J. Obstet. Gynecol.*, **29**, 181–91
2. Cohen, J. and Leal de Meirelles, H. (1983). Fertilité après biopsie ovarienne percoelioscopique. A propos de 477 cas en stérilité. *J. Gynecol. Obstet. Biol. Reprod.*, **12**, 73–9
3. Cohen, J. and Audebert, A. J. M. (1989). De la mécanique au fonctionnel: place des traitements chirurgicaux in endoscopiques dans les dystrophies ovariennes. In *Dystrophies Ovairennes*, pp. 183–94. (Paris: Masson)
4. Gjoannaess, H. (1989). The course and outcome of pregnancy after ovarian electrocautery with PCOS: the influence of body weight. *Br. J. Obstet. Gynaecol.*, **96**, 714–19
5. Greenblatt, E. and Casper, R. F. (1987). Endocrine changes after laparoscopic ovarian cautery in polycystic ovarian syndrome. *Am. J. Obstet. Gynecol.*, **42**, 517–18
6. Pellicer, A. and Remohi, J. (1992). *Management of the PCOS by Laparoscopy.* (Basel: Karger)
7. Cohen, J., Audebert, A., De Brux, J. and Giorgi, H. (1972). Biopsie ovarienne d'une grossesse. *Nouv. Presse. Med.*, **1**, 1294
8. Palmer, R. and Cohen, J. (1965). Biopsies percoelioscopiques. *Minerva Gynecol.*, **17**, 238–9
9. Cohen, J., Audebert, A., De Brux, J. and Giorgi, H. (1972). Les stérilités pour dysovulation: rôle pronotisque et thérapeutique et thérapeutique de la biopsie ovarienne percoelioscopique. *J. Gyn. Obstet. Reprod.*, 657–71
10. Diquelou, J. Y., Boyer, S. and Cicquel, J. M. (1988). Therapeutic role of ovarian biopsy done by laparoscopy in polycystic ovarian and unexplained infertility. *Hum. Reprod.*, **3** (Suppl.), Abstr. 80

11. Gjoannaess, H. (1984). Polycystic ovarian syndrome treated by ovarian electrocautery through the laparoscope. *Fertil. Steril.*, **41**, 20–5

12. Gjoannaess, H. (1994). Ovarian electrocautery in the treatment of women with PCOS. *Acta Obstet. Gynecol. Scand.*, **73**, 407–12

13. Sumioki, H., Korencaga, M., Utsunomyiya, T., Kadota, T. and Matsuoka, K. (1988). The effect of laparoscopic multiple punch resection of the ovary on hypothalamo–pituitary axis in PCOS. *Fertil. Steril.*, **50**, 567–72

14. Armar, N. A. and Lachelin, G. (1993). Laparoscopic ovarian diathermy: an effective treatment for antioestrogen resistant anovulatory infertility in women with PCOS. *Br. J. Obstet. Gynecol.*, 161–4

15. Campo, S., Felli, A. *et al.* (1993). Endocrine changes and clinical outcome after laparoscopic ovarian resection in women with PCO. *Hum. Reprod.*, **8**, 359–63

16. Kovacs, G., Buckler, H. *et al.* (1991). Treatment of anovulation due to PCOS by laparoscopic ovarian cautery. *Br. J. Obstet. Gynaecol.*, **98**, 30–5

17. Abdel Gadir, A., Mowafi, R. *et al.* (1990). Ovarian electrocautery versus pure FSH therapy in the treatment of PCOD. *Clin. Endocrinol.*, **33**, 585

18. Balen, A. and Jacobs, H. (1994). A prospective study comparing unilateral laparoscopic ovarian diathermy in women with PCOS. *Fertil. Steril.*, **62**, 921–5

19. Huber, J., Hosmann, J. and Spona, J. (1988). Polycystic ovarian syndrome treated by laser through the laparoscope. *Lancet*, **ii**, 215

20. Daniell, J. M. and Brown, D. H. (1982). Carbon dioxide laser laparoscopy: initial experience in experimental animals and humans. *Obstet. Gynecol.*, **159**, 761–5

21. Daniell, J. F. (1989). Polycystic ovaries treated by laparoscopic laser vaporization. *Fertil. Steril.*, **51**, 232–6

22. Ostrzenski, A. (1992). Endoscopic carbon dioxide laser wedge resection in resistant PCO. *Int. J. Fertil.*, **37**, 295–9

23. Donesky, B. and Adashi, E. (1995). Surgically induced ovulation in the PCO syndrome: wedge resection revisited in the age of laparoscopy. *Fertil. Steril.*, **63**, 439–63

24. Dabirashrafi, H., Mohamad, K., Behjatnia, Y. *et al.* (1991). Adhesion formation after ovarian electrocauterization on patients with PCO syndrome. *Fertil. Steril.*, **55**, 1200–1

25. Gurgan, T., Yarali, H. and Urman, B. (1994). Laparoscopic treatment of PCO disease. *Hum. Reprod.*, **9**, 573–7

26. Sakata, M., Tasaka, K. *et al.* (1990). Changes of bio-active LH laser laparoscopic ovarian cautery in patients with PCOS. *Fertil. Steril.*, **53**, 610–13

27. Mio, Y., Toda, T. *et al.* (1991). Transvaginal ultrasound guided follicular aspiration in the management of anovulatory infertility associated with polycystic ovaries. *Fertil. Steril.*, **56**, 1060–5

28. Cohen, B. M. (1989). Laser laparoscopy for polycystic ovaries. *Fertil. Steril.*, **52**, 167

6

IVF technology: clinical aspects

Non-responsive patients: characteristics of patients

50

L. Mettler, A. Salmassi, A. Brandenburg and N. Lutzewitch

Introduction

Just as ovulation stands in the center of reproductive life for women, it is the central feature in any ovarian stimulation program for *in vivo* and *in vitro* fertilization. The pregnancy outcome of any stimulation protocol for *in vivo* and *in vitro* fertilization and embryo transfer (IVF–ET) is influenced by various factors:

(1) The reason for sterility[1];

(2) The number of follicles or oocytes retrieved[2];

(3) The number of developing or transferred embryos[2–4];

(4) Oocyte maturity and quality[3, 5, 6];

(5) Plasma hormone levels[7, 8];

(6) Endometrial receptivity[5, 6];

(7) Sperm quality and bacteriology.

It is difficult to identify a single factor that is responsible for the success or failure of a desired *in vivo* fertilization or the success of pregnancy in an IVF program, but there is no doubt that ovarian stimulation and oocyte maturation are an important step in fertilization which has a profound impact on the success of these procedures. The successful treatment of women who respond poorly to ovarian stimulation is a perennial problem of IVF–ET and ovulation stimulation[9–11].

Low-response cycles within a hyperstimulation program are defined as cycles with serum estradiol levels on the day of the human chorionic gonadotropin (hCG) administration lower than 1000 pg/ml with growth of one or two or even no follicles. These patients are characterized as poor responders. Many factors could cause this poor response.

(1) Age of patients; numerous studies clearly state that there is an age-dependent regression in ovarian response to stimulation in hormonally-active elderly patients[12–14];

(2) Presence of antibodies to various endocrine organs[15];

(3) Latent or premature ovarian failure[16];

(4) Anatomical alterations influencing ovulation such as adhesions or a frozen pelvis[4, 17];

(5) Obesity[12];

(6) Smoking.

Materials and methods

From December 1992 to April 1995, 483 cycles in 348 patients were included in the Kiel IVF program. Out of 77 patients treated in the months of January–April 1955, 15 patients were described to be poor responders. In two patients, no follicle punctures were performed. Thirteen women with poor response were recruited to this study. All patients were stimulated according to our 'long protocol' of programmed oocyte retrieval – down-regulation was performed using subcutaneous daily injections of 100–500 mg D-TRP-6 luteinizing hormone releasing hormone (LHRH) Decapeptyl®) or the transnasal daily application of 900 mg nafaralin acetate (Synarela®) which were administered from day 21 of the natural

361

menstrual cycle until hCG application. Individu-alized follicle stimulating hormone (FSH) or human menopausal gonadotropin (hMG) stimulations were started on the second day of the cycle according to the estradiol reaction of patients. During stimulation, daily serum levels of luteinizing hormone (LH), FSH, estradiol and inhibin were determined. The day of hCG administration was chosen when at least one follicle with a diameter of more than 18 mm could be observed during the ultrasound exami-nations. The Siemens ultrasound machine (Sonoline SL-1) with 5.0 and 7.5 MHz trans-ducers was used. Ovarian puncture was per-formed 34–36 h after hCG injection. The re-trieved oocytes were inseminated *in vitro* 2–5 h later[18,19]. Additional serum samples were taken on the days of ovum pick-up, embryo transfer, on days 4, 8, 10 and 14 after embryo transfer. Serum levels of progesterone, estradiol, LH and inhibin were determined. The follicular fluid from the first follicle of each patient was col-lected for the measurements of estradiol, LH, inhibin, immunoglobulin, IgA and IgG. The data of poor responders were correlated to the age of the patient, the number of hCG ampules used, the size of follicles on ultrasound and the volume of the follicular fluid aspirated.

Results

Report on 406 IVF–ET cycles in 271 patients

The 271 patients with transvaginal follicular aspirations in 406 cycles represented an age range of between 21 and 44 years. In 2198 follic-ular punctures, a mean of 5.4 oocytes per cycle

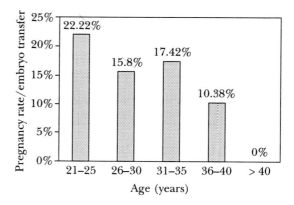

Figure 1 Pregnancy rate per embryo transfer cycle and patient's age

were retrieved; 61 pregnancies resulted from which there were 34 spontaneous deliveries, ten abortions, eight ectopics, six premature deliver-ies and three Cesarean sections. The pregnancy rate per cycle was estimated to be 15%, and per embryo transfer 20.3%.

The six investigated factors gave the follow-ing results in respect to pregnancy rates. Fig-ure 1 shows the patient's age correlated with the resulting pregnancy rates. In terms of etiology of sterility, tubal factor as an indication for IVF–ET showed the highest pregnancy rates per cycle (19.8%) and per embryo transfer (22.3%) (Figure 2).

Disappointing results were obtained in patients with reduced sperm parameters. Fertil-ization rates in relation to the stimulation scheme are detailed in Table 1. In 80 cycles the bacteriological sperm analysis gave positive results. The influence of bacteria on pregnancy rates in IVF–ET was striking (in negative

Table 1 Stimulation schemes for IVF–ET treatment

	hMG/FSH–hMG	GnRH 'short' protocol	GnRH 'long' protocol	Spontaneous
Pregnancy rate per IVF–ET cycle (%)	16.2	21.6	15.8	
Number of cycles	83	300	21	2
Number of IVF–ET cycles	62	218	19	2
Fertility rate per cycle (%)	74.7	72.7	90.5	
Number of pregnancies	10	47	3	1
Pregnancy rate per cycle (%)	12	15.7	14.3	

Table 2 Pregnancy and fertilization rates correlated to previous pregnancies

	No previous pregnancies	Secondary sterility	Total
Pregnancy rate per IVF–ET cycle (%)	21.6	19.7	20.3
Number of cycles	197	209	406
Number of IVF–ET cycles	134	167	301
Fertility rate per cycle (%)	68	78	74.1
Number of pregnancies	29	32	61
Pregnancy rate per cycle (%)	14.8	15.3	15

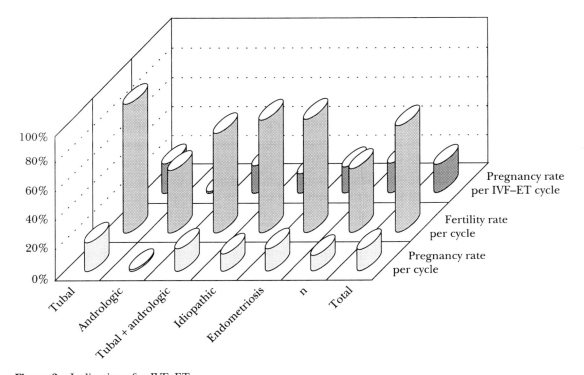

Figure 2 Indications for IVF–ET

cultures, 23.2%, in positive cultures, 8.5%). As regards the number of pregnancies in the patient's personal history, a slightly higher pregnancy rate was observed in patients with secondary sterility compared to those with no previously existing pregnancies (Table 2).

Report on a group of poor responders

Out of 77 patients, 15 were described as poor responders and, in two of these, cycles were cancelled prior to follicular puncture. Out of 75 patients punctured, the pregnancy rate was 31.3% per embryo transfer. The 13 poor responder patients showed significantly different IgA and estradiol values in follicular fluid compared to normal responders (Figure 3). In the 13 poor responders, a comparison to 13 normal patients resulted in three pregnancies: two ongoing and one missed abortion. Table 3 gives the comparative results regarding age, follicular fluid and serum hormone levels of estradiol, LH

Table 3 Some characteristics of poor responders versus normal responders in the hyperstimulation program

| | n | Age (years) | Follicular fluid | | | | | Serum | | Number of ampules |
			Inhibin (U/ml)	Estradiol (pg/ml)	LH (U/ml)	IgA (mg/dl)	IgG (mg/dl)	Inhibin (U/ml)	Estradiol (pg/ml)	
Poor responders	13	35	3513.40	294 342	152.3	68.47	817.4	8.80	950.0	74.6
Normal responders	13	32	3450.75	396 115	125.0	94.40	737.4	12.46	2020.5	32.3
Significance		NS	NS	$p < 0.01$	NS	$p < 0.01$	NS	$p < 0.01$	$p < 0.01$	$p < 0.01$

NS, not significant

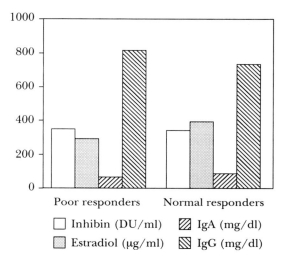

Figure 3 Follicular fluid measurements of inhibin, estradiol, IgA and IgG in poor and normal responders

and inhibin, as well as ampules needed until the day of the hCG administration. Figure 4 shows the difference of serum levels of estradiol, inhibin and LH between normal and poor responders during the follicular phase of the stimulation. The normal responders showed a parallel curve of rising or falling of hormonal levels, which we refer to as a synchronized hormonal reaction. The average levels of inhibin at the day of hCG administration were 12.5 U/ml. The poor responders have no synchronized reaction of their inhibin (8.8 U/ml) or estradiol levels. Thus, the characteristics of poor responders in an ovarian hyperstimulation program for oocyte retrieval are (1) less than three oocytes, (2) serum estradiol less than 1000 pg/ml, and (3) serum inhibin levels less than 8 U/ml.

Discussion

Fertilization depends on the maturation of valuable oocytes. Non-responsive patients should be excluded from follicular punctures. However, as pregnancies even occur in low responders, a withdrawal of these patients, once already stimulated, is difficult. This study seems to confirm that upon hyperstimulation poor responding patients in an IVF–ET program show abnormality of hormonal and immunological functions[15,20]. Nevertheless, there was no difference between inhibin and IgG levels in follicular fluid from normal and poor responders, but there was a significant difference in follicular fluid estradiol and IgA levels.

The law in Germany only permits the transfer of three embryos and cryopreservation is only allowed for pronuclear stages. In our department, a mild hyperstimulation program was applied. Gonadotropin releasing hormone (GnRH) applied in this study did not show any differences in the evaluated low responders. Like Barri and co-workers[9], we also found in the group of patients he calls 'bad responders' much lower estradiol levels compared to normal responders. Inhibin levels characterize mature follicles at levels more than 12.5 U/ml in serum and more than 3500 U/ml in follicular fluid.

Poor-responder patients, however, showed only a statistically lower serum inhibin level of < 8 U/ml. As a certain characteristic of patients responding poorly to the hMG/hCG stimulation protocol, we propose the unsynchronized

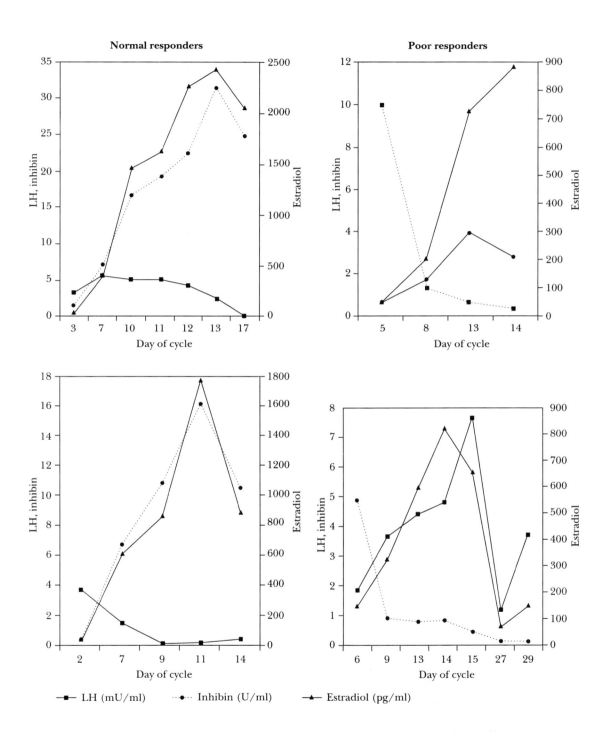

Figure 4 The levels of estradiol, LH and inhibin in serum during the follicular phase of hyperstimulation in normal and poor responders

reaction of serum estradiol and inhibin levels, which could depend on different regulation of inhibin and estradiol production[21,22]. These patients should be excluded from follicular puncture procedures and be stimulated in a consecutive cycle without GnRH analogs. In these patients, Kondaveeti and Gordon[11] tried a combined ovulation stimulation with growth hormones and gonadotropins.

Summary

In a retrospective analysis of pregnancy rates in 348 patients to various factors, the dependency on sperm quality, stimulation method, patient's age, etiology of sterility and bacterial contamination of sperm were revealed. In a subgroup of 77 patients treated in 1995, we looked only at the pregnancy rates per embryo transfer and the percentage of poor responders, of which only two were not submitted to follicular puncture. The pregnancy rate of poor responders was 19.8% (15 out of 77 cycles). The investigation of 13 poor-responder patients undergoing ovarian hyperstimulation revealed three characteristics of poor responders:

(1) The serum levels of estradiol and inhibin and the number of oocytes had the following values:
    (a) Estradiol levels < 1000 pg/ml;
    (b) Serum inhibin level < 8 U/ml;
    (c) Number of oocytes < 3.

(2) In follicular fluid, IgA and estradiol were found to be lower compared to normal responders, and this may influence follicular maturation.

(3) Only poor responders showed unsynchronized estradiol and inhibin reactions of serum levels during the follicular phase.

References

1. Harward, W. and Jones, J. R. (1988). Recent advances in *in vitro* fertilisation (IVF). *Hum. Reprod.*, 65–79
2. Aboulghar, M. A. (1994). The prognostic value of successful *in vitro* fertilisation in subsequent trials. *Hum. Reprod.*, **9**, 1932–4
3. Caspi, E. (1989). Early, late and sequential embryo transfer in *in vitro* fertilisation program. *Fertil. Steril.*, **52**, 146–8
4. Imoedemhe, D. A. G. (1988). *In vitro* fertilisation in women with 'frozen pelvis'. *Fertil. Steril.*, **49**, 268
5. Paulson, R. J., Sauer, M. V. and Lobo, R. A. (1991). *Am. J. Obstet. Gynecol.*, **165**, 1896–7
6. Tesarik, J. (1989). Viability assessment of preimplantation concept: a challenge for human embryo research. *Fertil. Steril.*, **52**, 364–6
7. Mouson, J., Lefevre, B. and Frydman, R. (1986). Factors affecting human *in vitro* fertilisation: a multifactorial study. *Fertil. Steril.*, **43**
8. Williams, K. A. (1989). Human chorionic gonadotrophin, estradiol and progesterone profiles in conception and non-conception cycles in an *in vitro* fertilisation program. *Fertil. Steril.*, **52**, 441–5
9. Barri, P. N., Coroleu, B. and Martinez, F. (1994). Management of bad responders in IVF. *Front. Endocrinol.*, **4**, 293–9
10. Nakamura, Y., Jinno, M., Ubukata, Y., Hanyu, I. and Yoshirmura, Y. (1994). Ovarian stimulation for *in vitro* fertilisation and embryo transfer in poor responders: application of pulsative hMG administration. *Perspect. Assist. Reprod.*, **4**, 363–9
11. Kondaveeti, U. and Gordon, A. C. (1994). Augmenting the ovarian response using adjuvant growth hormone. Presented at *The 2nd International Meeting of the BSF*, Glasgow
12. Crosignani, P. G. and Ragni, G. (1994). Induction of ovulation in 'poor responders'. *Front. Endocrinol.*, **4**, 457–63
13. Meldrum, D. R. (1993). Female reproductive aging – ovarian and uterine factors. *Fertil. Steril.*, **59**, 1–5
14. Segal, S. and Casper, R. F. (1990). The response to ovarian hyperstimulation and *in vitro* fertilisation in women older than 35 years. *Hum. Reprod.*, **5**, 255–7
15. Tung, S. K. and Teuscher, C. (1995). Mechanism of autoimmune disease in the testis and ovary. *Hum. Reprod. Update*, **1**, 35–50

16. Tanbo, T., Abyholm, Th., Bjoro, T. and Dale, P. O. (1990). Ovarian stimulation in previous failures from *in vitro* fertilisation: distinction of two groups of poor responders. *Hum. Reprod.*, **5**, 811–15

17. Diamond, M. P. (1988). The effect of periovarian adhesions on follicular development in patients undergoing ovarian stimulation for IVF–ET. *Fertil. Steril.*, **49**, 100–3

18. Mettler, L. and Michelmann, H. W. (1987). Estradiol values under gonadotrophin stimulation in relation to the outcome of pregnancies in *in vitro* fertilisation and embryo transfer. *J. In Vitro Fertil. Embryo Transfer*, **4**, 303–6

19. Michelmann, H. W., Tinneberg, H. R., Weisner, D. and Mettler, L. (1984). Die transvaginale ultraschallkontrolierte Follikelpunktion im Rahmen der menschlichen *in vitro* Fertilisation. *Geburtshilfe Frauenkunde*, **9**, 587–682

20. Pellicer, A., Lightmann, A., Diamond, M. P., Russel, J. B. and DeCherney, A. (1987). Outcome of *in vitro* fertilisation in women with low response to ovarian stimulation. *Fertil. Steril.*, **47**, 812–15

21. Hee, J. P., MacNaughton, J. and Baugdan, M. (1993). FSH induces dose-dependent stimulation of immunoreactive inhibin secretion during the follicular phase of the human menstrual cycle. *J. Clin. Endocrinol. Metab.*, **76**, 5

22. Dionission, A. A., Drakakis, P. and Loutradis, D. (1993). Follicular fluid inhibin levels in relation to age in patients in an *in vitro* fertilisation and embryo transfer programme. *Eur. J. Obstet. Gynaecol. Reprod. Biol.*, **51**, 55–61

367

Management of the non-responsive patient

51

S. H. Sohn and A. DeCherney

Introduction

As more *in vitro* fertilization (IVF) cycles are being completed across the world, the diagnosis and management of 'poor responders' or 'non-responders' become increasing important. Regardless of the type of stimulation protocol, the collection of a suitable number of mature oocytes is a prerequisite for IVF and other assisted reproductive technologies.

In the poor responder, stimulation cycles frequently end in cancellation with poor follicular recruitment and an inadequate or inappropriate estradiol response. Different indices have been used to define poor ovarian responsiveness to stimulation: peak estradiol level, suboptimal estradiol rise, poor follicular development and fewer retrieved oocytes. Regardless of the different end-points used, poor responders can be defined as showing a response with fewer follicles and/or less than normal estradiol when stimulated with a standard dose of human menopausal gonadotropin (hMG). More significant than the response of stimulation is the poor outcome associated with the poor responders. The fertilization rate is noted to be significantly lower per oocyte retrieved[1] and the rate of embryo cleavage is noted to be slower[2]. All these observations support the notion that poor-responder patients produce oocytes of poor quality, leading to failure in IVF cycles.

Possible causes

Age may be a possible cause of poor response; it is well known that fertility potential decreases significantly in older women. As women approach 40 years of age and beyond, the preg-

nancy rate in assisted reproductive techniques drops precipitously. This is probably due both to depletion of the oocyte pool and decrease in oocyte quality. The average age of menopause in the United States is 51 years, with two standard deviations being age 39 years. Since menopause is generally preceded by declining fecundity, this could account for some 'younger' women having a poor response to stimulation. Poor responders are noted to be older, on average, than normal responders, but the difference is not significant enough by itself to account for the poor response. A second possibility is premature ovarian failure and occult ovarian failure associated with antiovarian antibodies and antibodies to other hormone-producing organs such as the thyroid[3]. Tubal disease is a third possible cause; extensive pelvic adhesions are thought to interfere with ovarian function[4]. Finally, other factors – body weight, cigarette smoking, history of ovarian surgery and endometriosis – have also been implicated as possible causes.

Methods for identifying poor responders

The following tests (as well as a history of poor response) may enable one to identify patients at risk for poor response and perhaps help to identify those who have very little chance of achieving a response or pregnancy:

(1) Follicle stimulating hormone (FSH) level on cycle day 3: shown to have predictive value of IVF outcome[5].

(2) Clomiphene challenge test[6]: an ovarian performance predictive test to discriminate between patients with a very low chance of success and those with a fair fertility potential.

(3) Estradiol variation with leuprolide acetate.

(4) EFORT (the exogenous FSH ovarian reserve test): administer 300 IU of Metrodin on cycle day 3, and measure serum FSH prior to administration and 24 h after. (A basal FSH level > 10 mIU/ml and estradiol increase < 30 pg/ml are considered abnormal[7].)

Management

Many empirical treatments have been proposed thus far. These include stimulation with clomiphene citrate with and without hMG, down-regulation with gonadotropin releasing hormone analogs (GnRH-a), co-treatment with growth hormone and short flare protocol, but there are many others. Of these, no single protocol has been shown conclusively to be more beneficial than any other.

Brief summaries of more recently published papers which address the problem of poor responders follow.

Feldberg and colleagues[8] published a retrospective review which investigated the effectiveness of minidose GnRH-a + hMG. Three dosage groups were compared:

(1) Single dose of 3.75 mg;

(2) 0.5 mg daily until menses, 0.1 mg daily;

(3) 0.1 mg daily until menses, followed by 0.05 mg daily.

The results showed higher estradiol levels and lower progesterone levels on the day of human chorionic gonadotropin (hCG) and a lower cancellation rate, with a higher number of oocytes, higher fertilization rate and higher number of embryo transfers. The trend showed improved pregnancy and implantation.

van Hooff and co-workers[9] published a randomized study of the effect of doubling the hMG dose, using a total of 46 patients (low responders. After 5 days, with less than three follicles and estradiol levels < 500 pg/ml, 22 patients continued with 225 IU hMG, whilst 24 patients increased to 450 IU hMG. The results showed that a doubling of the hMG dose had no effect on the length of ovarian stimulation, peak estradiol level, number of follicles and number of cancelled cycles.

Dor and associates[10] published a retrospective study of 880 cycles with estradiol levels < 501 pg/ml on the day of hCG administration. The three treatments investigated, with resultant pregnancy rates in parentheses, were: clomiphene citrate (CC)/hMG (27%); hMG alone (15.1%; $p < 0.005$) and GnRH-a, hMG (20.8%, not significant).

The pregnancy rate was significantly lower in cycles with less than three follicles compared with cycles with four or more follicles (10.8% vs. 23.8%; $p < 0.0005$). It was concluded that the number of follicles retrieved is of greater prognostic value than estradiol levels, and that stimulation with GnRH-a, hMG does not appear to be superior to that with CC/hMG.

Jenkins and colleagues[2] investigated a group of 61 patients with a 'poor response' and 250 'good' responders and found the poor-response group to be significantly older ($p < 0.001$). There was no significant difference between the groups with regard to indication for IVF. In the poor-response group, the following was evident. A higher dose of hMG was required; it took longer for follicles to reach maturity; treatment resulted in 8.9 oocytes per retrieval vs. 11.8 oocytes ($p < 0.01$); the fertilization rate was lower than in the 'good' responders ($p < 0.01$); the rate of cell division was slower ($p < 0.01$); the pregnancy rate was 9% (vs. 29%, $p < 0.01$); and the implantation rate was 4.4% (vs. 16.1%, $p < 0.01$).

Check and associates[11] reported on their use of gonadotropin suppression and human menopausal gonadotropins to induce ovulation in women with hypergonadotropic amenorrhea in 100 women. In the majority of cases, estrogen was used to decrease the elevated luteinizing hormone (LH) and FSH levels with hMG to boost the follicle to maturation. The ovulation rate was 19% (68/361), the pregnancy rate per cycle was 5.2% (19/361) and the viable pregnancy rate was 2.2% (8/361).

Rosen and colleagues[12] published results from a prospective, cross-over study, carried out on eight women with idiopathic premature ovarian failure and secondary amenorrhea. Two protocols were used: first, protocol A: GnRH-a (Lupron®, 1 mg/l) to decrease FSH level to baseline; when FSH < 25 mIU/ml, Lupron was stopped, and followed with estradiol and FSH, with ultrasound examination for signs of ovulation; second, protocol B: the same except hMG treatment was started the day after stopping GnRH-a. The resultant average duration of GnRH-a use was 33.2 days; two women ovulated under protocol A, and two women also ovulated under protocol B. (One woman ovulated in both protocols.)

Several recent publications have reported ovulation induction in conjunction with growth hormone[13-17]; all the papers concluded that follicular recruitment, estradiol secretion by mature follicles, and oocyte yield and quality were uninfluenced by growth hormone treatment.

As evidenced by the papers cited, there is no protocol which has been shown to be superior. In managing poor responders, one must assess the patient's response to clomiphene, hMG, CC/hMG, leuprolide acetate/hMG (short and long protocols), etc. to find the best protocol for the individual patient. Few patients who continue to show a poor response in a stimulated cycle do well in a natural cycle. For the patients who persist in attempts at pregnancy without success, oocyte donation is a viable option available to the patient.

References

1. Rysselberge, M. V., Puissant, F., Barlow, P., Lejeune, B., Delvigne, A. and Leroy, F. (1989). Fertility prognosis in IVF treatment of patients with cancelled cycles. Hum. Reprod., 4, 663–6
2. Jenkins, J. M., Davies, D. W., Devonport, H., Anthony, F. W., Gadd, S. C., Watson, R. H. and Masson, G. M. (1991). Comparison of 'poor' responders with 'good' responders using a standard buserelin/human menopausal gonadotrophin regime for in-vitro fertilisation. Hum. Reprod., 6, 918–21
3. Alper, M. M. and Garner, P. R. (1985). Premature ovarian failure: its relationship to autoimmune disease. Obstet. Gynecol., 66, 27–30
4. Molloy, D., Martin, M., Seirs, A., Lopata, A., Clarke, G., McBain, J., Ngu, A. and Johnston, I. H. (1987). Performance of patients with a frozen pelvis in an in vitro fertilization program. Fertil. Steril., 47, 450–5
5. Scott, R. T., Toner, J. F., Muasher, S. J., Oehninger, S. C., Robinson, S. and Rosenwaks, Z. (1989). FSH levels on cycle day 3 are predictive of IVF outcome. Fertil. Steril., 51, 651
6. Navot, D., Rosenwaks, Z. and Margalioth, E. J. (1987). Prognostic assessment of female fecundity. Lancet, 2, 645–7

7. Olivennes, F., Fanchin, R., DeZiegler, D. and Frydman, R. (1993). Poor responders: screening and treatment possibilities. J. Assist. Reprod. Genet., 10, 115–17
8. Feldberg, D., Farhi, J., Ashkenazi, J., Dicker, D., Shalev, J. and Ben-Rafael, Z. (1994). Minidose gonadotropin-releasing hormone agonist is the treatment of choice in poor responders with high follicular-stimulating hormone levels. Fertil. Steril., 62, 343–6
9. van Hooff, M. H., Alberda, A. T., Huisman, G. J., Zeilmaker, G. H. and Leerentveld, R. A. (1993). Doubling the human menopausal gonadotropin dose in the course of an in-vitro fertilization treatment cycle in low responders: a randomized study. Hum. Reprod., 8, 369–73
10. Dor, J., Seidman, D. S., Ben-Shlomo, I., Levran, D., Karasik, A. and Mashiach, S. (1992). The prognostic importance of the number of oocytes retrieved and estradiol levels in poor and normal responders as in vitro fertilization treatment. J. Assist. Reprod. Genet., 9, 228–32
11. Check, J. H., Nowroozi, K., Chase, J. S., Nazari, A., Shapse, D. and Vaze, M. (1990). Ovulation induction and pregnancies in 100 consecutive women with hypergonadotropic amenorrhea. Fertil. Steril., 53, 811–16

12. Rosen, G. F., Stone, S. C. and Yee, B. (1992). Ovulation induction in women with premature ovarian failure: a prospective, crossover study. *Fertil. Steril.*, **57**, 448–9

13. Hughes, S. M., Huang, Z. H., Morris, I. D., Matson, P. L., Buck, P. and Lieberman, B. A. (1994). A double-blind cross-over controlled study to evaluate the effect of human biosynthetic growth hormone on ovarian stimulation in previous poor responders to *in-vitro* fertilization. *Hum. Reprod.*, **9**, 13–18

14. Levy, T., Limor, R., Villa, Y., Eshel, A., Eckstein, N., Vagman, I., Lidor, A. and Ayalon, D. (1993). Another look at co-treatment with growth hormone and human menopausal gonadotropins in poor responders. *Hum. Reprod.*, **8**, 834–9

15. Levron, J., Lewit, N., Erlik, Y. and Itskovitz-Eldor, J. (1993). No beneficial effects of human growth hormone therapy in normal ovulatory patients with a poor ovarian response to gonadotropins. *Gynecol. Obstet. Invest.*, **35**, 65–8

16. Jacobs, H. (1992). Growth hormone and ovulation: is there an indication for treatment of infertile women with growth hormone? *Horm. Res.*, **38** (Suppl. 1), 14–21

17. Shaker, A. G., Fleming, R., Jamieson, M., Yates, R. W. S. and Coutts, J. R. T. (1992). Absence of effect of adjuvant growth hormone therapy on follicular responses to exogenous gonadotropins in women: normal and poor responders. *Fertil. Steril.*, **58**, 919–23

Ovarian challenge tests

52

E. Loumaye

Introduction

Female fertility generally starts to decline about 20 years before the menopause. Evidence has now been accumulated which indicates that aging of follicle/oocyte complexes plays a significant role in this process of decline. There are two important aspects to this alteration of the ovarian reserve:

(1) The time of decline is highly variable – some women will have difficulty conceiving in their late twenties and others will conceive and deliver in their late forties; and

(2) Ovarian aging cannot be diagnosed using standard parameters such as cycle length or levels of progesterone during the mid-luteal phase.

Assessment of ovarian follicular reserve, however, could prove of clinical interest in this respect. This article reviews the endocrine tests that are currently available for this purpose.

Ovarian aging is a progressive process

Ovarian aging is a progressive process that actually starts during fetal life. This has been demonstrated by the following observations.

(1) The ovarian follicular reserve starts to decline through atresia at week 16 of fetal life. When menopause is established, the ovarian follicular reserve, although very diminished, is not zero – a few thousand follicles/oocytes may still be found in the ovary[1]. This indicates that the ovary's ability to respond to gonadotropin stimuli is not exclusively related to the presence of follicles, but also to an intrinsic ability of these follicles to respond.

(2) Female fertility declines significantly around the fourth decade, about 20 years before the establishment of menopause-related amenorrhea[2].

(3) The widespread use of assisted reproductive technologies (ART) for human infertility has led to the observations that oocytes produced by an aging ovary have a lower ability to become fertilized, embryos have a reduced implantation ability, and an implanted embryo is more prone to miscarriage. Oocyte/embryo donations from young donors have implantation and ongoing pregnancy rates that are similar in both aging women and younger recipients. This strongly suggests that follicle/oocyte complex aging is the principal cause of impaired fertility rather than an alteration of the endometrium or of the uterus[3].

Fecundity is reduced before becoming clinically evident through changes in menstrual cycle characteristics

Two observations have suggested that subtle alteration of the ovarian follicular reserve contributes to female infertility.

Navot and colleagues studied 51 patients of 35 years of age or more suffering from unexplained infertility. Eighteen patients showed an exaggerated follicle-stimulating hormone (FSH) response (measured on day 10 of their cycle) after administration of 100 mg clomiphene citrate for 5 days. Only one patient became pregnant in this group. Thirty-three patients presented low FSH levels after clomiphene citrate administration, measured on day 10 of the cycle. Fourteen of these (42%) subsequently became pregnant[4].

Some of the patients undergoing controlled ovarian hyperstimulation for ART, develop very few mature follicles despite appropriate stimulation. This blunted response to stimulation does not appear to be exclusively related to patient clinical characteristics such as age, cause of infertility, menstrual cycle length, or body mass index (BMI)[5]. An endocrine assessment of these patients revealed elevated serum FSH levels, despite an otherwise normal ovulatory cycle in terms of estradiol and progesterone levels. Serum FSH levels appear, therefore, to be a potential marker of an early alteration of the ovarian follicular reserve.

Serum FSH level as a diagnostic test for diminished ovarian follicular reserve

During a normal menstrual cycle, recruitment of a cohort of growing follicles, which will ultimately lead to ovulation of a dominant follicle, results from a late-luteal phase surge in FSH[6]. A decrease in both serum progesterone and inhibin levels during this period lead to an increase in FSH levels which culminates during menstruation. The resulting follicular growth then leads to an increase of serum estradiol and inhibin which subsequently causes a decrease in FSH levels. The luteo–follicular transition during the menstrual cycle appears to be an optimal stage for assessing ovarian sensitivity to FSH. Measurement of serum FSH to diagnose incipient ovarian failure is therefore made during this transition phase. In practice, three approaches have been evaluated for using FSH as a parameter to determine the ovarian follicular reserve.

Basal serum FSH levels (cycle day 3)

Serum FSH concentration on day 3 of the cycle has been negatively correlated with the outcome of *in vitro* fertilization–embryo transfer (IVF–ET). Scott and co-workers have measured basal serum FSH levels, prior to any medication administration, in 758 IVF cycles performed in 441 patients[7]. The highest pregnancy rate was recorded in patients in whom basal FSH levels were low (< 15 IU/l), intermediary in patients with a basal FSH level of 15–24.9 IU/l, and the lowest in patients with an elevated basal FSH level (> 25 IU/l). Pregnancy rates were 17.0, 9.3 and 3.6%, respectively. Basal FSH levels were also inversely correlated with the number of aspirated follicles during the ovum pick-up procedure and with the number of recovered oocytes.

Scott and colleagues looked at basal FSH levels on day 3 during three consecutive cycles in 81 patients[8]. Patients who presented FSH levels < 15 IU/l in each cycle, had very constant FSH levels (as assessed with the standard error of the mean). By contrast, those who had basal FSH levels above 15 IU/l on at least one occasion presented much larger variations in FSH, with FSH levels fluctuating between low and elevated values. In this last group of patients, the response to controlled ovarian hyperstimulation was impaired whether or not basal FSH was elevated at the start of the cycle. This indicates that fluctuations between normal and elevated FSH levels are observed in some patients, but once a patient has shown an elevated FSH level, it is very likely that she has an impaired ovarian follicular reserve and a reduced probability of conception.

More recently, this group has confirmed this observation in a study including 1748 cycles. They have shown that basal FSH level is a prognostic parameter for ovarian follicular reserve, independent of a patient's age[9].

Urinary excretion of FSH

Marcus and associates have compared serum FSH levels and urinary FSH concentrations on day 3 of the cycle. Urinary samples were collected in the morning and urinary concentrations were expressed as FSH IU per mmol of creatinine. This assessment was performed in 50 patients presenting with various causes of infertility. The correlation between serum FSH and urinary FSH was found to be good, suggesting that urinary FSH could be used for future screening of patients[10].

Serum FSH levels after administration of an ovarian challenge test

Navot and colleagues' initial observation[4] suggests that the difference in serum FSH levels between normal patients and patients with an impaired ovarian reserve is more marked after clomiphene citrate administration than at baseline. Patients with impaired ovarian reserve had a mean basal serum FSH level that was twice as high when compared with controls; after clomiphene citrate administration, however, serum FSH levels were three times higher in patients with impaired ovarian follicular reserve (both differences being statistically significant; $p < 0.02$ and $p < 0.001$, respectively)[4]. This observation combined with Scott and co-workers' observations[8] on fluctuating FSH levels in patients with elevated FSH led to the development of a clomiphene citrate challenge test.

We applied this test to 114 patients prior to receiving ART[11]. The sum of the serum FSH concentrations before (day 2) and after (day 10) administration of 100 mg clomiphene citrate/ day from day 5 to day 9 of the cycle correlates better with the number of growing follicles, the number of retrieved oocytes and the number of embryos than did basal serum FSH levels. In addition, when the sum was > 26 IU/l, no pregnancy was obtained.

A similar observation was reported by Tanbo and co-workers who evaluated the clomiphene citrate challenge test in 91 patients aged 35 years or more to be treated with ART[12]. An abnormal clomiphene citrate challenge test gave a positive predictive value, in terms of poor outcome of controlled ovarian hyperstimulation, of 85%, and a negative predictive value of 72%. In practice, out of every ten IVF cycles performed in a patient with an abnormal clomiphene citrate challenge test, eight to nine of the cycles will be cancelled due to insufficient ovarian response.

More recently, Scott and co-workers completed a long-term prospective evaluation of clomiphene citrate challenge test screening in women from the general infertility population[13]. Approximately 10% of the 236 patients had an abnormal clomiphene citrate challenge test . The incidence of abnormal tests rose with age and was < 3% in women < 30 years of age and 26% for women > 40 years of age. The pregnancy rate in the patients with diminished ovarian follicular reserve was markedly lower (9%) than the pregnancy rate in those with adequate reserve (43%). The pregnancy rates were still significantly decreased after controlling for age. Only seven of the 23 patients with abnormal tests had an elevated day 3 FSH level, again suggesting that the clomiphene citrate challenge test may be more sensitive than assessment of basal FSH levels.

The GnRH agonist stimulation test (GAST)

Pretreatment of patients undergoing ART with a gonadotropin releasing hormone (GnRH) agonist is now widely used. The estradiol secretion in response to the flare-up effect of the agonist on the pituitary secretion of FSH and LH has been used as a putative indicator of IVF outcome[14,15]. Four estradiol secretion patterns have been identified. A prompt elevation of estradiol was found to be associated with a pregnancy rate of 46% whereas absence of estradiol elevation was associated with a pregnancy rate of 6%. More recently, the GnRH agonist challenge test has been evaluated further in patients pretreated with a progestogen[16]. In this study, the estradiol response to the GnRH agonist also appeared to be a good indicator of IVF outcome.

Exogenous FSH test (EFORT)

Recently, an additional test of the ovarian follicular reserve has been reported[17]. In the test, the patient receives 300 IU FSH on day 3 of a spontaneous cycle. Serum estradiol is measured on the following day. So far, 52 patients have

Table 1 Summary of literature regarding incidence of impaired ovarian reserve. CCT, clomiphene citrate challenge test; GAST, GnRH agonist challenge test

Study	Patients/ cycles (n)	Test	Population	Patients with abnormal test (%)	Pregnancy rate (%) Abnormal test	Normal test
Scott (1989)[7]	758	basal FSH	IVF	7.6	3.6	25.2*
Toner (1991)[9]	1451	basal FSH	IVF	5.5	0.0	18.0*
Navot (1987)[4]	51	CCT	> 35 years, unexplained infertility	37.0	5.6	42.4**
Tanbo (1989)[20]	165	CCT	IVF	32.7	0.0	32.7*
Loumaye (1990)[11]	114	CCT	IVF	17.5	0.0	17.5*
Tanbo (1992)[12]	91	CCT	> 35 years, abnormal pelvis	41.0	0.0	20.0**
Scott (1993)[13]	236	CCT	infertility	11.0	8.7	43.2**
Padilla (1990)[14]	97	GAST	IVF	18.5	6.0	46.0*
Winslow (1991)[15]	228	GAST	IVF	7.9	6.0	24.6

*Pregnancy rate per treated cycle; **pregnancy rate per patient

been tested prior to undergoing IVF. These preliminary data indicate that the test could have a better predictive value than basal serum FSH levels.

Incidence of impaired follicular ovarian reserve

The various tests have been applied to different patient populations to assess the incidence of impaired ovarian follicular reserve in infertile women. The estimated incidences are summarized in Table 1.

Through use of the different tests, a highly significant proportion of the infertile patient population has been diagnosed as having an impaired ovarian reserve and have, therefore, a poor prognosis in terms of fertility treatment outcome. The incidence is about 10% in the general infertile population and is up to 40% when considering patients above 35 years of age. Unexplained infertility and patients with a history of pelvic surgery appear to have a high incidence of abnormal test results. In an IVF population, the clomiphene citrate challenge test appears to detect a higher incidence of impaired ovarian follicular reserve than the GAST test.

Conclusion

Published figures on the incidence of impaired ovarian follicular reserve strongly suggest that testing should be performed in all patients undergoing treatment for infertility. This is particularly applicable for patients over 35 years of age. To date, the clomiphene citrate challenge test has been best documented and appears to be the most sensitive. Other tests will require further evaluation, and will need to be compared with the clomiphene citrate challenge test prior to their use in clinical practice. Such testing, however, provides only a probability value with regard to infertility treatment outcome[18,19]. The clinical interest for performing an assessment of ovarian follicular reserve is threefold. First, it will provide couples with useful and additional information on their probability of achieving a pregnancy. Second, it should help avoid postponing treatment for infertility of short duration if the test proves abnormal. Finally, it helps clinicians and couples consider oocyte or embryo donation for solving the couple's infertility.

References

1. Speroff, L., Glass, R. H. and Kase, N. G. (1984). The ovary from conception to senescence. In *Clinical Gynecologic Endocrinology and Infertility*, pp. 101. (Baltimore: Williams and Wilkins)
2. Federation CECOS, Schwartz, D. and Mayaux, B. A. (1982). Female fecundity as a function of age: results of artificial insemination in 2193 nulliparous women with azoospermic husbands. *N. Engl. J. Med.*, **306**, 404–6
3. Sauer, M. V., Paulson, R. J. and Lobo, R. A. (1992). Reversing the natural decline in human infertility. *J. Am. Med. Assoc.*, **268**, 2175–321
4. Navot, D., Rozenwaks, Z. and Margalioth, E. (1987). Prognostic assessment of female fecundity. *Lancet*, **2**, 645–7
5. Cameron, I. T., O'Shea, F. C., Rolland, J. M., Hughes, E. G., De Kretser, D. M. and Healey, D. (1988). Occult ovarian failure: a syndrome of infertility regular menses, and elevated follicle-stimulating hormone concentrations. *J. Clin. Endocrinol. Metab.*, **67**, 1190–4
6. Roseff, S. J., Bangah, M. L., Kettel, L. M., Vale, W., Rivier, J., Burger, H. G. and Yen, S. S. (1989). Dynamic changes in circulating inhibin levels during the luteal follicular transition of the human menstrual cycle. *J. Clin. Endocrinol. Metab.*, **69**, 1033–9
7. Scott, R. T., Toner, J. S., Muasher, S. J., Oehninger, S., Robinson, S. and Rosenwaks, Z. (1989). Follicle-stimulating hormone levels on cycle day 3 are predictive of *in vitro* outcome. *Fertil. Steril.*, **51**, 651–4
8. Scott, R., Hofmann, G., Oehninger, S. and Muasher, S. (1990). Intercycle variability of day 3 follicle-stimulating hormone levels and its effect on stimulation quality in *in vitro* fertilization. *Fertil. Steril.*, **54**, 297–302
9. Toner, J. P., Philput, C. B., Jones, G. S. and Muasher, S. J. (1991). Basal follicle stimulating hormone level is a better predictor of *in vitro* fertilization performance than age. *Fertil. Steril.*, **55**, 784–91
10. Marcus, M., Grunfeld, L., Berkowitz, G., Kaplan, P. and Godbold, J. (1993). Urinary follicle-stimulating hormone as a biological marker of ovarian toxicity. *Fertil. Steril.*, **59**, 931–3
11. Loumaye, E., Billion, J., Mine, J., Psalti, I., Pensis, M. and Thomas, K. (1990). Prediction of individual response to controlled ovarian hyperstimulation by means of clomiphene citrate challenge test. *Fertil. Steril.*, **53**, 295–301
12. Tanbo, T., Dale, P. O., Lunde, O., Norman, N. and Abyholm, T. (1992). Prediction of response to controlled ovarian hyperstimulation: a comparison of basal and clomiphene citrate stimulated follicle stimulating hormone levels. *Fertil. Steril.*, **57**, 819–24
13. Scott, R. T., Leonardi, M. R., Hofmann, G. E., Illions, E. H., Neal, G. S. and Navot, D. (1993). A prospective evaluation of clomiphene citrate challenge test screening in the general infertility population. *Obstet. Gynecol.*, **82**, 539–45
14. Padilla, S. L., Bayati, J. and Garcia, J. E. (1990). Prognostic value of the early serum estradiol response to leuprolide acetate in *in vitro* fertilization. *Fertil. Steril.*, **53**, 288–94
15. Winslow, K. L., Toner, J. P., Brzyski, R. G., Oehinger, S. C., Acosta, A. A. and Muasher, S. J. (1991). The gonadotropin-releasing hormone agonist stimulation test – a sensitive predictor of performance in the flare-up in *in vitro* fertilization cycle. *Fertil. Steril.*, **56**, 711–17
16. Hugues, J. N., Attalah, M., Herve, F. and Kottler, M. L. (1992). Effects of short-term GnRH agonist – human menopausal gonadotropin hyperstimulation in progesterone-treated patients. *Hum. Reprod.*, **7**, 1079–84
17. Fanchin, R., De Ziegler, D., Olivennes, F., Taieb, J., Dzik, A. and Frydman, R. (1994). Exogenous follicle stimulating hormone ovarian reserve test (EFORT): a simple and reliable screening test for detecting "poor responders" in *in vitro* fertilization. *Hum. Reprod.*, **9**, 1607–11
18. Scott, R. T. and Hofmann, G. E. (1995). Prognostic assessment of ovarian reserve. *Fertil. Steril.*, **63**, 1–11
19. Wallach, E. E. (1995). Pitfalls in evaluating ovarian reserve. *Fertil. Steril.*, **63**, 12–14
20. Tanbo, T., Dale, P. C., Abyholm, T. and Stokke, K. T. (1989). Follicle-stimulating hormone as a prognostic indicator in clomiphene citrate/human menopausal gonadotrophin-stimulated cycles for *in-vitro* fertilization. *Hum. Reprod.*, **4**, 647–50

377

Women's age and assisted medical procreation

53

B. Hedon, F. Galtier-Dereure and H. Dechaud

Introduction

After a peak reached around the age of 20, fertility decreases steadily[1,2]. The phenomenon becomes statistically sensible after the age of 30. It can be estimated that the fertility of a 35-year-old woman is only half of what it was during her twenties. By the age of 40, it will have been halved once again to reach the level of zero at the time of menopause. This decline is made up of a reduction in the conception rate, and an increase in the spontaneous abortion rate. It is also associated with an increase in fetal chromosomal malformation rates.

All population studies, based on demographic data, are in agreement on this point[3]. When nothing is done to limit the size of a family, the average time to become pregnant increases with age and the average age of the mother during her last pregnancy is 41 years[4]. When marriage and the subsequent decision to have a child are delayed, the risk of remaining infertile is more than 60% when the woman is over 40 years of age. The decline in fertility with increasing age can be related to a number of factors among which are reduction in intercourse frequency, increased frequency of ovulatory defects, poorer quality of ovulated ovocytes as well as an increase in ovocyte chromosomal abnormalities, decreased endometrial receptivity and increased frequency of gynecological and extra-gynecological diseases. The age of the woman's partner can also have a negative influence.

Infertility becomes more frequent with increasing female age. Around the age of 40, when a woman desires a child, she tends to become anxious and very often seeks medical advice and access to assisted medical procreation techniques in the hope that they will help to obtain a quick result. The demand from 40-year-old patients is growing with the development of these techniques and the information appearing in the media about their successes. There is also a social trend to delay pregnancy and more women desire to become mothers after the age of 40.

Age of women participating in an IVF program

The average age of women participating in an *in vitro* fertilization (IVF) program is between 33 and 34 years of age[5]. This figure varies widely in different IVF programs, depending on the selection criteria. The proportion of women over 40 years old is between 10 and 15%. This proportion is increasing and reflects both the growing demand from older women and the greater tendency to accept these demands by the

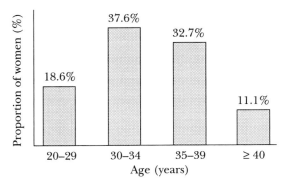

Figure 1 Age of women attending the IVF program (Montpellier University Hospital, 1985–92)

Men

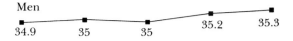

34.9   35   35   35.2   35.3

Women

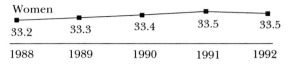

33.2   33.3   33.4   33.5   33.5

1988   1989   1990   1991   1992

Figure 2 Average age (years) of patients participating in an IVF program (FIVNAT)

medical community (Figures 1 and 2). The age of the women's partners, slightly higher than their spouses, follows the same pattern.

IVF results depending on age

The success of IVF is constantly reported to be adversely affected by increasing age. For example, in our IVF unit, the clinical pregnancy rate per egg retrieval decreases from 20.1% in patients under 35 years of age to 11.8% when the woman is over 40 (personal data, Montpellier University Hospital, 1990–94). This success rate would be even lower if each started stimulation cycle is considered, as age increases significantly the frequency of cycle cancellation. In fact, every stage of the IVF procedure, but fertilization *in vitro* itself, is affected: lower ovarian response to stimulation, less eggs retrieved, less embryos and lower implantation rate. Moreover, the clinical pregnancy rate reflects only imperfectly the performance of older women, because the spontaneous abortion rate can be as high as 50% of pregnancies. The take-home baby rate is less than 10%[5] (Table 1).

There are numerous reports which demonstrate similar data. The ongoing pregnancy rate (12%) is lower and the total abortion rate (60%) higher in patients 40 years of age or older in comparison with patients 39 years of age or younger[6]. Linear regression analysis of the effect of women's age on the ongoing pregnancy rate per embryo transfer shows a highly significant negative correlation: 26% for patients younger than 30 years of age, as compared with 9% for patients aged 37 years. Patients aged 40 years or more had a 50% miscarriage rate, compared with 29% in patients under the age of 40[7].

There are conflicting reports concerning the effect of female age on ovarian response to stimulation. Two consecutive IVF cycles were assessed in 25 women more than 35 years of age and their response was compared to a control group of 48 women less than 35 years of age who conceived in the IVF program. In the older women, the maximal estradiol response was proportional to the number of human menopausal gonadotropin (hMG) ampules used and did not differ from the response of younger women. Similarly, the number of follicles of diameter > 1 cm, the number of ovocytes recovered and the number of embryos which cleaved did not differ between the older and the younger women. However, conception rates were markedly lower in the older women[8].

Success rates decrease from 19.8% per attempt below the age of 25 years to 9.1% per attempt at 40 years or more. The effect is due to a reduction in ovocyte production and to a reduced implantation rate per embryo[9].

The influence of women's age on the results of IVF was analyzed in 1801 women undergoing the procedure. Advancing age was found to be

Table 1 Results of IVF according to age of the woman (FIVNAT)

	Woman's age (years)				
	≥ 35	36–37	38–39	40–41	≥ 42
Pregnancy rate/retrieval (%)	19.4	17.8	13.8	12.3	7.1
Spontaneous abortions (% of pregnancies)	16.1	17.2	29.3	28.7	52.0
Live childbirth/retrieval	15.9	12.7	8.4	7.5	2.8
twins (% of pregnancies)	24.8	21.2	19.0	13.0	5.4
triplets (% of pregnancies)	5.4	1.7	1.0	0.0	0.0

related to significantly reduced success rates, from an average of 30.1% per transfer below the age of 36 years to 15.9% per transfer at 37 years or more. The decrease is related to a reduction in ovocyte production (five at 25 years or less, four below the age of 40 years, three at 40 years of age or more, and two in the 43–37-year group) and is probably due to reduced implantation[10].

Age had a significant effect on the discharge rate during stimulation, changing from 5.6% in women under 30 years to 31.4% in women over 40 years. There was also an effect of age on the number of eggs retrieved, declining from an average of 9.1 for women under 30 years to 5.4 in women over 40 years. Fertilization and embryo transfer rates were not influenced by age, but pregnancy rates per transfer declined significantly from 17.5% in women under 30 years to 7% in women between 37 and 40 years. In women having the gamete intrafallopian transfer (GIFT) procedure, the pregnancy rate declined accordingly, from 35.5% in women under 30 years to 12.2% in women over 40 years[11].

In a series of 77 patients who underwent 210 treatment cycles of ovarian stimulation and intrauterine insemination after the age of 40, Frederick and colleagues obtained 11 pregnancies (5% per cycle), of which only three delivered. Compared with the success rates of the same technique obtained in younger women, one has to conclude that the success rate in women above 40 years of age is very poor[12].

Comparing two age groups ($\leq$ 35 and > 35 years of age), a British group found that the selection criteria used in their program for abandoning treatment cycles led to significantly more older patients being excluded from oocyte collection, but the patients from both groups that progressed to ovocyte collection and embryo transfer showed no significant difference in embryo implantation[13].

Ovum donation in aging women

Ovum donation has proven to be successful even in older women[14,15]. Comparing the results obtained in patients 45 years of age and older with standard IVF therapy and ovocyte donation. Yaron and colleagues could obtain no pregnancy in 52 treatment cycles in standard IVF, whereas 33 clinical pregnancies were obtained after 220 ovocyte donation cycles (17.5% per transfer)[16]. The same kind of comparison by Sauer and colleagues in patients 40 years of age and above leads to the same conclusion: improved outcomes are observed with regard to fertilization rates *in vitro*, number of embryos transferred, embryo implantation rate, clinical pregnancy rates and ongoing or successfully completed pregnancy rates. Moreover, results with ovum donation are similar in the different age groups. No age-related decline in fertility can be demonstrated when ovocyte donation is used[17].

The same author, reviewing retrospectively 300 cycles of ovocyte donation, concluded similarly: the establishment of pregnancy utilizing ovocyte donation is not adversely affected by the chronological age of the recipient. This implies that the age-related decline in fertility is due primarily to ovocyte aging, and not to loss of endometrial receptivity[18]. Similar conclusions are drawn by Abdalla and colleagues[19].

Mechanism of the age-related decline in fertility in women

Assisted medical procreation techniques, and in particular those utilizing donor gametes, offer a good model to study the factors responsible for the female age-related decline in fertility. Artificial insemination offering an appropriate timing for sperm injection alleviates the influence of coitus frequency. The use of donor sperm suppresses the influence of the husband's age. The lowering of pregnancy rates, despite the use of donor sperm, shows that there are other contributing factors directly related with the woman herself[20]. With IVF, it has become possible to investigate the different stages of the reproductive process (ovulation, fertilization and implantation).

The ovary

It has quickly become apparent that the first effect of age on the IVF procedure is to reduce the intensity of the ovarian response to stimulation. Despite the use of a higher daily dosage of gonadotropins, and whatever the nature of these gonadotropins (hMG, purified follicle stimulating hormone (FSH) from urinary extraction, or even recombinant FSH), less growing follicles can be seen on ultrasound and estradiol levels are lower in older women. The risk of developing a functional cyst or an empty follicle or of undergoing an atretic process is higher. The number of ovocytes retrieved is decreased (seven ovocytes are retrieved on average in patients under 36 years of age, and this number is less than four when the patient is over 40) and these women are more at risk than others to have no ovocyte at all.

The fecundation process is not altered. The fertilization rate of ovocytes is similar to that obtained in younger women and in more responsive patients. The diminished number of embryos produced by IVF is the direct consequence of the low number of ovocytes retrieved (3.4 embryos before 36, 2.6 between 38 and 39, and 2.2 over 40).

In fact, the number of embryos transferred is not very different from that in younger women because it is influenced by the transfer policy limiting the number of transferred embryos in younger women. But the implantation rate per embryo is decreased, and the resulting pregnancy rates per induced cycle, per ovocyte retrieval or per embryo transfer are reduced.

Many of these results can be explained by an alteration of follicular development and subsequent ovocyte quality. Aging of the ovary is associated with a reduction in the follicular population, affecting growing as well as reserve follicles[21]. On the other hand, the atretic process is accelerated. The rate of depletion of ovocytes in the ovaries is accelerated exponentially around the age of 37[22]. The number of potentially recruitable ovocytes is lowered. This quantitative impact of aging on the ovary is also accompanied by a qualitative alteration. The follicular phase of the cycle is shortened and preovulatory follicles are smaller. Above all, there are increasingly frequent chromosomal defects in the ovocyte. This could account for the lower implantation rate of embryos and the higher risk of miscarriage and chromosomal birth defect.

It is possible that the prolonged meiotic arrest renders the ovocyte more vulnerable to aging and to environmental influences. However, it is also possible that defective ovocytes are less responsive to recruitment than healthy ones. They can be recruited only when the latter have disappeared. This is shown experimentally in mice when removal of one ovary leads to shortening of reproductive life and earlier rise in aneuploidy[23].

The endometrium

Alteration of uterine receptivity can also be a factor explaining the age-related decline of fertility. The uterus undergoes dramatic modifications with advancing age and pathologies frequency develop. But uterine receptivity is a parameter difficult to analyze, mainly due to the lack of knowledge of specific tests and variables that determine successful implantation of the embryo. In fact, ovocyte donation offers a model with the use of which it becomes possible to obtain an evaluation of endometrial capabilities, independently of ovocyte age and quality. Reports are still conflicting, and if some are in favor of a reduced endometrial receptivity[24], others conclude that it is a negligible factor[25].

FSH as an indicator of age-related poor IVF prognosis

The period preceding the menopause is characterized by an increase in basal FSH, as measured before day 3 of the cycle[26]. This increase can start very early, long before any clinical manifestation, and tends to accelerate around the age of 42[27]. Moreover, menopause is associated with a structural change of ovaries[28]. This period is also characterized by an important intercycle variability[29,30].

On the clinical side, there is usually no symptom. A shorter duration of the cycle, and in particular of the follicular phase, can however, be present[31], as well as a smaller diameter of the preovulatory follicle just before its rupture[32]. Granulosa cell cultures exhibit a diminution of the proliferative index in patients with elevated FSH[33].

The appearance of these modifications is associated with ovarian aging. In non-responding patients, Cameron and colleagues isolated a group of patients with elevated FSH levels identifying occult ovarian insufficiency[34]. In a series of 758 cycles in 441 patients, Scott and colleagues demonstrated a correlation between basal FSH, ovarian response to stimulation and the pregnancy rate[35]. This has been confirmed in a series of 1478 cycles and a correlation has been found with every parameter of the ovarian response to stimulation (cancellation rate, peak estradiol levels, number of ovocytes, number of embryos and pregnancy rate). This predictive value of basal FSH has been found to be more accurate than age[36]. More studies have shown the value of FSH determination in various ovarian stimulation protocols[37] as well as for induction of ovulation[38].

The value of FSH measurement has been further refined by dynamic testing. Several tests have been defined in order to challenge the 'ovarian reserve' (clomiphene challenge test, gonadotropin challenge test). Others try to reveal an incipient rising FSH level (gonadotropin releasing hormone agonist stimulation test, luteinizing hormone releasing hormone test). But none of these tests has proved to be more valuable than basal FSH determination at the beginning of the cycle.

Conclusion

The social trend of increasing the age at which women want to have children is an important factor of infertility. In regard to the age-related decline in fertility, medicine, in general, and assisted medical procreation techniques have limited possibilities. The medical attitude must:

(1) Encourage couples to have their children while there is still time (the prescription of a contraceptive is a good opportunity to inform and favor reflection);

(2) Offer appropriate counselling to couples seeking help;

(3) Not engage in costly explorations and treatments whose results would be questionable;

(4) Have the humility to recognize that none of the actual treatments can possibly overcome the physiological evolution of declining fertility;

(5) Exert caution towards the use of donor gametes, the experience in of which is too recent and is disputed in many aspects.

Beyond medicine (what we can do), there are economy (what it is possible to do) and ethics (what we ought to do).

References

1. Menken, J., Trussel, J. and Larsen, U. (1986). Age and infertility. *Science*, **233**, 1389–94
2. Brock, D. and Holloway, S. (1990). Fertility of older women. *Lancet*, **335**, 1470
3. Mineau, G. and Trussel, J. (1982). A specification of marital fertility by parent's age, age at marriage, and marital duration. *Demography*, **19**, 335–50
4. Tietze, C. (1957). Reproductive span and rate of reproduction among Hutterite women. *Fertil. Steril.*, **8**, 89–97
5. FIVNAT (1993). Fécondation in vitro après 40 ans. *Contracept. Fertil. Sex.*, **21**, 367–70
6. Romeu, A., Muasher, S. J., Acosta, A., Veeck, L., Diaz, J., Jones, G., Jones, H. and Rosenwacks, Z. (1987). Results of *in vitro* fertilization attempts in women 40 years of age and older; the Norfolk experience. *Fertil. Steril.*, **47**, 130–6

7. Padilla, S. L. and Garcia, J. E. (1989). Effect of maternal age and number of *in vitro* fertilization procedures on pregnancy outcome. *Fertil. Steril.*, **52**, 270–3

8. Segal, S. and Casper, R. F. (1990). The response to ovarian hyperstimulation and *in-vitro* fertilization in women older than 35 years. *Hum. Reprod.*, **5**, 255–7

9. Piette, C., De Mouzon, J., Bachelot, A. and Spira, A. (1990). IVF: influence of women's age on pregnancy rates. *Hum. Reprod.*, **5**, 56–9

10. Dicker, D., Goldman, J. A., Ashkenazi, J., Feldberg, D., Shelef, M. and Levy, T. (1991). Age and pregnancy rates in *in vitro* fertilization. *J. In Vitro Fertil. Embryo Transfer*, **8**, 141–4

11. Wood, C., Calderon, I. and Crombie, A. (1992). Age and fertility: results of assisted reproductive technology in women over 40 years. *J. Assist. Reprod. Genet.*, **9**, 482–4

12. Frederick, J. L., Denker, M. S., Rojas, A., Horta, I., Stone, S. C., Asch, R. H. and Balmaceda, J. P. (1994). Is there a role for ovarian stimulation and intra-uterine insemination after age 40? *Hum. Reprod.*, **9**, 2284–6

13. Arthur, I. D., Anthony, F. W., Masson, G. M. and Thomas, E. J. (1994). The selection criteria on an IVF program can remove the association between maternal age and implantation. *Acta Obstet. Gynecol. Scand.*, **73**, 562–6

14. Borini, A., Bafaro, G., Violini, F., Branchi, L., Casadio, V. and Flamigni, C. (1995). Pregnancies in postmenopausal women over 50 years old in an oocyte donation program. *Fertil. Steril.*, **63**, 258–61

15. Check, J. H., Nowroozi, K., Barnea, E. R., Shaw, K. J. and Sauer, M. V. (1993). Successful delivery after age 50: a report of two cases as a result of oocyte donation. *Obstet. Gynecol.*, **81**, 835–6

16. Yaron, Y., Amit, A., Brenner, S. M., Peyser, M. R., David, M. P. and Lessing, J. B. (1995). *In vitro* fertilization and oocyte donation in women 45 years of age and older. *Fertil. Steril.*, **63**, 71–6

17. Sauer, M., Paulson, R. and Lobo, R. (1993). Pregnancy after age 50: application of ovocyte donation to women after natural menopause. *Lancet*, **341**, 321–3

18. Sauer, M. V., Paulson, R. J., Ary, B. A. and Lobo, R. A. (1994). Three hundred cycles of oocyte donation at the University of Southern California: assessing the effect of age and infertility diagnosis on pregnancy and implantation rates. *J. Assist. Reprod. Genet.*, **11**, 92–6

19. Abdalla, H. L., Burton, G., Kirkland, A., Johnson, M. R., Leonard, T., Books, A. A. and Studd, J. W. W. (1993). Age, pregnancy and miscarriage: uterine versus ovarian factors. *Hum. Reprod.*, **8**, 1512–17

20. Schwartz, D. and Mayaux, M. J. (1982). Female fecundity as a function of age. *N. Engl. J. Med.*, **307**, 404–8

21. Gougeon, A. and Chainy, G. B. N. (1987). Morphometric studies of small follicles in ovaries of women at different ages. *J. Reprod. Fertil.*, **81**, 433–42

22. Faddy, M. J., Gosden, R. G., Gougeon, A., Richardson, S. J. and Nelson, J. F. (1992). Accelerated disappearance of ovarian follicles in mid-life, implications for forecasting menopause. *Hum. Reprod.*, **7**, 1342–6

23. Zheng, C. and Byers, B. (1992). Oocyte selection: a new model for the maternal age dependence of Down syndrome. *Hum. Genet.*, **90**, 1–6

24. Meldrum, D. R. (1993). Female reproductive aging – ovarian and uterine factors. *Fertil. Steril.*, **59**, 1–5

25. Balmaceda, J., Bernardini, L., Ciuffardi, I., Felix, C., Ord, T., Sueldo, C. and Asch, R. (1994). Oocyte donation in humans: a model to study the effect of age on embryo implantation rate. *Hum. Reprod.*, **9**, 2160–3

26. Lenton, E., Sexton, L., Lee, S. and Cooke, I. (1988). Progressive changes in LH and FSH and LH : FSH ratio in women throughout reproductive life. *Maturitas*, **10**, 35–43

27. McNaughton, J., Banah, M., McCloud, P., Hee, J. and Burger, H. (1992). Age related changes in FSH, LH, estradiol and immunoreactive inhibin in women of reproductive age. *Clin. Endocrinol.*, **36**, 339–45

28. Mason, M., Fonseca, E., Ruiz, J., Moran, C. and Zarate, A. (1992). Distribution of FSH and LH isoforms in sera from women with primary ovarian failure compared with that of normal reproductive and postmenopausal women. *Fertil. Steril.*, **58**, 60–5

29. Sherman, B., West, J. and Korenman, S. (1976). The menopausal transition: analysis of LH, FSH, estradiol, and progesterone concentrations during menstrual cycles of older women. *J. Clin. Endocrinol. Metab.*, **42**, 629–36

30. Scott, R., Hofmann, G., Oehninger, S. and Muasher, S. (1990). Intercycle variability of day 3 FSH levels and its effects on stimulation quality in IVF. *Fertil. Steril.*, **54**, 297–302

31. Sherman, B. and Korenman, S. (1975). Hormonal characteristics of the human menstrual cycle throughout reproductive life. *J. Clin. Invest.*, **55**, 699–706

32. Fitzgerald, C., Seif, M., Killick, S. and Bennett, D. (1994). Age related changes in the female reproductive cycle. *Br. J. Obstet. Gynaecol.*, **101**, 229–33

33. Seifer, D., Charland, C., Berlinksy, D., Penzias, A., Haning, R., Naftolin, F. and Barker, B.

(1993). Proliferative index of human luteinized granulosa cells varies as a function of ovarian reserve. *Am. J. Obstet. Gynecol.*, **169**, 1531–5

34. Cameron, L., O'Shea, F., Rolland, J., Hughes, E., De Krester, D. and Healy, D. (1988). Occult ovarian failure: a syndrome of infertility, regular menses, and elevated FSH concentrations. *J. Clin. Endocrinol. Metab.*, **67**, 1190–4

35. Scott, R., Toner, J., Muasher, S., Oehninger, S., Robinson, S. and Rosenwacks, Z. (1989). FSH levels on cycle day 3 are predictive of IVF outcome. *Fertil. Steril.*, **51**, 651–4

36. Toner, J., Philput, C., Jones, G. and Muasher, S. (1991). Basal FSH is a better predictor of IVF performance than age. *Fertil. Steril.*, **55**, 784–91

37. De Geyter, C., De Geyter, M., Castro, E., Balspratsch, M., Hanker, J., Schlegel, W., Nieschlag, F. and Schneider, H. (1993). Predictive parameters for ovarian response to hyperstimulation with exogenous gonadotrophins after suppression of gonadotropin secretion of the pituitary using a long-acting GnRH agonist. *Eur. J. Obstet. Gynecol. Reprod. Biol.*, **51**, 139–47

38. Pearlstone, A., Fournet, N., Gambone, J., Pang, S. and Buyalos, R. (1992). Ovulation induction in women age 40 and older: the importance of basal FSH level and chronological age. *Fertil. Steril.*, **58**, 674–9

Long-term follow-up after assisted reproduction

54

G. Kovacs

Donor sperm insemination

The first report in the literature of the long-term follow-up of children born after reproductive technology was in 1968, in Japan, when Iizuka and colleagues[1] reported on the physical and mental development of 54 children conceived from donor sperm. They found that these offspring were in no way inferior to the controls. They further enlarged their series[2] and presented their data at the first International Workshop on Donor Insemination and Sperm Cryopreservation in Paris, France in 1979. Also presented here were data from two centers in France, reporting qualitatively in an uncontrolled fashion on 30[3] and 75[4] families, with overall reassuring results.

In Australia, a retrospective study of 50 artificial insemination donor (AID) families when the children were between one- and three-years-old[5] found that there were no apparent major obstetric, pediatric or emotional problems.

Another reassuring survey of AID families was reported from Wisconsin, USA in 1990, by Amuzu and colleagues[6]. They contacted 362 families when the children were between 3 months and 15 years of age (mean 5 years), and found that birth weight and length were comparable to that in the general population. Similarly milestones such as rolling over, pulling to stand, walking alone, first words and phrases had a distribution not significantly different from the general population. Information on school performance was available on 171 of 189 school attenders, with ten children (5.8%) with learning disability and 18 (10.5%) in gifted school programs. In this study when asked about telling the children about their origins, 47% said that they 'definitely would not', and 13% 'probably not tell' the children. Fifty-four per cent of couples felt that AID treatment had improved their marriage whereas 3% thought that it had had a detrimental effect. Twenty-six divorces amongst 357 couples (7.2%) were identified, a result which was significantly less than the 12.9% expected for an age and racially matched group over the same period.

A report from CECOS-Lyon of 108 children conceived by donor insemination (DI) that compared illness rates, doctors visits, pediatrician visits and hospitalizations to the population of Rhome-Alpes, and found no difference.

The first controlled study of the psychosocial development of children conceived by DI was reported from the Prince Henry's Institute, Melbourne, in 1993[7]. Twenty-two children conceived by DI were studied between 6 and 8 years of age, compared to 20 matched controls conceived naturally and ten children who were adopted. The children were assessed by the Achenbach Child Behaviour Checklist and psychometric scores were derived. There were no significant differences between any of the three groups studied.

In a study of 354 couples who had undergone DI at four clinics in New South Wales, Australia, Durna and colleagues (personal communication) had a 78% response rate, with 76% claiming a positive personal effect on them, and only 0.8% having regrets. Forty-seven per cent felt that the DI child had a positive, whilst only 3% felt it had a negative effect, on their marriage, a finding similar to that of Azumu and colleagues[6]. Again the incidence of marriage breakdown was lower than expected from the general population being only 3.6%. Seventy-four per cent felt that the child resembled their father. They concluded that prospective couples can be reassured that having a child by DI will have a positive effect on both themselves and their marriage.

In the most detailed study of families and emotional development of children conceived by the new reproductive technologies, Golombok and colleagues[8], in London, compared 45 families with a DI child, 41 families with an IVF child to 43 control (naturally conceived with no recognized problems) families and 55 families with an adopted child. Children were aged between 4 and 8 years of age, and assessment included interview with the mother, questionnaires by both parents, and a questionnaire completed by the teacher if the child was at school. The children were also assessed by a battery of standardized tests. Factors assessed included parents' marital and psychiatric state, quality of parenting, and the children's emotions, behaviour and relationships. They concluded that despite the concerns raised regarding the potential negative consequences of the new reproductive technologies for family functioning and child development, their results indicated that the quality of parenting is superior to that with a naturally conceived child, even when donor gametes were used. No significant differences were found between DI and IVF families.

It would therefore appear from the available data, that the long-term development for families created by donor insemination have not had any significant problems identified.

Ovum donation

With respect to ovum donation, the first pregnancy using donor oocytes was reported only in 1983, and a survey of donor oocyte clinics around the world, in 1991, identified only just over 200 pregnancies[9]. The report on follow-up of donor oocyte children published so far appears to be limited to that of the Monash group[10].

From a total of 36 couples who conceived children using donor oocytes, between 1983 and 1991, 29 took part in a follow-up study which consisted either of a semistructured interview or the completion of a questionnaire. Although 40% of couples using an anonymous donor would have liked more information on the donor, they were unanimous in never wanting to meet the donor. Keeping in mind that the children were from 12 weeks to 8 years, only one family had told the child of its genetic origins. There was unanimous agreement amongst couples in that they would recommend ovum donation to other couples. Further studies will have to be carried out on the long-term outcome of ovum donation before any conclusions can be made.

In vitro fertilization

Although the first successful birth following IVF was in Oldham, England, the first cohort of IVF children was delivered by the Monash unit in 1980–81. It is of little surprise therefore that initial reports on the follow-up of IVF children came from Monash[11]. A conscious decision was also made to have, if possible, the same pediatrician involved with all the IVF children. The initial report was published in 1985[11], on the first 52 children conceived by IVF. Forty-nine children were seen for a developmental assessment at birth and 10 months of age. In addition, 33 children had a psychosocial assessment at 1–3 years of age. The principal finding from this uncontrolled study was that the Cesarean section rate was much higher (37%) than in the community, with preterm children being four times the expected rate, and very-low-birth weight being 10 times more common, with twins 20 times as often as expected. Four of the families had a clinically significant issue. In three families the child had significant clinical problems, in the fourth family the mother had significant problems in adapting to her parental role. The incidence of less significant clinical problems, e.g. colic, asthma, were similar to that in the general population. The scores on the Bayley Scales of Infant Development fell within the normal range. They concluded that the families studied did not yield an increase in psychosocial problems above that which may be expected in the population at large. However, these conclusions came from uncontrolled studies, and the need for a controlled study was obvious. Such a study was subsequently carried out between 1991 and 1993[12].

Another early report on 20 IVF children at their first birthday came from Perth, Australia in 1986[13]. This study found an increased rate of preterm birth, intrauterine growth retardation and Cesarean section. However, only one child was slightly under expected development at 1 year of age on Griffith Developmental Scales.

A controlled study on 83 IVF children and 93 matched non-IVF controls was reported from Norfolk, Virginia in 1989[14]. The authors carried out a physical examination, neurological and developmental examination, echo- and electrocardiography, abdominal and cranial ultrasound examination on all children. The children were carefully matched for socio-economic factors, and a multidisciplinary 'blinded' team did the assessments. There was no significant difference in major malformations (IVF, 2; controls, 1), or in Mental Development Index scores (IVF, 115 ± 13; controls, 111 ± 13). With respect to Psychomotor Development Index scores, again there was no difference (IVF, 114 ± 14; controls, 108 ± 15).

A similar controlled study was carried out in Israel on 116 IVF children and 116 matched controls at 12 to 45 months of age[15]. The developmental indices were assessed by interview and examination, and the conclusion was that IVF children grow and develop similarly to non-IVF controls. They concluded that when and IVF pregnancy is carried to term yielding an apparently healthy infant, the infant can be expected to develop and thrive similarly to his non-IVF conceived peer. However, they point out that babies from multiple pregnancy score lower on average, both on physical and mental scales.

Another controlled, albeit small study on the psychological development of children born by *in vitro* fertilization was published in France, in 1993[16]. A group of 33 IVF children were compared to two control groups; infertile women having children after ovulation induction (OI), and a control group of children without medical intervention. In the early postpartum period both IVF and OI groups experienced more (but not significantly so) difficulties. At 9 months the OI group had slightly (not significantly) more minor illnesses, and insomnia and feeding difficulties were slightly more common in the IVF group. By 18 months these small differences had decreased further, and totally disappeared by 3 years. They concluded that there are no significant differences between IVF, OI or natural children concerning their relationship with their mother.

A study on the social repercussions of success from IVF was studied by Munro and colleagues, from the Monash group, in 1992[17]. They studied 40 sets of IVF twins and compared them to 25 sets of spontaneous twins and 15 couples who had infertility workup only prior to twin pregnancy. They concluded after a questionnaire study using 'Schedule for Social Interaction' that IVF twin parents had deficient social relationships, with mothers more so than fathers. They recommended a specific support group for IVF twin parents should be formed.

The largest and best designed report is from the Halasz and co-workers study[12]. This was published as a 247-page publication plus 24 appendices. The study is based on 314 IVF and 150 matched control children and their families. Families were assessed at 2 years of age with a battery of tests including 'Short Temperament Questionnaire for Toddlers', 'Family Environment Scale', 'General Health Questionnaire', 'Dyadic Adjustment Scale', 'Interview Schedule for Social Interaction', and the 'Monash Family Interview'. Conclusions were that cognitive and motor development of IVF children falls within the normal range, and there was no difference in perceived temperament at 2 years of age. Pediatric analysis found no difference in neonatal problems, medical follow-up, physical outcomes, including disabilities or congenital malformations, parental concerns or patterns of child care between IVF parents and controls.

There was, however, an increased rate of obstetric interference with a higher rate of Cesarean section in IVF pregnancies. On assessing the parents, they found that probably psychiatric disturbance in terms of abnormal results did not differ between IVF parents and controls, but IVF couples differed from controls in expressing greater satisfaction with their relationship. They conclude by highlighting that although these results are reassuring, a long-term national study of offspring and families should be established. This is a daunting and difficult task fraught with logistic and ethical difficulties.

Recently, a French study of DI offspring had to be suspended at the request of the National Commission for Information Science and Freedom (CNIL) for the ethical aspects to be studied[18].

A report by Olivennes and Frydman[19], in Clamart Cedex, found from a multicenter French study that the reported increased incidence of prematurity, intrauterine growth retardation and raised perinatal mortality was due to multiple pregnancy rather than IVF technology in itself.

In 1992, the National Health and Medical Research Council of Australia[20] established a working party to examine the long-term health effects on women of assisted conception. Subsequently, the brief was extended to include children and men/families. This working party actually raised more questions than it answered. It has recommended that a number of studies be established to try to answer some questions. It recommended a retrospective study to investigate whether assisted conception is associated with an increase in breast, ovarian or other cancers.

A retrospective study on the incidence of cancers in women having undergone IVF treatment, in Melbourne between 1979 and 1994, is being carried out at the moment. Results should be available for presentation by late 1995.

In summary, no deleterious long-term effects of reproductive technology have been demonstrated on either the offspring, on women treated or their families. IVF has been subjected to more scrutiny than any other medical treatment. Nevertheless, long-term studies should continue.

References

1. Iizuka, R., Swada, Y. and Nishina, Ohi, M. (1968). The physical and mental development of children born following artificial insemination. *Int. J. Fert.*, **13**, 24–32
2. Mochimaru, F., Sato, H., Kobayashi, T. and Iizuka, R. (1980). Physical and mental development of children born through AID. In David, G. and Price, W. S. (eds.) *Human Artificial Insemination and Semen Preservation*, pp. 277–82. (New York, London: Plenum Press)
3. Semenov, G., Mises, R. and Bissery, J. (1980). Attempt at follow-up of children born through AID. In David, G. and Price, W. S. (eds.) *Human Artificial Insemination and Semen Preservation*, pp. 474–7. (New York, London: Plenum Press)
4. Manuel, C. and Czyba, J. (1980). Follow-up study on children born through AID. In David, G. and Price, W. S. (eds.) *Human Artificial Insemination and Semen Preservation*, pp. 467–74. (New York, London: Plemun Press)
5. Clayton, C. E. and Kovacs, G. T. (1982). AID offspring. Initial follow-up study of 50 couples. *Med. J. Aust.*, **1**, 338–9
6. Amuzu, B., Laxova, R. and Sander, S. (1990). Pregnancy outcome, health of children, and family adjustment after donor insemination. *Obstet. Gynecol.*, **75**, 899–905
7. Kovacs, G. T., Mushin, D., Kane, H. and Baker, H. W. G. (1993). A controlled study of the psychosocial development of children conceived following insemination with donor semen. *Hum. Reprod.*, **8**, 788–90
8. Golombok, S., Cook, R., Bish, A. and Murray, C. (1995). Families created by the new reproductive technologies: quality of parenting and social and emotional development of the children. *Child Dev.*, **64**, 285–98
9. King, C. M. and Kovacs, G. T. (1992). Oocyte donation: survey of results. In *Oocyte Donation, Reprod. Fertil. Dev.*, **4**, 119–24

10. Munro, J., Leeton, J. and Horsfall, T. (1992). Psychosocial followup of families from a donor oocyte programme: an exploratory study. In *Oocyte Donation, Reprod. Fertil. Dev.*, **4**, 125–30

11. Mushin, D. N., Spensley, J., Barreda-Hanson, M. (1985). Children of *in vitro* fertilization. *Clin. Obstet. Gynecol.*, **12**, 865–76

12. Halasz, G., Munro, J., Saunders, K., Astbury, J. and Spensley, J. (1993). The growth and development of children conceived by IVF. Report to Commonwealth Department of Health, Housing, Local Government and Community Services, and Victorian Health Promotion Foundation, Melbourne

13. Yovich, J. L., Parry, T. S., French, N. P. and Grauaug, A. A. (1986). Development assessment of twenty *in vitro* fertilization (IVF) infants at their first birthday. *J. in Vitro Fertil. Embryo Transfer*, **4**, 253–7

14. Marin, N., Wirth, F., Johnson, D. H., Frank, L. M., Presburg, H., Van de Water, V., Chee, E. M. and Mills, J. L. (1989). Congenital malformations and psychosocial development in children conceived by *in vitro* fertilization. *J. Paediatr.*, **115**, 222–7

15. Brandes, J. M., Scher, A., Itzkovits, J., Thaler, I., Sarid, M. and Gershoni-Baruch, R. (1992). Growth and development of children conceived by *in vitro* fertilization. *Pediatrics.*, **90**, 424–9

16. Raoul-Duval, A., Bertrand-Servais, M. and Frydman, R. (1993). Comparative prospective study of the psychological development of children born by *in vitro* fertilization and their mothers. *J. Psychosom. Obstet. Gynecol.*, **14**, 117–26

17. Munro, J. M., Ironside, W. and Smith, G. C. (1992). Successful parents of *in vitro* fertilization (IVF): the social repercussions. *J. Assist. Reprod. Genet.*, **2**, 170–6

18. Patel, T. (1993). Ethical doubts halt psychology study on children. *New Scientist*, **137**, 6

19. Olivennes, F. and Frydman, R. (1993). Les complications pediatriques des grossesses apres PMA. *Jobgyn*, **1**, 332–42

20. National Health and Medical Research Council (1995). *Long-term Effects on Women from Assisted Conception.* Consultation document

7

IVF technology: biological aspects

Microinsemination

55

A. Van Steirteghem, J. Liu, P. Nagy, H. Joris, C. Staessen, J. Smitz, H. Tournaye,
M. Camus, I. Liebaers and P. Devroey

Introduction

In the last two decades, *in vitro* fertilization (IVF) has been successful in the treatment of long-standing infertility due to tubal disease, idiopathic and male factor infertility. It is a well documented fact that the results of IVF in male infertility are not as good as those in patients with normal semen parameters. In andrological infertility only 20–30% of the inseminated cumulus–oocyte complexes are normally fertilized, which is much lower than the 60–70% fertilization rate in patients with tubal infertility[1]. Absence of fertilization may occur in about one-third of the cycles. It has been the experience of all centers for reproductive medicine, including our own, that a certain number of patients with andrological infertility cannot be helped by standard IVF treatment. Furthermore, a sizeable number of couples cannot be accepted for IVF if the number of progressively motile spermatozoa with normal morphology available for insemination is below a certain threshold number, such as 500 000.

In the past 6 years, assisted fertilization procedures have been developed to circumvent the barriers that prevent sperm access to the ooplasma, namely the zona pellucida and the ooplasmic membrane. Successful fertilization, embryo development, pregnancies and births have been reported after partial zona dissection (PZD) and subzonal insemination (SUZI)[2–4].

In 1992, the first pregnancies and births obtained by a novel procedure of assisted fertilization, intracytoplasmic sperm injection (ICSI), were reported by our group[5]. In rabbits and cattle, embryos obtained by ICSI have been transferred to recipient mothers and live offspring have resulted[6]. Very recently, ICSI was also successful in the mouse when a piezo-driven micropipette was used instead of a mechanically driven conventional pipette[7]. The results of the first 600 cycles of assisted fertilization by SUZI and ICSI at the Brussels Free University Center, as well as a controlled comparison on 144 oocytes in 11 cycles, indicated that the normal fertilization rate after ICSI is substantially higher than after SUZI, while the further *in vitro* development to transferable or freezable embryos is quite similar for the two procedures. The higher fertilization rate and similar cleavage rate resulted in more embryos for replacement after ICSI and high implantation rates have been obtained[8–11].

This report describes a 4-year survey on 2853 cycles in 1953 couples treated by ICSI between January 1991 and December 1994. ICSI was not carried out in 33 cycles (1.2%) because there were:

(1) No cumulus–oocyte complexes in 19 cycles;

(2) No metaphase II oocytes in seven cycles; and

(3) No spermatozoa in seven cycles.

ICSI was carried out in 2820 cycles.

Patient selection and management

ICSI can be carried out in couples who have undergone at least one but usually more cycles of standard IVF procedure; after juxtaposition of the cumulus–oocyte complexes with 200 000 or more progressively motile spermatozoa per ml, fertilization did not occur or occurred in fewer than 5% of the oocytes. ICSI can also be carried out in couples with semen parameters too impaired to be accepted for standard IVF because, after semen preparation, fewer than, for example, 500 000 progressively motile spermatozoa with normal morphology were present in the total ejaculate.

ICSI can also be carried out with epididymal or testicular spermatozoa in couples with obstructive azoospermia due to congenital bilateral absence of the vas deferens or failed vasovasectomy and vasoepididymostomy[12–15]. ICSI can also be carried out in some couples with non-obstructive azoospermia due to Sertoli-cell only syndrome or maturation arrest, for example.

The couples were fully informed about the novelty of the ICSI procedure and about its many unknown aspects. After extensive counselling, they agreed and signed a consent form to have prenatal diagnosis and to participate in a prospective follow-up study of the children born after ICSI[16–18].

Oocytes for intracytoplasmic sperm injection

Ovarian stimulation was carried out by a combination of gonadotropin releasing hormone agonist and human menopausal gonadotropins. The ovulation was induced with human chorionic gonadotropins when at least three follicles measured 18 mm or more in diameter and when serum estradiol concentration was at least 1000 ng/l. The luteal phase was supplemented with intravaginally administered micronized progesterone[19–21].

Oocyte retrieval was carried out by vaginal ultrasound-guided follicular puncture 36 h after hCG. In all, 36 425 cumulus–oocyte complexes were retrieved in these 2820 cycles, i.e. a mean of 12.9 complexes per cycle. Inspection of these complexes under the inverted microscope revealed that in almost all cases the cumulus and corona cells were well dispersed. These complexes were transferred into 5-ml Falcon tubes with 1 ml of pre-equilibrated Earle's medium and transported in a thermobox at 37°C to the microinjection laboratory, which is located at a distance of about 500 m.

The cells of the cumulus and corona cells were removed by a combination of an enzymatic and mechanical procedure: incubation for about 1 min in HEPES-buffered Earle's medium with about 60 IU hyaluronidase/ml and then aspiration of the cumulus–corona–oocyte complexes in and out of hand-drawn glass pipettes with two different diameters, first with an opening of 250–300 μm and then with an opening of 200 μm. Afterwards the oocytes were rinsed several times in droplets of HEPES-buffered Earle's and B_2 medium and then carefully observed under the inverted microscope at × 200 magnification. This included an assessment of the zona pellucida and the oocyte as well as noting the presence or absence of a germinal vesicle or the first polar body. Of the 36 425 complexes, 34 572 (95%) contained an intact oocyte with an intact zona pellucida and clear cytoplasm. Analysis of the nuclear status revealed 81% of the cumulus–oocyte complexes contained metaphase II oocytes which had extruded the first polar body, 10% germinal-vesicle stage oocytes and 4% metaphase I oocytes which had undergone breakdown of the germinal vesicle but had not yet extruded the first polar body. The oocytes were then incubated in 25 μl microdrops of B_2 medium covered by mineral oil at 37°C in an atmosphere of 5% O_2, 5% CO_2 and 90% N_2. ICSI was carried out on all metaphase II oocytes.

Spermatozoa for intracytoplasmic sperm injection

Before the start of the treatment cycle, semen analysis and a semen selection procedure were carried out to verify whether enough spermatozoa were present to carry out ICSI. Semen analysis included the assessment of conventional semen characteristics by the procedures recommended by the World Health Organization[22] except for sperm morphology, which was assessed by strict Tygerberg criteria after Shorr staining[23]. Semen values were considered normal if:

Table 1 Sperm characteristics of freshly ejaculated semen in 2524 ICSI treatment cycles

	Cycles	%
Normal semen	175	7
Single sperm defect	377	15
oligozoospermia	91	
asthenozoospermia	119	
teratozoospermia	167	
Double sperm defects	731	29
oligoteratozoospermia	339	
asthenoteratozoospermia	217	
ologoasthenozoospermia	175	
Triple sperm defects		
oligoasthenoteratozoospermia	1241	49

(1) Sperm concentration was at least 20×10^6/ml;

(2) Progressive sperm motility was at least 40%; and

(3) Normal sperm morphology was at least 14%.

The distribution of the semen characteristics of freshly ejaculated semen used for ICSI in 2524 cycles was analyzed and revealed that:

(1) Normal semen parameters were present in 7% of the cycles;

(2) A single sperm defect was present in 15% of the cycles;

(3) A double sperm defect was present in 29% of the cycles; and

(4) Oligoasthenoteratozoospermia was present in 49% of the cycles (Table 1).

The preparation of the ejaculated sperm for ICSI involved the following steps:

(1) Removal of the seminal fluid by washing with medium, by centrifugation at $1800 \times g$ for 5 min and removal of the supernatant;

(2) A passage through two or three layers of a discontinuous Percoll gradient; and

(3) A final centrifugation step just prior to microinjection[24].

Epididymal sperm was usually recovered by microsurgery from the most proximal part of the caput of the epididymis. During the microsurgical epididymal sperm aspiration, several sperm fractions were collected into separate tubes. Sperm fractions with similar concentration and motility were pooled and then treated in the same way as ejaculated semen. Whenever possible, a part of the freshly recovered sperm was frozen for later use to avoid surgery in subsequent cycles[12,13,25,26]. After thawing, epididymal sperm were put on a discontinuous Percoll gradient and thereafter treated as ejaculated semen.

Testicular spermatozoa were isolated from a testicular biopsy specimen. The testicular biopsy tissue was transferred into a Petri dish with HEPES-buffered Earle's medium and shredded into small pieces with sterile microscope slides on the heated stage of a stereomicroscope. The presence of spermatozoa was assessed on the inverted microscope. The pieces of the biopsy tissue were removed and the medium was centrifuged at $300 \times g$ for 5 min. The pellet was then resuspended for the intracytoplasmic sperm injection procedure[14,15,26,27].

Intracytoplasmic sperm injection procedure

The details of microtool preparation and microinjection procedure have been described in detail[9,10]. Holding and injection pipettes were made from washed borosilicate glass capillary tubes which were first pulled on a horizontal microelectrode puller and then with the help of a microgrinder and microforge a sharp opening was made at the end of the injection pipette. The injection pipette had a 5–6 μm inner and 7–8 μm outer diameter, respectively. Both needles were bent to an angle of about 40°.

The injection dish contained eight droplets of 5 μl HEPES-buffered Earle's medium surrounding a central droplet of medium with 10% polyvinylpyrrolidone and 1 μl of the resuspended sperm droplet. The intracytoplasmic sperm injection procedure was carried out on the heated stage of an inverted microscope at × 400 magnification using the Hoffman Modulation Contrast system. The holding and injection pipettes were fixed into a tool holder and were connected to a micrometer-type microinjector. The movement of the pipettes was coordinated by two coarse positioning manipulators and with two three-dimensional hydraulic remote-control micromanipulators.

A single, living, immobilized spermatozoon was aspirated tail first into the injection pipette. The oocyte was fixed on the holding pipette in such a way that the polar body was situated at the 6 o'clock position while the injection pipette was pushed through the zona pellucida at the 3 o'clock position and into the cytoplasm, where the sperm was delivered together with the smallest possible amount of medium.

After injection, the oocytes were washed and stored in 25 μl microdrops of B_2 medium in a Petri dish and stored at 37°C in an incubator containing 5% CO_2, 5% O_2 and 90% N_2.

Oocyte damage and fertilization after intracytoplasmic sperm injection

Oocytes were inspected for intactness and fertilization 16–18 h after microinjection[27]. The number and aspect of polar bodies and pronuclei were recorded. Oocytes were considered to be normally fertilized when two individualized or fragmented polar bodies were present together with two clearly visible pronuclei. In these 2820 cycles, ICSI was carried out on 29 415 metaphase II oocytes, i.e. a mean of 10.4 oocytes per cycle. The number of intact oocytes after ICSI was 26 228, i.e. 89.2% of the injected oocytes. The mean number of successfully injected oocytes was 9.3 per treatment cycle. The num-

ber of normally fertilized oocytes was 18 364, i.e. 70% of the successfully injected oocytes, 62.4% of the injected metaphase II oocytes and 50.4% of the retrieved cumulus–oocyte complexes. The number of abnormally fertilized oocytes was 991 one-pronuclear oocytes (3.8% of the intact oocytes) and 1194 three-pronuclear oocytes (4.6% of the intact oocytes). One-pronuclear oocytes were reassessed for their pronuclear status a few hours after the initial observation. In contrast to our standard IVF program, no change in pronuclear status was observed at the time of the second microscopic observation[28]. If these abnormally fertilized oocytes cleave, they are not transferred. This parthenogenetic activation may be due to mechanical or chemical factors. It may come as a surprise to observe three-pronuclear oocytes after the injection of only one spermatozoon into the ooplasm. We carefully observed the polar bodies at the time of fertilization and it is obvious that the three pronuclei were mostly due to non-extrusion of the second polar body at the time of fertilization.

Table 2 summarizes the damage and normal fertilization rates after ICSI for the three types of sperm used to carry out ICSI. The percentage of intact oocytes was 89 or 90% and the normal fertilization rate varied from 58 to 71% of the intact oocytes. The percentage of normally fertilized oocytes was significantly higher with ejaculated semen than with fresh or frozen-thawed epididymal sperm or testicular sperm.

The exceptional circumstances in which none of the injected oocytes were normally fertilized occurred when:

(1) Only one metaphase II oocyte was available for ICSI;

Table 2 Sperm origin and normal fertilization after ICSI

	Ejaculated	Epididymal	Testicular
Cycles	2572	128	120
Oocytes injected	26343	1628	1444
Intact after ICSI (%)	89	90	89
Intact two-pronuclear oocytes (%)	71*	58*	60*

*; $p = 0.0001$ by χ^2 contingency table

Table 3 Sperm origin and embryo development after ICSI

	Ejaculated	Epididymal	Testicular
Two-pronuclear embryos	16 758	844	767
Transferable embryos (%)	74*	67*	71*
Embryos transferred or frozen (%)	65	63	68

*; $p = 0.0001$ by χ^2 contingency table

Table 4 Sperm origin and embryo quality after ICSI

	Ejaculated (%)	Epididymal (%)	Testicular (%)
Type-A embryos (0% fragmentation)	8	7	9
Type-B embryos (1–20% fragmentation)	53	46	49
Type-C embryos (20–50% fragmentation)	13	14	13

(2) Only totally immotile spermatozoa were available for the injection;

(3) Gross abnormalities were present in the oocytes;

(4) Round-headed spermatozoa were injected; and

(5) When all oocytes were damaged by the injection procedure.

Some of these patients achieved fertilization in a subsequent cycle.

Embryo development and replacements after intracytoplasmic sperm injection

The embryo cleavage of the two-pronuclear oocytes was evaluated after a further 24 h of *in vitro* culture. The cleaving embryos were scored according to the equality of size of the blastomeres and the number of anucleate fragments. These embryos were classified into three categories according to the percentage of anucleate fragments:

(1) Excellent type-A embryos (without anucleate fragments);

(2) Good-quality type-B embryos (between 1 and 20% of the volume filled with anucleate fragments); and

(3) Fair-quality type-C embryos (between 21 and 50% anucleate fragments).

Cleaved embryos with less than half of their volume filled with anucleate fragments were eligible for transfer. Up to two, three or, exceptionally, four embryos were loaded with a few microliters of Earle's medium into a Frydman catheter and transferred into the uterine cavity. Embryo replacement was usually performed about 48 h after the microinjection procedure. If supernumerary embryos with less than 20% anucleate fragments were available, they were cryopreserved on day 2 or day 3 after oocyte retrieval using the slow-freezing protocol with dimethylsulfoxide[29,30].

The total number of embryos of sufficient quality to be transferred, i.e. those with less than 50% anucleate fragments, was 13 479, i.e. 73.4% of the two-pronuclear oocytes, 51.4% of the successfully injected oocytes, 45.8% of the injected metaphase II oocytes and 37.0% of the retrieved cumulus–oocyte complexes.

The percentages of two-pronuclear oocytes which developed to transferable embryos and which were actually transferred or frozen when ICSI was carried out with ejaculated, epididymal and testicular spermatozoa are summarized in Table 3.

Table 4 shows that there was no difference in the distribution of excellent-quality type-A embryos, good-quality type-B embryos and fair-

Table 5 ICSI and number of embryos transferred in relation to the ejaculated sperm parameters

| Sperm parameters | Cycles | Transfers n % | | Number of embryos | | | | | | | |
| | | n | % | 1 | | 2 | | 3 | | > 3 | |
				n	%	n	%	n	%	n	%
Normal	175	162	93	18	11	45	28	87	54	12	7
One anomaly	377	350	93	22	6	115	33	192	55	21	6
Two anomalies	731	685	94	52	8	236	35	360	53	37	5
Three anomalies	1241	1139	92	105	9	405	36	575	51	54	5

Table 6 Sperm origin and embryo transfer after ICSI

	Ejaculated	Epididymal	Testicular
Cycles	2572	128	120
Transfers (%)	2382 (93)	117 (91)	108 (90)
Pregnancies/transfers (%)	21/204 (10)	1/7 (14)	2/14 (14)
1 embryo	78/321 (24)	3/15 (20)	4/13 (32)
2 embryos	218/488 (45)	3/14 (21)	3/12 (25)
2 embryos (elective)	253/694 (36)	17/37 (46)	10/12 (48)
3 embryos	254/544 (47)	17/24 (71)	11/20 (55)
3 embryos (elective)	47/131 (36)	9/20 (45)	13/28 (46)
> 3 embryos			
Total	871/2382 (37)	50/117 (43)	43/108 (40)
Pregnancies/cycle (%)	34	39	36

quality type-C embryos when ICSI was carried out with ejaculated, epididymal or testicular spermatozoa.

The total number of embryos which were actually transferred or frozen (less than 20% anucleate fragments) was 11 983, i.e.. 65.3% of the two-pronuclear oocytes, 45.7% of the successfully injected oocytes, 40.7% of the injected metaphase II oocytes and 32.9% of the retrieved cumulus–oocyte complexes.

An embryo replacement was possible in 2608 of the 2820 treatment cycles (92.6%). This is a high transfer rate for couples with previous fertilization failure in standard IVF, with ejaculated sperm too poor to be included in IVF or with obstructive or non-obstructive azoospermia. As indicated in Table 5, the percentage of transfers was similar in the four groups of ejaculated semen parameters; the transfer rate varied from 92 to 94% of the cycles. The distribution of transfers with one, two, three or more than three embryos was also similar in the four groups of semen parameters. Except for some patients older than 40, the number of embryos replaced was limited to a maximum of two or three embryos[31].

The number of patients with positive serum hCG was 964, i.e. a 36.9% pregnancy rate per transfer and 34.2% per started cycle. As indicated in Table 6, the pregnancy rates were similar for ICSI with ejaculated, epididymal and testicular sperm. The pregnancy rate was especially high when an elective transfer of two or three embryos could be carried out.

The main features of these 2853 cycles planned for intracytoplasmic sperm injection are summarized in Table 7. ICSI could not be carried out in only 1% of the started cycles. Of the 29 415 injected metaphase II oocytes, 11% were damaged during the ICSI procedure. Of the intact oocytes, 70% became normally fertilized after injection with ejaculated, epididymal

Table 7 Summary of intracytoplasmic sperm injection treatment cycles

	n	%
Cycles with ICSI/started cycles	2820/2853	99
Metaphase II oocytes injected	29 415	
Intact oocytes	26 228	89
Two-pronuclear oocytes	18 364	70
Embryos transferred	6744 ⎱	65
Embryos frozen	5239 ⎰	
Transfers	2608	91
Pregnancies	964	34% per cycle

or testicular spermatozoa. Of the normally fertilized oocytes, 65% developed into embryos which were either transferred or frozen in view of eventual later use. A replacement of fresh embryos was possible in 91% of the started cycles and a positive serum hCG was observed in 34% of the cycles.

Prenatal diagnosis and follow-up of children

Because of the novelty and the many unknown aspects of ICSI, the couples were asked after extensive counselling to adhere to the follow-up conditions, which include genetic counselling, agreement to prenatal testing and participation in a prospective clinical follow-up study of the children[16–18].

As of 1 March 1995, the number of positive serum hCG after ICSI embryos were replaced was 1160, including 64 pregnancies after replacement of frozen-thawed embryos. After chorionic villus sampling or amniocenteses, 491 fetal karyotypes were obtained. The sex ratio was close to the expected 50/50 distribution. There were six abnormal karyotypes, two cases of 47,XXY, and one of each of the following 47,XXX, 47,XYY, 46,XX/47,XXX and 47,XY + 21. Two pregnancies were interrupted at 12 and 14 weeks of gestation. Three intrauterine deaths occurred at around 38 weeks of gestation with no apparent reason. So far, 669 children have been born. The 18 major congenital malformations are listed in Table 8; this corresponds to a malformation rate of 2.7%, a percentage not different from the percentages

Table 8 Major malformations in 699 children born after ICSI, in whom 18 major congenital malformations (2.7%) were detected

Singleton pregnancies (seven children)
Cleft lip and palate and duplication of pyelum of kidney
Hypospadias with unilateral cryptorchidism
Malformation of left hip and left leg
Preaxial polydactyly of toes
Pseudo-arthrogryposis and Pierre–Robin sequence
Cleft lip and palate and malformation of foot and hand
Hypotrophy of left ventricle

Twin pregnancies (ten children in nine pregnancies)
Two children with cleft palate
Tetralogy of Fallot
Femur–fibula–ulna syndrome
Two children with hypospadias
Hernia diafragmatica
Down syndrome
Situs inversus
Spina bifida and hydrocephaly

Triplet pregnancy (one child)
Holoprosencephaly, two other children are well

of abnormalities observed after natural conception or after standard IVF treatment. Eleven of these 18 malformations occurred in multiple pregnancies: ten in twin pregnancies and one in a triplet pregnancy.

Although there is no indication of an increase in major congenital malformations after replacement of embryos obtained after ICSI, it is important to continue this careful prospective follow-up study of the children in different centers practising ICSI. This is one of the goals of the 'Task Force on ICSI' established by the

European Society of Human Reproduction and Embryology (ESHRE).

Acknowledgements

The authors are indebted to their many colleagues of the Centre for Reproductive Medicine and the Center for Medical Genetics. Special thanks to Geertrui Bocken, An Vankelecom, Heidi Van Ranst, Bart Desmet and Nadine Franceus of the microinjection team. Research nurses Marleen Magnus, Andrea Buysse and Pascale Dekoninck for collecting the data on pregnancy and pediatric follow-up, Viviane De Wolf for typesetting the manuscript and Michael Whitburn of the Language Education Center for correcting the manuscript. This work is supported by grants from the Belgian Fund for Medical Research and from Organon International.

References

1. Tournaye, H., Devroey, P., Camus, M., Staessen, C., Bollen, N., Smitz, J. and Van Steirteghem, A. C. (1992). Comparison of *in-vitro* fertilization in male and tubal infertility: a 3-year survey. *Hum. Reprod.*, **7**, 218–22

2. Cohen, J., Alikani, M., Adler, A., Berkely, A., Davis, O., Ferrara, T. A., Graf, M., Grifo, J., Liu, H. C., Malter, H. E., Reing, A. M., Suzman, M., Talansky, B. E., Trowbridge, J. and Rosenwaks, Z. (1992). Microsurgical fertilization procedures: the absence of stringent criteria for patient selection. *J. Assist. Reprod. Genet.*, **9**, 197–206

3. Fishel, S., Timson, J., Lisi, F. and Rinaldi, L. (1992). Evaluation of 225 patients undergoing subzonal insemination for the procurement of fertilization *in vitro*. *Fertil. Steril.*, **57**, 840–9

4. Ng, S. C., Bongso, A. and Ratnam, S. S. (1991). Microinjection of human oocytes: a technique for severe oligoasthenoteratozoospermia. *Fertil. Steril.*, **56**, 1117–23

5. Palermo, G., Joris, H., Devroey, P. and Van Steirteghem, A. C. (1992). Pregnancies after intracytoplasmic injection of single spermatozoon into an oocyte. *Lancet*, **340**, 17–18

6. Iritani, A. (1991). Micromanipulation of gametes for *in vitro* assisted fertilization. *Mol. Reprod. Develop.*, **28**, 199–207

7. Kimura, Y. and Yanagimachi, R. (1995). Intracytoplasmic sperm injection in the mouse. *Biol. Reprod.*, **52**, 709–20

8. Palermo, G., Joris, H., Derde, M.-P., Camus, M., Devroey, P. and Van Steirteghem, A. C. (1993). Sperm characteristics and outcome of human assisted fertilization by subzonal insemination and intracytoplasmic sperm injection. *Fertil. Steril.*, **59**, 826–35

9. Van Steirteghem, A. C., Liu, J., Joris, H., Nagy, Z., Janssenswillen, C., Tournaye, H., Derde, M.-P., Van Assche, E. and Devroey, P. (1993). Higher success rate by intracytoplasmic sperm injection than by subzonal insemination. Report of a second series of 300 consecutive treatment cycles. *Hum. Reprod.*, **8**, 1055–60

10. Van Steirteghem, A. C., Nagy, Z., Joris, H., Liu, J., Staessen, C., Smitz, J., Wisanto, A. and Devroey, P. (1993). High fertilization and implantation rates after intracytoplasmic sperm injection. *Hum. Reprod.*, **8**, 1061–6

11. Van Steirteghem, A. C., Liu, J., Nagy, Z., Joris, H., Tournaye, H., Liebaers, I. and Devroey, P. (1993). Use of assisted fertilization. *Hum. Reprod.*, **8**, 1784–5

12. Silber, S. J., Nagy, Z. P., Liu, J., Godoy, H., Devroey, P. and Van Steirteghem, A. C. (1994). Conventional *in-vitro* fertilization versus intracytoplasmic sperm injection for patients requiring microsurgical sperm aspiration. *Hum. Reprod.*, **9**, 1705–9

13. Tournaye, H., Devroey, P., Liu, J., Nagy, Z., Lissens, W. and Van Steirteghem, A. C. (1994). Microsurgical epididymal sperm aspiration and intracytoplasmic sperm injection: a new effective approach to infertility as a result of congenital bilateral absence of the vas deferens. *Fertil. Steril.*, **61**, 1045–51

14. Devroey, P., Liu, J., Nagy, Z., Torunaye, H., Silber, S. J. and Van Steirteghem, A. C. (1994). Normal fertilization of human oocytes after testicular sperm extraction and intracytoplasmic sperm injection. *Fertil. Steril.*, **62**, 639–41

15. Silber, S. J., Van Steirteghem, A. C., Liu, J., Nagy, Z., Tournaye, H. and Devroey, P. (1995). High fertilization and pregnancy rate after intracytoplasmic sperm injection with spermatozoa obtained from testicle biopsy. *Hum. Reprod.*, **10**, 148–52

16. Bonduelle, M., Desmyttere, S., Buysse, A., Van Assche, E., Schiettecatte, J., Devroey, P., Van Steirteghem, A. and Liebaers, I. (1994). Prospective follow-up study of 55 children born after subzonal insemination and intracytoplasmic sperm injection. *Hum. Reprod.*, **9**, 1765–9

17. Wisanto, A., Magnus, M., Bonduelle, M., Liu, J., Camus, M., Tournaye, H., Liebaers, I., Van Steirteghem, A. C. and Devroey, P. (1995). Obstetric outcome of 424 pregnancies after intracytoplasmic sperm injection (ICSI). *Hum. Reprod.*, in press

18. Bonduelle, M., Legein, J., Derde, M. P., Buysse, A., Schiettecatte, J., Wisanto, A., Devroey, P., Van Steirteghem, A. and Liebaers, I. (1995). Comparative follow-up study of 130 children born after ICSI and 130 children born after IVF. *Hum. Reprod.*, in press

19. Smitz, J., Devroey, P., Camus, M., Deschacht, J., Khan, I., Staessen, C., Van Waesberghe, L., Wisanto, A. and Van Steirteghem, A. C. (1988). The luteal phase and early pregnancy after combined GnRH-agonist/hMG treatment for superovulation in IVF or GIFT. *Hum. Reprod.*, **3**, 585–90

20. Smitz, J., Devroey, P., Faguer, B., Bourgain, C., Camus, M. and Van Steirteghem, A. C. (1992). A prospective randomized comparison of intramuscular or intravaginal progesterone as a luteal phase and early pregnancy supplement. *Hum. Reprod.*, **7**, 168–75

21. Smitz, J., Bourgain, C., Van Waesberghe, L., Camus, M., Devroey, P. and Van Steirteghem, A. C. (1993). A prospective randomized study on oestradiol valerate supplementation in addition to intravaginal micronized progesterone in buserelin and hMG induced superovulation. *Hum. Reprod.*, **8**, 40–45

22. World Health Organization (1992). *WHO Laboratory Manual for the Examination of Human Semen and Sperm Cervical Mucus Interaction*. (Cambridge: Cambridge University Press)

23. Kruger, T. F., Menkveld, R., Stander, F. S. H., Lombard, C. J., Van der Merwe, J. P., van Zyl, J. A. and Smith, K. (1986). Sperm morphologic features as a prognostic factor in *in vitro* fertilization. *Fertil. Steril.*, **46**, 1118–23

24. Liu, J., Nagy, Z., Joris, H., Tournaye, H., Devroey, P. and Van Steirteghem, A. C. (1994). Intracytoplasmic sperm injection does not require special treatment of the spermatozoa. *Hum. Reprod.*, **9**, 1127–30

25. Devroey, P., Silber, S. J., Nagy, Z., Liu, J., Tournaye, H., Joris, H., Verheyen, G. and Van Steirteghem, A. C. (1995). Ongoing pregnancies and birth after intracytoplasmic sperm injection with frozen-thawed epididymal spermatozoa. *Hum. Reprod.*, **10**, 903–6

26. Nagy, Z., Liu, J., Janssenswillen, C., Silber, S., Devroey, P. and Van Steirteghem, A. C. (1995). Using ejaculated, fresh and frozen-thawed epididymal and testicular spermatozoa gives rise to comparable results after intracytoplasmic sperm injection. *Fertil. Steril.*, **63**, 808–15

27. Nagy, Z. P., Liu, J., Joris, H., Devroey, P. and Van Steirteghem, A. (1994). Time-course of oocyte activation, pronucleus formation and cleavage in human oocytes fertilized by intracytoplasmic sperm injection. *Hum. Reprod.*, **9**, 1743–8

28. Staessen, C., Janssenswillen, C., Devroey, P. and Van Steirteghem, A. C. (1993). Cytogenetic and morphological observations of single pronucleated human oocytes after *in-vitro* fertilization. *Hum. Reprod.*, **8**, 221–3

29. Van Steirteghem, A. C., Van der Elst, J., Van den Abbeel, E., Joris, H., Camus, M. and Devroey, P. (1994). Cryopreservation of supernumerary multicellular human embryos obtained after intracytoplasmic sperm injection. *Fertil. Steril.*, **62**, 775–80

30. Van der Elst, J., Camus, M., Van den Abbeel., E, Maes., R, Devroey, P. and Van Steirteghem, A. C. (1995). Prospective randomized study on the cryopreservation of human embryos with dimethylsulfoxide of 1,2-propanediol protocols. *Fertil. Steril.*, **63**, 92–100

31. Staessen, C., Janssenswillen, C., Van den Abbeel, E., Devroey, P. and Van Steirteghem, A. C. (1993). Avoidance of triplet pregnancies by elective transfer of two good quality embryos. *Hum. Reprod.*, **8**, 1650–3

Microfertilization techniques: choice of correct indications

56

L. Hamberger, A. Sjögren and K. Lundin

Introduction

During the last 5 years of clinical applications, more invasive techniques for fertilization have been applied, such as zona drilling, partial zonal dissection, subzonal sperm injection and, more successful than the others, intracytoplasmic sperm injection[1,2]. Techniques that promote hatching have also been utilized, either in isolation or combined with intracytoplasmic sperm injection. Assisted hatching can be carried out either mechanically or enzymatically[3]. This could also mean a difference in risk, since acid Tyrode solution, which is generally used for enzymatically induced assisted hatching, may be teratogenic. Moreover, when these microsurgical fertilization techniques are applied, the zona pellucida no longer has the same protective role as *in vivo* or in conventional *in vitro* fertilization (IVF). This fact increases the demand for culture media of high purity (pharmaceutical grade) with reference to DNA content and the presence of endotoxins or other potential teratogenic agents. At present, both intracytoplasmic sperm injection and assisted hatching are undertaken under culture conditions which, generally, do not differ from those applied in conventional IVF. Until these problems have been solved and until more knowledge is gathered concerning the potentially greater risks with the new techniques, it seems advisable to apply the techniques only in situations where conventional IVF cannot be used, or has very low success rates. We here report our own policy in the different situations.

Intracytoplasmic sperm injection in the next cycle following failed IVF

During the last 2 years in our IVF program, we have developed the policy of performing conventional IVF and intracytoplasmic sperm injection in a 1/1 proportion after one trial with a poor fertilization rate (< 15%), in routine IVF or when sperm parameters are below our criteria for standard IVF (< 0.5 million progressive motile sperm after preparation). In 2/3 of the cases with poor or no fertilization in the first routine IVF cycle, the following cycle showed good fertilization and pregnancy rates with conventional IVF (see Table 1), while in 1/3 of the cases the poor outcome persisted. This means that the majority of cases in this group do not need to be shifted to intracytoplasmic sperm injection. It is our impression, however, that many centers switch all of these patients to intracytoplasmic sperm injection provided they have

Table 1 Outcome of combined *in vitro* fertilization (IVF) and intracytoplasmic sperm injection (ICSI) due to suspected sperm and/or oocyte factors

	IVF failed (n = 23)		IVF poor (n = 42)	
	IVF	ICSI	IVF	ICSI
No. of oocytes	186	212	344	413
Fertilization rate (%)	0	58	51	70
No. of replacements	0	23	11*	21*
No. of pregnancies	0	7	3	5
Pregnancy rate (%)	0	30	27	24
Implantation rate (%)	0	19	12	10

*All embryos were frozen in eight patients because of threatened ovarian hyperstimulation syndrome

Table 2 Intracytoplasmic sperm injection of oocytes with various degree of maturity following controlled ovarian stimulation. Time between follicular aspiration and injection varied between 4 and 6 h

	GV	Metaphase I	Metaphase II	Uncertain maturity
No. of oocytes	77	101	2089	207
%	3	4	84	8
No. of fertilized 2PN	8/77	31/101	1379/2089	113/207
%	10	31	66	54
Cleavage rate	7/8	31/31	1301/1379	105/113
%	88	100	94	93

GV, germinal vesicles; PN, pronuclear

this technique, or 2–3 routine IVF trials are often made prior to referral to an IVF unit with the possibility of performing intracytoplasmic sperm injection.

Intracytoplasmic sperm injection on 1-day-old unfertilized oocytes after conventional IVF

In certain cases of unexplained infertility, the sperm in the ejaculate may have a qualitative disorder and fail to fertilize the oocytes. In such cases, intracytoplasmic sperm injection may be tried on the following day. We recently reported two such pregnancies[4]. Even if both the children were healthy with normal karyotypes and no malformations, we have become hesitant to continue this practice other than for diagnostic purposes, since it has been claimed that a principal increased genetic risk may prevail in these somewhat postmature oocytes. It is also possible that a 2 pronuclear phase can be overlooked and that, in fact, a polyspermic embryo will be obtained with this practice.

Immature oocytes

In gonadotropin-stimulated cycles, a proportion of the retrieved oocytes are not in the metaphase II stage at the time of oocyte collection. However, the majority of metaphase I oocytes and also a high proportion of oocytes with germinal vesicles (50%) will undergo full maturation *in vitro* within 24 h (unpublished observa-

tions). In conventional IVF, fertilization is most likely to be somewhat delayed in these immature oocytes. With intracytoplasmic sperm injection, it is possible to fertilize at least the metaphase I oocytes without delay but at a lower fertilization rate (Table 2). It has not been evaluated whether such a procedure has any advantages or may, on the contrary, involve increased risks.

Anti-sperm antibodies

Six to eight per cent of all men produce antibodies against their own spermatozoa. These antibodies are mainly of the IgG and/or IgA type and can be directed against the head, midpiece or tail of the spermatozoa. Dependent on the position and the concentration of the anti-sperm antibodies, various degrees of agglutination and immobilization can occur. In the past, men with anti-sperm antibodies were often refused treatment with IVF because of expected low chances for success. However, recently published results from our IVF program demonstrate that high success rates can be achieved with conventional IVF in this group of patients, but that intracytoplasmic sperm injection needs to be applied in some of the more serious cases[5]. In the first gonadotropin-stimulated cycle, we always try to perform IVF and intracytoplasmic sperm injection on a 1/1 ratio in these couples. If good fertilization and cleavage rates are obtained with IVF, intracytoplasmic sperm injection is not utilized in the following cycle.

Intracytoplasmic sperm injection or IVF in association with microepididymal sperm aspiration and testicular sperm extraction

In the past, a few pregnancies have been reported in which microepididymal sperm aspiration was combined with either an IVF or a gamete intrafallopian transfer (GIFT) procedure[6,7]. However, in a majority of these cases, only a small number of spermatozoa can be found, thereby making intracytoplasmic sperm injection the most effective option. Furthermore, if a high percentage of the spermatozoa lack or have low motility, and if abnormal forms are frequent, intracytoplasmic sperm injection improves the chance of choosing the spermatozoa and this can be one reason for the higher fertilization rate. So far, 67 such cycles (45 couples) have been studied in our IVF program. A satisfactory ongoing clinical pregnancy rate (38%) was achieved in this group, in fact, slightly higher than in the total intracytoplasmic sperm injection program (31%). It seems wise, therefore, to use intracytoplasmic sperm injection exclusively in these patients, since, even if abundant spermatozoa can occasionally be aspirated from the epididymis, the remaining material can be frozen and utilized in a later cycle. When using testicular spermatozoa, which are often not motile at all, the intracytoplasmic sperm injection technique is, of course, an absolute necessity.

IVF or intracytoplasmic sperm injection in connection with preimplantation genetic diagnosis

In the first cases of preimplantation genetic diagnosis, the oocytes were fertilized by conventional IVF[8]. As pointed out by us and others, the risk is obvious for contamination by sperm caught in the zona pellucida and not clearly visible in the microscope, especially when the polymerase chain reaction (PCR) is performed. This, of course, is particularly deleterious in connection with sexing. It thus seems reasonable to recommend only intracytoplasmic

sperm injection in combination with preimplantation genetic diagnosis.

Intracytoplasmic sperm injection in combination with assisted hatching

The intracytoplasmic sperm injection procedure can in itself be regarded as a form of assisted hatching. However, the injection needles used are of such a small size that they are probably insufficient, in most cases, to create a permanent opening. Thus, the same indications for assisted hatching may remain as for conventional IVF. A recent communication at the *World Congress on IVF and Alternate Assisted Reproduction*[9], supported the view that a combination of intracytoplasmic sperm injection and assisted hatching leads to a higher clinical pregnancy rate (28.8% vs. 18.5% in the control group). However, larger randomized comparisons are needed before a general recommendation can be made concerning this combination of microsurgical techniques.

Conclusions

As is evident from the short summary of indications above, both intracytoplasmic sperm injection and IVF can be used in parallel in a number of situations where the outcome is most likely to be similar. It has been claimed by a few enthusiasts that intracytoplasmic sperm injection should perhaps always be used instead of standard IVF, although the majority of centers are more cautious at present. The main reason for their caution, naturally, is their concern for adverse effects introduced by the new techniques. As mentioned in the introduction, the use of more pure and well-defined media and culture conditions can be one way of avoiding such increased risks. It cannot be excluded that, for some sperm factors (e.g. anti-sperm antibodies), an intact zona pellucida can constitute an important 'natural' barrier. On the other hand, it must be stressed that the statistical evaluations presented to date (ESHRE) have not indicated any increased risk for chromosomal aberrations or malformations when intracytoplasmic sperm injection is applied. In our present experience of intracytoplasmic sperm injection, 100 deliveries with 122 children have been carefully examined. Only one major malformation (aortic valve stenosis) has, so far, been found, where the child did not need any surgical correction. In conclusion, it seems likely that conventional IVF in stimulated cycles will remain the technique of choice for the majority of infertile couples.

References

1. Palermo, G., Joris, H., Devroey, P. and Van Steirteghem, A. C. (1992). Pregnancies after intracytoplasmatic injection of single spermatozoon into an oocyte. *Lancet*, **340**, 17–18
2. Van Steirteghem, A. C., Nagy, Z., Joris, H., Staessen, C., Smitz, J., Wisanto, A. and Devroey, P. (1993). High fertilization and implantation rates after intracytoplasmic sperm injection. *Hum. Reprod.*, **8**, 1061–6
3. Cohen, J., Elsner, C., Kort, H., Malter, H., Massey, J., Pat Mayer, M. and Wiemer, K. (1990). Impairment of the hatching process following IVF in the human and improvement of implantation by assisting hatching using micromanipulation. *Hum. Reprod.*, **5**, 7–13
4. Sjögren, A., Lundin, K. and Hamberger, L. (1995). Intracytoplasmic sperm injection of 1-day old oocytes after fertilization failure. *Hum. Reprod.*, 974
5. Lundin, K. and Hamberger, L. (1995). Antisperm antibodies and assisted reproduction. *Assist. Reprod. Rev.*, in press
6. Temple-Smith, P. D., Southwick, G. J., Yates, C. A., Trounson, A. O. and de Kretser, D. M. (1985). Human pregnancy by IVF using sperm aspirated from the epididymis. *J. In Vitro Fertil. Embryo Transfer*, **2**, 119–22
7. Sibler, S., Balmaceda, J., Borrero, C., Ord, T. and Asch, R. (1988). Pregnancy with sperm aspiration from the proximal head of the epididymis: a new treatment for congenital absence of the vas deferens. *Fertil. Steril.*, **50**, 525–8
8. Handyside, A. H., Kontogianni, E H., Hardy, K. and Winston, R. M. L. (1990). Pregnancies from biopsied human preimplantation embryos sexed by Y-specific DNA amplification. *Nature (London)*, **344**, 768–70
9. Jun, J. H., Lee, H. J., Kim, J. W., Park, Y. S., Lee, Y. S., Hong, J. Y., Son, I. P. and Jun, J. Y. (1995). Fertilization and pregnancy rate of ICSI and ICSI with AHA procedure. Presented at the *World Congress on IVF and Alternate Assisted Reproduction*, April, Vienna, abstr. *J. Assist. Reprod.*, **12**, 240

Follow-up of children born after intracytoplasmic sperm injection

57

I. Liebaers, M. Bonduelle, J. Legein, A. Wilikens, E. Van Assche, A. Buysse, A. Wisanto, P. Devroey and A. C. Van Steirteghem

Introduction

A number of mainly retrospective follow-up studies of children born after _in vitro_ fertilization and embryo transfer (IVF–ET) or other assisted reproductive technologies (ART) have been published and are ongoing[1–11]. The results showed that, compared to data obtained from population-based studies, no increased risk for congenital malformations was observed[12–15]. In 1992, IVF after intracytoplasmic sperm injection (ICSI) was described as a novel approach to alleviate severe male infertility[16–19]. Within the frame of our prospective study of children born after different methods of assisted reproduction started in 1983, data on prenatal karyotypes and on congenital malformations in children born after subzonal insemination (SUZI) and ICSI were and are being compiled[20,21]. This contribution reports on 491 prenatal karyotypes and 460 children born mostly after ICSI with ejaculated sperm[16–19] or with sperm retrieved from the epididymis or the testes[22–25].

Materials and methods

Before starting the appropriate assisted reproductive treatment, couples are asked to participate in the follow-up study, including prenatal diagnosis and genetic counselling[20,21]. The couples are seen at the Center for Medical Genetics before starting the treatment if the woman is over 35 years of age, if after karyotyping one of the parents is a carrier of a chromosomal aberration, if the family history is positive for a possible genetic disease or if the man has congenital bilateral absence of the vas deferens.

All other couples are seen by a geneticist when the woman is 7–8 weeks pregnant after ICSI. The possible indication for prenatal diagnosis in relation to this novel ICSI procedure is again discussed, stressing the risk of possible miscarriage. If agreed upon, an appointment for chorionic villus sampling (in most cases of twin pregnancy) or an amniocentesis (in most cases of singleton pregnancies) is scheduled. The child follow-up study is discussed during the same session and parents are asked to visit the pediatrician-geneticist with their baby at birth or at 2 months of age and subsequently at 1 and 2 years of age. If impossible (for example, if the family is living abroad), data on the child will be obtained from the parents, the gynecologist and the pediatrician.

By the end of February 1995, 1160 pregnancies, including 64 after transfer of frozen–thawed embryos, were established after SUZI or ICSI with ejaculated sperm[16–19] or sperm retrieved from the epididymis[22,23] or the testes[24,25]. From these pregnancies, 491 prenatal karyotypes were performed. Not all pregnancies progressed, a number were not yet at term for prenatal diagnosis and, finally, only 73% of the patients agreed to have a prenatal test. From the 1160 pregnancies, 669 children have been born at the time of writing. Data on congenital malformations from all of these were recorded, based on reports by the referring gynecologist and pediatrician and our own observations. On 460 of these children, additional information on the frequency of singletons, twins and triplets, on the sex ratio, on their weight, length and head circumference was processed. Our definition of major malformation is those malformations that generally cause functional impairment or require surgical correction.

Results

Of the 491 prenatal karyotypes, 479 (97.6%) were normal 46,XX or 46,XY. Six (1.2%) were benign structural aberrations such as inversions or translocations inherited from the father. Another six (1.2%) were abnormal: 47,XXY ($n = 2$: one after transfer of fresh embryos and one after transfer of frozen–thawed embryos), 47,XXX ($n = 1$), 47,XYY ($n = 1$), 46,XX/ 47,XXX ($n = 1$) and 47,XY + 21 ($n = 1$).

Two of the 1160 pregnancies were terminated and one twin pregnancy was selectively reduced because of malformations seen on ultrasound examination. They were, respectively, a gastroschisis and body stalk anomaly in one fetus and a hygroma colli in the second fetus, both seen at 12 weeks of gestation. One of the twins presented with an encephalocele at 14 weeks of gestation. Five pregnancies ended between 26 and 40 weeks of gestation with an intrauterine death. Three of these showed normal pathology, while in one twin pregnancy a placental problem was observed, and the fetus who died at 26 weeks presented with major growth retardation.

From the first 460 children, 250 (54.5%) were singletons, 198 (43%) were twins and 12 (2.5%) were triplets. The sex ratio was 241 boys to 219 girls, which is 1.1. The mean birth weight was 2.803 kg with a range from 0.610 to 4.500 kg. The mean length was 47.5 cm and the mean head circumference was 32.3 cm. Among the total of 669 children born at the time of writing, 18 (2.7%) presented with a major malformation (Table 1). Seven of these children were from singleton pregnancies, ten were from twin pregnancies and one from a triplet pregnancy.

Discussion

The major contribution of this paper is to give a report on the number and the type of chromo-

Table 1 List of major malformations (18/669) or 2.7% in children born after ICSI

Singleton pregnancies (seven children)
Cleft lip and palate and duplication of pyelum of kidney
Hypospadias with unilateral cryptorchidism
Malformation of left hip and left leg
Preaxial polydactyly of toes
Pseudo-arthrogryposis and Pierre–Robin sequence
Cleft lip and palate and malformation of foot and hand
Hypotrophy of left ventricle

Twin pregnancies (ten children in nine pregnancies)
Two children with cleft palate
Tetralogy of Fallot
Femur–fibula–ulna syndrome
Two children with hypospadias
Hernia diafragmatica
Down syndrome
Situs inversus
Spina bifida and hydrocephaly

Triplet pregnancy (one child)
Holoprosencephaly, two other children are well

somal aberrations observed prenatally in pregnancies established after SUZI and mostly after ICSI as well as the number and type of congenital malformations in the children born after this novel procedure.

Most (97.6%) of the prenatal karyotypes were normal 46,XX or 46,XY. The six (1.2%) paternally transmitted structural aberrations were most probably related to the fertility problem of these men, but were not related to the ICSI procedure itself. The remaining six (1.2%), from which five of the six were sex chromosome anomalies, may be related to the procedure since the population incidence of these aneuploidies is normally less than 0.3–0.4%[26] and even less when compared to data in the literature concerning results in large series of results of prenatal diagnoses[27–30].

An incidence of 2.7% major malformations is comparable to the figures of other studies after ART[1–11] or in population registries[12–15]. A still small comparative study between the outcome of children born after IVF or ICSI does not show any increase in malformations after ICSI[21]. Some of the observed malformations are quite common in general, such as cleft palates and lips or neural tube defects; others are more rare. Certainly, no particular type of malformation seems to occur in this still small number of children.

To confirm these observations which are encouraging and reassuring, continuing efforts should be made by all centers involved to evaluate their own short-term results and to contribute to the efforts made at different levels (national and international) to collect as many data as possible, in order to increase the numbers and enable the medical and scientific community to accept the technique as a safe routine procedure as far as major malformations and chromosomal aberrations are concerned.

Moreover, short- and long-term follow-up studies have to be started or continued with

regard to the risk of transmitting infertility. Certainly, new possibilities to gain more insight into fertility regulating genes[31,32] are emerging at the molecular level, and, before they are fully understood, patients should be told about this possible risk.

Acknowledgements

The authors thank all their colleagues from the Center of Medical Genetics and Center for Reproductive Medicine. Special thanks go to Marleen Magnus, Pascale DeConinck and Johan Schiettecatte for collecting and processing the data and to Jolanda Heulaerts for typing the manuscript. This work is supported by grants from the Belgian Fund for Medical Research and from Organon.

References

1. Australian in-vitro fertilization collaborative group (1988). In-vitro fertilization pregnancies in Australia and New Zealand. *Med. J. Aust.*, **148**, 429–36

2. Medical Research International, Society for Assisted Reproductive Technology (SART) and The American Fertility Society (1992). *In vitro* fertilization–embryo transfer (IVF–ET) in the United States: 1990 results from the IVF–EF Registry. *Fertil. Steril.*, **57**, 15–24

3. Morin, N. C., Wirth, F. H., Johnson, D. H., Frank, L. M., Presburg, H. J., Van de Water, V. L., Chee, E. M. and Mils, J. L. (1989). Congenital malformations and psychosocial development in children conceived by *in vitro* fertilization. *J. Pediatr.*, **115**, 222–7

4. National Perinatal Statistics Unit and The Fertility Society of Australia (1988). *IVF and GIFT pregnancies, Australia and New Zealand, 1987.* Sydney National Perinatal Statistics Unit (NPSU)

5. Rufat, P., Oliviennes, F. *et al.* (1994). Task force report on the outcome of pregnancies and children conceived by *in vitro* fertilization (France: 1987 to 1989). *Fertil. Steril.*, **61**, 324–30

6. Ron-El, R., Lahat, E., Golan, A. *et al.* (1994). Development of children born after ovarian superovulation induced by long-acting gonadotrophin-releasing hormone agonist and meno-

tropins, and by *in vitro* fertilization. *J. Pediatr.*, **125**, 734–7

7. Cohen, J., Mayaux, M. J. and Guihard-Moscato, L. (1988). Pregnancy outcomes after *in vitro* fertilization. A collaborative study on 2342 pregnancies. *Ann. N. Y. Acad. Sci.*, **541**, 1–6

8. Beral, V. and Doyle, P. (1990). Report of the MRC Working Party on Children Conceived by In Vitro Fertilization. Births in Great Britain resulting from assisted conception, 1978–1987. *Br. Med. J.*, **300**, 1229–33

9. Rizk, B., Doyle, P., Tan, S. L., Rainsbury, P., Betts, J., Brinsden, P. and Edwards, R. G. (1991). Perinatal outcome and congenital malformations in in-vitro fertilization babies from the Bourn–Hallam group. *Hum. Reprod.*, **6**, 1259–64

10. Andrews, M. C., Muasher, S. J., Levy, D. L. *et al.* (1986). An analysis of the obstetric outcome of 125 consecutive pregnancies conceived *in vitro* and resulting in 100 deliveries. *Am. J. Obstet. Gynecol.*, **154**, 848–54

11. Yovich, L. J., Parry, T. S., French, N. P. and Grauaug, A. A. (1986). Developmental assessment of twenty *in vitro* fertilization (IVF) infants at their first birthday. *J. In Vitro Fertil. Embryo Transfer*, **3**, 253–7

12. Marden, P. M., Smith, D. W. and McDonald, M. J. (1964). Congenital anomalies in the new-

born infant including minor variations. A study of 4412 babies by surface examination for anomalies and buccal smear for sex chromatin. *J. Pediatr.*, **64**, 357–71

13. Leppig, K. A., Werler, M. M. *et al.* (1987). Predictive value of minor anomalies association with major anomalies. *J. Pediatr.*, **110**, 531–7

14. Liverpool Congenital Malformations Registry from Rizk *et al.*, 1991, reference 9

15. Congenital Malformation Notification Scheme of the Office of Population Censuses and Surveys (OPCS) of England and Wales (1985) from Rizk *et al.* (1991), reference 9

16. Palermo, G., Camus, M., Joris, H., Derde, M.-P., Devroey, P. and Van Steirteghem, A. (1993). Sperm characteristics and outcome of human assisted fertilization by subzonal insemination and intracytoplasmic sperm injection. *Fertil. Steril.*, **59**, 826–35

17. Van Steirteghem, A. C., Liu, J., Joris, H., Nagy, Z., Janssenswillen, C., Tournaye, H., Derde, M.-P., Van Assche, E. and Devroey, P. (1993). Higher success rate by intracytoplasmic sperm injection than by subzonal insemination. Report of a second series of 300 consecutive treatment cycles. *Hum. Reprod.*, **8**, 1055–60

18. Van Steirteghem, A. C., Nagy, Z., Joris, H., Liu, J., Staessen, C., Smitz, J., Wisanto, A. and Devroey, P. (1993). High fertilization and implantation rates after intracytoplasmic sperm injection. *Hum. Reprod.*, **8**, 1061–6

19. Van Steirteghem, A., Nagy, Z., Liu, J., Joris, H., Janssenswillen, C., Tournaye, H., Smitz, J., Bonduelle, M. and Devroey, P. (1993). Intracytoplasmic sperm injection. *Assisted Reprod. Rev.*, **3**, 160–3

20. Bonduelle, M., Desmyttere, S., Buysse, A. *et al.* (1994). Prospective follow-up study of 55 children born after subzonal insemination and intracytoplasmic sperm injection. *Hum. Reprod.*, **9**, 1765–9

21. Bonduelle, M., Legein, J., Buysse, A., Devroey, P., Van Steirteghem, A. and Liebaers, I. (1994). Comparative follow-up study of 130 children born after ICSI and 130 children born after IVF. *Hum. Reprod.*, **9** (Suppl. 4), 38

22. Silber, S. J., Nagy, Z. P., Liu, J., Godoy, H., Devroey, P. and Van Steirteghem, A. C. (1994). Conventional in-vitro fertilization versus intracytoplasmic sperm injection for patients requiring microsurgical sperm aspiration. *Hum. Reprod.*, **9**, 1705–9

23. Tournaye, H., Devroey, P., Liu, J., Nagy, Z., Lissens, W. and Van Steirteghem, A. C. (1994). Microsurgical epididymal sperm aspiration and intracytoplasmic sperm injection: a new effective approach to infertility as a result of congenital bilateral absence of the vas deferens. *Fertil. Steril.*, **61**, 1045–51

24. Devroey, P., Liu, J., Nagy, Z., Tournaye, H., Silber, S. J. and Van Steirteghem, A. C. (1994). Normal fertilization of human oocytes after testicular sperm extraction and intracytoplasmic sperm injection. *Fertil. Steril.*, **62**, 639–41

25. Silber, S. J., Van Steirteghem, A. C., Liu, J., Nagy, Z., Tournaye, H. and Devroey, P. (1995). High fertilization and pregnancy rate after intracytoplasmic sperm injection with spermatozoa obtained from testicle biopsy. *Hum. Reprod.*, **10**, 148–52

26. Jacobs, P. A., Broune, C., Gregson, N., Joyce, C. and White, H. (1992). Estimates of the frequency of chromosome anomalies detectable using moderate levels of banding. *J. Med. Genet.*, **29**, 103–8

27. Ammala, P., Hiilesmaa, V., Liukkonen, S., Saista, T., Teramo, K. and von Koskull, H. (1993). Randomized trial comparing first-trimester transcervical chorionic villus sampling and second-trimester amniocentesis. *Prenat. Diagn.*, **13**, 919–27

28. Ledbetter, D., Zachary, J., Simpson, J., Golbus, M., Pergament, E., Jackson, L., Mahoney, M., Desnick, R., Schulman, J., Copeland, K., Verlinsky, Y., Yang-Feng, T., Schonberg, S., Babu, A., Tharapel, A., Dorfmann, A., Lubs, H., Rhoads, G., Fowler, S. and de la Cruz, F. (1992). Cytogenetic results from the US collaborative study on CVS. *Prenat. Diagn.*, **12**, 317–45

29. Lippman, A., Tomkins, D., Shime, J. and Hamerton, J. (1992). Canadian multicentre randomized clinical trial of chorion villus sampling and amniocentesis. *Prenat. Diagn.*, **12**, 385–476

30. Palo, P., Piiroinen, O., Honkonen, E., Lakkala, T. and Aula, P. (1994). Transabdominal chorionic villus sampling and amniocentesis for prenatal diagnosis: 5 years' experience at a university centre. *Prenat. Diagn.*, **14**, 157–62

31. Vest, P., Chandley, A. C., Hargreave, T. B., Keil, R., Ma, K. and Sharbey, A. (1992). Micro deletions in interval 6 of the Y chromosome of males with idiopathic sterility points to disruption of AZF, a human spermatogenesis gene. *Hum. Genet.*, **89**, 491–6

32. Chandley, A. C. and Cooke, H. J. (1994). Human male infertility-Y-linked genes and spermatogenesis. *Hum. Mol. Genet.*, **3**, 1449–52

Culture and co-culture techniques

58

Y. Menezo, M. Dumont, A. Hazout, B. Nicollet, J. L. Pouly and L. Janny

Introduction

In the culture of embryos of most mammalian species, the embryo is submitted *in vitro* to developmental arrests, most frequently at the time of genomic activation. Moreover, embryo metabolism is obviously depressed in simple culture media[1], even that enriched with serum. In order to overcome this cell block and to improve (or at least maintain) embryo viability, several co-culture assays have been developed. In farm animals, this is especially important, as embryo transfer cannot be performed before the morula/blastocyst stage, when the embryo is normally (chronologically) in the uterus. The human is a special model, as very early embryos can be transferred into the uterus. To explain the failures, it is considered that a motility effect is in some cases associated with the effect of uterine hostility.

Co-culture experiments have been developed first with trophoblastic cells[2] and then with oviduct cells[3]. In non-human primates, successful attempts were realized by using uterine epithelial cells[4,5]. In the human, attempts to culture oviduct cells were successful, as for other species[6], and the first co-cultures on oviduct epithelial cells were achieved by Bongso and associates[7]. In all cases for the same developmental stage, co-cultured embryos have higher numbers of cells and a full cohesive inner cell mass, when compared to embryos cultured, even for shorter times, in simple liquid media.

Co-culture with fibroblasts leads to loss of viability[3], and has not been found to overcome the cell block. Most human embryos in *in vitro* fertilization (IVF) are also submitted to developmental arrest[8]. However, blastocysts can be obtained[9] in simple culture media containing serum, but their quality is not optimum with regards to the pregnancy rates obtained with these embryos. It can be postulated that the so-called 'embryotropic factors' are neither hormone-dependent nor tissue-specific, but rather dependent on the transport epithelium. This was confirmed by the use of kidney cell lines[10,11]. In all cases, the incidence and the quality of blastocyst formation is highly dependent on the co-culture medium[12]. This explains the discrepancies observed between experiments, especially in overcoming the cell block.

Preliminary results concerning the regulation of blastocyst formation and some clinical data on IVF programs with Vero cells are presented here.

Setting up of co-cultures

In most experiments with cells, the cells suddenly loose their vigor after several generations *in vitro*. For mammalian oviduct cells, this degeneration process starts after 5–15 sub-passages[6]. The cells exhibit unusual morphology, with vacuoles. At the end, they usually become bi-nucleated, with no further multiplication. The use of this type of non-established cell line leads to the setting up of primary cultures, generally obtained from organs collected from abattoirs and is associated with much work in controlling the safety of the cells. Cells derived from these cultures are often contaminated with adventitious agents, and must be discarded.

The Vero cell line has become a standard tool in biology. The cells come from the WHO library: reference Vero, 6758, at passage 134, with the label 'Non hazardous to Human' (Public Health Laboratory Service, European Collection of Animal Cell Culture, Salisbury, UK).

These cells are not tumorigenic before passage 162[13], there are no extraneous viruses, and uniform cell lots can be securely produced using large-scale cultivation.

All the protocol for our own experiment has already been described[10,14,15]. It is necessary to organize the cell culture system very carefully. From the frozen cells, flasks are set up. When the seeding is 2–3 millions cells, confluence is reached within 4 days (6–8 million cells per flask). After trypsinization of the flask, the cells are split into three portions: one to seed a new flask, one to be frozen, and the remaining to seed wells at 100 000 cells per well. Confluence is reached in wells within 3 days. Cells must not be repeatedly passed from flasks: we observed that after four sub-passages, the growth was slower. It is better to freeze these cells and to take cells previously frozen to seed another flask. For cell freezing and thawing, see reference 6. The cells are controlled after four sub-passages for *Chlamydia* (BioMérieux Kit 5532/1) and for *Mycoplasma* (BioMérieux Kit 4240/2) as an internal standard of laboratory quality. We never trypsinize our cells more than seven times; we do not use them after passage 142, to stay far below the putative limit of tumorigenicity.

The co-culture medium is the B2 medium[16] France: CCD/rue P. Charron, Paris; USA: Fertility Technologies; Canada: Pharmasciences), largely used for human and zootechnical purposes in biotechnologies related to IVF.

The wells seeded for co-culture on a Friday are used for all the following week. Whatever the day they are used, the wells are rinsed only once: 1 h before the cells are used, the medium is removed and replaced with new medium. Each patient has their own plates, whatever the number of embryos co-cultured, to avoid any mistake or possible cross-contamination. The embryos are set in co-culture either on day 1 at the time of rinse, or at the pronuclear stage (delayed transfer at the blastocyst stage). In our experience, freezing at the blastocyst stage gives better and more reliable results; the supernumerary embryos to be frozen after transfer at early stages can be put on co-culture at day 2, at the 2–4-cell stage. In both cases, it is not neces-

sary to change the medium during this co-culture period. In a first approach we used to change the medium once, 2 days after the beginning of co-culture. Our last experience with no medium renewal does not support this necessity. After use, all the plates are discarded: wells must never be re-used for different patients.

The blastocyst formation in our control without cells has always been low, never reaching 20% of true blastocysts. With the use of Vero cells, the overall blastocyst formation rate was 48–60%. In smaller experiments, Hazout and Dumont (1991, unpublished) gave the same type of results with MDBK cells as were observed with Vero cells, with high pregnancy rates after transfer. This type of result is similar with bovine or human oviduct epithelial cells[7,17]. There is no difference in blastocyst formation when the embryos are co-cultured with or without serum.

Factors affecting blastocyst formation

Maternal effect

In two different IVF centers, blastocyst formation was controlled in patients submitted to long or ultrashort analog treatments. The blastocyst formation (56 vs. 61%) was the same with long (> 30 days) and ultrashort (7–8 days) treat-

Table 1 The effect of maternal age on blastocyst formation

	Maternal age (years)			
	< 30	30–35	35–40	> 40
Patients (*n*)	62	107	89	31
Embryos, day 2 (*n*)	555	774	518	156
Blastocysts (*n*)	254	267	169	49
(%)	46	35	33	31

Table 2 The effect of sperm quality on blastocyst formation

	Normal sperm	Impaired sperm
Patients (*n*)	144	95
Embryos, day 2 (*n*)	1387	560
Blastocysts (*n*)	621	194
(%)	45	35

ment with gonadotropin releasing hormone (GnRH).

We found a strong maternal effect in relation to the age of the patient. Age did not impair the fertilization rate, but it impaired the blastocyst formation and the blastocyst expansion rates (Table 1). Women over 40 years showed a significant reduction ($p < 0.001$).

Paternal effect

In IVF programs, we compared blastocyst formation in patients with frozen donor sperm and other patients with normal or impaired sperm. Blastocyst formation was impaired in patients with very low quality sperm as well as with frozen sperm[18] (Table 2). The difference was significant ($p < 0.001$).

Clinical aspects

Transfer at the blastocyst stage after repeated failure of embryo transfer

A group of 183 patients with repeated failures of embryo transfer ($n > 4$), with their agreement, were systematically transferred, at day 5, at the blastocyst stage, if this stage was obtained in co-culture. Blocked embryos were not transferred. The age of these patients was below 40, and all had a normal hysteroscopy and no known ovarian dysfunction. All had already produced embryos in their previous IVF attempts.

In this small experimental protocol, 172/183 obtained at least one blastocyst and were trans-

ferred (94%). The mean number of embryos transferred was 2.6. Seventy-two patients became pregnant with a total of 112 implantations. The overall pregnancy rate per transfer was 42%. The yield per embryo obtained was 112/447 (25%). Whatever the indication, the implantation rate per blastocyst was close to 20%.

Prevention of multiple pregnancies

Transfers at the blastocyst stage should lessen the likelihood of multiple pregnancies (rank > 3) by replacing only two blastocysts, without impairing the pregnancy rates (Table 3).

Freezing co-cultured blastocysts

For freezing at the blastocyst stage, we reached a final concentration of 10% glycerol in two steps[19]. The cooling protocol was: room temperature to $-7°C$ at $-1°C$ per min, followed by seeding induction with cold forceps; then cooling to $-37°C$ at a rate of $-0.3°C$ per min, followed by immediate cooling at $-196°C$.

The embryos were first of all thawed quickly at room temperature in air. Then followed six steps, with decreasing concentrations of glycerol. Before transfer, the embryos recovered for 3 h in B2 medium + serum.

With this protocol, out of 467 cycles, 428 had embryo replacement (91%). A total of 870/1051 (83%) embryos recovered from the freezing and thawing process; 89 patients became pregnant (21% per transfer; ongoing 81,

Table 3 Pregnancy results of transferring two or three embryos at the early or blastocyst stage

	Embryos transferred at early stage		Embryos transferred at blastocyst stage	
	Two	Three	Two	Three
Transfers (n)	191	311	236	245
Embryo implantation (n)	54	129	100	123
(% of embryos transferred)	14.1	13.8	21.2	16.7
Ongoing pregnancy (n)	46	94	79	87
(% of transfers)	24.1	30.2	33.5	35.5
Twin pregnancies (n)	8	27	21	20
(% of pregnancies)	17.4	28.7	26.6	23.0
Triplet pregnancies (n)	—	4	—	8
(% of pregnancies)		4.2		9.2

19%); 111 embryos implanted. The overall implantation rate was 13% per embryo. The comparison between stimulated cycles, natural cycles and artificial cycles showed a clear tendency in favor of the artificial (substitution) cycles. In preliminary experiments, we found a pregnancy per transfer rate of 6/47 (13%) in the natural cycle group, 27/257 (11%) in the stimulated group and 56/214 (26%) in the substituted group ($p < 0.05$ between natural cycles and substitution cycles).

Discussion

According to these preliminary experiments, blastocyst formation does not strictly depend upon the cell support used for co-culture. The success is mainly related to transport epithelia. In our experiment, serum addition is not necessary. This seems logical, as otherwise culture in complex media with high levels of serum should be an answer to these developmental problems *in vitro*, and this is not the case. Moreover, as observed[20], complex mixtures of growth factors are generally poorly efficient. The specificity rather than the quantity is more important. If we can conclude that the stimulation regimen does not influence blastocyst formation, a maternal effect is more than probable, as for some patients, this process seems impossible. However, this should be confirmed for these patients, by changes in the maturation protocols.

As suggested by our results with frozen sperm and severely impaired semen obtained in IVF, a paternal effect drives blastocyst formation. It seems to be an 'all or nothing' law, as the number of patients with blastocysts is severely lowered, but the yield per successful patient is the same. It is clear that severe morphological defects in sperm should interfere with early embryonic development. One should consider at least DNA packaging, centrosome and centriole duplication and formation of the first spindle. The centriole is brought by the spermatozoon: a defect of this organelle will severely impair the formation of the first spindle, and in consequence, the quality of the first division.

Alteration of sperm (that can occur by breaks of DNA strands, through the formation of uric acid) may impair early embryonic development, especially if the degraded area corresponds to an important coding region.

Transfer at the blastocyst stage could improve the IVF results by two different means: (1) a selection process, as suggested by the implantation rates per embryo in the pregnant women. This selection process is mainly related to cytogenetic problems. In our experience, 40–50% of the embryos arrested in co-culture have chromosomal anomalies; (2) a lower sensitivity of the genital tract to manipulation at day 5 (due to the higher level of progesterone at this time?), diminishing the expulsion of embryos. Freezing these blastocysts is feasible, with good yields, as more than 2/3 of the embryos recover after freezing and thawing.

Mechanism of action of the feeders

Removal of toxic compounds from the culture medium (heavy metal divalent cations and metabolic inhibitors) and/or a contribution of embryotropic regulating compounds, such as lipids (this is less credible) and growth factors are the more probable methods of action. However, the embryo is submitted to metabolic blocks[21,22]. One positive effect of the co-culture could be to provide metabolites downstream of the block, avoiding any delay in the embryonic development: a misfit can occur at the time of genomic activation. Due to the turnover of the maternal mRNA and proteins, if a delay occurs, the cleaving machinery stops before enough new molecules are neosynthesized. This is also more than probable in humans[8]. This positive effect should be strengthened by the contribution of growth factors at the time when the *ad hoc* receptors are present[23]. The overall beneficial effect of the co-culture technique should be demonstrated, whatever the cell support, with a double-blind randomized study, taking the results obtained with freezing into account. It is not clear that progress can be assessed for all the indications, but the final goals are:

(1) A selection of the best embryos;

(2) A better synchronization of embryo development and the surrounding environment;

(3) A reduction of the number of embryos transferred, to avoid multiple pregnancies (of > 3); and

(4) A provision of biopsies for genetic diagnosis.

It is clear that this technology is temporary: progress in culture and culture media technology should lead in the near future to an avoidance of the use of cells.

Acknowledgements

Annick Carneiro, Nathalie Cassara, Veronique Durhone and Karin Hermannsonn are acknowledged for their skilful technical assistance.

References

1. Jung, T. (1989). Protein synthesis and degradation in non-cultured and *in vitro* cultured rabbit blastocysts. *J. Reprod. Fertil.*, **86**, 507–12

2. Camous, S., Heyman, Y., Meziou, W. and Ménézo, Y. (1984). Cleavage beyond the block stage and survival after transfer of early embryos cultured with trophoblastic vesicles. *J. Reprod. Fertil.*, **72**, 479–85

3. Gandolfi, F. and Moor, R. M. (1987). Stimulation of early embryonic development in the sheep by co-culture with oviduct epithelial cells. *J. Reprod. Fertil.*, **81**, 23–8

4. Goodeaux, L. L., Voelkel, S. A., Anzalone, C. A., Ménézo, Y. and Graves, K. H. (1989). The effect of rhesus epithelial cell monolayers on *in vitro* growth of rhesus embryos. *Theriogenology*, **39**, 197

5. Goodeaux, L. L., Thibodeaux, J. K., Voelkel, S. A., Anzalone, C. A., Roussel, J. D., Cohen, J. C. and Ménézo, Y. (1990). Collection, co-culture and transfer of Rhesus preimplantation embryos. *ARTA*, **1**, 370–9

6. Ouhibi, N., Ménézo, Y., Benet, G. and Nicollet, B. (1989). Culture of epithelial cells derived from the oviduct of different species. *Hum. Reprod.*, **4**, 229–35

7. Bongso, A., Ng, S. C., Sathanathan, H., Ng, P. L., Rauff, M. and Ratnam, S. S. (1989). Improved quality of human embryos when co-cultured with human ampullary cells. *Hum. Reprod.*, **4**, 706–13

8. Hardy, K., Winston, R. M. L. and Handyside, A. H. (1993). Binucleate blastomeres in preimplantation human embryos *in vitro*: failures of cytokinesis during early cleavage. *J. Reprod. Fertil.*, **98**, 349–58

9. Bolton, V. N., Wren, M. E. and Parsons, J. H. (1991). Pregnancies after *in vitro* fertilization and transfer of human blastocysts. *Fertil. Steril.*, **55**, 830–2

10. Ménézo, Y., Guérin, J. F. and Czyba, J. C. (1990). Improvement of human early embryo development *in vitro* by coculture on monolayers of Vero cells. *Biol. Reprod.*, **42**, 301–6

11. Ouhibi, N., Hamidi, J., Guillaud, J. and Ménézo, Y. (1990). Coculture of 1-cell mouse embryos on different cell supports. *Hum. Reprod.*, **5**, 537–43

12. Xu, K. P., Yadav, B. R., Rorie, R. W., Plante, L., Betteridge, K. J. and King, W. A. (1992). Development and viability of bovine embryo derived from oocytes matured and fertilized *in vitro* and co-cultured with bovine epithelial cells. *J. Reprod. Fertil.*, **94**, 33

13. Levenbook, I. S., Petricianni, J. C. and Elisberg, B. L. (1984). Tumorigenicity of Vero cells. *J. Biol. Standard*, **12**, 391

14. Ménézo, Y., Janny, L. and Khatchadourian, C. (1994). Embryo quality and coculture. In Mastroianni, L., Coelingh Bennink, H. J. T., Suzuki, S. and Vemer, H. M. (eds.). *Gamete and Embryo Quality*, pp. 139–55. (Carnforth, UK: Parthenon Publishing)

15. Ménézo, Y. (1994). Laboratory aspects of embryo co-cultures. *50th American Fertility Society Meeting*, San Antonio

16. Ménézo, Y., Testart, J. and Perronne, D. (1984). Serum is not necessary in human *in vitro* fertilization, early embryo culture, and transfer. *Fertil. Steril.*, **42**, 750–5

17. Wiemer, K. E., Hoffman, D. I., Maxson, W. S., Eager, S., Muhlberger, B., Fiore, I. and Cuervo, M. (1993). Embryonic morphology and rate of implantation of human embryos following coculture on bovine oviductal epithelial cells. *Hum. Reprod.*, **8**, 97

18. Janny, L. and Ménézo, Y. (1994). Evidence for a strong paternal effect on blastocyst formation in human. *Mol. Reprod. Dev.*, **38**, 36–42

19. Ménézo, Y., Nicollet, B., Herbaut, N. and André, D. (1992). Freezing cocultured human blastocysts. *Fertil. Steril.*, **58**, 977–81

20. Russer-Long, J. A., Dickey, J. F., Richardson, M. E. and Ivey, K. W. (1991). Culture of ovine embryos in the absence of bovine serum albumin. *Theriogenology*, **35**, 383–91

21. Schini, S. A. and Bavister, B. D. (1988). Two cell block to development of cultured hamster embryos is caused by phosphate and glucose. *Biol. Reprod.*, **39**, 1183–92

22. Ménézo, Y. and Khatchadourian, C. (1990). Involvement of glucose 6 phosphate isomerase (EC 5319) in the mouse embryo 2-cell block *in vitro*. *C.R. Acad. Sci.*, **310**, 297–301

23. Werb, Z. (1991). Expression of EGF and TGF-alpha genes in early mammalian development. *Mol. Reprod. Dev.*, **27**, 10–15

Embryo freezing in humans: an overview

59

J. Mandelbaum

Introduction

Mammalian embryos have been successfully frozen and stored since 1972 when Whittingham and colleagues[1] obtained live mice after the transfer of freeze–thawed morulae[1]. In humans, the first birth from a frozen embryo occurred in 1984 in Australia[2] and this cryotechnology, derived from rodent and cattle routines, became a necessary part of *in vitro* fertilization programs owing to the optimization and simplification of the biological procedures[3]. Ten years later, we must ask what is the contribution of human embryo cryopreservation to assisted reproduction? Moreover, are improvements and/or new developments still possible or even necessary?

Are there new trends in human embryo freezing technology?

Cryoprotectants and technical parameters

It is now well documented that human embryos can be successfully cryopreserved by protocols using 1,2-propanediol (PROH)[3], dimethylsulfoxide (DMSO)[1] or glycerol[4]. Each of these cryoprotectants gives an optimal efficacy when used at a particular embryo developmental stage: PROH for zygotes or early cleaved embryos; DMSO for cleaved stages; and glycerol for blastocysts, depending on the permeability of blastomere membranes.

The protocol using PROH (1.5 mol/l) and sucrose (0.1 mol/l) was reported to be quite successful when embryos were slow-cooled (0.3°C/min) to −30°C and was especially suitable for pronucleated and 2- or 3-day-old embryos at the time of IVF transfer[5,6,7]. This protocol was, therefore, the most widely employed throughout the world, despite it still remaining difficult to determine which method produces the best results. A recent randomized study by Van der Elst and co-workers[8] on 2220 multicellular supernumerary embryos reported a higher chance of survival and implantation after cryopreservation when DMSO had been used. So, at present, one may conclude that it is possible to use either DMSO or PROH as a cryoprotectant from the pronucleate to the eight-cell stage, except for blastocysts which should, by common consent, be exposed to glycerol[4,9,10]. Attempts to try new molecules (polymers, antifreeze proteins) have just emerged in humans[11].

The efficiency of the ice-seeding technique is also of major importance[12] and may be impaired in some freezers with automatic seeding, thus leading to a failure of the whole freezing program. A serum supplementation to the medium is usual in preparing freezing and thawing solutions. The serum source varies (human fetal, individual autologous or pooled maternal samples, fetal calf serum or human serum albumin fraction) but has the disadvantage, especially for pooled and cord sera, of an incomplete security toward virus transmission. Substitutes are also used but there are no studies on the necessity and comparative efficiency of these compounds.

Slow or fast cooling

Some papers[13,14] have confirmed the report by Trounson and Sjoblom[13] that human embryos might survive a simple ultrarapid procedure where, after a brief exposure to DMSO and sucrose at high concentrations, embryos are directly plunged into liquid nitrogen, thus avoiding the need for programable freezers. However, in fact, ultrarapid freezing has not produced the same performances as slow procedures and has not been widely developed; and neither has vitrification, despite many animal reports[15].

Storage time

Supernumerary embryos are cryopreserved with the aim of optimizing the chances of every couple entering an IVF procedure obtaining one birth or more from each oocyte recovery, even after long periods of storage. However, we need to ask whether this extended storage affects the outcome of thawing cycles. In an earlier study, we have observed no impairment in the viability of surviving transferred embryos[16], despite a light but significant decrease in survival rates after the 4th year of storage, but on a rather small series of 977 embryos. Recent papers have come to the same conclusions on embryo viability and even survival[17,18]. Human embryos can, therefore, afford at least 5 years of cryopreservation.

From zygote to blastocyst: what is the best embryo to freeze?

A matter of developmental stage?

From the available data, it does not seem that developmental stage is a key factor in freezing ability of embryos. Pronucleated eggs can be successfully frozen using PROH and sucrose and give similar results to early cleaved embryos (2 or 3 days old, from two to eight cells), with implantation rates per thawed embryo reaching 6.3 and 6%, respectively, according to published data[16]. Precise timing appears to be important for optimal zygote freezing in order to avoid the risks of cooling a single cell with spindle structures or during DNA synthesis[19] – the best time should be 20–22 h after insemination. There are

few reports of advantages to using zygote cryopreservation[20] and these are the counterbalancing of time constraints and the inability to allow the selection of embryos for the fresh transfer on developmental criteria. Nevertheless, zygote freezing is applied routinely in many IVF centers, especially in Germany, for ethical reasons.

A new controversy has emerged recently about whether to freeze embryos at early or late developmental stages, such as blastocysts[10]. Blastocyst cryopreservation, despite initial good results[4], was forsaken because of suboptimal culture conditions which led to a poor ability for human embryos to be cultured *in vitro* to these late stages[9]. Co-culture on feeder cells drastically improved this ability with 50–60% of cultured embryos developing into blastocysts. After freezing and thawing, embryos such as these were able to implant at high rates (8.8–18%)[10,21]. Nevertheless, there are no conclusive data showing a significant improvement in the results when comparing blastocyst and multicellular embryo freezing and, furthermore, co-culture is time-consuming. Another option could be to combine, on day 2 postinsemination, fresh embryo transfer and cryopreservation of good embryos while co-culturing the poorest ones. Those poor embryos able to develop to the blastocyst stage of day 5 or 6 could, therefore, be 'rescued' and frozen, thus optimizing the chances for each patient.

A matter of aspect?

For zygotes, selection on morphological grounds is not a problem and survival is easy to assess on this single cell and its ability to further cleave. For blastocysts, all studies have demonstrated that good expanded blastocysts have the best cryopreservability[4,9,10], although survival prospects are not so easy to appraise, except upon the re-expansion of the collapsed blastocelic cavity in culture.

For early cleaved embryos, parameters affecting their ability to survive cryopreservation and implant are well documented and are essentially represented by their morphologic aspect before freezing[22] as we confirmed on a series of 598 transfers of single freeze–thawed embryos[16]. Indeed, good embryos survived in 80% of cases as compared to 66% for those presenting cytoplasmic fragments ($\leq 40\%$) or unequally sized blastomeres ($p < 0.001$). However, the birth rate per singly surviving and transferred embryo did not differ significantly between the good embryos (5.8%) and the others (4.6%).

Other embryonic parameters have no effect on freezing ability. These parameters include (1) the age of cleaved embryos (day 2 or 3), (2) the number of cells before freezing, (3) the stimulation regimen of the recovery cycle (whether comprising gonadotropin-releasing hormone (GnRH) analogs or not)[12], and (4) the size of the oocyte cohort from which they were issued[23]. Even micromanipulated embryos have the same potential as intact ones to afford the freeze–thaw process[24]. However, the survival rate – i.e. percentage of initial blastomeres surviving at thawing – is essential, and below 50% of intact blastomeres the reported pregnancies are exceptional. In routine programs, and in large series, thawed embryos survive in 70% of the cases, allowing almost 90% of patients attempting embryo thawing to have a transfer, and leading to a birth rate of 10–15% among different groups throughout the world[16,24–26].

What is the contribution of embryo freezing to IVF programs?

The major aim of embryo cryopreservation was to provide further possibilities for conception in addition to those obtained through the initial cycle and fresh transfer. This goal was achieved with an increase in birth rate of 8% for the women who had embryos cryopreserved and by 5% for the overall program[16,23,25–27]. Embryo freezing has also contributed to lowering the risks of severe ovarian hyperstimulation by cancelling the fresh transfer[28] and to simplifying oocyte donation[29]. In the latter case, embryo freezing could become, as in France, an obligatory step to limit the risks of viral transmission. In well-trained centers, cryopreservation could also offer the possibility for transporting embryos for pre-implantation diagnosis which, presently, is performed on fresh embryos only.

The ultimate objective: the babies

A recent report of a study in mice on the long-term effects of embryo freezing confirmed that this procedure did not induce major anomalies, even in senescence, but could be responsible for small differences, such as a 15% increase in body weight in males at senescence, depending on genotype, sex or age[30]. This study highlighted the importance of large surveys on the condition of human babies conceived by the use of cryopreserved embryos. Until now, comparative analysis with pregnancies issued from fresh embryo transfers have not found any differences, particularly in respect to the rate of congenital anomalies[16,31,32].

Embryo freezing in humans is definitely a well-established procedure. Improvements will be difficult even though 20–30% of cryopreserved embryos do not survive thawing. Perhaps improvements may arise from cryotechnology (new molecules, new procedures) or from better strategies in embryo culture and selection. If new freezing procedures can emerge, they will rather be derived from the search for an optimal way to cryopreserve the oocyte.

References

1. Whittingham, D. G., Leibo, S. P. and Mazur, P. (1972). Survival of mouse embryos frozen to −196°C and −269°C. *Science*, **178**, 411–14
2. Trounson, A. and Mohr, L. (1983). Human pregnancy following cryopreservation, thawing and transfer of an eight-cell embryo. *Nature (London)*, **305**, 707–9
3. Lassalle, B., Testart, J. and Renard, J. P. (1985). Human embryo features that influence the

success of cryopreservation with the use of 1,2-propanediol. *Fertil. Steril.*, **44**, 645–51

4. Cohen, J., Simons, R. F., Edwards, R. G., Fehilly, C. B. and Fishel, S. B. (1985). Pregnancies following the frozen storage of expanding human blastocysts. *J. In Vitro Fertil. Embryo Transfer.*, **2**, 59–64

5. Testart, J., Lassalle, B., Belaisch-Allart, J., Hazout, A., Forman, R., Rainhorn, J. D. and Frydman, R. (1986). High pregnancy rate after early human embryo freezing. *Fertil. Steril.*, **46**, 268–72

6. Mandelbaum, J., Junca, A. M., Plachot, M., Alnot, M. O., Salat-Baroux, J., Alvarez, S., Tibi, C., Cohen, J., Debache, C. and Tesquier, L. (1988). Cryopreservation of human embryos and oocytes. *Hum. Reprod.*, **3**, 117–19

7. Van der Auwera, I., Meuleman, C. and Koninckx, P. R. (1994). Human menopausal gonadotrophin increases pregnancy rate in comparison with clomiphene citrate during replacement cycles of frozen/thawed pronucleate ova. *Hum. Reprod.*, **8**, 2068–74

8. Van der Elst, J., Camus, M., Van den Abbeel, E., Maes, R., Devroey, P. and Van Steirteghem, A. C. (1995). Prospective randomized study on the cryopreservation of human embryos with dimethylsulfoxide or 1,2-propanediol protocols. *Fertil. Steril.*, **63**, 92–100

9. Hartshorne, G. M., Elder, K., Crow, J., Dyson, H. and Edwards, R. G. (1991). The influence of *in vitro* development upon post-thaw survival and implantation of cryopreserved human blastocysts. *Hum. Reprod.*, **6**, 136–41

10. Menezo, Y., Nicollet, B., Herbaut, N. and Andre, D. (1992). Freezing cocultured human blastocysts. *Fertil. Steril.*, **58**, 977–80

11. Dumoulin, J., Bergers-Janssen, J. M., Pieters, M., Enginsu, M., Geraedts, J. and Evers, J. (1994). The protective effects of polymers in the cryopreservation of human and mouse zonae pellucidae and embryos. *Fertil. Steril.*, **62**, 793–8

12. Mandelbaum, J. (1990). Human embryo cryopreservation. *Contracept. Fertil. Sex.*, **18**, 341–53

13. Trounson, A. and Sjoblom, P. (1988). Cleavage and development of human embryos *in vitro*, after ultrarapid freezing and thawing. *Fertil. Steril.*, **2**, 373–6

14. Feichtinger, N., Hochfellner, C. and Ferstl, U. (1991). Clinical experience with ultra-rapid freezing of embryos. *Hum. Reprod.*, **6**, 735–6

15. Ali, J. and Shelton, J. N. (1993). Vitrification of preimplantation stages of mouse embryos. *J. Reprod. Fertil.*, **98**, 459–65

16. Mandelbaum, J., Plachot, M., Junca, A. M., Alvarez, S., Alnot, M. O., Antoine, J. M., Salat-Baroux, J., Belaisch-Allart, J. and Cohen, J. (1994). Human embryo cryopreservation in an IVF program. Limits, facts, prospects. In Mori, T., Aono, T., Tominaga, T. and Hiroi, M. (eds.) *Frontiers in Endocrinology*, Ares Serono Symposia Publ., **4**, 505–12

17. Lin, Y. P., Cassidenti, D. L., Chacon, R. R., Soubra, S. S., Rosen, G. F. and Yee, B. (1995). Successful implantation of frozen sibling embryos is influenced by the outcome of the cycle from which they were derived. *Fertil. Steril.*, **63**, 262–7

18. Avery, S., Marcus, S., Spillane, S., Macnamee, M. and Brinsden, P. (1995). Does the length of storage time affect the outcome of frozen embryo replacement? *J. Assist. Reprod. Genet.*, **12**, 67S

19. Wright, G., Wiker, S., Elsner, C., Kort, H., Massey, J., Mitchell, D., Toledo, A. and Cohen, J. (1990). Observations on the morphology of pronuclei and nucleoli in human zygotes and implications for cryopreservation. *Hum. Reprod.*, **5**, 109–15

20. Demoulin, A., Jouan, C., Gerday, C. and Dubois, M. (1991). Pregnancy rates after transfer of embryos obtained from different stimulation protocols and frozen at either pronucleate or multicellular stages. *Hum. Reprod.*, **6**, 799–804

21. Hazout, A., Nathan-Abbou, C., Cohen-Bacrie, P. and Dumont, M. (1995). Results of replacement cycles in patients with frozen cocultured supernumeraries blastocysts. *J. Assist. Reprod. Genet.*, **12**, 67–8S

22. Mandelbaum, J., Junca, A. M., Plachot, M., Alnot, M. O., Alvarez, S., Debache, C., Salat-Baroux, J. and Cohen, J. (1987). Human embryo cryopreservation, intrinsic and extrinsic parameters of success. *Hum. Reprod.*, **2**, 709–15

23. Toner, J. P., Brzyski, R. G., Oehninger, S., Veeck, L. L., Simonetti, S. and Muasker, S. J. (1991). Combined impact of the number of preovulatory oocytes and cryopreservation on IVF outcome. *Hum. Reprod.*, **6**, 284–9

24. Van Steirteghem, A. C., Van der Elst, J., Van den Abbeel, E., Joris, H., Camus, M. and Devroey, P. (1994). Cryopreservation of supernumerary multicellular human embryos obtained after intracytoplasmic sperm injection. *Fertil. Steril.*, **62**, 755–80

25. Kahn, J. A., von Düring, V., Sunde, A., Sodal, T. and Molne, K. (1993). The efficacy and efficiency of an *in-vitro* fertilization programme including embryo cryopreservation: a cohort study. *Hum. Reprod.*, **8**, 247–53

26. Wang, X. J., Ledger, W., Payne, D., Jeffrey, R. and Matthews, C. D. (1994). The contribution of embryo cryopreservation to *in-vitro* fertilization/gamete intra-fallopian transfer: 8 years' experience. *Hum. Reprod.*, **9**, 103–9

27. Van Steirteghem, A. C., Van den Abbeel, E., Van der Elst, J., Camus, M., Maes, R., Van Waesberghe, L. and Devroey, P. (1994). Human embryo cryopreservation. In Mori, T., Aono, T., Tominaga, T. and Hiroi, M. *Frontiers in Endocrinology*, Ares Serono Symposia Publ., **4**, 475–80

28. Pattinson, H. A., Hignett, M., Dunphy, B. C. and Fleetham, J. A. (1994). Outcome of thaw embryo transfer after cryopreservation of all embryos in patients at risk of ovarian hyperstimulation syndrome. *Fertil. Steril.*, **62**, 1192–6

29. Salat-Baroux, J., Cornet, D., Alvarez, S., Antoine, J. M., Tibi, C., Mandelbaum, J. and Plachot, M. (1988). Pregnancies after replacement of frozen-thawed embryos in a donation program. *Fertil. Steril.*, **49**, 817–21

30. Dulioust, E., Toyama, K., Busnel, M. C., Moutier, R., Carlier, M., Marchaland, C., Ducot, B., Roubertoux, P. and Auroux, M. (1995). Long-term effects of embryo freezing in mice. *Proc. Natl. Acad. Sci. USA*, **92**, 589–93

31. FIVNAT (1994). Pregnancy outcome after replacement of frozen-thawed embryos and after transfer of fresh embryos in French IVF registry. *Contracept. Fertil. Sex.*, **22**, 287–91

32. Wada, I., Macnamee, M. C., Wick, K., Bradfield, J. M. and Brinsden, P. R. (1994). Birth characteristics and perinatal outcome of babies conceived from cryopreserved embryos. *Hum. Reprod.*, **9**, 543–6

Fluorescent *in situ* hybridization in human blastomeres

60

S. Munné, M. Alikani, J. Levron, G. Tomkin, G. Palermo, J. Grifo and J. Cohen

Introduction

The reduced implantation rate of morphologically and/or developmentally abnormal cleavage-stage human embryos is well known, but the causes are still largely unknown. Factors implicated in embryonic impairment range from culture conditions, hormonal stimulation, gamete immaturity or aging, to chromosome abnormalities. This chapter discusses the relationship between chromosome abnormalities and embryonic impairment. Most of the data presented here have been obtained at the Department of Obstetrics and Gynecology of The New York Hospital – Cornell University Medical College by using fluorescent *in situ* hybridization (FISH) to analyze multiple chromosomes simultaneously.

Advantages and limitations of FISH analysis

Several conditions are needed to study numerical chromosome abnormalities in single cells of preimplantation human embryos. First, interphase assessments are necessary to evaluate embryos whose cells no longer divide (arrested) and consequently cannot be observed at metaphase. Second, comparison between cells of individual chromosomes is necessary in order to determined differences in specific aneuploidy rates. Third, all the blastomeres of an individual embryo must be analyzed to distinguish mosaicism from other abnormalities. Chromosome studies on early human embryos have mostly been performed by classical cytogenetic techniques[1-8]. Karyotype analysis, however, has limitations. It must be performed at the metaphase stage; not all the cells of cleaving embryos produce metaphases, and optimal banding of blastomere metaphase chromosomes is difficult to achieve. Therefore, cleavage-arrested embryos, which may constitute up to 20% of all embryos, cannot be properly studied by using karyotype analysis. Recent studies involving karyotyping of human blastomeres have shown that only a small proportion of the embryos (24–29%) could be analyzed[7,8], and less than 25% of those had all their cells karyotyped.

Fluorescent *in situ* hybridization with multiple probes has been used successfully to differentiate polyploidy, mosaicism and aneuploidy in arrested human embryos[9,10]. When most or all cells of an embryo are analyzed, mosaicism can be distinguished from FISH or fixation failure, as well as from aneuploidy. FISH also provides a mechanism for assessing the exact formation of the chromosomal anomaly[11]. By use of FISH analysis and multiple probes, results can be obtained for nearly all embryos (depending on whether a single cell is biopsied or all blastomeres are analyzed) and for 85–90% of their blastomeres[9,12-15]. Furthermore, the typical loss of chromosomes occurring during the fixation of metaphase nuclei does not allow the differentiation of aneuploidy from mosaicism, much less determination of the mechanisms of mosaicism formation. FISH has the obvious disadvantage of supplying information on only chromosomes for which specific probes are used.

The following criteria have been used in all our FISH studies to classify an embryo as chromosomally abnormal. In these studies, at least two chromosome pairs were analyzed, and most or all of the cells of each embryo were assessed. An embryo was considered to be aneuploid when all cells showed an extra (trisomic) or missing (monosomic) signal for one kind of chromosome, while showing two for the remaining chromosomes analyzed. An embryo was considered to be polyploid when every cell had $3 + n$ signals for each chromosome, where n was equal to or larger than 0 and constant for each chromosome and cell analyzed in that embryo. Similarly, when each cell of an embryo had a single chromosome of each kind, the embryo was classified as haploid. However, one of the most common abnormalities in human embryos is mosaicism. An embryo was classified as mosaic when two or more groups of cells from that embryo had different chromosome complements. The combinations could be normal/aneuploid, normal/polyploid, normal/haploid, aneuploid/polyploid, or more complex combinations. The problem of distinguishing mosaicism from FISH failure has been addressed previously[9].

Morphological traits and chromosome abnormalities

Karyotyping has shown that morphologically abnormal monospermic embryos (dysmorphic embryos) have a higher rate of chromosome abnormalities than morphologically normal embryos[3–8]. However, chromosomally normal and abnormal human embryos cannot necessarily be distinguished morphologically[16]. It is unlikely that chromosome abnormalities detected at the 2–8-cell stage would not induce dysmorphisms, since embryonic translation has not yet commenced[18,19], but the mechanism producing embryonic dysmorphisms may also generate chromosome abnormalities.

Individual morphological abnormalities have been specifically studied by means of FISH. These dysmorphisms and their corresponding chromosome abnormalities are summarized in Table 1. Embryos derived from polyspermic fertilization have been found to be very abnormal mosaics, although they are seldom purely triploid[20]. In contrast, tri-pronuclear embryos derived from intracytoplasmic sperm injection are invariably triploid and seldom triploid mosaics[20]. Another typical morphological abnormality is the occurrence of unipronuclear zygotes. Normally cleaving embryos derived from these zygotes are mostly normal and diploid when obtained by standard insemination[21], and mostly haploid when obtained by intracytoplasmic sperm injection[22]. This is because in the first case the two pronuclei have fused[23], whereas in the second case the oocyte has been activated by the sperm injection but the spermatozoa have failed to produce a pronucleus.

The study of other morphological abnormalities such as fragmentation has produced results that are not informative, at least as a tool to select normal embryos. Although fragmentation has been associated with chromosome abnormalities[4,7,8], in particular mosaicism, highly

Table 1 Morphological abnormalities that are related to chromosomal abnormalities

4–8-Cell embryo morphology	Chromosomal status	Reference
Normal morphology	23% mosaic and/or polyploid	Munné et al. (1995)[30]
3PN after regular IVF	100% mosaic or triploid	Cohen et al. (1995)[20]
3PN after ICSI	triploid	Cohen et al. (1995)[20]
Cleaving 1PN after regular IVF	normal	Munné et al. (1994)[21]
Cleaving 1PN after ICSI	haploid	Sultan et al. (1995)[22]
Giant embryos (> 220 mm)	triploid	Munné et al. (1994)[32]
Dominant single blastomere	polyploid	Munné et al. (1994)[32]
> 20% fragments, normal development	56% mosaic and/or polyploid	Munné et al. (1995)[30]
Multinucleated	74% mosaic and/or polyploid	Kligman et al. (1995)[31]

PN, pronuclei; IVF, *in vitro* fertilization; ICSI, intracytoplasmic sperm injection

fragmented embryos can still be chromosomally normal.

Multinucleation is another common morphological abnormality described frequently in cleaving embryos; it can apparently occur at any time between the first cleavage division and the blastocyst stage. Multinucleated blastomeres have been described in embryos developing *in vitro* as well as *in vivo*, and in arrested, slow or normally developing embryos, and their frequency ranges from 17 to 69% in normally developing embryos[9,24–29]. In a recent study involving more than 500 embryos, significantly fewer normally developing embryos (34.4%) contained multinucleated cells than did dysmorphic embryos (47.2%)[30]. Studies by Hardy and co-workers[28] suggested that multinucleation may reduce developmental competence of the embryo, since dinucleated cells are usually arrested. FISH studies on multinucleated blastomeres have been performed to assess these as a source of misdiagnosis when preimplantation genetic diagnosis is carried out[9,29]. For instance, these studies showed that the chromosomal content of each nucleus of a multinucleated blastomere was not always the same as the chromosomal content of the nuclei of the sibling blastomeres. These studies, however, were performed on cells identified after embryo biopsy on day 4 of development. A more recent study has found that the presence of multinucleated cells in non-arrested human embryos of day 2 or day 3 is indicative in 74% of the cases of extensive mosaicism and/or polyploidy[31]. According to these results, day 2 of the development appears to be a critical stage for multinucleation, since, by definition, half or more of the cells would be abnormal and the embryo seriously affected. This differs from previous analyses in which multinucleated blastomeres were detected on day 4 after biopsy. In those studies, morphologically normal embryos with a single or few multinucleated blastomeres were mostly chromosomally normal[9,29].

In contrast to fragmented embryos or embryos containing multinucleated blastomeres, which could still be chromosomally normal and develop to term, we have detected two instances in which monospermic embryos with a particular morphological abnormality were chromosomally abnormal in all cases[32]. These two groups of monospermic embryos were: (a) embryos ($n = 13$) with only one large cell surrounded by smaller blastomere-sized extracellular fragments. These embryos were polyploid and frequently polyploid mosaic. Some of these embryos showed ploidies of up to 20n, and the single cell was normally multinucleated; (b) embryos ($n = 6$) developing from larger than normal oocytes, with diameters of 220 mm or more, and zygotes displaying two polar bodies and two pronuclei. These embryos were invariably triploid or triploid mosaics, with XXX or XXY gonosome constitutions, which suggested a higher contribution of maternal genomes. These large eggs were most likely to be derived from diploid oocytes. The occurrence of giant digynic triploid eggs has also been reported in the Chinese hamster[33]. Atypical morphology was not seen in other polyploid monospermic embryos.

Abnormal development and chromosome abnormalities in monospermic embryos

Classical cytogenetic techniques cannot analyze arrested embryos because, by definition, non-cleaving cells cannot produce metaphase chromosomes to karyotype. In addition, only a proportion of blastomeres in non-arrested embryos show metaphases. To avoid this problem, FISH has been used[9,11,30] to assess embryos with different developmental rates. Embryos were classified into three large groups: those with 'arrested', 'slow or fragmented' and 'normal' development. Arrested embryos were considered to be those that did not develop beyond the eight-cell stage on their 4th day of development and had not cleaved during a 24-h period. Slow/fragmented embryos were those that had not reached the eight-cell stage on their 4th day of development but had cleaved during a 24-h period, or embryos cleaving at a normal pace but with more than 20% fragmentation. Normal embryos were those that had normal development. Normally developing monospermic embryos were donated by a group of patients with a mean maternal age of 40, who had repeatedly failed *in vitro* fertilization (IVF), or were embryos from any maternal age, which after preimplantation genetic diagnosis, were considered at a high risk of being affected.

For this study, a total of 524 monospermic embryos were included; 283 were analyzed with X, Y, 18 and 13/21 probes and the remainder with X, Y and 18 probes. They were classified into three maternal age groups: 20–34, 35–39 and 40–47 years.

The frequencies of these groups among IVF-obtained embryos included in our database were 13.8% for 'arrested', 33.0% for 'slow or fragmented' and 53.2% for 'normal' embryos, respectively. (The EggCyte relational database used Parabase and Sybase on NeXT, and was based on 5751 monospermic embryos from 1388 women undergoing IVF at Cornell University Medical College between 1993 and 1994.) These data also showed that 36% were 20–34 years old, 40% were 35–39 years old and 24% were 40–47 years old. Since the embryos analyzed by FISH did not correspond to our general IVF population, the raw data[30] are here normalized according to the IVF maternal age distributions (Table 2).

The major chromosomal abnormality detected in arrested embryos was polyploidy (43%). The origin of polyploidy in arrested embryos has been discussed in a recent publication[9]. Polyspermic fertilization was unlikely, since only two pronuclei were observed after insemination. It may be that for polyploid

monospermic embryos, their DNA synthesis continued, although cellular division had stopped. In some instances they also continued karyokinesis, producing multinucleation in almost half their cells. That DNA synthesis is not prevented by cleavage arrest has been demonstrated by Artley and associates[34]. According to Winston and colleagues[35], even if karyokinesis and gene activation do not fail, impaired cytokinesis may arrest the embryo, because there are insufficient cells to produce a functional inner-cell mass. Since most polyploid embryos became arrested before the onset of genome activation, which occurs around the 4–8-cell stage[18,19], oocyte quality or embryo culture conditions may have been the cause of their arrest.

The observation that aneuploid embryos became arrested less frequently than normally developing embryos can be explained by the same argument. Since aneuploidy occurs in the gametes, and the embryo has not reached the onset of genome activation, aneuploidy cannot produce cleavage arrest, and morphologically normal embryos with aneuploid complements can go on cleaving normally. That aneuploidy is less detected in arrested embryos may be related to the fact that, in many cases, polyploid embryos are mosaics with very different numbers of individual chromosomes per cell. An aneuploid zygote could be difficult to identify once it became a polyploid mosaic embryo. In total, 71% of arrested embryos were chromosomally abnormal.

Slow and/or fragmented embryos were chromosomally abnormal in 57% of cases, with aneuploidy (23%) followed by extensive mosaicism

Table 2 Abnormal development and chromosome abnormalities detected by FISH and normalized for maternal age. The percentage of aneuploid embryos was calculated by adding individual aneuploidy rates for each chromosome studied, since not all embryos were studied with the same probes. For the total, embryos with two or more kinds of chromosomal abnormality were counted only once

Development	n	Polyploid (%)	Haploid (%)	2n-extensive mosaicism (%)	Aneuploid (%)	Total (%)
Arrested	182	43.4[a]	2.6	22.5[d]	6.4[g]	71.5[j]
Slow or fragmented	154	13.1[b]	1.9	22.1[e]	22.9[h]	57.4[k]
Normal	188	2.3[c]	3.9	13.3[f]	10.6[i]	28.8[l]

Significance: ab = $p < 0.001$; ac = $p < 0.001$; df = $p < 0.05$; ef = $p < 0.05$; gh = $p < 0.001$; hi = $p < 0.005$; jk = $p < 0.025$; jl = $p < 0.001$; kl = $p < 0.001$

Table 3 Aneuploidy, maternal age and developmental competence

	Maternal age groups (years)			Differences between maternal age groups
	20–34	35–39	40–47	
Total aneuploidy (%)				
arrested	5.5	5.6	10.4[e]	NS
slow/fragmented	6.0[a]	15.6	29.5[f]	af:$p < 0.025$
normal	4.0[b]	9.4	37.2[g]	bg:$p < 0.005$
total (normalized for morphology)	5.4[c]	10.3[d]	27.7[h]	ch,dh:$p < 0.001$
Differences between morphological groups	NS	NS	eg:$p < 0.05$	

Aneuploidy and total abnormality significances were calculated with the Mantel–Haenszel test to take into account that aneuploidy for 13/21 could only be detected in embryos analyzed with the 13/21 probe. Mosaicism and polyploidy significance were calculated with the χ^2 test

Table 4 Individual chromosome aneuploidies detected by FISH in human embryos, regardless of morphology or maternal age

Chromosome	n	Monosomy	Trisomy	Reference
XY	524	10	2	Munné et al. (1995)[30]
18	524	14	10	Munné et al. (1995)[30]
13 and 21	283	16	17	Munné et al. (1995)[30]
16	64	2	1	Munné et al. (1995)[37]

(22%) and polyploidy (13%). High rates of mosaicism have also been described in these embryos by some karyotyping studies[5]. The rate of mosaicism can be calculated as the number of embryos with at least one cell being different from the other cells of that embryo, or as the number of embryos with a percentage of chromosomally abnormal cells high enough to jeopardize the viability of the embryo. Based on totipotency evaluations from embryo biopsy[36] and freeze/thaw data, embryos that have lost three out of eight cells are able to develop normally to term. If abnormal cells have suboptimal proliferation, embryos with a low number of abnormal cells may still mostly develop into normal embryos. Using either classification of mosaicism, 'arrested' and 'slow or fragmented' embryos had similar rates of diploid mosaicism, but double the rate of normally developing embryos (Table 3). Since many polyploid arrested embryos were in addition mosaics, it can be argued that arrested embryos have more

mosaicism than slowly developing ones. Pellestor and colleagues[7] analyzed a group of embryos (grade IV) that could be similar to our 'slow and/or fragmented' group. They found that only 10% of these embryos were chromosomally normal, while 27.1% were hypodiploid, 3.4% hyperdiploid, 10.7% mosaics, 11.8% haploid, 10.2% polyploid and 12.7% contained structural abnormalities. However, the differences between hypo- and hyperdiploidy suggest that most hypodiploidy was caused by artifactual loss. As Table 4 shows, we detected as many monosomies as trisomies[30,37]; Jamieson and co-workers[8] detected the same by karyotyping all chromosomes. The fact that only 0–25% of the embryos analyzed in the most recent karyotype studies[7,8] had all their cells analyzed, indicates that mosaicism was either underestimated or erroneously classified in some instances as aneuploidy.

We were able to determine the cell division at which chromosome mosaicism occurred, by assessing the number of blastomeres of each cell type[11]. This could be accomplished when the majority of embryonic cells had been analyzed. Blastomeres, regardless of their karyotype, were assumed to have the same chance of development, because previous studies of human embryos have suggested that abnormal cells can in fact cleave[9]. All blastomeres of monospermic embryos were abnormal, when the chromosome abnormality occurred during the first embryonic division. When one-half or one-fourth of the blastomeres were abnormal, mosaicism arose at the second and third division, respectively. According to these criteria, it was found that polyploid and haploid mosaic embryos usually originated at the first division, whereas monospermic diploid mosaics were generated in 97% of the cases at the second or later division[11] (Table 5). These differences may be explained by events taking place during the first and second embryonic divisions. During the first cleavage, two pronuclei with replicated DNA enter syngamy and then continue to karyokinesis, but the first time that a diploid nucleus undergoes a mitotic division is during the sec-

Table 5 Number of observed mosaic embryos according to their onset of mosaicism and ploidy. From reference 11

	Monospermic			
Cleavage	Diploid	Polyploid	Haploid	Dispermic
First	1	9	3	17
Second	17	15	1	11
Third or later	17	3	1	0
Total	35	27	5	28

Table 6 Types of mosaicism and mechanisms in monospermic diploid embryos (%). From reference 11

Aneuploid mosaics	46
by mitotic non-disjunction	24
by random division	10
by anaphase lag	2
by endoreduplication of a single chromosome	2
by other mechanism	8
2n/4n mosaics	41
2n/n mosaics	13

ond division. The results suggest that in diploid embryos, pronuclear syngamy occurs correctly, whereas mosaicism is generated by ensuring mitotic aberrations. Triploid dispermic zygotes, in contrast, may have problems distributing their chromosomes equally between two nuclei, because of the presence of several paternal centrosomes, with a resulting disarrangement of chromosomes[38-40].

Mosaicism in monospermic diploid embryos was mostly caused by mitotic non-disjunction or by tetraploidization of one or two cells[11] (Table 6). Giant polyploid cells are a frequent phenomenon in the trophoblastic tissue of many animals, including humans[41-44]. The presence of similar cells on day 3 of development may indicate early differentiation, although the present data do not prove that there is a direct link between the two events. More than half of the monospermic polyploid embryos were a combination of two cell types of different ploidy levels, most of them having one type with twice the ploidy of the other. This suggests endoreduplication or karyokinesis failure. The remainder were mostly complex mosaics whose origin was unknown[11].

Our results for normally developing embryos showed very few polyploid or mosaic embryos, but the highest rate of aneuploidy was detected in this group. Polyploidy was very rare in normally developing embryos, and mosaicism and aneuploidy were also lower than in slow embryos. In total, 29% of morphologically normal embryos were chromosomally abnormal for the chromosomes studied.

It may be important to perform embryo transfer on day 3. By that time, some arrested embryos may have been distinguished, since developmentally abnormal 2–4-cell embryos have been selected. The difference between arrested and normally developing embryos was 71% and 29% of mostly lethal chromosomal abnormalities, respectively. Previous studies comparing day 2 and day 3 transfers have not shown significant differences in pregnancy rates. In our laboratory only 15% of embryos were arrested by day 3, and therefore pure transfers of arrested embryos were rare, explaining the difficulty in showing differences between transfers on day 2 or day 3.

Maternal age and chromosome abnormalities in monospermic embryos

Genetic analysis of abortuses and live offspring has shown that older women are at a higher risk of delivering trisomic fetuses. Most of this aneuploidy is the result of non-disjunction in maternal meiosis-I[45-50]. Several theories, which have been reviewed by Warburton[51], have tried to explain this phenomenon, and the most accepted theory is that aged oocytes are more prone to non-disjunction during meiosis-I. Another hypothesis, called 'relaxed selection', suggests that the increase in trisomy is the result of the failure of older women spontaneously to abort an abnormal embryo[52]. As far as we know, no unequivocal relationship between maternal age and oocyte aneuploidy has yet been shown. Oocytes and cleavage-stage embryos have been examined by karyotyping, but only two reports among many demonstrated a slight correlation between aneuploidy and maternal age[53,54]. Most other studies failed to show any significant difference[55,56]. This may be largely due to problems inherent in unrepresentative patient populations and karyotyping. These problems can be avoided by using FISH in patients with a large maternal age spectrum.

Our most recent study[30] shows that aneuploidy increases significantly ($p < 0.001$) with maternal age (Table 3). This corroborates the hypothesis that oocytes of older women are more prone to non-disjunction caused by meiotic errors at the gamete level. The risk of conceiving a fetus has been estimated to increase from 1.9% of clinically recognized pregnancies in women 25–29 years old, to 19.1% in women over 39 years of age[45]. For chromosomes 18, 13 and 21, aneuploidy in clinically recognized pregnancies increased from 1.3% in the 35–39-year-old group to 4.3% in the 40–45 group[57]. However, in cleavage-stage embryos, we found that aneuploidy rates for chromosomes XY, 18, 13 and 21 increased from 5.4% and 10.3% in the

20–34 and 35–39 years groups, respectively, to 27.7% in the 40–45-year-old group[30] (Table 3). If only normally developing embryos are considered, the differences were even greater, increasing from 4% in the 20–34-year-old group, to 37.2% in the 40–45 group. The differences between aneuploidy in cleavage-stage embryos and clinically recognized pregnancies may be that many aneuploid embryos are being eliminated before a pregnancy is clinically recognized. For instance, the data in this study show that the rate of monosomy was equal to or more frequent than trisomy (Table 4), while with the exception of monosomy 21 (1/1000 karyotyped abortions), the other autosomal monosomies were normally undetected in clinically recognized pregnancies. Since non-disjunction produces disomic and nullisomic gametes with the same frequency, monosomic embryos must be the ones eliminated during the first days or weeks of pregnancy. The fact that most aneuploid embryos develop normally to the eight-cell stage is not in contradiction with the high mortality rate at later stages. The embryonic genome may not be activated until to 4–8-cell stage[18,19], and consequently, any detrimental effect caused by aneuploidy could not be detected until later. Similarly, because the genome is not activated, the aneuploid embryonic genome cannot be actively producing dysmorphisms. The decrease of aneuploidy with embryonic dysmorphism observed in this study remains puzzling. One explanation may be the difficulty of detecting aneuploid zygotes once these become polyploid mosaic. Since arrested aneuploid embryos have a 21% chance of being polyploid-mosaic, an aneuploid zygote is often very difficult to identify once it becomes a polyploid mosaic embryo.

The fact that 37.2% of 'normal' embryos from women 40 or older were aneuploid for four chromosome pairs may suggest that for 23 pairs the number of aneuploid embryos may exceed 100%. However, other chromosomes may be less commonly involved in aneuploidy, or double or multiple aneuploidies may occur. For example, taking all the morphological groups together, the number of double aneuploidies accounted for 19.1% (9/47) of all aneuploidies in embryos from women 40 or older, compared to only 4.5% (1/22) for women of 39 or younger[30].

Regarding individual aneuploidy rates per specific chromosome, we have found[30,37] that these range from 2.1% for gonosomes to 5.1% for chromosome 16, and 10.4% for 13 and 21 chromosomes combined. Since chromosomes 13 and 21 were detected by using the same probe[13], their aneuploidy frequency is given as the sum of both aneuploidy rates (Table 5).

FISH for preimplantation genetic diagnosis of aneuploidy

From the results above, the selection on day 3 of development of IVF-human embryos according to morphological and developmental traits has been shown to be effective in selecting against embryos with higher chances of carrying lethal chromosome abnormalities. Therefore, when available, only morphologically and developmentally normal embryos should be transferred.

However, in women of advanced maternal age, we found that morphologically and developmentally normal embryos had equally or higher chances of being aneuploid[30]. Therefore, morphological and developmental criteria are not suitable to prevent the transfer of these embryos. For that purpose, we have proposed preimplantation diagnosis for aneuploidy. Two approaches have been suggested: the first, to biopsy one cell of a day-3 embryo, and analyze it by FISH[13]; the second, to biopsy the first polar body or both polar bodies before insemination, and perform FISH or chromosome analysis[58–61]. The okadaic acid treatment suggested by Dyban and associates[60] to allow karyotyping of polar body chromosomes has not yet been applied to human polar bodies. As FISH analysis can analyze only a few chromosomes at a time, only those involved in trisomies at risk of arriving to term (XY, 13, 18, 21) have been targeted. Actually, preimplantation diagnosis of aneuploidy is intended to achieve two purposes: the first, to prevent the transfer of embryos that may result in the conception of a trisomic baby; the second,

to increase pregnancy rates by transferring only embryos normal for these chromosomes. Even though monosomy-X and trisomies for these chromosomes can arrive to term, all autosomal monosomies and most of these trisomies will die or spontaneously abort. For instance, in women 40 or older, 37% of cleavage-stage normally developing embryos are aneuploid for these chromosomes, but at birth, only 2.7% are still aneuploid. The rest did not implant or spontaneously aborted. In theory, by transferring only embryos normal for these chromosomes, embryo wastage would be reduced, and pregnancy rates increased in the event that enough chromosomally normal embryos are available for transfer.

The first objective, screening for the most common aneuploidies, has been accomplished. FISH has been shown to screen successfully for 90–95% of these aneuploidies, in a time frame compatible with IVF. The efficiency of the technique has been tested in blastomeres from embryos unsuitable for transfer[13], in first polar bodies[61] and by re-analysis of the non-trans-

Table 7 Efficiency assessment of the preimplantation diagnosis of aneuploidy by re-analysis of the non-transferred embryos from 18 cases

---

58 normal
  54 transferred
  4 re-analyzed
    3 confirmed
    1 error (undetected trisomy 13/21)

49 abnormal
  5 transferred (monosomy 13/21)
  44 re-analyzed
    19 aneuploid
    3 polyploid
    4 haploid
    17 mosaics (80–100%) abnormal
    1 error (false trisomy 13/21)

10 no results (due to 13/21 unclear, multinucleation or no nuclei)
  4 aneuploid
  2 mosaic
  4 normal

Total error rate 4% (2/48)
Aneuploidy rate 25% (29/117)
Other abnormalities 22% (26/117)

---

ferred embryos after 18 clinical cases of preimplantation diagnosis of aneuploidy (Table 7).

Regarding the second objective of the study, 18 cycles of preimplantation diagnosis of aneuploidy by FISH have been performed at the Department of Obstetrics and Gynecology of The New York Hospital – Cornell University Medical Center between August 1993 and March 1995, using a previously described protocol[13]. The average maternal age was 41.1 years, and the average number of embryos transferred was three. We obtained five pregnancies, which resulted in a singleton and twin spontaneous abortions, two ongoing twin pregnancies, and one delivery of a healthy and chromosomally normal baby. Therefore, the delivery rate could be estimated to be around 17% (3/18) which is not different from that expected (17.2%) for a group of patients with similar maternal ages. While more cases should be diagnosed for confirmation of these figures, and similar results from Verlinsky and colleagues[59] are more encouraging, our preliminary data suggest that the pregnancy rate does not increase after preimplantation diagnosis of these aneuploidies. This could be due to the fact that other aneuploidies could also be as common as the ones with a risk of arriving to term. If that is the case, other approaches should be taken to screen for aneuploid embryos. For instance, preimplantation diagnosis could be performed at the blastocyst stage after co-culture[62]. FISH analysis of blastocysts has been successfully applied for a few chromosomes[44,63]. However, if enough cells are biopsied, subgroups of cells could be analyzed for different chromosomes, and information obtained for all possible aneuploidies. Another approach, suggested by Mark Hughes, is to perform comparative genome hybridization[64] on single blastomeres from cleavage-stage embryos. This technique, however, has not yet been shown to be ready for clinical use in preimplantation genetics.

Acknowledgements

The authors would like to acknowledge the embryological skills of John Garrisi, Alexis Adler, Adrienne Reing, Toni Ferrara, Cindy Anderson, Elena Kissin and Sasha Sadowy. We would like to thank Drs Michael Bedford, Zev Rosenwaks and William Ledger, for their support of this work.

References

1. Angell, R. R., Aitken, R. J., van Look, P. F. A., Lumsden, M. A. and Templeton, A. A. (1983). Chromosome abnormalities in human embryos after in-vitro fertilization. Nature (London), 303, 336–8

2. Zenzes, M. T., Belkier, L., Kan, I., Schneider, H. P. G. and Nieschlag, E. (1985). Cytologic investigation of human in vitro fertilization failures. Fertil. Steril., 43, 883–91

3. Angell, R. R., Templeton, A. A. and Aitken, R. J. (1986). Chromosome studies in human in vitro fertilization. Hum. Genet., 72, 333–9

4. Plachot, M., Junca, A. M., Mandelbaum, J., De Grouchy, J., Salat-Baroux, J. and Cohen, J. (1987). Chromosome investigations in early life. II. Human preimplantation embryos. Hum. Reprod., 2, 29–35

5. Bongso, A., Fong, C. H., Ng, S. C., Ratman, S. and Lim, J. (1991). Preimplantation genetics: chromosomes of fragmented human embryos. Fertil. Steril., 56, 66–70

6. Zenzes, M. T., Wang, P. and Casper, R. F. (1990). Chromosome analyses in human preimplantation embryos. J. In-vitro Fert. Embryo Transfer, 7, 45

7. Pellestor, F., Dufour, M. C., Arnal, F. and Humeau, C. (1994). Direct assessment of the rate of chromosomal abnormalities in grade IV human embryos produced by in-vitro fertilization procedures. Hum. Reprod., 9, 293–302

8. Jamieson, M. E., Coutts, J. R. T. and Connor, J. M. (1994). The chromosome constitution of human preimplantation embryos fertilized in vitro. Hum. Reprod., 9, 709–15

9. Munné, S., Grifo, J., Cohen, J. and Weier, H. U. G. (1994). Chromosome abnormalities in

human arrested preimplantation embryos: a multiple-probe FISH study. *Am. J. Hum. Genet.*, **155**, 150–9

10. Harper, J. C., Coonen, E., Handyside, A. H., Winston, R. M. L., Hopman, A. H. N. and Delhanty, J. D. A. (1995). Mosaicism of autosomes and sex chromosomes in morphologically normal, monospermic preimplantation human embryos. *Prenat. Diagn.*, **15**, 41–9

11. Munné, S., Weier, H. U. G., Grifo, J. and Cohen, J. (1994). Chromosome mosaicism in human embryos. *Biol. Reprod.*, **51**, 373–9

12. Griffin, D. K., Wilton, L. J., Handyside, A. H., Winston, R. M. L. and Delhanty, J. D. A. (1992). Dual fluorescent *in situ* hybridization for simultaneous detection of X and Y chromosome-specific probes for the sexing of human preimplantation embryonic nuclei. *Hum. Genet.*, **89**, 18–22

13. Munné, S., Lee, A., Rosenwaks, Z., Grifo, J. and Cohen, J. (1993). Diagnosis of major chromosome aneuploidies in human preimplantation embryos. *Hum. Reprod.*, **8**, 2185–91

14. Delhanty, J. D. A., Griffin, D. K., Handyside, A. H., Harper, J., Atkinson, G. H. G., Pieters, M. H. E. C. and Winston, R. M. L. (1993). Detection of aneuploidy and chromosomal mosaicism in human embryos during preimplantation sex determination by fluorescent *in situ* hybridization (FISH). *Hum. Mol. Genet.*, **2**, 1183–5

15. Harper, J. C., Coonen, E., Ramaekers, F. C. S., Delhanty, J. D. A., Handyside, A. H., Winston, R. M. L. and Hopman, A. H. N. (1994). Identification of the sex of human preimplantation embryos in two hours using an improved spreading method and fluorescent *in-situ* hybridization (FISH) using directly labelled probes. *Hum. Reprod.*, **9**, 721–4

16. Zenzes, M. T. and Casper, R. F. (1992). Cytogenetics of human oocytes, zygotes, and embryos after *in-vitro* fertilization. *Hum. Genet.*, **88**, 367–75

17. Angell, R. R., Templeton, A. A. and Aitken, R. J. (1986). Chromosome studies in human *in vitro* fertilization. *Hum. Genet.*, **72**, 333–9

18. Braude, P., Bolton, V. and Moore, S. (1988). Human gene expression first occurs between the four- and eight-cell stages of preimplantation development. *Nature (London)*, **333**, 459–61

19. Tesarik, J., Kopecny, V., Plachot, M. and Mandelbaum, J. (1988). Early morphological signs of embryonic genome expression in human preimplantation development as revealed by quantitative electron microscopy. *Dev. Biol.*, **128**, 15–20

20. Cohen, J., Levron, J., Palermo, G., Munné, S., Adler, A., Alikani, M., Schattman, G., Sultan, K. and Willadsen, S. (1995). Atypical activation and fertilization patterns in humans. *Theriogenology*, in press

21. Munné, S., Tang, Y. X., Grifo, J. and Cohen, J. (1994). Origin of single pronucleated human zygotes. *J. Assist. Reprod. Genet.*, **10**, 276–9

22. Sultan, K. M., Munné, S., Palermo, G. D., Alikani, M. and Cohen, J. (1995). Ploidy assessment of embryos derived from single-pronucleated human zygotes obtained by regular IVF and intra-cytoplasmic sperm injection (ICSI). *Hum. Reprod.*, **10**, 132–6

23. Levron, J., Willadsen, S., Munné, S. and Cohen, J. (1995). Formation of male pronuclei in partitioned human oocytes. *Biol. Reprod.*, **53**, 209–13

24. Hertig, A. T., Rock, J., Adams, E. C. and Mulligan, W. J. (1954). On the preimplantation stages of the human ovum: a description of four normal and four abnormal specimens ranging from the second to the fifth day of development. *Contrib. Embryol.*, **35**, 201–20

25. Lopata, A., Kohlman, D. and Johnston, I. (1983). The fine structure of normal and abnormal human embryos developed in culture. In Beier, H. M. and Lindner, H. R. (eds.) *Fertilization of the Human Egg In-vitro*, pp. 189–210. (Heidelberg: Springer Verlag)

26. Plachot, M. (1985). *Contribution l'étude de la fécundation et du développement* in vitro *de l'oeuf humain*. Doctoral thesis, pp. 1–114, University of Paris

27. Tesarik, J., Kopecny, V., Plachot, M. and Mandelbaum, J. (1987). Ultrastructural and autoradiographic observations on multinucleated blastomeres of human cleaving embryos obtained by *in-vitro* fertilization. *Hum. Reprod.*, **2**, 127–36

28. Hardy, K., Winston, R. M. L. and Handyside, A. H. (1993). Binucleate blastomeres in preimplantation human embryos *in-vitro*: failure of cytokinesis during early cleavage. *J. Reprod. Fertil.*, **98**, 549–58

29. Munné, S. and Cohen, J. (1993). Unsuitability of multinucleated human blastomeres for preimplantation genetic diagnosis. *Hum. Reprod.*, **8**, 1120–5

30. Munné, S., Alikani, M., Tomkin, G., Grifo, J. and Cohen, J. (1995). Embryo morphology, developmental rates and maternal age are correlated with chromosome abnormalities. *Fertil. Steril.*, in press

31. Kligman, I., Alikani, M., Cohen, J. and Munné, S. (1995). The presence of multinucleated blastomeres correlates with chromosomal abnormalities in human embryos. *J. Assist. Reprod. Genet.*, **12**, 27S

32. Munné, S., Alikani, M., Grifo, J. and Cohen, J. (1994). Monospermic polyploidy and atypical embryo morphology. *Hum. Reprod.*, **9**, 506–10

33. Funaki, K. and Mikamo (1980). Giant diploid oocytes as cause of digynic triploidy in mammals. *Cytogenet. Cell Genet.*, **28**, 158–68

34. Artley, J. K., Braude, P. R. and Johnson, M. H. (1992). Gene activity and cleavage arrest in human pre-embryos. *Hum. Reprod.*, **7**, 1014–21

35. Winston, N. J., Braude, P. R., Pickering, S. J., George, M. A., Cant, A., Currie, J. and Johnson, M. H. (1991). The incidence of abnormal morphology and nucleocytoplasmic ratios in 2-, 3- and 5-day human pre-embryos. *Hum. Reprod.*, **6**, 17–24

36. Hardy, K., Martin, K. L., Leese, H. J., Winston, R. M. L. and Handyside, A. H. (1990). Human preimplantation development *in-vitro* is not adversely affected by biopsy at the 8-cell stage. *Hum. Reprod.*, **5**, 708–14

37. Munné, S., Sultan, K. M., Weier, H. U. G., Grifo, J., Cohen, J. and Rosenwaks, Z. (1995). Assessment of numerical abnormalities of X, Y, 18 and 16-chromosomes in preimplantation human embryos prior transfer. *Am. J. Obstet. Gynecol.*, **172**, 1191–201

38. Sathananthan, A. H., Kola, I., Osborne, J., Trounson, A. O., Ng, S. C., Bongso, A. and Ratnam, S. S. (1991). Centrioles in the beginning of human development. *Proc. Natl. Acad. Sci. USA*, **88**, 4806–10

39. Long, C. R., Pinto-Correia, C., Duby, R. T., Ponce-de-Leon, F. B., Boland, M. P., Roche, J. F. and Robl, J. M. (1993). Chromatin and microtubule morphology during the first cell cycle in bovine zygotes. *Mol. Reprod. Devel.*, **36**, 23–32

40. Palermo, G., Munné, S. and Cohen, J. (1994). The human zygote inherits its mitotic potential from the male gamete. *Hum. Reprod.*, **9**, 1220–5

41. Hare, W. C. D., Singh, E. L., Betteridge, K. J., Eaglesome, M. D., Randall, G. C. B., Mitchell, D., Bilon, R. J. and Trouson, A. O. (1980). Chromosomal analysis of 159 bovine embryos collected 12 to 18 days after estrus. *Can. J. Genet. Cytol.*, **22**, 615–26

42. Murray, J. D., Moran, C., Boland, M. P., Nancarrow, C. D., Sutton, R., Hoskinson, R. M. and Scaramuzzi, R. J. (1986). Polyploid cells in blastocysts and early fetuses from Australian Merino sheep. *J. Reprod. Fertil.*, **78**, 439–46

43. Long, S. E. and Williams, C. V. (1982). A comparison of the chromosome complement of inner cell mass and trophoblast cells in day-10 pig embryos. *J. Reprod. Fertil.*, **66**, 645–8

44. Benkhalifa, M., Janny, L., Vye, P., Malet, P., Boucher, D. and Menezo, Y. (1993). Assessment of ploidy in human morulae and blastocysts using co-culture and fluorescent *in-situ* hybridization. *Hum. Reprod.*, **8**, 895–902

45. Hassold, T. and Chiu, D. (1985). Maternal age-specific rates of numerical chromosome abnormalities with special reference to trisomy. *Hum. Genet.*, **70**, 11–17

46. Hassold, T., Jacobs, P. A., Leppert, M. and Sheldon, M. (1987). Cytogenetic and molecular studies of trisomy 13. *J. Med. Genet.*, **24**, 725–32

47. Warburton, D., Kline, J., Stein, Z. and Strobino, B. (1986). Cytogenetic abnormalities in spontaneous abortions of recognized conceptions. In Porter, I. H. and Willey, A. (eds.) *Perinatal Genetics: Diagnosis of Treatment*, pp. 133–48 (New York: Academic Press)

48. May K. M., Jacobs, P. A., Lee, M., Ratclffe, S., Robinson, A., Nielsen, J. and Hassold, T. J. (1990). The parental origin of the extra X chromosome in 47,XXX females. *Am. J. Hum. Genet.*, **46**, 754–61

49. Antonorakis, S. E., Lewis, J. G., Adelsberg, P. A., Peterson, M. B., Schinzel, A. A., Binkert, F., Schmid, W. *et al.* (1991). Parental origin of the extra chromosome in trisomy 21 revisited: DNA polymorphism analysis suggests maternal origin in 95% of cases. *N. Engl. J. Med.*, **324**, 872–6

50. Nothen, M. M., Eggermann, T., Erdmann, J., Eiben, B., Hofmann, D., Propping, P. and Schwanitz, G. (1993). Retrospective study of the parental origin of the extra chromosome in trisomy 18 (Edwards syndrome). *Hum. Genet.*, **92**, 347–9

51. Warburton, D. (1989). The effect of maternal age on the frequency of trisomy: change in meiosis or *in utero* selection? In *Molecular and Cytogenetic Studies of Non-disjunction*, pp. 165–81. (New York: Alan R. Liss)

52. Ayme, S. and Lippman-Hand, A. (1982). Maternal-age effect in aneuploidy: does altered embryonic selection play a role?. *Am. J. Hum. Genet.*, **34**, 558–65

53. Plachot, M., De Grouchy, J., Junca, A. M., Mandelbaum, J., Salat-Baroux, J. and Cohen, J. (1988). Chromosome analysis of human oocytes and embryos: does delayed fertilization increase chromosome imbalance? *Hum. Reprod.*, **3**, 125–7

54. Macas, E., Floersheim, Y., Hotz, E., Imthurn, B., Keller, P. J. and Walt, H. (1990). Abnormal chromosomal arrangements in human oocytes. *Hum. Reprod.*, **5**, 703–7

55. Plachot, M., Veiga, A., Montagut, J., De Grouchy, J., Calderon, G., Lepretre, J. S., Junca, A. M., Santalo, J., Carles, E., Mandelbaum, J., Barri, P., Degoy, J., Cohen, J., Egozcue, J., Sabatier, J. and Salat-Baroux, J. (1988). Are clinical and biological IVF parameters correlated with chromosomal disorders in early life: a multicentric study. *Hum. Reprod.*, **5**, 627–35

56. Pellestor, F. (1991). Frequency and distribution of aneuploidy in human female gametes. *Hum. Genet.*, **86**, 283–8

57. Snijders, R. J. M., Holzgreve, W., Cuckle, H. and Nicolaides, K. H. (1994). Maternal age-specific risks for trisomies at 9–14 weeks' gestation. *Prenat. Diagn.*, **14**, 543–52

58. Verlinsky, Y., Ginsberg, N., Lifchez, A., Valle, J., Moise, J. and Strom, C. M. (1990). Analysis of the first polar body: preconception genetic diagnosis. *Hum. Reprod.*, **5**, 826–9

59. Verlinsky, Y., Cieslak, J., Freidine, V., Ivakhnenko, G., Wolf, G., Kavalinskaya, L., White, M., Lifchez, A., Kaplan, B., Moise, J., Valle, J., Strom, C. and Kuliev, A. (1995). Pregnancies following preconception diagnosis of common aneuploidies by FISH. *J. Assist. Reprod. Genet.*, **12**, 89S

60. Dyban, A. P., De Sutter, P., Dozortsev, D. and Verlinsky, Y. (1992). Visualization of second polar body chromosomes in fertilized and artificially activated mouse oocytes treated with okadaic acid. *J. Assist. Reprod. Genet.*, **9**, 572–9

61. Munné, S., Dailey, T., Sultan, K. M., Grifo, J. and Cohen, J. (1995). The use of first polar bodies for preimplantation diagnosis of aneuploidy. *Hum. Reprod.*, **10**, 1015–21

62. Weimer, K. E., Cohen, J., Amborski, G. F., Wiker, S., Wright, G., Munyakazi, L. and Godke, R. A. (1989). *In vitro* development and implantation of human embryos following culture on fetal bovine uterine fibroblast cells. *Hum. Reprod.*, **4**, 595–600

63. Muggleton-Harris, A. L., Glazier, A. M., Pickering, S. and Wall, M. (1995). Genetic diagnosis using polymerase chain reaction and fluorescent *in-situ* hybridization analysis of biopsied cells from both the cleavage and blastocyst stage of individual cultured human preimplantation embryos. *Hum. Reprod.*, **10**, 183–92

64. Kallioniemi, A., Kallioniemi, O. P., Sudar, D., Rutovitz, D., Gray, J. W., Waldman, F. and Pinkel, D. (1992). Comparative genomic hybridization for molecular cytogenetic analysis of solid tumors. *Science*, **258**, 818–21

8

Ethics

Fate of disposable embryos

61

W. *Thompson*

Introduction

It is now 17 years since the first child was born following *in vitro* fertilization (IVF). Since then, at least 150 000 children in more than 36 countries world-wide have resulted from IVF and other assisted conception techniques.

Unfortunately, such treatments are still considered a luxury in most health-care programs. Availability, to the majority of infertile couples, is limited by inadequate funding and resources. Although scientists and physicians view developments in assisted reproduction as important, advances in the treatment of the infertile couple have aroused, and continue to arouse, a storm of public controversy. Governments have established Committees of Enquiry into the social, legal and ethical aspects of assisted reproduction. Based on their recommendations, several countries have subsequently enacted legislation. However, there remains little international agreement on even fundamental questions[1].

One of the major issues which still engender fierce public debate is the fate of the so-called 'disposable' or 'spare' embryos and their use in research programs. Internationally, professional and legal regulations on embryo handling range from the generally permissive (as in the United Kingdom's Human Fertilisation and Embryology Act) to the totally prohibitive (as in the German Embryo Protection Act of 1990).

Source of disposable embryos

In today's typical IVF cycle, of the oocytes collected, perhaps only 66% will fertilize and perhaps of these only 75% will continue to divide and grow prior to transfer. However, these figures can range from 0% to 100%. Of the embryos which go on to transfer, in optimal circumstances the success (or pregnancy) rates are rarely in excess of 30% per transfer. Therefore, to address this high wastage, current IVF practice almost universally employs ovarian hyperstimulation to produce a potential surplus of eggs, and, following culture with sperm, a potential surplus of embryos. Most authorities accept that no more than three embryos should be transferred in view of the risk of high multiple pregnancy. However, in view of the above figures, it is unreasonable to suggest that only three eggs are fertilized. This would almost certainly result in less than the optimal number of embryos being available for transfer, and, therefore, a significantly decreased pregnancy rate.

Embryo research, through the use of the surplus embryos from these treatment cycles, is in general directed at medical and scientific enquiry relevant to human reproduction. Therefore, at least potentially, it may serve to benefit the larger population of human embryos in the future but obviously at the cost of the specific embryos used as research subjects. It could be argued that it is morally unjust not to undertake research on embryos if the overall low success rate of IVF is to be addressed in the patient's interest.

It is natural to believe that human embryo research is both immoral and unnecessary. However, it is this very lack of success of IVF that has produced the possibility of spare embryos for research. Few scientists or clinicians would propose the creation of embryos specifically for research – a sort of 'sub-culture' of human life.

In this presentation, some of the advantages of human embryo research are reviewed.

439

Uses of disposable embryos

The birth of the first IVF baby was the result of many years of embryo research[2]. More recently, research has centered on the concept of human embryo freezing. Human embryos are different from the embryos of other animals. They require different culture conditions and are notoriously brittle in their response to freezing. However, the success of work comparing different cryopreservatives and staged temperature-lowering protocols has lead us to the situation where some centers are reporting better pregnancy rates with frozen embryos than with fresh ones[3].

In this research, it has become obvious that transient cooling of oocytes during IVF may induce abnormalities of the meiotic spindle. This may lead to chromosomal defects at fertilization and thus be incompatible with embryonic survival or, even worse, result in an abnormal conceptus[4]. Thus, the significance of temperature control when handling human oocytes is an example of an important advance in IVF research made possible through the study of disposable embryos.

Fifty per cent of infertility (at least) is due to male factor causes. Some are so severe that, even with IVF, conception is not possible. With the availability of human oocytes, the intracytoplasmic sperm injection (ICSI) techniques have been developed. This had had, and will continue to have, a profound effect on the practice of IVF. Although the animal model was used in some of the earlier experiments and is still used to train personnel for this technique, it is only the availability of human material which has made the research a clinical reality.

Although a potential treatment is now available through human embryo research for practically all cases of male infertility, the area of 'unexplained' infertility is still obviously unanswered. Aberrations of the subtle mechanisms of human embryo growth, differentiation and implantation may well explain some of these cases. The identification and functional analysis of embryonic growth factors and chemical messengers is therefore of intense scientific interest.

Preliminary research has begun to reveal some answers for these unfortunate patients.

Fundamental research is also necessary to ascertain the mechanism and necessary conditions for successful implantation of the embryo in the uterine wall. This remains, probably, the single most important factor in the failure of IVF treatment. Does the problem, however, lie with the mother or with the embryo? Animal models of implantation are useful in determining some of the basic concepts of implantation. However, human implantation and placentation differ quite significantly from most animal models and only work with human embryos can produce the definitive answers.

Human embryo research, though, is not only of value to infertile couples. In an ideal world, we would like to diagnose hereditary abnormalities before conception. It is heart-breaking for parents to face the diagnosis of a fatal abnormality in their newborn child, and it is even more tragic to watch it happen to a subsequent child. Human embryo research has given rise to the concept of preimplantation genetic diagnosis[5]. In this technique, one cell is removed from the eight-cell embryo prior to freezing. If subsequent DNA analysis shows this cell to be negative for a particular genetic condition, the embryo can then be thawed and replaced in the uterus. The parents are then secure in the knowledge that their child will not have the abnormality they so fear and the much more emotive procedures of amniocentesis and termination of pregnancy in the early second trimester are avoided.

The use of disposable embryos in the development of several contraceptive methods is another important area of research. Henderson and colleagues[6] have demonstrated the potential of a contraceptive device based on an antibody that reacts with the human zona pellucida. Although the method is effective in marmosets, it will be necessary to test the ability of the antibody to prevent *in vitro* spermatozoal penetration of the human zona pellucida before field trials on the human can be undertaken.

It is a common misconception to believe that research on human disposable embryos advances only the practice and success of assisted reproductive methods. Clearly this is not so. It is also a common misconception that animal models are entirely satisfactory for the development and assessment of new techniques. To a point this is true. However, the fragility of the human embryo and the differences in its behavior and responses to its mother make research with human material essential. Without this research we would not have had Louise Brown and the thousands of other IVF pregnancies.

Ethical issues

The major limiting factor to embryo research continues to be the scarcity of human embryos for any purpose other than attaining pregnancy. The increasing use of cryopreservation in clinical practice will exacerbate this situation. A major ethical debate, as yet unresolved, centers around the creation of embryos for the specific purpose of research where donors consent to their gametes and embryos being used in this way.

There are others who view research on disposable embryos in an entirely different way, and central to this is the status of the human embryo. Scientists may view this as merely a group of totipotential cells but cannot ignore the view of fundamentalists who adhere to the absolutist position, namely that, as soon as a human egg is fertilized, it becomes a human being and must not be used for research. In the USA, this controversy has focused public attention on the question of when human life begins, and has placed research on disposable embryos at the center of the abortion debate. It has resulted in a restriction of funding for such research. In support of this ban on embryo research, they refer to the *Helsinki Declaration* which states that 'In research on man the interests of science and society should not take precedence over consideration to the well-being of the subject'.

Unfortunately, there is public misinformation about the aims of embryo research and this is particularly the fault of scientists and clinicians. The fears remain that such research will lead to genetic manipulation of fertilized eggs or to the production of identical individuals by cloning, or of 'designer' babies. In fact research in any of these areas is specifically prohibited in most countries[7]. It could be argued that to ban embryo research would mean that the woman undergoing IVF treatment becomes the focus of the research.

References

1. Eser, A. (1992). The legal status of the embryo in comparative perspective. *Med. Law.*, **11**, 579–90
2. Edwards, R. G., Steptoe, P. C. and Purdy, J. M. (1970). Fertilisation and cleavage *in vitro* of preovulatory human oocytes. *Nature (London)*, **227**, 1307–9
3. Seibel, M. M. (1988). A new era in reproductive technology: IVF, GIFT and donated embryos and gametes'. *N. Engl. J. Med.*, **318**, 828–34
4. Sathananthan, A. H., Trounson, A. O., Freeman, L. and Brady, T. (1988). The effects of cooling human oocytes. *Hum. Reprod.*, **3**, 968–77
5. Handyside, A. H., Kontogianni, E. H., Hardy, K. and Winston, R. M. L. (1990). Pregnancies from biopsied human preimplantation embryos sexed by Y-specific DNA amplification. *Nature (London)*. **344**, 768–70
6. Henderson, C. J., Hulme, M. J. and Aitken, R. J. (1988). Contraceptive potential of antibodies to the zona pellucida. *J. Reprod. Fertil.*, **83**, 325–43
7. McLaren, A. (1990). Research on the human conceptus and its regulation in Britain today. *J. R. Soc. Med.*, **83**, 209–13

First-trimester selective termination in multiple pregnancies

62

P. Boulot, H. Dechaud, M. Ermini-Peirera, P.-L. Giacalone, F. Laffargue and B. Hedon

Introduction

The deliberate reduction of the number of fetuses in a desired high-order multiple pregnancy is an alternative to the abortion of all the fetuses. Selective fetocide in the first trimester is performed in multiple pregnancies in order to decrease the chance of complications (i.e. early or late miscarriages, immaturity, fetal growth retardation, *in utero* fetal death[1-3]). Only a few papers dealing with the obstetrical outcome following fetal reduction are available and the risks of these procedures for both the surviving fetuses and their mothers have not yet been well assessed. The aims of this paper are, firstly, to analyze the obstetric data from a series of 100 consecutive reductions performed on high-order multiple pregnancies or triplets and, secondly, to evaluate the need for embryonic reduction in triplet pregnancies.

Obstetric data from 100 first-trimester selective terminations

Patients and methods

Patients   The study included 100 women who consulted between 1 April 1986 and 31 January 1994. They were referred to our institution for first-trimester selective fetocide. The mean age of the women was 31.1 years (standard deviation (SD) 3.9) with a range of 21–42 years. Among the 100 pregnancies, there were 63 triplets, 29 quadruplets, six quintuplets, one heptuplet and one twin pregnancy. A total of 61 pregnancies (61%) were achieved as a result of *in vitro* fertilization (IVF) procedures: 36 (36%) by ovulation induction and three (3%) occurring spon-

taneously. Some pregnancies had poor prognosis factors such as a scarred uterus (eight cases, all with triplets), with uterine malformation (two), with diabetes (two: one was insulin-dependent, the other not). In four pregnancies (three triplets and one quadruplet) there were monoamniotic pairs of fetuses; one of these monoamniotic pairs was conjoined and had been diagnosed by vaginal scan at 10 weeks of gestation.

Methods   Couples were allowed 10 days in which to make a decision on fetal reduction; precise information concerning the risks of the method was given and couples gave informed consent for the procedure; the retention of twins was the aim of the procedure in the majority. All the women had preliminary abdominal or transvaginal scans to confirm the exact number of embryos and to determine the type of placentation (monochorionic or dichorionic). The first method used was sac perforation by vaginal route: a trophoblast biopsy forceps (Storz biopsy forceps, 8591 A) was inserted through the undilatated cervix until it contacted with the membranes, which were then perforated widely. The embryo was crushed with the forceps if size permitted (< 8 weeks' gestation). The second method used the transabdominal route; this involved the percutaneous puncture of the embryo using a 22-gauge spinal needle inserted into the sac nearest the maternal wall. The needle was pushed into the fetal pericardiac area and a small volume (2–3 ml) of a potassium chloride solution or hypertonic sodium chloride solution was injected. The needle was then removed and the operation was repeated with an adjacent sac after a new introduction of the needle. The transcervical approach was used in 26 and the transabdominal route in 74 pregnancies. When using the transabdominal approach, we selected the fundal fetus(es) in order to avoid rupture of the membranes and the probability of amniotitis. The choice of the fetuses for reduction was based only on technical accessibility. After the procedures, the women remained in the unit for a few hours. Antibiotic prophylaxis was used in all except a few cases at the beginning of the study (amoxicilline-clavulanic acid, 1 g immediately before the procedure). All the pregnancies underwent a scan in the hours following. Subsequently, a scan was performed every 15 days until the end of the first trimester, and then every month until the end of pregnancy. Outcome data were available for all the pregnancies and all the infants, although not all received their obstetric care in our unit.

Statistics Data of the two parts of this paper are presented as means with SDs. Length of gestation was established from the date of *in vitro* fertilization or ovulation induction or, with spontaneous conception, from the first day of the last menstrual period and checked by ultrasound examination. The duration of pregnancies is presented as completed weeks of gestation. Delivery at term was after 37 completed weeks. Fetal weights were assessed from French curves drawn for singletons. The perinatal mortality rate included deaths that occurred from the beginning of the 24th week to the 7th day after birth. The χ^2 test was used to test for significant differences.

Results

Pregnancies after reduction included five singletons, 91 twins and four triplets. The reasons for the five singletons were: a severe maternal depressive reaction that might have necessitated abortion of all the fetuses if a singleton had not been obtained; in another pregnancy, our decision was influenced by uterine scars with a risk of rupture during the pregnancy; in another, conjoined twins were associated with a singleton in a triplet pregnancy; lastly, the association of monoamniotic twins with a singleton led to reduction. Four triplets were also obtained in four quadruplet pregnancies on the specific request of the couples.

Mean gestational age The mean gestational age at reduction was 9.6 (SD, 1.3) weeks, ranging from 7.0 to 15.5 weeks. Only one procedure was performed at 15.5 weeks', because a quadruplet pregnancy was diagnosed late, after ovulation induction.

Unplanned fetal loss Complete miscarriages occurred in 11 pregnancies (11%). Two of these occurred within 8 days after the fetal reduction and nine others more than 3 weeks after the procedure (two at 12; two at 14; two at 18; and three at 21 weeks' gestation). Four partial miscarriages affecting only one fetus occurred 2 and 3 weeks after the procedure and these pregnancies continued without any other complication. These women experienced vaginal bleeding, and repeated scans demonstrated the disappearance of these sacs. Table 1 shows the distribution of births among the 76 deliveries.

Outcome of pregnancies Of the five singleton pregnancies, two were complicated by complete miscarriage, two were delivered at 36 and 37 weeks', respectively, and one had not yet been delivered at the time of writing. As regards the twin pregnancies, eight were complicated by complete miscarriage, 71 were delivered, and 12

Table 1 Distribution of deliveries from 100 reduced pregnancies

Gestational age at birth (weeks)	Deliveries	
	n	%
24–28	0	0
28–30	4	5.2
31–32	9	11.8
33–34	11	14.5
35–37	19	25
> 37	33	43.5

are ongoing. Of the four triplet pregnancies, one was complicated by complete miscarriage, and three were delivered.

In utero death   *In utero* death (IUD) occurred in four twin pregnancies, at 28, 30, 31 and 34 weeks' gestation. Each fetus was growth-retarded. Three of these pregnancies continued without complications while maternal coagulation remained normal and cerebral scans of the surviving twins did not reveal any anomaly. In the third pregnancy, preterm labor associated with rupture of membranes of the lowest sac containing the dead fetus occurred, at 31 weeks'.

Preterm labor   The preterm labor rate was determined for all 76 deliveries. The rate of preterm labor (before 37 completed weeks' gestation) was 56.5% (43/76). The mean gestational age at term for twin pregnancies was 35.7 ± 3 weeks (extremes ranging from 28 to 41 weeks. The mean gestational age at term for triplets was 35.5 ± 2.2 weeks (range, 33–36.5 weeks). The distribution of births is reported in Table 1.

Outcome for the infants   A total of 137 infants were born, of whom 134 were alive at birth. Of the 126 infants from twin pregnancies, 57 (45%) were not growth-retarded; 46 (36.5%) were growth-retarded (below the tenth centile), and 23 (18.3%) were severely growth-retarded (below the third centile). Of the 134 infants, four died within 8 days of life. All the deaths were of infants born after gestations from 29 to 31 weeks. Except for an infant with Peina-Shoker's syndrome, the other deaths were due to respiratory distress syndrome or intracranial hemorrage. Three infants born before 32 weeks' had problems: two have mild mental retardation; the other, who had hydrocephalus, was successfully treated. The perinatal mortality rate was 5.8% (8/137).

No fetal injury was noted during the neonatal examination. The mean weight at birth for twins was 2228 ± 606 g for twin 1 and 2236 ± 527 g for twin 2.

Maternal complications   No maternal complications, (e.g. massive hemorrhage, septicemia or uterine perforation) occurred.

Discussion

These results suggest that selective fetocide has some risks for the remaining fetuses but reduces the rate of preterm delivery that would have occurred had the high multiple pregnancies been left intact. However, there was still a risk of very early preterm labor (between 28 and 32 weeks').

The rate of subsequent miscarriage in this series was similar to that observed when we reported the first 34 of these pregnancies, and is comparable to the rate previously reported by others (Lynch[6], Timor-Tritsch[11], Berkowitz[10]; Salat-Baroux[3] and respective colleagues, but higher than the rate reported by Wapner and colleagues[5] or Tabsh[7], who only used the transabdominal approach) (Table 2). Dommergues and co-workers[8] have recently reported a higher miscarriage rate (30%). Although there are no conclusive statistical data to determine the choice of technique, we prefer the transabdominal approach. We consider that there would probably be an increase of infection associated with the more extensive perforation of the membranes which could lead to ascending infection from the vagina when the transcervical approach is used. The very low miscarriage rate reported by Wapner and associates[5] seems to confirm this point of view. The study of Evans and colleagues[2] shows that the transabdominal approach is the most widely accepted technique; they did not find statistical differences in term of fetal losses before 24 weeks' gestation between 846 transabdominal approaches and 238 transvaginal approaches (respectively, 16.2% vs. 13.1%). Fetal losses are related to the confidence of operators using one technique since there was a decrease in miscarriages during two periods throughout which the same transabdominal technique was used: 16.2% of fetal losses between 1986 and 1991 and only 8.8% from 1991 to 1993. Performing selective fetocide as late as 10 weeks' allows the phenom-

Table 2 Obstetrical data from reports of first-trimester selective terminations over the period 1988–95

Author(s)	Year	Number of cases	Miscarriage (%)	Overall pre-maturity rate* (%)	Preterm births[†] (%)	Perinatal mortality (%)
Salat-Baroux et al.[3]	1988	42	12	ND	6	2
Shalev et al.[4]	1989	20	25	36	ND	2
Wapner et al.[5]	1990	38	3	51	12	3
Lynch et al.[6]	1990	85	15	65	9	0
Tabsh[7]	1990	40	0	64	7	3.5
Dommergues et al.[8]	1991	58	31	47	24	5
Boulot et al.[9]	1993	61	13	57	13	11
Berkowitz et al.[10]	1993	200	9.5	45	9	1.8
Timor-Tritsch et al.[11]	1993	134	14	38	15	2.5
Dommergues et al. (French study)[12]	1994	262	16	48	15.5	ND
Evans et al. (international study)[2]	1994	1084	14	50	15.8	3.8
This study	1995	100	11	56.5	17	5.8

ND = not determined; *after the completed 37th week; [†]≤ 32 weeks' gestation

enon of vanishing twins to occur; indeed, spontaneous losses have been reported to occur frequently in multiple pregnancies[1,13]. In pregnancies in which reduction was performed before 9 or 10 weeks', it would be difficult to distinguish iatrogenic from spontaneous losses. After 10 weeks of gestation, spontaneous losses are much less likely. The risk of miscarriage should be explained to the couples who ask for the procedure because of the problem these infertile couples would have in achieving another pregnancy. The decision to perform a fetocide is so important that a period of reflection is necessary, to minimize later regrets if the pregnancy is lost. As the miscarriage rate after the procedure among our infertile and older women (mean age: 31.1 years) is comparable with the clinical miscarriage rate in the general population, and less than the rates of miscarriages reported after the use of clomiphene citrate, gonadotropins or IVF procedures, we suggest that the procedure we used did not considerably increase the early fetal loss[9].

We believe the preterm labor rate for the reduced pregnancies to be a reliable index of the efficacy of the procedure, as preterm labor is the most important complication of multifetal gestations. Preterm labor occurred at a high rate (57%), and the mean gestation at delivery in our series was 35.6 weeks, which is consistent with results reported from other studies dealing with selective reductions (see Table 2). This result is due principally to the large number of twin pregnancies in our series. It should be noted that the preterm labor rate among the 71 twins is similar to that generally reported for twins. Although special attention was given to these women to minimize preterm labor (i.e. early diagnosis, leave from work, antenatal management at home by a midwife, monitoring of uterine activity) very early preterm labor was not avoided and 17% of deliveries occurred between 28 and 32 weeks', leading to all the neonatal deaths reported. The characteristics of our cohort of mainly subfertile women must be taken in account; their pregnancies are at greater risk of preterm labor as well as growth retardation. In Evans and colleagues' study[2], 10% of births (between 29 and 32 weeks' gestation) occurred among reduced pregnancies and 5.4% of births were noted from 25 to 28 weeks'[3].

The mean gestational age at birth for the 71 twins obtained after the reduction of triplets was 35.6 (SD, 3) weeks, whereas the mean gestation at delivery of triplets managed without reduction has been reported to be 33–34 weeks. This suggests that the gain in maturity from the reduction of triplets in our series was about 2 weeks. These data confirm our preliminary results[19] and selective fetocide appears to have been effective in the reduction of preterm labor in triplet pregnancy. The death of immature fetuses explains the high perinatal mortality (5.8%).

There is a need to consider the number of embryos that should be suppressed. To some extent, four recommendations can be made without major ethical consideration as follows.

Firstly, multiple pregnancies with more than three embryos should be reduced, and twins, rather than singletons, should be the aim of the reduction. Without reduction, it is unlikely that such pregnancies would continue without significant risk of fetal loss and neonatal morbidity and mortality. A review of the literature in such cases shows a high perinatal mortality rate[14]. These risks seem to us to be important and we suggest the possibility of fetal reduction to couples who have conceived more than three viable fetuses. In our series, twins were our intention in this type of pregnancy, except in the case of four couples who asked for triplets – they were afraid that the risk of miscarriage would be greater if more than one fetus was suppressed: as there were no reliable data at the time concerning this point, their requests were granted.

Secondly, pregnancies occurring in a scarred or malformed uterus should also be reduced to obtain twins or singletons, according to the number of scars or to the type of uterine malformation. Selective fetocide performed on twin pregnancies associated with a scarred uterus has been previously reported, although the risk of uterine rupture in such cases had not yet been assessed (there is a lack of data in the literature).

A third recommendation is that pregnancies associated with maternal disease (e.g. diabetes in our series) should be considered for reduction, with the aim of reducing both fetal and maternal complications.

Finally, if one considers that the aim of the procedure is to obtain a low-risk pregnancy, reducing the multiple pregnancy to obtain a singleton remains possible. However, there is a relationship between the number of reduced embryos and the subsequent rate of miscarriage. Prevention of prematurity is best achieved when a single embryo is left at the cost of a significant increase of pregnancy loss-rate[2].

First-trimester selective termination in triplet pregnancies

Although the selective fetocide indication poses no problems when dealing with high-order multiple fetal gestations (quadruplet pregnancies or higher), the same is not true when considering triplets where the indications have not been clearly established. With the introduction of ovulation-inducing agents and *in vitro* fertilization procedures, the incidences of triplets has reached a high frequency and important series of data collected over several years are now available for analysis. A national collection of data from French IVF centers (FIVNAT) over a 4-year-period showed a triplet incidence rate of 3.2% (206/6345 pregnancies)[1]. A review of papers dealing with triplet gestations shows a high rate of preterm deliveries or extreme preterm deliveries (between 24 and 32 weeks' gestation), an important proportion of small-for-age fetuses, and a high rate of perinatal mortality[1,14–17]. Lastly, some severe maternal complication during gestation or labor have been reported[15]. To date, we need to evaluate the effect of selective termination in triplet gestations. In this work, we compare obstetrical data (i.e. abortions, preterm labor, *in utero* death, *in utero* growth retardation, perinatal mortality rate and maternal complications) from 65 triplet pregnancies managed without selective fetocide, with data from 73 reduced triplet pregnancies, to determine whether selective fetocide improves the obstetrical outcome.

Materials and methods

A total of 138 women with triplets were referred to our institution between 1 January 1985 and 1 January 1995. During the first consultation, patients were informed of all of the risks in these pregnancies. To respect ethical concerns, patients in the two groups were not randomized. Sixty-five women (group I) wished to continue their pregnancies whereas 73 couples (group II)

Table 3 Origin of triplets from groups I and II

	Group I		Group II	
	n	%	n	%
In vitro fertilization	45	69	54	74
Ovulation induction	12	19	17	23
Spontaneous	8	12	2	3
Total	65		73	

requested selective termination, mostly to obtain twins. Group I was the control group. The mean age of patients was 30 ± 3.9 years for group I (range, 20–38 years) and 32.1 ± 4 years for group II (range, 21–42 years). There was no significant difference concerning maternal age and origin of pregnancies (Table 3).

Management of group I Pregnancies were all managed in our fetal medicine unit as follows. Leave from work was systematically imposed, as well as a substantial reduction in maternal physical activity, once the diagnosis was established. Management at home began at 20 weeks' by a midwife; cervical cerclage was not performed. In cases of cervical change or increased uterine activity, women were referred to our center immediately. Women were examined by obstetricians monthly until the 5th month and then every 15 days. Serial ultrasound scans were performed every month by the same practitioner. In cases of threatened preterm labor, magnesium sulfate was administered intravenously, whilst β-agonists (salbutamol, Salbumol™, Glaxo, Paris, France) were used more rarely. β-Methasone was given to accelerate fetal lung maturation from 30 to 34 weeks' gestation, and in cases of important cervical changes, thyrotropin releasing hormone (TRH) was administered from 26 to 30 weeks'. Delivery was planned by means of Caesarean section under spinal anesthesia, and was decided when possible as the mother reached the completed 36th week of gestation. However, in many cases, delivery was determined either when the patient went into labor or when major tocolysis was unable to prevent preterm labor. For each

delivery, three experienced neonate obstetricians were present in the delivery room. In both groups, infants underwent follow-up until 6 months of age.

Management of group II Before reduction, couples were allowed at least 10 days to decide, and all patients were informed of the risks of the method. The procedure was carried out under strong sedation for our first attempts and then under local anesthesia, as previously described[9]. Two techniques were used as described above. The procedures were performed between 8 and 13.5 weeks' (the mean gestational age was 9.5 ± 1.1 weeks. A total of 16 transcervical approaches were employed until 1988, followed by 57 transabdominal approaches during the period 1988–95). Scans were then performed monthly until the end of pregnancy. Patients in group II underwent the same procedures to prevent prematurity (similar tocolysis and similar modified activities) as in group I. Women were followed by different obstetric teams specialized in high-risk pregnancies. Reduction led to 68 twins and five singletons. In three cases, there were poor prognosis factors (uterine scar, malformed uterus and a triplet pregnancy, including monoamniotic twins and singleton). The remaining two singletons were obtained on the specific request of the couples.

Results

All pregnancies reached term with follow-up of children ranging from age 6 months to 7 years. For uniformity, infant follow-up refers to follow-up to 6 months of age for both populations.

Miscarriages before 24 weeks' gestation In Group I, five (7.7%) miscarriages were noted, three before 15 week's two at 21 and 23 weeks'. In Group II, seven (9.6%) complete abortions occurred. A partial abortion occurred once and the remaining embryo developed normally.

Prematurity in groups I and II The results are reported in Table 4. The rate of prematurity is

Table 4 Impact of selective termination on preterm deliveries

	Group I (n = 65)	Group II (n = 73)
Prematurity rate (%)	93.4	50*
Mean term (weeks) proportion at:	33.8	36.4*
24–28 weeks (%)	6.6	0**
29–32 weeks (%)	21.6	11.3**
33–34 weeks (%)	18.3	11.3**
35–37 weeks (%)	46.6	24.5**
≥ 37 weeks (%)	6.6	52.8**

$*p \leq 0.05; **p \leq 0.001$

Table 5 Fetal and neonatal data

	Group I (n = 65)	Group II (n = 73)
Infants	180	141
Mean weight (g)	1816	2377*
< 3rd centile (%)	21.2	9.3
500–1000 g (%)	6.6	1[†]
1000–1500 g (%)	17.7	5.3[†]
1500–2000 g (%)	37.7	13[†]
2000–2500 g (%)	29.4	39[†]
> 2500 g (%)	8.3	41[†]
In utero deaths	2	3[†]
Neonatal deaths	10	2[†]
Perinatal mortality (%)	5.5	3.5
Maternal complications	6	0

*values in groups I and II are significantly different, $p < 0.0001$; [†]the difference in distribution of weights in five classes for the two groups is significant for the whole ($p < 0.0005$)

higher in group I (93.4%) than group II (50%). The mean gestational age at birth was 33.8 weeks in group I vs. 36.4 weeks in group II. No birth occurred before 28 weeks' gestation in the reduced group, while 6.6% of all the births of the unreduced group occurred before 28 weeks'. Lastly, 28.2% of all births occurred before 32 weeks' in group I vs. 11.3% in group II.

In utero *fetal death* In group I, intrauterine death of one fetus occurred in two cases: one case, at 31 weeks', remains unexplained even after birth since the autopsy did not reveal any anomaly because of maceration. The other case occurred at 34 weeks' and was related to severe, early and well-balanced fetal growth retardation with a normal karyotype. In group II, intrauterine death occurred in three cases: two of these deaths were related to severe growth restriction evident between 30 and 34 weeks' gestation. The third case was related to a cerebral malformation in one of the surviving twins which led to a successful selective fetocide on the malformed twin.

Birth and outcome In group I, Caesarean section was performed in 57 cases and three patients were vaginally delivered respectively at 25.5, 27 and 27 weeks'. In this group I, 180 fetuses were delivered: 178 alive and two dead. The mean weight of newborns (excluding *in utero* deaths) was 1840 ± 505 g with extremes from 590 to 3180 g. There were ten neonatal deaths before the 7th day of life (one with renal dysplasia, one with acute hepatitis and the others related to extreme prematurity). One child died between the 7th and the 24th day of life. The perinatal mortality rate in this group was 5.5% (10/180).

In group II, birth occurred by means of vaginal delivery or Caesarean section according to cervical conditions, course of the labor, fetal distress, or fetal presentation. A total of 141 infants were delivered: 138 alive and three dead. The mean weight of newborns (excluding *in utero* deaths) was 2377 ± 50 g with extremes from 810 to 3530 g. Two deaths occurred: one was related to extreme prematurity, the other to a difficult breech extraction of the second twin, which was performed in another center. Comparison of fetal weights are reported in Table 5. Lastly, one child died between the 7th and the 24th day of life. The perinatal mortality rate in this group was 3.5% (5/141).

Maternal complications In group I, six life-threatening maternal complications arose. The first was a spontaneous rupture of the liver, complicated by severe pre-eclampsia with a hemolysis elevated liver enzymes and low plate-let (HELLP) syndrome at 34 weeks' gestation. Hemostasis was obtained by ligature of the right hepatic artery. In the second case, one hemiple-gia occurred during the 6th month and the mother's recovery is currently incomplete. In the third, massive pulmonary embolism oc-curred 2 days after a Caesarean section, despite preventive anticoagulant treatment. The out-come was favorable in the cardiac intensive care unit. In the fourth and fifth cases two massive postpartum hemorrhages occurred a few hours after a Caesarean section. The outcome was favorable with prostaglandin treatment. A mas-sive pulmonary embolism occurred, in the sixth case, 2 days after a Caesarean section, despite preventive anticoagulant treatment. The out-come was favorable in the cardiac intensive care unit.

In group II, maternal complications included severe depression observed in two cases after the birth of a singleton and a pair of twins, and was treated by psychotherapy.

Discussion

Two essential results from our study suggest that selective termination may be helpful, in the management of triplet pregnancies:

(1) The rate of prematurity before 32 weeks', the fetal growth and the perinatal mortality rate were more favorable in group II than in group I.

(2) No life-threatening maternal complication occurred in the reduced-pregnancy group (II).

Some methodological aspects of our monocen-tric study, which is one of the largest published, should be detailed. First, patients were not ran-domized, otherwise this would have been an unethical and unacceptable approach. Second, our two groups were similar (same maternal age, same proportion of IVF and ovulation-induced pregnancies). Only multicenter studies enable the inclusion of a large number of couples, but

such studies would be difficult to perform be-cause of the wide variety of management tech-niques used in the various centers, and because of the rarity of triplets. To date, Lipitz' study[13] (including 140 triplets of which 34 were reduced mostly to twins and 106 expectantly managed) has led to the same conclusions. Porreco's study[18] gave similar results, although included smaller cohorts.

The comparison between group I and group II showed no significant differences concerning the miscarriage rate. The rate of spontaneous embryo loss in triplets remains difficult to eval-uate. Lipitz' study[13] reported 20.7% spon-taneous losses vs. 8.7% in the reduced-pregnancy group. The risk of iatrogenic abor-tion following the procedure varies from 8 to 14%, according to the largest series (see Table 2), depending principally on the opera-tor's experience[2]. A complete fetal loss follow-ing reduction in these infertile women should be considered when counselling the parents, since further pregnancies would be difficult or impossible to achieve.

One important challenge in triplet pregnan-cies is the high rate of premature delivery, which ranges from 87.5 to 91.6%, while the mean age at delivery is 34 weeks in all important series[1,14–18]. Preterm birth before 32 weeks' var-ies from 6.6% (in Newmann and colleagues' study[16]) to 35% in the French multicenter sur-vey[12]. The mean gestational age at delivery (34.4 weeks) in group I was comparable to that re-ported in the literature concerning the manage-ment of triplets. There was a significant decrease in prematurity in group II compared to group I, since pregnancies of the reduced population continued for an average of 2 weeks longer. More important is the dramatic decrease of the extreme prematurity between 28 and 32 weeks' and the absence of preterm birth before 28 weeks' in group II. These data are consistent with those reported in three similar stu-dies[13,18,19]. Lastly, it should be noted that reduc-tion does not seem to be effective for avoiding premature births. They occurred at the same rate in the reduced group than in the cases of twins spontaneously obtained.

Concerning the rate of small-for-gestational-age infants, there was a significant and important weight-gain among the reduced pregnancies: the birthweight of infants in the reduced group was 560 g higher. It would thus appear that embryonic reduction does improve fetal growth. Indeed, there were significant differences in infant weight distributions in the two groups. However, the data should be interpreted with caution since no growth curves were available for triplets in our center, and since the data were only compared to singleton curves, this could bias the results. These data are similar to those from Lipitz' study[13], where the incidence of very low birthweights among the reduced-pregnancy group was dramatically decreased, as compared to the expectantly-managed group. The weight gain revealed the absence of any detrimental effects of selective reduction on the growth of the surviving twins. However, we consider that the increase in birthweight may be explained partially by the avoidance of placental functional insufficiency in triplet cases and by the increase in gestational age at delivery, since birthweight and gestational age are linked.

Perinatal mortality rate was lower in group II. Indeed, reducing the extreme prematurity rate and improving fetal growth by means of reductions in group II logically have led to a lower perinatal mortality rate as compared to the rate in group I. The mortality rate observed in group I is similar to those previously reported in papers dealing with triplets. Over the last 2 years, other reports on new trends in the management of such pregnancies have also shown favorable outcomes. The data collected from 24 regional centers (including 98 triplet pregnancies over 3 years and reported by Newman and co-workers[16]) indicate a perinatal mortality rate of 5%. It should be noted that a rate of 5.5%, though satisfactory, is still six times higher than the rates observed in the management of singletons. The perinatal mortality rate in group II is in agreement with rates previously reported for twins. Our results suggest that the perinatal outcome for twins obtained after selective reductions in triplets does not differ (in terms of prematurity, fetal growth or perinatal mortality rate) from results for naturally-managed twins.

The incidence of maternal complications was very different in groups I and II; this is one of the most important results of our study. There were no serious maternal complications in the reduced-pregnancy group, yet six life-threatening complications occurred in the group continuing with triplets. These maternal complications were difficult or impossible to prevent, since liver rupture is a very rare complication of pre-eclampsia with HELLP syndrome. Maternal complications of β-mimetic therapy for preterm labor have been reported and it is well known that women with multiple pregnancies, in comparison to these with singleton pregnancies, have an increased blood volume which can lead to cardiac failure and pulmonary edema. As three out of six maternal complications occurred in the first triplets we managed, we considered it necessary to inform the couples of all the risks involved in these pregnancies. Under these conditions, it is not surprising that 73 of the 138 couples with triplets chose selective fetocide. Two mothers had depressive reactions when their pregnancies were reduced. Some women worried because they felt that they would be unable to give enough attention, tenderness and love to each triplet, so some of them asked for partial abortion. We assume that this major dilemma, in addition to the important risk of whole (and iatrogenic) abortion, can lead some women who choose selective fetocide to depression[20–22]. After having listened to these depressive women, psychological attention (by means of interviews) was given by a child psychiatrist throughout gestation and after birth to other women.

Indications of reduction in triplet pregnancies remain controversial. However, reduced triplet pregnancies account for an important part of all reduced pregnancies. A total of 445 (42%) of the 1084 fetocides collected by Evans and colleagues[2] were performed on triplets. In the French study[12], 107 out of the 262 cases (41%) of reductions were performed on triplets. Among the monocentric series reported in the literature, approximately 40% of the procedures of reductions are done on triplets: 44% (Wapner et al.[15]), 43% (Salat-Baroux et al.[3]), 26% (Dommergues et al.[18]), 57.5% (Tabsh[7]), 33% (Lynch et al.[16]), 24% (Lipitz et al.[13]), 50% (Timor-Tritsch et al.[11]), 44% (Berkowitz et al.[10]) but only 5% in the study of Shalev et al.[4]. With regards to triplets, there is no consensus among specialists concerning the indication of selective termination. In the light of the clinical data and according to our experience, we aimed to find a compatible position between selective termination, ethical principles, and respect for the moral status of embryos and fetal life. Some authors consider that the procedures, when applied to triplets, is an unethical approach to the problem and can be criticized because the medical risks related to these gestations do not systematically justify reduction. Indeed, the recently reported perinatal mortality rate of triplets in some series are quite similar to the corresponding rate amongst twins[23]. Another fear is the possible impact of these interventions performed at an early stage of gestation, which could lead to malformations or delayed fetal growth. However, Evans and colleagues study[2] reported that the rate of malformed newborns from more than 1000 reduced pregnancies was less than the expected rate (probably due to the selective tendency to reduce embryos at higher risk of having a congenital malformation). Lastly, there is an objective because of the strong paradox of wishing to reduce such wanted pregnancies which themselves were often difficult to achieve. Theoretically, the information received and the acceptance of the risk of a multiple pregnancy by a couple requesting an IVF procedure should encourage the acceptance of a triplet pregnancy if it should occur. In other words, a fully informed couple should accept a triplet gestation. Here is the main point of the discussion: should triplet pregnancies be considered as a success or as a complication of infertility treatments? If one considers triplet pregnancy as a success, it is not surprising that the procedure will be rejected. Conversely, if a triplet pregnancy is considered as an iatrogenic complication of infertility treat-

ment, it seems logical to perform reduction if requested by the couple.

The acceptance of the procedure in cases of triplets is dependent on many factors. We propose that selective termination in triplets (resulting in twins, and less often in singletons) should be considered in triplet cases when there is a scarred or malformed uterus, because uterine overdistension can lead to scar rupture or to early miscarriage. This procedure should also be considered in cases of pregnancies associated with serious maternal disease (i.e. heart disease) in order to avoid maternal complications (cardiac failure). Nevertheless, fetocide has been performed in twin pregnancies associated with a scarred uterus, or for psychiatric reasons[3,22]. Our results indicate that reduction of triplets improves some obstetrical parameters and avoids serious maternal complications. Consequently, the couples referred with triplets should be informed of the possibility of performing reduction and the associated risks, as well as the risks of triplet gestation. We consider, therefore, that the ultimate decision should be made by the woman and her spouse.

Couples may have additional reasons for requesting selective terminations, such as financial and social problems; working women are obliged to stop their professional activities, there is anticipation of a poor quality of life after the birth of triplets and, finally, there is woman's right to decide what to do with her pregnancy within the legal period, in accordance with laws on voluntary abortion. Some couples in our series demanded partial abortion, resulting in a singleton, based on this law. This unexpected request was granted in order to avoid complete abortion after long and difficult antifertility treatments (despite the fact that all couples before beginning such treatments received full information on the risks of multiple pregnancies).

In conclusion, first-trimester selective terminations improve the prognosis of triplets. Information on the risks (miscarriage) and advantages (gain in fetal growth and prematurity, decrease of maternal complications) of fetocide should be supplied to all couples with triplet pregnancies by an obstetrician experienced in dealing with multiple pregnancies. Reduction seems necessary for triplet pregnancies when there are poor prognosis factors, such as scarred uterus or severe maternal disease. Psychologi-cal, social and financial assistance should be provided for couples who decline selective ter-mination. For ethical reasons, efforts should be made to prevent these difficult situations, which are side-effects of infertility treatments.

References

1. Boulot, P., Hedon, B., Pellicia, G., Rousseau, O., Molenat, F., Laffargue, F. and Viala, J. L. (1992). Grossesses triples et plus – interruptions sélec-tives de grossesses *Mises à jour en Gynécologie – Obstétrique*, pp. 379–413. (Paris: Vigot Ed)

2. Evans, M. I., Dommergues, M., Wapner, R. J., Lynch, L., Dumez, Y., Goldberg, J. D., Ni-colaides, K. H., Johnson, M. P., Golbus, M. S., Boulot, P., Aknin, A. J., Monteagudo, A. and Berkowitz, R. L. (1994). Transabdominal versus transcervical and transvaginal multifetal preg-nancy reduction: International collaborative ex-perience of more than thousand cases. *Am. J. Obstet. Gynecol.*, **170**, 902–9

3. Salat-Baroux, J., Aknin, J., Antoine, J. M. and Alamowitch, R. (1988). The management of multiple pregnancies after induction for super-ovulation. *Hum. Reprod.*, **3**, 399–401

4. Shalev, J., Frenkel, Y., Goldenberg, M., Shalev, E., Lipitz, S., Barkai, G., Nebel, L. L. and Maschi-ach, S. (1989). Selective reduction in multiple gestations: pregnancy outcome after transvagi-nal and transabdominal needle-guided proce-dures. *Fertil. Steril.*, **52**, 416–20

5. Wapner, R. J., Davis, G. H., Johnson, A., Wein-blatt, V. J., Fischer, R. L., Jackson, L. G., Cher-venak, F. A. and McCullough, L. B. (1990). Selective reduction of multifetal pregnancies. *Lancet*, **335**, 90–4

6. Lynch, L., Berkowitz, R. L., Chitkara, U. and Alvarez, M. (1990). First-trimester transabdomi-nal multifetal pregnancy reduction: a report of 85 cases. *Obstet. Gynecol.*, **75**, 735–8

7. Tabsh, K. A. (1990). Transabdominal multifetal pregnancy reduction: report of 40 cases. *Obstet. Gynecol.*, **75**, 739–41

8. Dommergues, M., Nisand, I., Mandelbrot, L., Isfer, E., Radunovic, N. and Dumez, Y. (1991). Embryo reduction in multifetal pregnancies fol-lowing infertility therapy: obstetrical risks and perinatal benefits are related to operative strategy. *Fertil. Steril.*, **55**, 801–11

9. Boulot, P., Hedon, B., Pelliccia, G., Lefort, G., Deschamps, F., Arnal, F., Humeau, C., Laf-fargue, F. and Viala, J. L. (1993). Multifetal preg-nancy reduction: a consecutive series of 61 cases. *Br. J. Obstet. Gynaecol.*, **100**, 63–8

10. Berkowitz, R. L., Lynch, I., Lapinski, R. and Bergh, P. (1993). First-trimester transabdominal multifetal pregnancy reduction: a report of two hundred completed cases. *Am. J. Obstet. Gynecol.*, **169**, 17–21

11. Timor-Tritsch, I. E., Peisner, B. D., Mon-teagudo, A., Lerner, J. P. and Sharma, S. (1993). Multifetal pregnancy reduction by transvaginal puncture: evaluation of the technique used in 134 cases. *Am. J. Obstet. Gynecol.*, **168**, 799–804

12. Dommergues, M., Aknin, J., Boulot, P., Nisand, I., Lewin, F., Oury, J. F., Herlicoviez, M., Dumez, Y. and Evans, M., pour le Club Francophone de Médecine foetale (1994). Réductions embryon-naires dans les grossesses multiples. Une en-quête multicentrique française. *J. Gynecol. Obstet. Biol. Reprod.*, **23** 415–18

13. Lipitz, S., Reichman, B., Uval, J., Shalev, J., Achiron, R., Barkai, G. and Maschiach, S. (1994). A prospective comparison of the out-come of triplet pregnancies managed expec-tantly or by multifetal reduction to twins. *Am. J. Obstet. Gynecol.*, **170**, 874–9

14. Seoud, M. A., Kruithoff, C. and Muasher, S. J. (1991). Outcome of triplet and quadruplet preg-nancies resulting from *in vitro* fertilization. *Eur. J. Obstet. Gynecol. Reprod. Biol.*, **41**, 79–84

15. Pons, J. C., Fernandez, H. P., Diochin, P., May-enga, J. M., Plu, G., Frydman, R. and Papiernick, E. (1989). Prise en charge des grossesses triples. *J. Gynecol. Obstet. Biol. Reprod.*, **18**, 72–8

16. Newman, R., Hamer, C. and Miller, M. (1989). Outpatient triplet management: a contem-porary review. *Am. J. Obstet. Gynecol.*, **161**, 547–53

17. Lipitz, S., Reichman, B., Paret, G., Modan, M., Shalev, J., Serr, D., Mashiach, S. and Frenkel, Y. (1989). The improving outcome of triplet preg-nancies. *Am. J. Obstet. Gynecol.*, **161**, 1279–84

18. Porreco, R. P., Burke, M. S. and Hendrix, M. L. (1991). Multifetal reduction of triplets and preg-nancy outcome. *Obstet. Gynecol.*, **78**, 335–9

19. Boulot, P., Hedon, B., Pelliccia, G., Peray, P., Laffargue, F. and Viala, J. L. (1993). The effects

of selective reduction in triplet gestations: a comparative study on 80 cases managed with or without this procedure. *Fertil. Steril.*, **60**, 497–503

20. Nanternoz, F., Molenat, F., Boulot, P., Hedon, B., Roy, J. and Visier, J. P. (1991). Implications psychologiques de la réductions embryonnaire sur grossesse multiple: reflexions préliminaires. *Neuropsychiatrie de l'enfance*, **39**, 594–7

21. Robin, M., Bydlowsky, M., Cahen, F. and Josse, D. (1991). Aspects psychologiques des naissances triples: de la grossesse triple à l'établisse-ment des premières relations. In *Les Grossesses Multiples*, pp. 269–81. (Paris: Doin Ed)

22. Molenat, F., Nantermoz, F., Balmès, C. and Boulot, P. (1994). Impact psychologique sur les parents de la réduction embryonnaire. Reflexions à partir de 45 cas. In *Les grossesses multiples*, pp. 46–52. (Paris: Doin Ed)

23. Sassoon, D. A., Castro, L. C., Davis, J. L. and Hobel, C. J. (1990). Perinatal outcome in triplet versus twin gestations. *Obstet. Gynecol.*, **7**, 817–20

Ethical aspects of surrogacy

63

S. A. Carson

Introduction

Advances in reproductive technology have invited more third party assistance into reproduction. Although sperm donors have assisted infertile couples for over half a century, only recently has the technology been available to conceive a child for a couple in which the woman is the partner unable either to conceive or gestate. Surrogacy, although not widely practiced, has become very visible in the public eye due to its legal, ethical and social consequences. Little clinical research is available to form scientifically based decisions on questions that arise regarding surrogacy, perhaps because surrogacy was introduced and continues to be performed by institutions outside most universities and is largely managed by lawyers and business men. The medical team, in most instances, are peripheral to all but the insemination. Nonetheless, they should be informed of the issues involved, so that they may advise patients in their decision to pursue surrogacy.

Although there is disagreement in the use and definition of the term *surrogate mother*, it is usually applied to the oocyte donor and gestational mother of a child conceived with the sperm of an infertile couple and later adopted by the wife of that couple. This is slightly different from the *gestational surrogate*, who accepts and gestates the embryos formed by the fertilization of the infertile couple's oocytes and sperm. Both surrogates undertake the medical risk of pregnancy and experience the responsibilities, joys and discomfort of gestation and delivery. In this discussion, *surrogate* will refer to both the surrogate mother and gestational surrogate unless otherwise stated.

Ethical issues

Ethical issues regarding surrogacy revolve around seven areas:

(1) The rights of the surrogate;

(2) The rights of the infertile parents;

(3) The rights of the child;

(4) The veracity of the informed consent;

(5) The threat and implications involved in paying a woman to provide a service uniquely possible only by women;

(6) The threat to the family unit and the implications of third-party reproduction;

(7) The violation of an intimate human right.

Proponents and opponents of surrogacy bring up different ethical viewpoints in each of these areas. The woman who volunteers to assume the medical risk for the benefit of others may be most analogous to the kidney donor who voluntarily incurs medical risk for the benefit of others. Pregnancy is different in that, first, the actual risk is spread out over a period of time and, second, perhaps more importantly, a psychological bonding is present between the growing fetus and the mother. The former may be analogous to harboring a foster child and then giving the child up after 9 months. Foster parents also psychologically bond while caring for a child who is destined to be raised by another in a relatively short period of time.

Adoption is not analogous to surrogacy in that the pregnancy in cases of adoption is not planned and the decision to permit one's child to be adopted incurs a different set of variables and considerations. Indeed, there is no one situation analogous to surrogacy.

The rights of the surrogate

It is the overlapping individual rights which make questions regarding surrogacy difficult to answer. Because surrogacy is truly a contracted gestator, we are forced to choose between the hired person, the employer and an innocent third party in situations which are emotional and challenge our most intimate and fundamental values. The conflict of overlapping rights is best demonstrated by the question, 'Should a surrogate be able to change her mind in the middle of pregnancy?' Not only is arriving at the answer difficult, so is knowing what to do if a consensus is reached. Lori Andrews[1], of the American Bar Association, queried the implications and repercussions of putting into law that the surrogate is not able to change her mind, questioning whether this would lead to the supposition by some that women are so flighty that they cannot be trusted to honor any business contract and their word must always be explicitly defined. The surrogate's rights also may overlap with the rights of the fetus if she is forced to undergo Cesarean section. If a surrogate is screened for α-fetoprotein and the test result is low, can she then be forced to undergo amniocentesis, even if it is against her wishes? As a corollary, what if the fetus has a genetic defect and the biological parents want to abort? Would the surrogate be able to refuse abortion? Proponents of surrogacy maintain that these issues may all be brought up before pregnancy is undertaken and possible conflicts resolved before any such event occurs. Although unlikely to imagine all possible conflicts, it is certainly possible to discuss the majority.

The rights of the infertile parents

Describing the rights of the infertile couple exemplifies the major dilemma of surrogacy because the emphasis is on contractual aspects rather than the fundamental values of reproduction which we all hold dear. Essentially, the couple is hiring a valuable employee to conceive, gestate and be delivered of their child. Except for the medical risk to the surrogate, this is little different to the couple than hiring a babysitter to care for their child while both parents work. Employers can ask their babysitter to avoid smoking, so a surrogate should be also made to avoid cigarettes, alcohol or teratogen exposure if the couple so desires. Proponents of surrogacy see this as no different. However, opponents argue that the behavioral change requested is continuous, for 9 months, with no time for individual freedom.

The rights of the child

It is the rights of the child that pose the most difficult questions. At first glance, there is little to suggest that the baby will be unwanted by a couple who were so desirous of it, that they were willing to pay high prices and undergo intense emotional risk for its birth. Clearly, this child will be born with the proverbial silver spoon. However, what if the baby is not that of the infertile father, but rather a child of the surrogate and another man? Opponents to surrogacy argue that another unplanned child is born and that a surrogate should not be forced to accept a child she did not want. Proponents, of course, retort that the problem can be easily solved by the abundance of couples waiting to adopt a baby.

The psychological issues which may affect the child are unknown. Many children of donor sperm have long been kept unaware of their biological parenting; the 'family secret' has generated much writing and opinions from psychologists. Similarly, adopted children may experience psychological trauma when they learn their biological parents are different from their rearing parents. Surrogacy is too new a procedure to make any conclusions or recommendations; however, it is unlikely to be psychologically different from that of either donor gametes or adoption. Even in children resulting from those procedures, there are no definite answers as to what trauma is induced by the procedures or what would have happened anyway. Thus, no concrete evidence exists as to what psychological effects are caused.

Other issues are not as easily solved by analogies: What if the surrogate develops a life-threatening disease while pregnant? Does her life supersede that of the fetus? May a woman at 32 weeks who develops a cervical cancer make different decisions about her therapy if the child were meant for her rather than another couple?

These questions pose the classical ethical dilemma of individual freedom (surrogate's rights) to beneficence (doing the right thing for the unborn).

The veracity of the informed consent

One tenet of ethics is that if the regulations regarding a procedure are unenforceable, then the procedure is inherently unethical. Proponents of surrogacy stress that most ethical issues may be answered by discussion and agreement beforehand through informed voluntary consent of both the infertile couple and the surrogate. Likewise, surrogacy's opponents hold that these issues are agreed upon, but are unenforceable and therefore unethical.

Proponents maintain that adult women are competent and fully capable of understanding what surrogacy entails including relinquishing the child. Feeling a child move within you and bonding to the fetus cannot be imagined until it is experienced. However, in the not too distant past, wet nurses were employed. Just like gestation, breast feeding is uniquely female. Women were hired to perform a vital service without which the baby would die. In many cases this was an excuse for the mother who could afford it to avoid the inconvenience. In other cases, it was because the mother had died. Nonetheless, the resultant child could not have continued to exist without the wet nurse. The surrogate is little different as the child could not exist without her. Maternal–child bonding is also significant during suckling. The baby is held close to the lactating woman, eye contact and affections are unavoidable. The health risks are fewer but not absent in the lactating woman and this probably comprises the major difference. Proponents argue that reproduction is a right and part of

having such a right is the ability to waive or sell it.

Opponents of surrogacy feel gestation is a powerful human right which is difficult to understand until experienced; deep-seated human emotions are brought into force which cannot be waived or relinquished before hand.

The threat and implications involved in paying a woman to provide a service uniquely possible only by women

Women are not incubators and those most critical of surrogacy warn us that wealthy women may hire surrogates to bear their children and avoid the medical risks and the cosmetic risks of pregnancy. Critics feel women may become victimized for money.

The American Fertility Society Ethics Committee[2] has recommended that surrogates be paid only for their inconvenience and expenses. This is an attempt to select women volunteering to surrogate for altruistic reasons rather than for monetary reasons. Organ donation experience has led to the practice of not paying organ donors to prevent victimization of the donors. Furthermore, organ donation has been found to work best if a family member volunteers to donate, not only for medical reasons but also for the alleviation of coercion. Much writing focuses on preventing surrogacy from seeking poor women to be the reproductive slaves of wealthier women who want a gestational surrogate rather than go through the inconvenience or medical risk of pregnancy. However, is this hypocritical? We hire young healthy men to risk their lives to guard the President of the United States. Many have been killed and maimed doing exactly that. Also, stunt men in Hollywood are paid to take inordinate risks as a substitute for the highly paid, talented actor who either does not have the skill or desire to perform a risky stunt required by the movie script. As long as adults are informed of the risks and freely under take the contract, how is reproduction different from any of the tasks for which adults are paid in order to assume risk for others? That some women see surrogacy as a possible source of income, for whatever reason, is offensive to some and quite logical to others.

Finally, the classic social role of the woman as the gestator of the family is removed by surrogacy. Indeed, a man no longer biologically needs a wife to have a family. However, this is only parallel to single women being artificially inseminated with donor sperm. Nonetheless, surrogacy may threaten many women who have no identity except as gestator and family caretakers; this too is a choice.

The threat to the family unit and implications of third-party reproduction

Many object to the surrogate interfering with the family unit. Adding a third party to reproduction may interfere with the intimacy of marriage. However, gamete donation alone has long been done without damage to the marital unit, except in occasional cases. Proponents of surrogacy state that children are a natural evolution of the marital unit and that raising the child is much more unifying than conceiving and proceeding through a pregnancy, since that is essentially done by only one parent anyway. In fact, it may be argued that surrogacy, especially gestational surrogacy, evens out the marital reproductive roles, as both parents will be solely gamete donors. No parent has the additional 'one-upmanship' of gestation. Wanted children are born to desiring couples, thus protecting the family unit. They argue that adoption is now

difficult and surrogacy allows infertile couples to have a family without baby selling or black market adoption. All is above board and can be regulated by laws if necessary.

Opponents' arguments revolve mostly around religious tenets regarding violations of the marital relationship. Besides religious objections, opponents argue that parental commitment to children is basic and moral and should never be contingent upon commercial obligations. Surrogacy undermines the long-standing social traditions and basic human urge for biological offspring.

The argument that surrogacy poses an asymmetric parental commitment, because only one parent is a genetic parent, either decries the decades of experience with donor sperm or denigrates the ability of women to care for children only if they gestate the child.

Summary

Surrogacy evokes more emotional and ethical dilemmas than medical ones. The opponents of surrogacy have no argument which supersedes society's intense feelings toward allowing everyone the opportunity of reproducing; no argument appears intense enough to allow reproductive choices to falter. Because ethics seem to be less a science than a field of organized common sense, it is unlikely that these issues will prevent individual choice and judgement by the physician–patient team.

References

1. The New York State Task Force on Life and the Law (1988). *Surrogate Parenting: Analysis and Recommendations for Public Policy*, p. 30. New York, USA, May

2. American Fertility Society Ethics Committee (1990). Ethical considerations of the new assisted reproductive technologies. *Fertil. Steril.*, **535**, 1–75

9

Research

Analysis of clinical research

64

J. Collins

Introduction

Clinical trials are the theme of this research session, and randomized clinical trials (RCTs) constitute the most refined clinical research designs. Nevertheless, it is worthwhile to describe briefly the broader context of clinical research domains in order to demonstrate the specific position that is filled by the randomized clinical trial. For this purpose clinical research constitutes studies which are based on human subjects and designed to improve medical care.

Research domains

A variety of research disciplines may contribute to improvements in medical care. A useful categorization groups these disciplines under the following headings: ethnographic, epidemiologic, agricultural and biological.

The ethnographic domain

Ethnographic research comprises observations on individuals, such as daily diaries, participant observer records, and open-ended questionnaires. Clearly this approach fosters diversity and makes use of this variability to guide practitioners. The ethnographic research disciplines demand an orderly and objective approach to the summarization and interpretation of such data.

The epidemiologic domain

Epidemiologic research typically studies groups of people in natural settings to evaluate causes and outcomes of human disease. The research methods focus on singular issues but accept variability among subjects and samples. The epi-

demiologic research disciplines focus on analyses that take into account the influence of variability on the question under study.

The agricultural domain

Randomized clinical trials are an evolution from the agricultural experiments of the 1920s and 1930s. The research methods involve random allocation in order to reduce variability to the minimum that is achievable among human subjects. The agricultural research disciplines minimize every possible source of bias that might affect the clinical question.

The biological domain

Biological research methods refine the question under study until it is isolated from any external influence. The research methods involve the use of controls for every potential influence and repetition to reduce experimental error. The biological research disciplines eliminate variability in order to address a single isolated question.

The common theme among all of the above research domains is the disciplined approach: formulate the question, devise an appropriate methodology, interpret the data, and place the interpretation within a framework of scientific knowledge. The most rudimentary difference among the domains lies in their approach to variability: the ethnographic domain fosters variability, the epidemiologic accounts for extrinsic variability; the agricultural domain randomizes to minimize extrinsic variability; and successful biological research designs eliminate external influences entirely.

Clinical research designs

The questions most often asked in clinical research concern issues of causation, prognosis, diagnosis and treatment effectiveness. The majority of research designs to address these clinical questions are based on the epidemiological or agricultural traditions.

(1) *Causation* The etiology or causation of a disease may be addressed by cohort studies, in which exposed and unexposed cohorts are followed to determine whether the disease frequency differs according to exposure. Unfortunately, many important diseases have such a low incidence that cohort studies would be impractical. Therefore case–control studies are employed for this purpose. In this design, cases of disease are compared with controls retrospectively for differences in exposures that might be linked to disease incidence.

(2) *Prognosis* Prognosis for a given disorder can best be ascertained by means of well-done case series. Consecutive cases are assembled at a similar stage in the evolution of the disease in question, and followed in a meticulous manner until all clinically relevant outcomes can be recorded.

(3) *Diagnosis* Diagnostic tests optimally are evaluated by means of clinical trials in which the diagnostic test allocates eligible subjects into cohorts with abnormal and normal results, who are then followed to determine whether the test result predicts the clinically important outcome.

(4) *Treatment effectiveness* To evaluate treatment, well-designed trials depend on random allocation and adequate concealment of the allocation sequence. The allocation should be double-blinded when that is ethical and feasible. The outcome assessment should be unarguable (such as a live-born delivery) or the outcome assessor should be blinded. In short, every possible care must be taken to ensure that bias was minimized.

Table 1 Nomenclature for randomized clinical trials

Authors	Variability minimized	Variability tolerated
Cochrane[2]	efficacy	effectiveness
Feinstein[3]	fastidious	pragmatic
Sackett and Gent[4]	explanatory	management

In the evaluation of treatment effectiveness, randomization is necessary in order to isolate the effects of treatment from the effects of other variables that might affect a patient's outcome. For example, prognostic variables were more often maldistributed in non-randomized studies than in randomized unblinded studies[1].

RCTs are generally designed either to eliminate all possible extraneous variability, or the design is permitted to tolerate normal clinical conditions. These two major design sub-types have been given different pairs of names by different authorities (Table 1). In general, trials designated by the last term in each pairing (effectiveness, pragmatic, management) take place in typical clinical settings and have more general clinical usefulness. Efficacy trials are usually designed to evaluate the isolated effect of a drug on a disease, and the subjects are highly selected to reduce variability. Thus, the results of these trials may not be generalizable in clinical practice.

The quality of clinical research

Several groups have taken on the task of assigning a ranking of quality to study designs for clinical research. The ranking shown in Table 2 is a detailed example. Although listed as class III evidence, the validity of cohort studies suggests that a true numeric ranking might be considerably lower.

Randomized clinical trials and the analysis of clinical research

RCTs might have been designed specifically for the evaluation of infertility therapy. There is an

Table 2 Levels of evidence for therapy effectiveness[5]

Level	Description relative to clinically significant benefit (CSB)
I +	Overview 95% CI exceeds CSB: trial results homogeneous
I	No overview: RCTs with low alpha and beta errors
I–	Overview 95% CI exceeds CSB: trial results heterogeneous
II +	Overview point estimate exceeds CSB: trial results homogeneous
II	No overview: RCTs with high alpha and beta errors
II–	Overview point estimate exceeds CSB: trial results heterogeneous
III	Non-randomized concurrent cohort studies
IV	Non-randomized historical cohort studies
V	Case series

CI = confidence interval; RCT = randomized clinical trial

untreated success rate, there is uncertainty and debate about the superiority of various approaches, and few, if any, interventions are free of cost or side-effects. Furthermore, each single cause may be co-existent with other contributing factors and there are numerous non-diagnostic prognostic factors, such as secondary infertility and female age. Pragmatic or management RCTs seem ideally suited to evaluate therapy under such conditions. Such trials address the problems of clinical practice in a realistic fashion, recognizing that the treatments are often empirical, and that much of the variability in pregnancy rates remains unexplained.

Issues in the design of management trials

The trial literature includes the following guides to pragmatic design issues.

(1) The question should be expressed in a simple manner. Because the design of trials is so intricate, it is essential to express the idea itself – the question which is being addressed – in a plain and lucid manner.

(2) Another practical guide is to keep the trial as short as possible. This has an effect on the power of the trial, because outcomes such as pregnancy are so infrequent. Nevertheless, it is in the long run better to complete a number of small trials than to have a single large cohort study or incomplete trial. The results of the small trials

can, at least, be combined in a meta-analysis to yield useful information.

(3) Consider basing the trial design on a surrogate outcome. The outcome of interest is, of course, live birth, but baseline live birth rates hover around 2% per cycle. Therefore hundreds of subjects may be needed in each arm of a trial to have a reasonable change of showing a doubling of the baseline rate. If one were to design a preliminary trial, however, and that trial showed an important effect on a surrogate outcome, then there would be more public and professional interest in a larger follow-up trial to evaluate the effect on the outcome of interest, live birth.

(4) Avoid complex designs. Cross-over trials and latin square designs were useful in crop experiments, but there are fundamental problems with their use when the outcome is an event. It is best, therefore, to use the straightforward parallel design.

(5) Do the trial in your own practice, if at all possible. This not only facilitates getting consent from patients, it also reduces cost.

(6) Consider a lag-time trial when a 'no treatment' arm is necessary. In lag-time trials, patients are randomized to receive the test treatment immediately or after a delay of 1 or 2 months. Experience has shown that a six month lag-time creates logistic difficulties that are best avoided by using shorter delays of 1 or 2 months.

References

1. Chalmers, I. (1989). Evaluating the effects of care during pregnancy and childbirth. In Chalmers, I., Enkin, E. and Keirse, M. J. N. C. (eds.) *Effective Care in Pregnancy and Childbirth*, pp. 3–38. (Oxford: Oxford University Press)

2. Cochrane, A. L. (1982). *Effectiveness and Efficiency: Random Reflections on Health Services.* (London: Nuffield Provincial Hospitals Trust)

3. Feinstein, A. R. (1983). An additional basic science for clinical medicine: II. The limitations of randomized trials. *Ann. Intern. Med.*, **99**, 544–50

4. Sackett, D. and Gent, M. (1979). Controversy in counting and attributing events in clinical trials. *N. Engl. J. Med.*, **301**, 1410–12

5. Cook, D. J., Guyatt, G. H., Laupacis, A. and Sackett, D. L. (1992). Rules of evidence and clinical recommendations on the use of antithrombotic agents. *Chest*, **102**, 305–11S

Evaluation of infertility treatment: multicenter trials or national registers?

65

P. A. L. Lancaster

Introduction

In evaluating benefits and risks of infertility treatment, the benefits of achieving pregnancies and of the births of healthy children are readily apparent, but assessing potential harm may not always be so clear-cut. Of the many different clinical approaches to treating infertility, only treatment by assisted conception will be considered here.

While some of the risks of treatment were predictable when *in vitro* fertilization (IVF) was first introduced, clinical trials and observational studies are essential to assess both anticipated and unanticipated outcomes. Based on earlier experience with fertility drugs[1], the risk of ovarian hyperstimulation was predictable but the higher doses of these drugs in assisted conception meant that the actual risks needed to be reappraised. Studies of infertile women treated in the pre-IVF era had already shown higher pregnancy losses than in the general population, so this outcome was also predictable. The transfer of more than one embryo into the uterus in assisted conception also meant that more multiple births were to be expected. Less predictable was the possibility that superovulation might increase the risk of ovarian cancer, although this hypothesis was current at the time IVF began[2]. Exposure of infertile women treated with human pituitary gonadotropins to any risk of Creutzfeldt–Jakob disease occurred mainly before IVF was introduced.

In Australia, it seems likely that there will be further broadening of scope in evaluating infertile women treated by assisted conception. The National Health and Medical Research Council has recently released a consultation document for public comment which includes recommendations for assessment of the psychosocial well-being of women and their families before, during and after any active intervention, irrespective of whether treatment is successful[3]. The consultation document also recommends that the effects on pregnancy rates of various psychological interventions for anxiety and depression should be evaluated by randomized controlled trials.

Since the initial success of a healthy child born after IVF, the major phases in the rapidly developing field of assisted conception have included (1) ovarian hyperstimulation, thus enabling fertilization of multiple oocytes collected in the same treatment cycle and subsequent transfer of more than one embryo to achieve higher pregnancy rates, (2) use of gonadotropin-releasing hormone analogs to induce ovulation, (3) ultrasound-guided oocyte retrieval, (4) cryopreservation of embryos, thus avoiding the need for hyperstimulation in every treatment cycle, (5) transfer of gametes and embryos to the Fallopian tubes, (6) refinements of laboratory procedures, (7) microinsemination techniques for treating male infertility, and (8) clinical trials of recombinant follicle-stimulating hormone[4–6]. Following study of the efficacy of these new techniques, many have been introduced into clinical practice without having their effectiveness compared with existing modalities of treatment in randomized controlled trials.

Strategies for evaluating treatment of infertility

Clinical pregnancy rates are the usual endpoints for studies that evaluate the effectiveness of new drugs and techniques. These studies often lack sufficient numbers of patients to assess the immediate risks of treatment or the outcomes of pregnancy. It is often not clear from published randomized trials in assisted conception how the sample size was determined, but the number of treated women in a trial seems to be based more on pregnancy rates than on pregnancy outcomes. In a major systematic review of randomized controlled trials of infertility treatment[7], fewer than 20% of the 51 trials of ovarian hyperstimulation in assisted conception had more than 100 patients. So, even an immediate adverse effect such as severe ovarian hyperstimulation syndrome, which occurs in less than 5% of treated women[8], could not be evaluated reliably in most of these studies. Other approaches are therefore needed to determine both short-term and long-term outcomes and risks associated with treatment.

Multicenter randomized trials provide one alternative approach but so far there have been very few such trials in assisted conception. As well as increasing sample size, multicenter trials have the advantage of reducing the possible selection bias that might be found among infertile couples treated in a particular IVF center, particularly those in tertiary institutions, and also improve the generalizability of the results by increasing the likelihood that patients in the trial have characteristics similar to all couples eligible for treatment. Nevertheless, these trials are often costly and require considerable organizational skills; problems, however, that have not proved insurmountable in other fields of clinical practice.

Once the effectiveness of new drugs or techniques has been established in well-conducted clinical trials, the risks of treatment can be evaluated by systematic and frequent analysis of overall results in an IVF center. Even then, subgroups of women who have varying causes of infertility and different requirements for fertil-

ity drugs may lack an adequate sample size for determining risks. More rapid appraisal can be achieved by combining the results of several IVF centers or by setting up population-based registers to monitor treatment cycles and pregnancy outcomes. As well as pregnancy rates and significant adverse effects such as ovarian hyperstimulation syndrome, other outcomes of particular interest include early pregnancy loss, preterm birth, low birthweight, perinatal mortality, multiple births, congenital malformations, the growth and development of children, and possible risks of cancer in treated women and their children. Insights into advantages or disadvantages of the various methods of treatment and procedures can also be gained by comparing results between countries, as has proved valuable in many other fields of clinical practice.

National registers and related data systems in an increasing number of countries complement continuing clinical evaluation and have an important role in analyzing adverse outcomes. These registers enable assessment of trends in the treatment of infertility by assisted conception; evaluation of the outcome of treated women, their pregnancies and their children; determination of risks associated with treatment; and development of policies for providing and funding clinical services. By analyzing pregnancy outcome in much larger numbers than occur in a single IVF center, unexpected outcomes such as the high rate of preterm birth in singleton pregnancies can be identified, posing new questions about possible causes and generating new hypotheses. The high perinatal mortality in multiple births reported to the register in Australia and New Zealand[9] was influential in changing national policy, resulting in a recommendation to reduce the number of embryos or oocytes transferred during assisted conception. The disadvantage, of course, was lower pregnancy rates. There are now distinct differences between countries in the number of embryos transferred and in the proportion of multiple births that follow assisted conception[10,11].

Strategies other than randomized trials and registers of pregnancy outcome are needed to evaluate possible risk of cancer in women treated by ovarian hyperstimulation. The usually long interval between any exposure to fertility drugs and diagnosis of ovarian cancer means that conventional case–control and cohort studies are more appropriate. Nevertheless, well-kept clinical records and registers of cohorts of treated women can be an invaluable resource, enabling linkage of these records to cancer registers when required[12]. Identifying cohorts of women treated with fertility drugs before assisted conception began, so that various hypotheses can be tested, is likely to be a much more difficult task. In case–control studies of ovarian cancer, there may be major problems in accurately documenting drug exposure that occurred many years previously.

Conclusions

Randomized controlled trials are essential in evaluating the effectiveness of new drugs and techniques and in assessing the benefits of treatment. Multicenter randomized trials can provide important information about relatively common adverse effects but need to be complemented by analysis of overall results in each IVF center and by population-based registers. Other useful approaches for evaluating the benefits and risks of treatment are international comparisons of outcomes and, when the need arises, linkage of records of treated infertile women and their children with records in cancer registries.

Looking to the future, areas in which randomized controlled trials should prove useful include (1) the transfer of embryos at the blastocyst stage of development, (2) the study of factors affecting uterine secretion and implantation, (3) the use of oocytes that mature *in vitro*, and (4) the effect on pregnancy rates of selecting for transfer embryos of differing quality, especially after embryo freezing.

It is exciting to be on the growing edge of developing new ways of treating infertile couples, especially when a sizable proportion of these couples have had little reason for joy until recent years. However, it should be remembered that over the centuries clinical practice has been littered by many apparent advances in treatment, only to see them eventually abandoned because they were ineffective. Already, treatment by assisted conception is starting to fill its own waste bins with failed treatments that were embraced enthusiastically but were not adequately evaluated in the first place.

References

1. Schenker, J. G. and Weinstein, D. (1978). Ovarian hyperstimulation syndrome: a current survey. *Fertil. Steril.*, **30**, 255–68
2. Fathalla, M. F. (1971). Incessant ovulation – a factor in ovarian neoplasia? *Lancet*, **2**, 163
3. National Health and Medical Research Council (1995). Long-term effects on women from assisted conception. Consultation document, January. (Canberra: National Health and Medical Research Council)
4. Edwards, R. G. and Craft, I. (1990). Development of assisted conception. *Br. Med. Bull.*, **46**, 565–79
5. Skakkebæk, N. E., Giverman, A. and de Kretser, D. (1994). Pathogenesis and management of male infertility. *Lancet*, **343**, 1473–9
6. Healy, D. L., Trounson, A. O. and Andersen, A. N. (1994). Female infertility: causes and treatment. *Lancet*, **343**, 1539–44
7. Vandekerckhove, P., O'Donovan, P. A., Lilford, R. J. and Harada, T. W. (1993). Infertility treatment: from cookery to science. The epidemiology of randomised controlled trials. *Br. J. Obstet. Gynaecol.*, **100**, 1005–36
8. Editorial. (1991). Ovarian hyperstimulation syndrome. *Lancet*, **338**, 1111–12
9. Assisted conception, Australia and New Zealand, 1991. (Sydney: Australian Institute of Health and Welfare National Perinatal Statistics Unit)
10. Lancaster, P. A. L. (1992). International comparisons of assisted reproduction. *Assist. Reprod. Rev.*, **2**, 212–21

11. Cohen, J., de Mouzon, J. and Lancaster, P. (1993). World collaborative report 1991. *VIIIth World Congress on In vitro Fertilization and Alternative Assisted Reproduction*, Kyoto, September

12. Rossing, M. A., Daling, J. R., Weiss, N. S., Moore, D. E. and Self, S. G. (1994). Ovarian tumours in a cohort of infertile women. *N. Engl. J. Med.*, **331**, 771–6

Index